ESSKA Instructional Course Lecture Book

Michael Tobias Hirschmann
Elizaveta Kon • Kristian Samuelsson
Matteo Denti • David Dejour
Editors

ESSKA Instructional Course Lecture Book

Milan 2021

Springer

European Society of Sports Traumatology, Knee Surgery & Arthroscopy
ESSKA

Editors
Michael Tobias Hirschmann
Department of Orthopaedic Surgery
and Traumatology
Kantonsspital Baselland
(Bruderholz, Liestal, Laufen)
Switzerland

Elizaveta Kon
Center of Functional and Biological
Reconstruction of the Knee
Humanitas University, Humanitas
Research Hospital
Milan
Italy

Kristian Samuelsson
Department of Orthopaedics
Sahlgrenska University Hospital
Gothenburg
Sweden

Matteo Denti
Istituto Ortopedico Galeazzi
Milano
Italy

David Dejour
Department of Orthopaedics
Lyon Ortho Clinic
LYON
France

Project Coordinator
Julie Agel
Department of Orthopaedic Surgery
University of Minnesota
2450 Riverside Avenue South, Suite # 200
Minneapolis, MN 55454, USA
agelx001@umn.edu

ISBN 978-3-662-61266-8 ISBN 978-3-662-61264-4 (eBook)
https://doi.org/10.1007/978-3-662-61264-4

This Springer imprint is published by the registered company Springer-Verlag GmbH, DE part of Springer Nature.
The registered company address is: Heidelberger Platz 3, 14197 Berlin, Germany

Preface

Dear all,

As you know, unfortunately the COVID-19 pandemic forced ESSKA to reschedule the Milan congress for May 2021. However, the production of this book started in 2019 with a very tight schedule in mind, in order to have it published for May 2020. When we were asked to approve the opening pages of the book, we decided to leave the below preface unchanged, as a testimony to the efforts made by all parties involved to meet the original congress deadline.

The volume editors

Dear readers, Dear ESSKA Members, Dear ESSKA Congress participants,

Milan 2020! The biannual meeting is a special edition with an outstanding program.

As a tradition we worked on delivering an ICL book to give you the flavor of the meeting and the best update on hot topics in the field of orthopedic, arthroscopy, sports, and science.

This edition will be special because we faced some terrific deadlines in terms of book production. All our ICL chairs who worked hard for you to make the best of the best ICL were given a very short time to collect, resume, and write one chapter for each ICL. It is a huge effort and investment to accept to chair an ICL; it is an even bigger investment in terms of time and energy to collect the material of their invited speakers and re-write a chapter following the rules and guidelines of a scientific book published by one of the best publishers in the medicine world (Springer).

Everybody tried to do the best, but the material that we received exceeded 1000 pages! This shows how ESSKA and especially the people who make ESSKA great were involved in their task.

Unfortunately, publishing a book of more than 1000 pages was impossible in terms of time, organization, and funding. We had to make a choice—having no book and upset many of you including authors or having a memory of our meeting and ICL sessions by making a selection from the number of articles we received. Of course, nothing was perfect, but the second option is what we decided upon. We know that it will give you only a part of the Milan 2020 Show, but it is yet a very good book for you to read.

You will find in it all the different aspects and pathology treatments; it will be definitely a very good help in your practice in 2020.

Take the time to go through the following chapters, and for the topic you cannot find in this book, we invite you to go to the ESSKA Academy, our online educational platform, where all material is available: https://academy.esska.org.

We would like to thank the faculty for their involvement and work to give you the best.

Bruderholz, Basel Land, Switzerland	Michael Tobias Hirschmann
Milan, Italy	Elizaveta Kon
Gothenburg, Sweden	Kristian Samuelsson
Milan, Italy	Matteo Denti
Lyon, France	David Dejour

Acknowledgements

ESSKA wishes to thank all the outstanding contributors of the 2021 ICL's in Milan:

Paolo Adravanti
Pontus Andersson
Peter Angele
Daisuke Araki
Jean-Noel Argenson
Paolo Arrigoni
Olufemi R. Ayeni
Corrado Bait
Ali Bajwa
Peter Balcarek
David Barastegui
Cecile Batailler
Zoran Bathtijarevic
Knut Beitzel
Pedro Belon
Kerem Bilsel
Hamid Rahmatullah
Bin Abd Razak
Nicolas Bonin
Kyle Borque
Gaetano Lo Bue
James Calder
Karen Caroline Cabral Castro
Haluk Celik
Panayiotis Christofilopoulos
Hakan Turan Çift
Davide Cucchi
Ramon Cugat
Francesco Della Villa
Covadonga Arraiz Diaz
Florian Dirisamer
Lutz Durselen
Felix Dyrna
Seper Ekhtiari
Rene El Attal
Tristan Fauchille
Marta Ferrari
Matthias J. Feucht
Christian Fink
Radu Fleaca
Benjamin Freychet
Karl-Heinz Frosch
Pablo E. Gelber
Alan Getgood
Stefano Ghirardelli
Antonio Giardella
Michele Giuntoli
Mark Glazebrook
Alli Gokeler
Nuno Gomes
Andreas H. Gomoll
Alberto Grassi
Vincenzo Guarrella
David Guenther
Stephane Guillo
Pedro Hinarejos
Anna Hirschmann
Michael Tobias Hirschmann
Christian Hoser
Yuichi Hoshino
Pier Francesco Indelli
Henrique Jones
Rahul Kakar
Etienne Kalk
Mustafa Karahan
Jon Karlsson
Eustathios Kenanidis
Raghbir S. Khakha

Peter P. Koch
Nanne Kort
Ladislav Kovacic
Volker Krutsch
Werner Krutsch
Ryosuke Kuroda
Adrian Z. Kurz
Lasse Lempainen
Ofer Levy
Manuel Leyes
Michael Liebensteiner
Franceso Luceri
Angelina Lukaszenkoi
Sebastien Lustig
Luca Macchiarola
Antonio Maestro
Fabrizio Margheritini
Oliver Marin-Pena
Frank Martetschlager
Kentaro Matsui
Takehiko Matsushita
Geert Meermans
Sean Meredith
Andrew Metcalfe
Giuseppe Milano
Hema Mistry
Volker Musahl
Kanto Nagai
Stefan Nehrer
Markus Neubauer
Cedric Ngbilo
Haruki Odagiri
Matthieu Ollivier
Geert Pagenstert
Sven Pal
Sebastien Parratte
Tom Patt
Christopher J. Pearce
Martin Pietsch
Boris Poberaj
Chad Purcell
Pietro Simone Randelli
Salvatore Risitano
James R Robinson
Mario Ronga
Claudio Rosso
André Sarmento
Andreas M. Seitz
Dexter Seow
Filipe Serralva
Elvire Servien
Vieira da Silva
Helen Simpson
Nick Smith
Bertrand Sonnery-Cottet
Tim Spalding
Joanna M. Stephen
Marc Jacob Strauss
Mark Tauber
Ettore Taverna
Andrea Tecame
Robert A. Teitge
Mathieu Thaunat
Philippe M. Tscholl
Ismail Turkmen
Ronald Van Heerwaarden
Francesca Vannini
Thais Dutra Vieira
Helen Vint
Bruno Violante
Tomislav Vlahovic
Norman Waugh
Andy Williams
Adrian J. Wilson
Matthias A. Zumstein
Nestor A. Zurita

Contents

1 Meniscus Allografts: How to Improve Clinical Results, Limit Chondral Degeneration?

Nicolas Pujol, Lukasz Lipinski, and Seong Hwan Kim

1.1 Introduction

Meniscus injury is the most frequent injury of the knee. Despite the increasing knowledge of the meniscus pathology and the importance of repairing repairable lesions, meniscectomy is still a way of treatment in symptomatic knee [1]. Meniscus allograft transplantation (MAT) is a favorable option in patients with a painful knee after a meniscectomy. It provides good improvements in function and symptoms [2].

Several techniques of meniscal transplantation have been reported. Most frequent used techniques are soft tissue fixation and bone plug fixation. Bone plug technique is technically demanding.

Soft tissue fixation leads to more extrusion when compared to bone block techniques, even if there is no clinical relevance [3].

There are a lot of data in the literature about the early extrusion of meniscal allografts [4–7]. This extrusion may worsen the chondral degeneration and might be responsible of failures and reoperations in the midterm.

We present a novel technique of soft tissue allograft meniscal transplantation with a double anterior anchorage involving a tenodesis of the intermeniscal ligament of the allograft in addition to the fixation of the anterior root. This technique is less complex than bone plug methods, it is less invasive but still provides stable and secure graft fixation. It will help surgeons to improve clinical results and to limit secondary extrusion.

1.2 Surgical Indications (Table 1.1)

The ideal indication for MAT is a young, nonobese patient with a history of prior meniscectomy, almost neutral alignment and no severe cartilage

Table 1.1 Indications of MAT

Indications:
Age: between 20 and 50 years old
BMI < 30
Intact ACL or ACL reconstruction
Symptomatic post meniscectomy syndrome
Cartilage lesions: Outerbridge classification less than 2 or 3
Kellgren–Lawrence grade I-II on radiographs
Favorable alignment (i.e., no valgus >3° for a lateral transplant, no varus >3° for a medial transplant) of the knee

N. Pujol (✉)
Department of Orthopedic Surgery, Centre Hospitalier de Versailles, Le Chesnay, France
e-mail: npujol@ch-versailles.fr

L. Lipinski
Department of Orthopedic Surgery, Centre Hospitalier de Versailles, Le Chesnay, France

Orthopedics and Pediatric Orthopedics Clinic, Medical University of Lodz, Lodz, Poland

S. H. Kim
Department of Orthopedic Surgery, Centre Hospitalier de Versailles, Le Chesnay, France

Department of Orthopedic Surgery, Chung-Ang University Hospital, Seoul, Republic of Korea

M. T. Hirschmann et al. (eds.), *ESSKA Instructional Course Lecture Book*,
https://doi.org/10.1007/978-3-662-61264-4_1

damage. ACL reconstruction is difficult to perform using a bone bridge for lateral meniscal transplantation due to the position of the tibial tunnel.

The classic contraindications for isolated meniscal allograft transplantation include malalignment and Outerbridge IV changes. There is little high-level evidence in the literature to guide treatment for combined lesions involving ACL, meniscus, malalignment, and cartilage.

Other potential contraindications to meniscal allograft transplantation include open physes, previous infection, and inflammatory arthropathy.

1.3 Meniscal Extrusion of Allografts

Numerous publications studying meniscus extrusion following MAT have been published [8–10]. Noyes and Barber-Westin [11] performed a systematic review of this literature to determine the incidence and clinical significance of meniscus extrusion following MAT. They found no significant association between extrusion and patient reported outcomes in the short term. In the long term, there is no data but results would be different. Extrusion of the native meniscus has a high association with the development of osteoarthritis. Therefore, extrusion following MAT may result in graft failure and the early development of osteoarthritis as well. So one of the goals of the technical improvements in MAT should be to decrease graft extrusion. Mid-body fixation of MAT to the tibia doesn't prevent extrusion under loading conditions [12]. Soft tissue fixation leads to a higher level of meniscal extrusion when compared to bone block fixation technique [3]. Bone block fixation keyhole technique may lead to greater extrusion when the keyhole tunnel is not perfectly placed in the axial plane [6]. So there is a need of additional technical improvements.

1.4 The Intermeniscal Ligament (IML)

The intermeniscal ligament is present in 54–94% of knees [13]. Nelson and LaPrade distinguished III types of anatomic variants of this ligament with I type being most frequent one [14]. It connects anterior horns of medial and lateral meniscus, preventing from excessive extrusion during knee flexion [15].

Potential positive effect of anterior intermeniscal ligament on meniscal allograft fixation and preventing extrusion has been neglected. We believe that it could increase stability if the MAT and prevent early extrusion (Fig. 1.1).

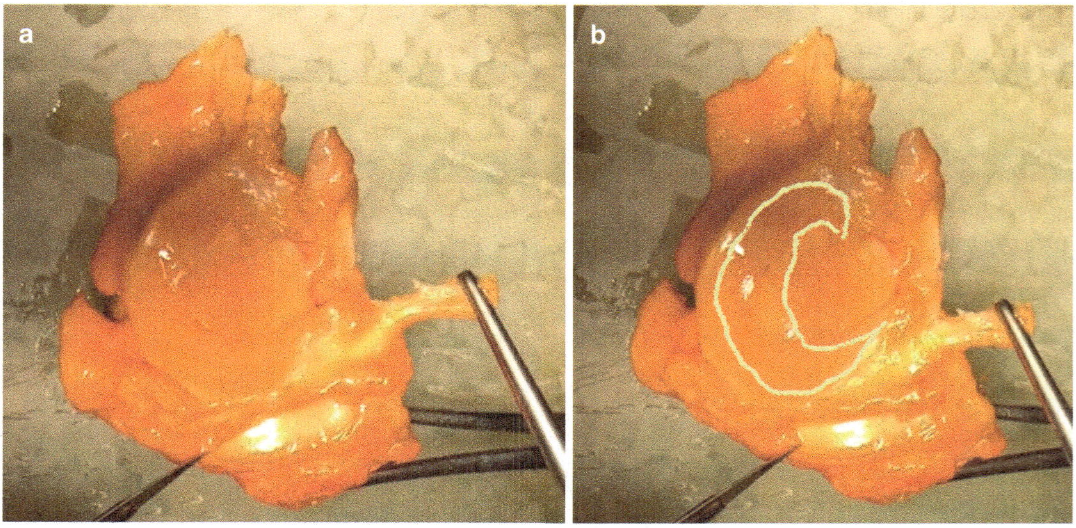

Fig. 1.1 Anatomic description of the ability of the IML to limit extrusion (**a**) under tension, (**b**) without tension

1.5 Preferred Surgical Technique

1.5.1 Knee Position

Patients under general anesthesia are positioned supine on a standard operating table.

The procedure commences with a diagnostic arthroscopy to evaluate the chondral surfaces to reconfirm that the patient is a candidate for meniscal allograft transplantation according to the aforementioned indications.

The medial portal is initially created so as to align the lateral portal with visualization over the anterior horn attachment site. On the medial side, superficial medial collateral ligament is released with a pie-crusting technique for better visualization of medial compartment [16]. Debridement of the meniscal remnant is carried out minimally to the peripheral capsule and a tuft of capsular attachment of meniscus is left to provide a reference for anchoring of the transplant, as well as provide some tissue to sew into peripherally.

The peripheral rim of the tibial plateau is abraded with a shaver or a 4 mm motorized burr, using the same principles of the glenoid preparation for Bankart repair. All osteophytes are removed [17].

1.5.2 Tibial Tunnel Preparation

Posterior root attachment is previously marked with a radiofrequency device.

Using an ACL tip guide, a 0.62 mm Kirschner wire is drilled to a position that would correspond to the posterior margin of the posterior root of the meniscus. The tunnel is overdrilled with a 4.5 mm reamer. A suture is pulled out by the tunnel.

1.5.3 Graft Preparation

Fresh-frozen grafts are being used in all cases and graft size is being determined by preoperative planning after proper measuring sagittal, coronal, and transverse planes on X-ray, CT, and MRI scans. Careful inspection of the graft is performed in terms of lesions and degeneration. Sterile marker is used to determine anterior to posterior orientation as well as estimated areas of sutures insertions. No 2 FiberWire® (Arthrex, Naples, FL, USA) is being used to anchor posterior root with several baseball stitches. No 2 TigerWire® (Arthrex, Naples, FL, USA) is being used to anchor anterior root in the same manner. The anterior aspect of the MAT is carefully dissected to determine the insertion of intermeniscal ligament (Fig. 1.2). Intermeniscal ligament remnant is secured with baseball stich with No 2 FiberWire®.

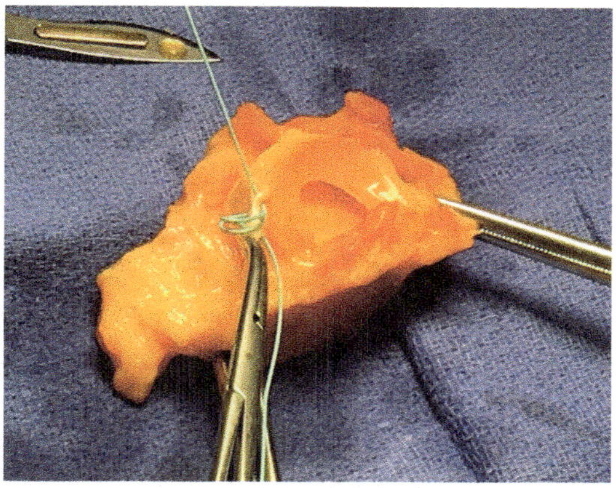

Fig. 1.2 Dissection of the IML of the allograft

The graft is being inserted into the joint by pulling suture through the previously prepared medial or lateral portal. When MAT is in place the posterior root pulling suture is secured temporarily with a clamp. Probe is used to allow smooth localization of the graft. MAT is sutured from posterior to anterior with Fastfix 360® (Smith and Nephew, UK) using combination of horizontal and perpendicular sutures located alternatively on the superior side or on the inferior side of the transplant. The anterior root is fixed with a SwiveLock® 4.75 mm (Arthrex, Naples, FL). The remnant of the intermeniscal ligament is fixed by using a SwiveLock® 4.75 mm near the anatomic insertion to anterior root of the native meniscus (Fig. 1.3). Posterior root pulling suture is secured to the tibia with a cortical button with the knee placed near full extension for a medial meniscus and in 70° of flexion for a lateral meniscus. Final inspection is performed to confirm proper graft position and tension on the whole meniscus.

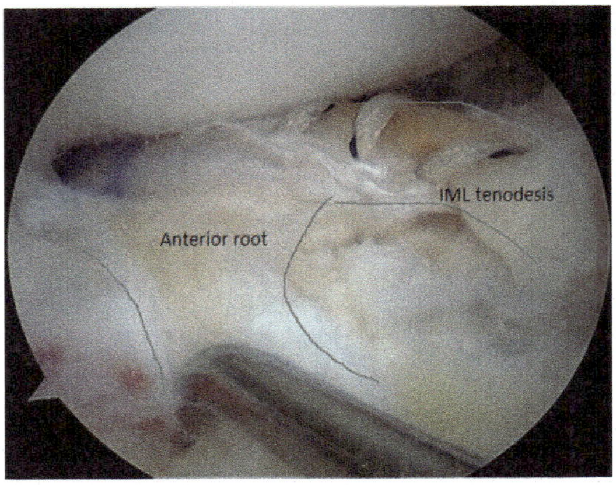

Fig. 1.3 Arthroscopic aspect of the two anterior fixations (example of a medial meniscus, left knee)

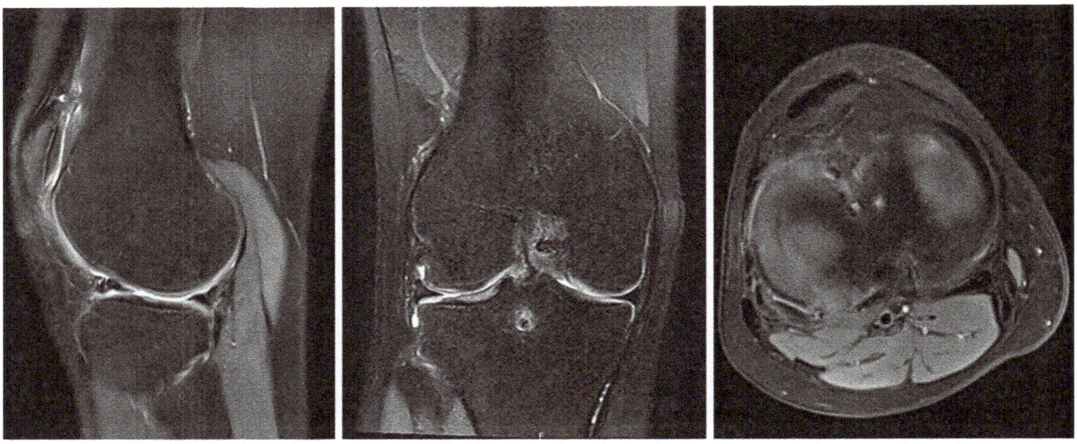

Fig. 1.4 MRI scans showing MAT with preservation of IML at 1 year

1.6 Conclusion

The purpose of this Technical Article was to describe a novel technique of arthroscopic soft tissue MAT with additional anterior fixation of the intermeniscal ligament. We performed this technique for more than 5 years. Mid-term results are encouraging (clinically and with MRI controls, Fig. 1.4). Previous soft tissue outcomes show less encouraging outcome in term of extrusion. This should be a way of research in order to improve our results and if possible decrease the rate of young patients knees converted into total knee replacements.

References

1. Jacquet C, Pujol N, Pauly V, Beaufils P, Ollivier M. Analysis of the trends in arthroscopic meniscectomy and meniscus repair procedures in France from 2005 to 2017. Orthop Traumatol Surg Res. 2019;105:677–82.
2. De Bruycker M, Verdonk PCM, Verdonk RC. Meniscal allograft transplantation: a meta-analysis. SICOT J. 2017;3:33.
3. Abat F, Gelber PE, Erquicia JI, Pelfort X, Gonzalez-Lucena G, Monllau JC. Suture-only fixation technique leads to a higher degree of extrusion than bony fixation in meniscal allograft transplantation. Am J Sports Med. 2012;40:1591–6.
4. Faivre B, Boisrenoult P, Lonjon G, Pujol N, Beaufils P. Lateral meniscus allograft transplantation: clinical

and anatomic outcomes after arthroscopic implantation with tibial tunnels versus open implantation without tunnels. Orthop Traumatol Surg Res. 2014;100:297–302.

5. Ha JK, Shim JC, Kim DW, Lee YS, Ra HJ, Kim JG. Relationship between meniscal extrusion and various clinical findings after meniscus allograft transplantation. Am J Sports Med. 2010;38:2448–55.
6. Lee DH, Kim JM, Lee BS, Kim KA, Bin SI. Greater axial trough obliquity increases the risk of graft extrusion in lateral meniscus allograft transplantation. Am J Sports Med. 2012;40:1597–605.
7. Lee SY, Yoon J, Cho YS, Son RC, Kim SK, Ahn SH, et al. Various factors contribute to graft extrusion in lateral meniscus allograft transplantation. Knee Surg Sports Traumatol Arthrosc. 2017;25:374–82.
8. Jang KM, Wang JH. Lateral meniscus allograft transplantation using a single-incision technique. Knee Surg Sports Traumatol Arthrosc. 2015;23:258–63.
9. Koh YG, Moon HK, Kim YC, Park YS, Jo SB, Kwon SK. Comparison of medial and lateral meniscal transplantation with regard to extrusion of the allograft, and its correlation with clinical outcome. J Bone Joint Surg Br. 2012;94:190–3.
10. Lee DH, Kim SB, Kim TH, Cha EJ, Bin SI. Midterm outcomes after meniscal allograft transplantation: comparison of cases with extrusion versus without extrusion. Am J Sports Med. 2010;38:247–54.
11. Noyes FR, Barber-Westin SD. A systematic review of the incidence and clinical significance of postoperative meniscus transplant extrusion. Knee Surg Sports Traumatol Arthrosc. 2015;23:290–302.
12. Hewison C, Kolaczek S, Caterine S, Berardelli R, Beveridge T, Lording T, et al. Peripheral fixation of meniscal allograft does not reduce coronal extrusion under physiological load. Knee Surg Sports Traumatol Arthrosc. 2019;27:1924–30.
13. Poh SY, Yew KS, Wong PL, Koh SB, Chia SL, Fook-Chong S, et al. Role of the anterior intermeniscal ligament in tibiofemoral contact mechanics during axial joint loading. Knee. 2012;19:135–9.
14. Nelson EW, LaPrade RF. The anterior intermeniscal ligament of the knee. An anatomic study. Am J Sports Med. 2000;28:74–6.
15. Ollivier M, Falguieres J, Pithioux M, Boisrenoult P, Beaufils P, Pujol N. Sectioning of the anterior intermeniscal ligament changes knee loading mechanics. Arthroscopy. 2018;34:2837–43.
16. Jeon SW, Jung M, Chun YM, Lee SK, Jung WS, Choi CH, et al. The percutaneous pie-crusting medial release during arthroscopic procedures of the medial meniscus does neither affect valgus laxity nor clinical outcome. Knee Surg Sports Traumatol Arthrosc. 2018;26:2912–9.
17. Jeon B, Kim JM, Lee CR, Kim KA, Bin SI. An osteophyte in the tibial plateau is a risk factor for allograft extrusion after meniscus allograft transplantation. Am J Sports Med. 2015;43:1215–21.

2 First-Time Patellar Dislocation: A Modern Treatment Strategy

Patellar Height as a Factor

M. Berruto and D. Tradati

Patellar height is one of the most important primary factors in patellar instability. At the time of the first patellar dislocation x-rays evaluation is performed in the majority of the cases, therefore patellar height assessment is largely feasible in daily practice. The evolving knowledge in patello-femoral instability mechanisms led to the introduction of further methods to characterize more precisely patellar height, including the use of other imaging sources like CT-scan and MRI. The importance of this parameter relies on the fact that patients with pathological patellar height could present an inadequate engagement of the patella with the femoral trochlea thus leading to an increased risk of dislocation.

Dejour and Walch [1] reported an incidence of abnormal patellar height in 24% of patients with primary lateral patellar dislocation (LPD) while only 3% in controls. Higher values were reported by Askenberger et al. [2] considering a population of 103 children under 14 years of age who underwent LPD and a control population of 69 patients. Patella alta was reported in 76% of the LDP patients and in 36% of the control group. Similarly Arendt et al. [3] reported an incidence of patella alta equal to 54%, analyzing a mixed population of 157 patients who underwent primary LPD.

Lower data were reported by Christensen et al. [4] in a cohort study including 584 patients with LPD and a mean age of 21.5 years. Only 14.6% of them had radiographic evidence of patella alta.

The variability of these data could be heavily affected by the age of the selected population. Patellar height measurements were initially developed on adult's knees. Since the patella ossification proceeds from proximal to distal and both the tibial and tibial tubercle profile could be not fully recognized, therefore higher patellar height values could be observed considering a younger population in comparison to a mixed one.

The most common methods in order to evaluate patellar height, based on plain X-rays, are represented by the Insall-Salvati Index (ISI) [5] and the Caton-Deschamps Index (CDI) [6].

The ISI represents the ratio between the length of the patellar tendon from the lower pole of the patella to its tibial insertion and the greatest pole-to-pole distance of the patella on a sagittal view.

The CDI is defined as the ratio between the distance from the antero-superior angle of the tibia to the lower edge of the joint surface of the patella and the length of the patellar joint surface. Patella alta is defined in the presence of a ISI greater than 1.2 or a CDI greater than 1.2.

Since the introduction of the MRI and CT, many authors tried to adapt these indexes to both

M. Berruto (✉) · D. Tradati
Department of Knee Surgery, University Clinic of Milan, ASST Pini-CTO, Milan, Italy
e-mail: massimo.berruto@fastwebnet.it

M. T. Hirschmann et al. (eds.), *ESSKA Instructional Course Lecture Book*,
https://doi.org/10.1007/978-3-662-61264-4_2

the methods. Current data seem to support the good correlation between these techniques, nevertheless a mean patellar height overestimation of +0.1 should be assumed for both the MRI and CT methods [7, 8].

Both ISI and CDI represent good and reliable too for patellar height assessment, nevertheless they lack information to describe the relationship between trochlea and patella.

Some subjects could present patella alta without experiencing instability due to the increased trochlear length improving the patellofemoral engagement. Conversely, other patients with nonpathological patellar height values could report patellar instability due to a short trochlea or a small patellar articular surface leading to an inadequate engagement. In order to overcome this problem, Biedert and Albrecht proposed a new method based on the MRI, the Patello-Trochlear Index (PTI) [9].

The PTI is defined as the ratio between articular cartilage of the patella and trochlear cartilage. The reference slice used to measure this index is represented by the one including the maximal patellar length and the cutoff values range from 0.125 to 0.28.

Nevertheless this technique could be unreliable in cases of patella instability, in which patella may be positioned more laterally than the center of the trochlea therefore lying on a different sagittal plane. In order to overcome this limitation, Dejour et al. [10] proposed the measurement of the Sagittal Patellofemoral Engagement (SPE), using two different slices for both the patellar and trochlear references.

The use of both PTI and SPE are not yet commonly spread therefore there are missing data in literature in order to consider them as standard tools in the assessment of patellar redislocation risk. Conversely, both CDI and ISI have been objects of many studies in literature in order to predict the risk of further dislocations.

Arendt et al. [11] reported a predicted probability of redislocation equal to 15.6% in patients with isolated patella alta, rising to 42.8–47.3% when in combination to open-growth-plate or sulcus angle >154° and equal to 78.5% when concomitant to both of them. The adjusted odds ratios for redislocation in patients with patellar alta was estimated in 3.00 (1.34–6.70).

According to these data, Christensen et al. [4] reported in patients with radiographic evidence of patella alta a 10.4-fold increased risk of new patellar dislocation and 8.9-fold increased risk of contralateral patellar dislocation. Moreover, time to recurrence was significantly decreased in patients with patella alta (16.4 months). Overlapping data regarding LDP reoccurrence were reported by Zhang et al. [12] using the MRI to determine patellar height (OR: 8.4).

Nevertheless there is no complete agreement in literature over this topic and some author reported no effect of patellar height over the risk of LPD reoccurrence. Population age and measurement techniques could highly impact the result of these studies and the comparison between them could be hardly managed.

The current data seem to suggest that patellar height could be a useful tool in predicting the risk of new patellar dislocation when associated to other factors of patellar instability, conversely should not be considered alone since it could be a normal variant of the knee anatomy.

References

1. Dejour H, Walch G, Nove-Josserand L, Guier C. Factors of patellar instability: an anatomic radiographic study. Knee Surg Sports Traumatol Arthrosc. 1994;2(1):19–26.
2. Askenberger M, Janarv PM, Finnbogason T, Arendt EA. Morphology and anatomic patellar instability risk factors in first-time traumatic lateral patellar dislocations: a prospective magnetic resonance imaging study in skeletally immature children. Am J Sports Med. 2017;45(1):50–8.
3. Arendt EA, England K, Agel J, Tompkins MA. An analysis of knee anatomic imaging factors associated with primary lateral patellar dislocations. Knee Surg Sports Traumatol Arthrosc. 2017;25(10):3099–107.
4. Christensen TC, Sanders TL, Pareek A, Mohan R, Dahm DL, Krych AJ. Risk factors and time to recurrent Ipsilateral and contralateral patellar dislocations. Am J Sports Med. 2017;45(9):2105–10.
5. Insall J, Salvati E. Patella position in the normal knee joint. Radiology. 1971;101(1):101–4.

6. Caton J, Deschamps G, Chambat P, Lerat JL, Dejour H. Patella infera. Apropos of 128 cases. Rev Chir Orthop Reparatrice Appar Mot. 1982;68(5):317–25.
7. Yue RA, Arendt EA, Tompkins MA. Patellar height measurements on radiograph and magnetic resonance imaging in patellar instability and control patients. J Knee Surg. 2017;30(9):943–50.
8. Lee PP, Chalian M, Carrino JA, Eng J, Chhabra A. Multimodality correlations of patellar height measurement on X-ray, CT, and MRI. Skelet Radiol. 2012;41(10):1309–14.
9. Biedert RM, Albrecht S. The patellotrochlear index: a new index for assessing patellar height. Knee Surg Sports Traumatol Arthrosc. 2006;14(8):707–12.
10. Dejour D, Ferrua P, Ntagiopoulos PG, Radier C, Hulet C, Remy F, et al. The introduction of a new MRI index to evaluate sagittal patellofemoral engagement. Orthop Traumatol Surg Res. 2013;99(8 Suppl):S391–8.
11. Arendt EA, Askenberger M, Agel J, Tompkins MA. Risk of redislocation after primary patellar dislocation: a clinical prediction model based on magnetic resonance imaging variables. Am J Sports Med. 2018;46(14):3385–90.
12. Zhang GY, Ding HY, Li EM, Zheng L, Bai ZW, Shi H, et al. Incidence of second-time lateral patellar dislocation is associated with anatomic factors, age and injury patterns of medial patellofemoral ligament in first-time lateral patellar dislocation: a prospective magnetic resonance imaging study with 5-year follow-up. Knee Surg Sports Traumatol Arthrosc. 2019;27(1):197–205.

Operative Techniques: Kinematic Alignment

3

Max Ettinger and Tilman Calliess

3.1 Introduction

Over the last years, the dogma of mechanical alignment (MA) was fading. With aligning the femoral and tibial component perpendicular to the mechanical axis in the coronal plane, long-term survivorship and the restoration of the patient's function was supposed to be superior compared to outliers beyond ±3° to the mechanical axis. Correcting the natural anatomy to neutral means to adapt the soft tissue envelop with the risk of instability and paradoxical kinematics, is referred to be a major reason for revision surgery. This might be a major reason why up to 25% of patients are dissatisfied with their TKA and 10% need revision within the first 10 years [1, 2]. Further, the natural constitution of the general population is not neutral [3], thus the correction of the limb to the mechanical axis requires several balancing steps [4].

Kinematic alignment (KA) recently emerged as a potential alternative. The biomechanical rationale for KA is based on Hollister's findings about the axes of rotation of the knee [5], as well as Eckoff's findings about the three-dimensional morphology and kinematics of the distal part of the femur [6]. Their findings indicate, that three kinematic axes are defined: (1) The primary flexion-and-extension axis about which the tibia flexes and extends is located in the distal femur condyles and defined by the shapes of those. Moreover, the axis is geometrically defined by the axis of a cylinder aligned to the articular surface of the distal and dorsal condyle. (2) The axis where the tibia internally and externally rotates is defined to be perpendicular to axis number one (femoral-tibial flexion-extension axis). Logically, the actual position of the tibia rotation axis is dynamic throughout the range of motion. This is mandatory in order to get femoral rollback and tibial pivoting. These findings are in line with biomechanical in vivo studies showing that the position of this tibial rotation axis is depending on different motor tasks and loading conditions [7, 8]. (3) The third axis is the axis about which the patella rotates. This axis is defined to be parallel to the primary femur axis and located anterior and proximal to it. Overall, the knee motion is defined by the femoral surface anatomy and guided by the soft tissue. In particular, the rollback of the femur and the rotation kinematics are driven by the soft tissue envelop.

Based on the biomechanical rationale, the concept of kinematic alignment is to restore the constitutional (healthy/pre-arthritic) anatomy and the physiological joint line orientation with the implant. This is done by aligning the

M. Ettinger (✉)
Department of Orthopaedic Surgery, Hannover Medical School, Hanover, Germany
e-mail: Max@ettinger.info

T. Calliess
Articon Bern, Bern, Switzerland
e-mail: Tilman@calliess.ch

M. T. Hirschmann et al. (eds.), *ESSKA Instructional Course Lecture Book*,
https://doi.org/10.1007/978-3-662-61264-4_3

prosthetic components with respect to the shape of the distal and dorsal femur. Therewith the flexion radius of the femoral prosthetic component is co-aligned to the physiological primary flexion-extension axis of the knee, enabling the restoration of the isometric stability of the medial compartment. The reconstruction of the flexion-extension axis automatically co-aligns the trochlea radius to the patella-rotation axis, as it is parallel. As mentioned before, aligning the tibia component with respect to the femur (parallel) also restores the perpendicular tibia rotation axis.

A key part of the KA concept is, that the pre-arthritic joint surface of the individual patient is the desired situation, which is to be reconstructed. Thus, the individual wear situation has to be analyzed in order to calculate the pre-arthritic situation and to restore it with the prosthetic components as close as possible.

With aligning the components parallel to the natural joint line orientation, this technique provides a more anatomic position of the implant, leading to no- or less-balancing steps [9]. Up to date, six randomized controlled trials (RCTs) compare KA versus MA with a follow up between 12 and 24 months [10–16]. Out of these six RCTs, two reported equality between KA and MA, whereas four studies are in favor of KA. The potential benefit of KA is concluded to the ability of a more central weight bearing in the knee during gait, combined with the ability to stand more parallel to the floor [16], as well as better pain relief and an increased range of motion (ROM).

3.2 Surgical Techniques

General: The primary goal in KA is to reproduce the physiological (natural/pre-arthritic) joint line surface of the distal and posterior femur in the first place. Thus a "true measured resection technique" is mandatory, in order to exactly resect the amount of bone and cartilage that is replaced by the implant thickness. The key issue is to take the wear that is present into account aiming for the pre-arthritic surface and to compensate for it during surgery. Several studies report data concerning the average cartilage thickness and typical wear patterns in knee osteoarthritis [17, 18], as well as the elasticity of the cartilage and meniscus by about 20–25% of the volume [19]. Both, thickness and elasticity have to be taken into account within the process of wear calculation, as the prosthetic implant shows no elasticity at all.

Based on this consideration, 2 mm have been established as a good average estimation for complete cartilage wear.

3.3 Manual Technique

After calculating the wear, it is compensated by the use of spacer blocks of 2 mm thickness adjusted to the distal cut. Different variants of the block are available in order to compensate for different wear patterns (Fig. 3.1).

The orientation of the distal cut is aligned to the physiological joint line orientation instead of the mechanical axis (Fig. 3.2). The femoral

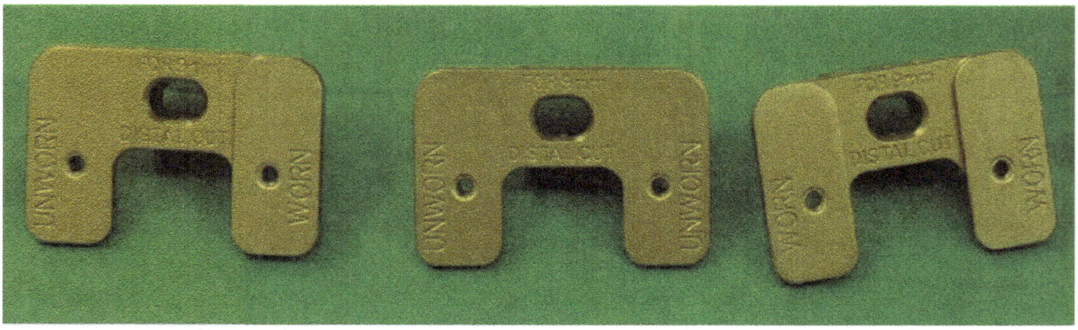

Fig. 3.1 Three different blocks are available in order to compensate for different wear patterns at the distal femur. Worn/unworn for isolated medial/lateral wear and worn/worn for complete wear medial and lateral

rotation is aligned to the posterior condylar line at 0° external rotation. In the concept of true measured resection, a strict posterior referencing for the component position and sizing is mandatory (Fig. 3.3).

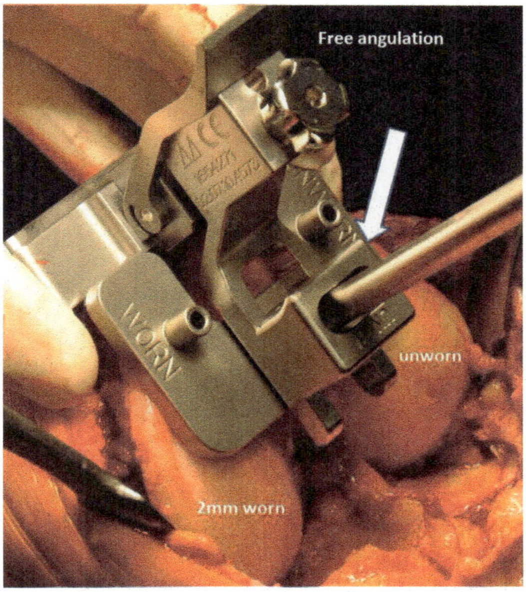

Fig. 3.2 The distal resection follows the natural valgus angle of the distal femur after compensating for the wear. This shows a worn side medial and an unworn lateral side

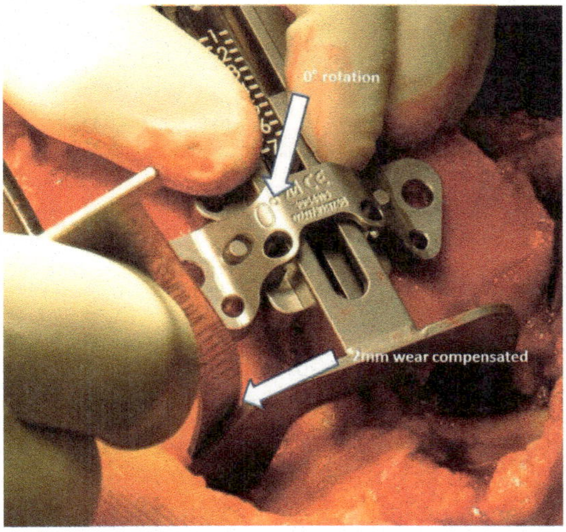

Fig. 3.3 The rotation is set to 0° with respect to the posterior condylar line after compensating for potential posterior wear. This is done in order to reconstruct the natural flexion-extension axis of the knee

Therewith already four of six degrees of freedom to position the femoral component are defined. The only two parameters left are about the mediolateral alignment of the component (which is of minor biomechanical impact), and the femoral flexion. The femoral flexion should be orientated with respect to the physiological flexion of the distal femur (distal ¼) as this influences patella tracking and sizing of the component [20]. To achieve that, an intramedullary alignment with respect to the distal portion of the femur has been described as a reliable technique [21]. In the standard technique a 10-cm-long intramedullary rod is inserted through a centered entrance hole a.p. and m.l. wise to set the femoral flexion (Fig. 3.4).

The resection height of every cut is measured using a caliper. The saw blade thickness is also taken into account, so that the typical resection is about 7 mm with no wear present and 5 mm with complete cartilage abrasion (for an 8 mm femoral component) (Fig. 3.5).

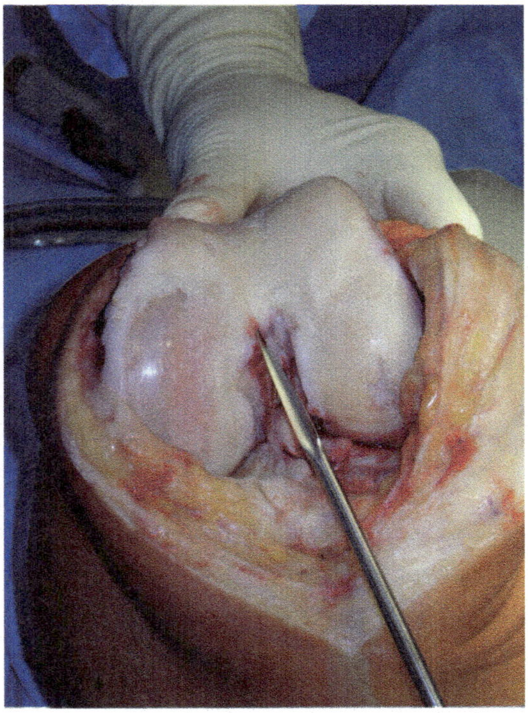

Fig. 3.4 A centered entrance hole a.p. and m.l. wise aligns the flexion of the femoral with respect to the anatomy of the distal femur

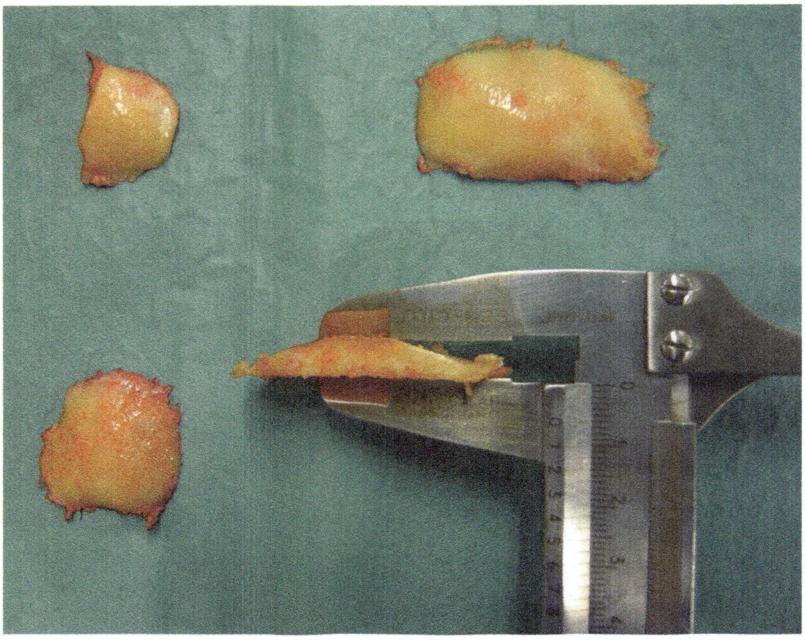

Fig. 3.5 All cuts have to be checked by a caliper. The thickness of the sawblade as well as the wear have to be taken into account when measuring the resection heights. Wear+ sawblade+ bone should equal the thickness of the femoral component

The tibia cut now follows the femur with the aim to produce a symmetrically balanced extension gap and an isometric balance on the medial compartment through the whole ROM. On the lateral side the physiological laxity in flexion is accepted accordingly. As the femoral surface is restored physiologically a mismatch of the flexion to the extension gap does not appear and the physiological isometry of the medial compartment can be reconstructed.

For alignment of the tibia, the femoral trial component is used in the first place. After clearing off the relevant osteophytes, it is placed onto the femur and the knee is brought to extension. Using spacer blocks analogue to unicompartmental knee arthroplasty, now the wear on the tibia side can be evaluated and the soft tissue can be brought to its natural length and tension. This determines the resection level on each side as well as the varus-valgus orientation of the tibia as the cut is parallel to the distal femur. With both cruciate ligaments still intact, even the tibia rotation can be determined with respect to the femur (Fig. 3.6).

The initial tibial cut should be conservative regarding the thickness and degree of posterior slope. Further, the initial cut should go into the direction of the tibial varus (Fig. 3.7).

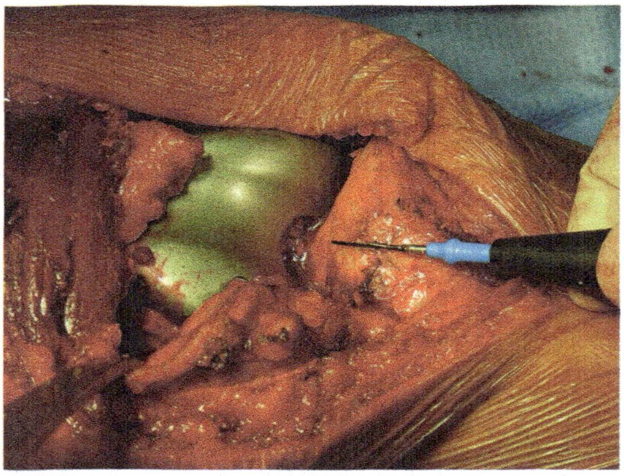

Fig. 3.6 With both cruciate ligaments still intact, the tibia rotation can be determined with respect to the femur and may be marked with an electric cautery

Further, the physiological rollback should be reconstructed with the prosthesis. If the later, during trial reduction, the knee shows pathological rollback, the slope needs to be adapted (if excessive rollback occurs) or the prosthesis could to be changed to a posterior stabilized design (in case of a paradoxical anterior contact point). Usually the native slope should be reduced in the first place to compensate for the loss of the anterior cruciate ligament.

Based on these parameters evaluated with the femoral trail in place, the tibial cut is aligned and conducted. The varus orientation can be visualized using an extramedullary alignment rod and a goniometer. After that, the joint balance is evaluated by the use of a balancer (Fig. 3.8). If there is an imbalance present, the tibial cut is adapted accordingly.

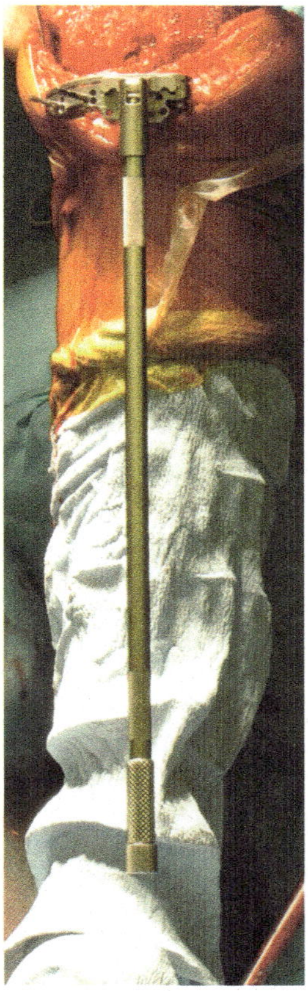

Fig. 3.7 The initial tibial cut is set in slight varus (left knee)

Adapting the tibial cut may be done by using correction blocks. Different correction blocks are available to adapt the alignment to more varus or valgus orientation, or to change the slope precisely (Fig. 3.9).

In general, this described technique can be carried out with standard instruments for TKA, independent from the TKA design or manufacturer. Only a few basic conditions have to be fulfilled: (1) ability to set the femoral valgus angle independent to the intramedullary guide, (2) strict posterior referencing of the femur size and rotation, and (3) extramedullary alignment of the tibia to reassemble the varus and slope independent from anatomical axis.

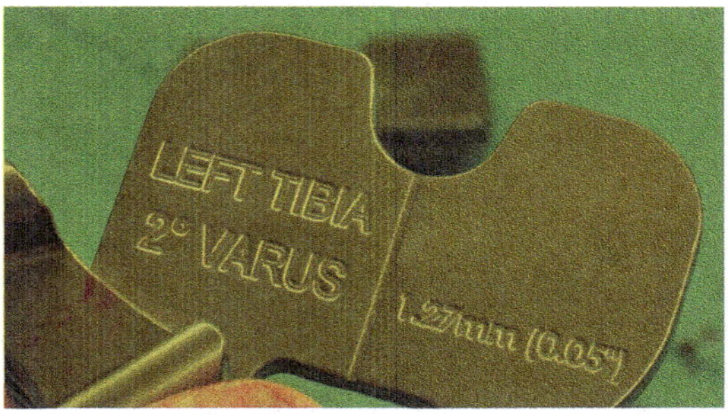

Fig. 3.9 The alignment may be adapted by precise correction blocks

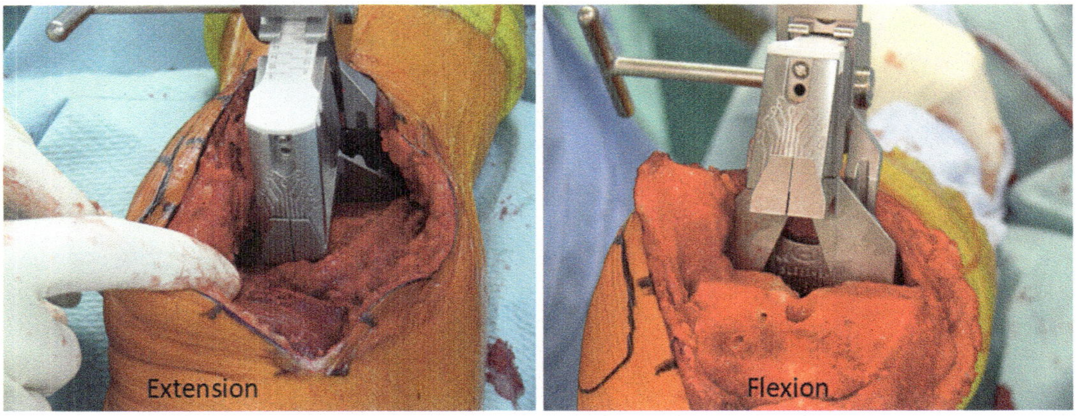

Fig. 3.8 The joint balance and kinematics are evaluated by the use of balancers

3.4 Patient-Specific Cutting Bocks (PSI)

CT-based PSI blocks may be used for KA as well. The major advantage of this technique is, that it relies on an image-based, segmented, three-dimensional (3D) model of the individual patient-derived CT scans. Thus, a precise reconstruction of the individual anatomy and joint surface is possible by positioning the implant in this 3D model (Fig. 3.10a–c). The resulting overall limb alignment can be displayed, the interaction between the actual joint geometry and the later prosthetic geometry can be visualized and parameters like the optimal component flexion can be determined. Further, all cutting angles and resection heights may individually planned (Fig. 3.11).

The operative plan is transferred in to the patient via PSI blocks (Fig. 3.12). The resection height of every cut has to be controlled with a caliper as well.

However, the drawback of the technique is that no soft tissue is included in the planning. This becomes a major limitation whenever compromises in the position of the prosthesis, for example in terms of the slope are to be made. Equal to the manual technique, a conventional balancer is used after the bony cuts in order to check the soft tissue balance. If there is an imbalance present, the tibial cut is adapted accordingly using "Cheating blocks" for varus/valgus or slope corrections, as described for the manual technique.

3.5 Image-Based Robotic Arm Assisted Surgery

This CT-based technique works with a preoperative reconstruction of the patient's individual anatomy as well. Figure 3.13 displays the patient's individual anatomy and the preoperative KA plan. This patient has an individual valgus of 1° in the femur and 4° of varus in the tibia (Fig. 3.14).

In contrast to the PSI, the surgeon has the feasibility to detect the soft tissue stability and tension at the beginning of the operation. Thus, the preoperative plan can be adapted to the individual situation of the patient, in order to achieve the

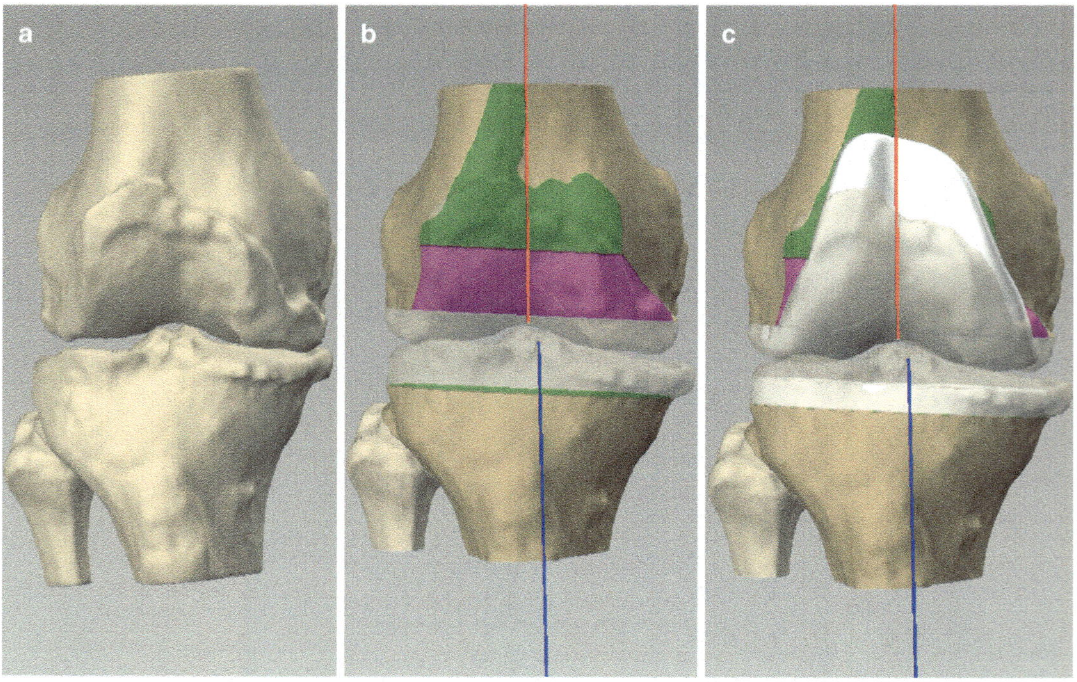

Fig. 3.10 (**a–c**) The CT-based PSI technique allows a precise reconstruction of the patient's individual anatomy

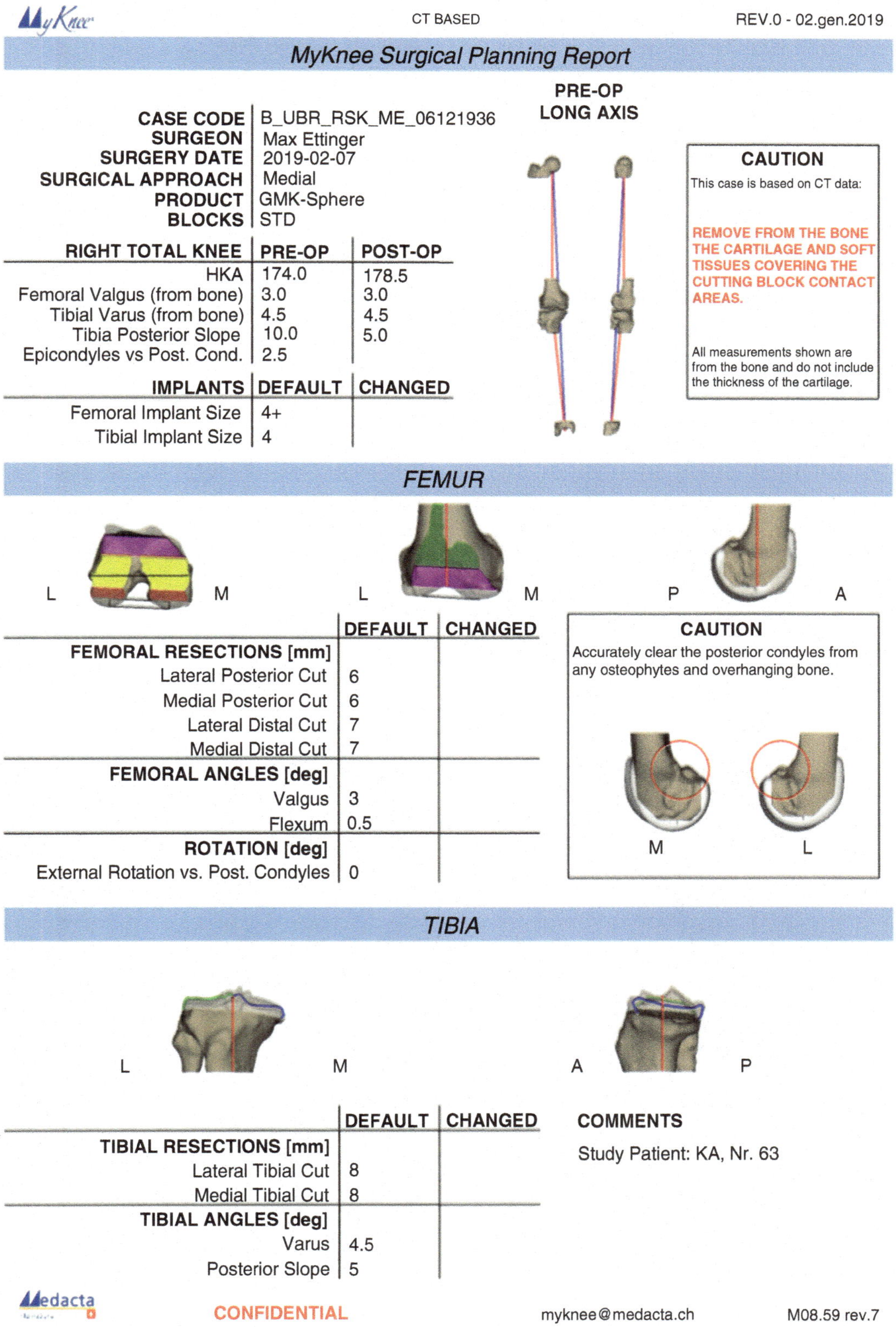

MyKnee CT BASED REV.0 - 02.gen.2019

MyKnee Surgical Planning Report

CASE CODE	B_UBR_RSK_ME_06121936
SURGEON	Max Ettinger
SURGERY DATE	2019-02-07
SURGICAL APPROACH	Medial
PRODUCT	GMK-Sphere
BLOCKS	STD

RIGHT TOTAL KNEE	**PRE-OP**	**POST-OP**
HKA	174.0	178.5
Femoral Valgus (from bone)	3.0	3.0
Tibial Varus (from bone)	4.5	4.5
Tibia Posterior Slope	10.0	5.0
Epicondyles vs Post. Cond.	2.5	

IMPLANTS	**DEFAULT**	**CHANGED**
Femoral Implant Size	4+	
Tibial Implant Size	4	

PRE-OP LONG AXIS

CAUTION
This case is based on CT data:
REMOVE FROM THE BONE THE CARTILAGE AND SOFT TISSUES COVERING THE CUTTING BLOCK CONTACT AREAS.
All measurements shown are from the bone and do not include the thickness of the cartilage.

FEMUR

L M L M P A

	DEFAULT	**CHANGED**
FEMORAL RESECTIONS [mm]		
Lateral Posterior Cut	6	
Medial Posterior Cut	6	
Lateral Distal Cut	7	
Medial Distal Cut	7	
FEMORAL ANGLES [deg]		
Valgus	3	
Flexum	0.5	
ROTATION [deg]		
External Rotation vs. Post. Condyles	0	

CAUTION
Accurately clear the posterior condyles from any osteophytes and overhanging bone.
M L

TIBIA

L M A P

	DEFAULT	**CHANGED**
TIBIAL RESECTIONS [mm]		
Lateral Tibial Cut	8	
Medial Tibial Cut	8	
TIBIAL ANGLES [deg]		
Varus	4.5	
Posterior Slope	5	

COMMENTS
Study Patient: KA, Nr. 63

Medacta CONFIDENTIAL myknee@medacta.ch M08.59 rev.7

Fig. 3.11 The patients individual anatomy preoperative and postoperative in the surgical planning screen: The femoral valgus, the tibial varus, the femoral flexion, the overall limb alignment, the posterior slope, the femoral rotation, the resection heights, and the implant size may individually be planned within the CT based KA planning algorithm best stability and kinematics with the implant in place. This allows the surgeon to adapt the plan for minor changes before the bone cuts are conducted. After cutting, a trial reduction is conducted in order to check the individual balance.

Figure 3.15 displays the real time situation. The software shows the postoperative situation with trial implants in place. This allows the surgeon to adapt the plan for minor changes if an imbalance occurs. Bony corrections may be conducted in 0.5 mm steps.

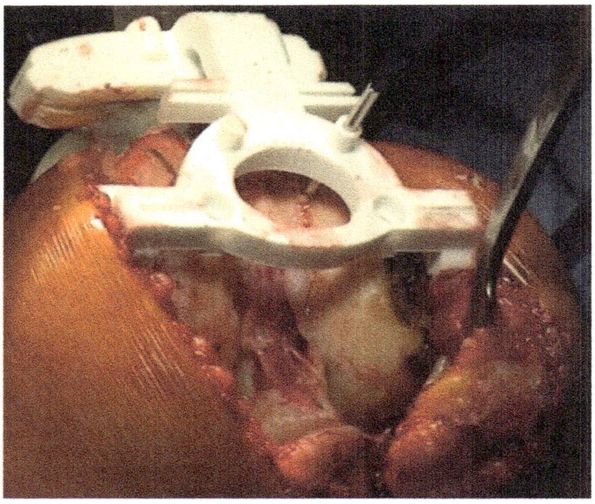

Fig. 3.12 PSI block for the preoperative KA plan

3.6 Image Less Robotic-Assisted Surgery

This image less technique works with an intraoperative reconstruction of the patient's individual anatomy. Compared to the CT-based techniques, the surgeon has to take the wear into account when using this technique, because a one-on-one surface reconstruction is done during the procedure using a pointer. Figure 3.16 demonstrates the image less reconstruction of the patient's individual anatomy calculated by the software at the beginning of the procedure. Equal to the PSI and image-based robotic techniques, the individual 3D reconstructed knee is the basis for the conduction of the KA plan.

With this technique, the surgeon has the feasibility to detect the soft tissue stability and tension at the beginning of the operation. Thus, the preoperative plan can be adapted to the individual situation of the patient, in order to achieve the best stability and kinematics with the implant in

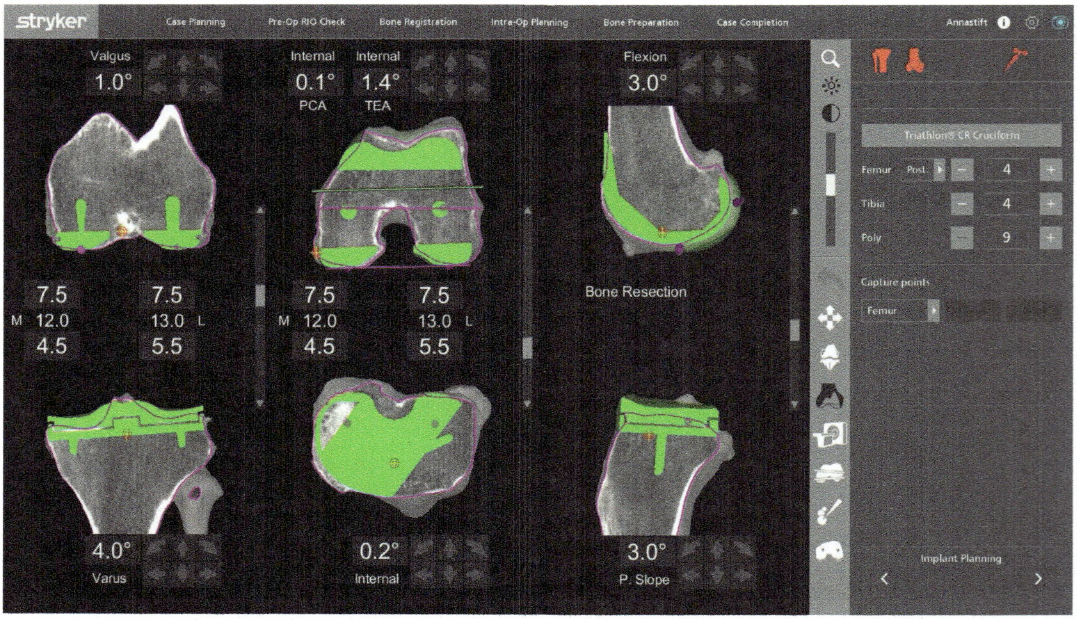

Fig. 3.13 Preoperative KA plan with image based robotics

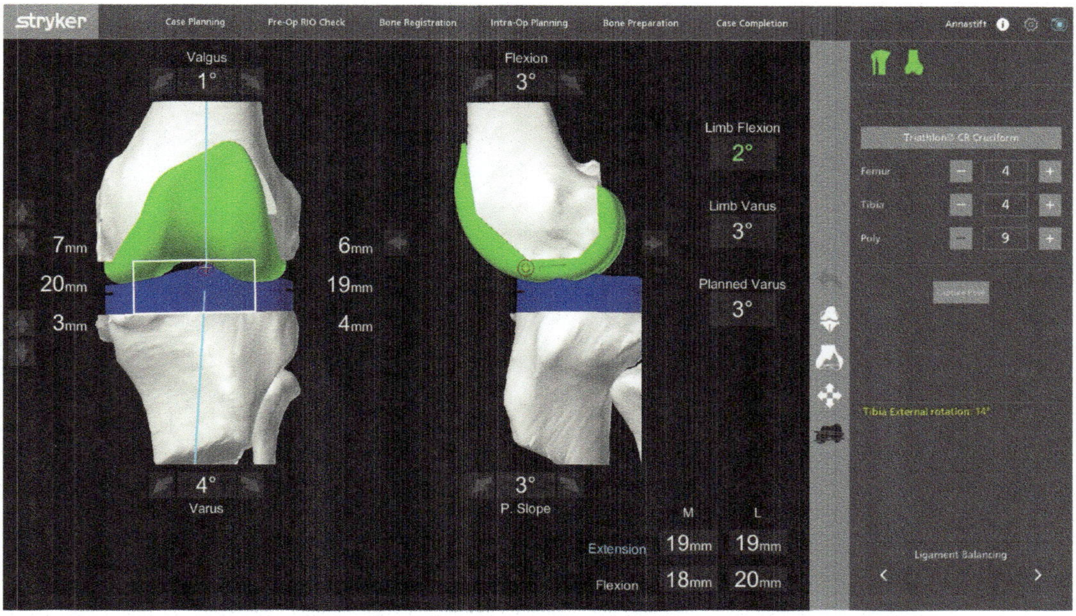

Fig. 3.14 (**a**–**c**) Image-based robotic arm assisted KA reconstruction. (**a**) Demonstrates a patient's individual valgus of 1° in the femur and 4° of varus in the tibia. (**b**) Demonstrates the individual reconstruction of the joint line obliquity and height. (**c**) Demonstrates the individual anatomy in the sagittal plane with 10° tibial slope and 11° of flexion of the distal femur with respect to the sagittal mechanical axis. (**d**) Demonstrates 0° of femoral flexion with respect to the distal femur anatomy and a reduced slope to 3°

place. Figure 3.17 shows the patients individual laxity (medial and lateral) throughout the whole range of motion.

Due to the detection of the individual soft tissue situation, the preoperative plan can be adapted to the individual situation of the patient, in order to achieve the best stability and kinematics with the implant in place. Figure 3.18 displays the virtual planning. The software simulates the postoperative situation. This allows the surgeon to adapt the plan for minor changes before the bone cuts are conducted.

Equal to the image-based robotic technique, a trial reduction is conducted in order to check the individual balance after the cutting with trial implants in place.

Figures 3.19 displays the real-time situation. The software shows the postoperative situation with trial implants in place. This allows the surgeon to adapt the plan for minor changes if an imbalance occurs. Bony corrections may be conducted in 0.5 mm steps (Fig. 3.20).

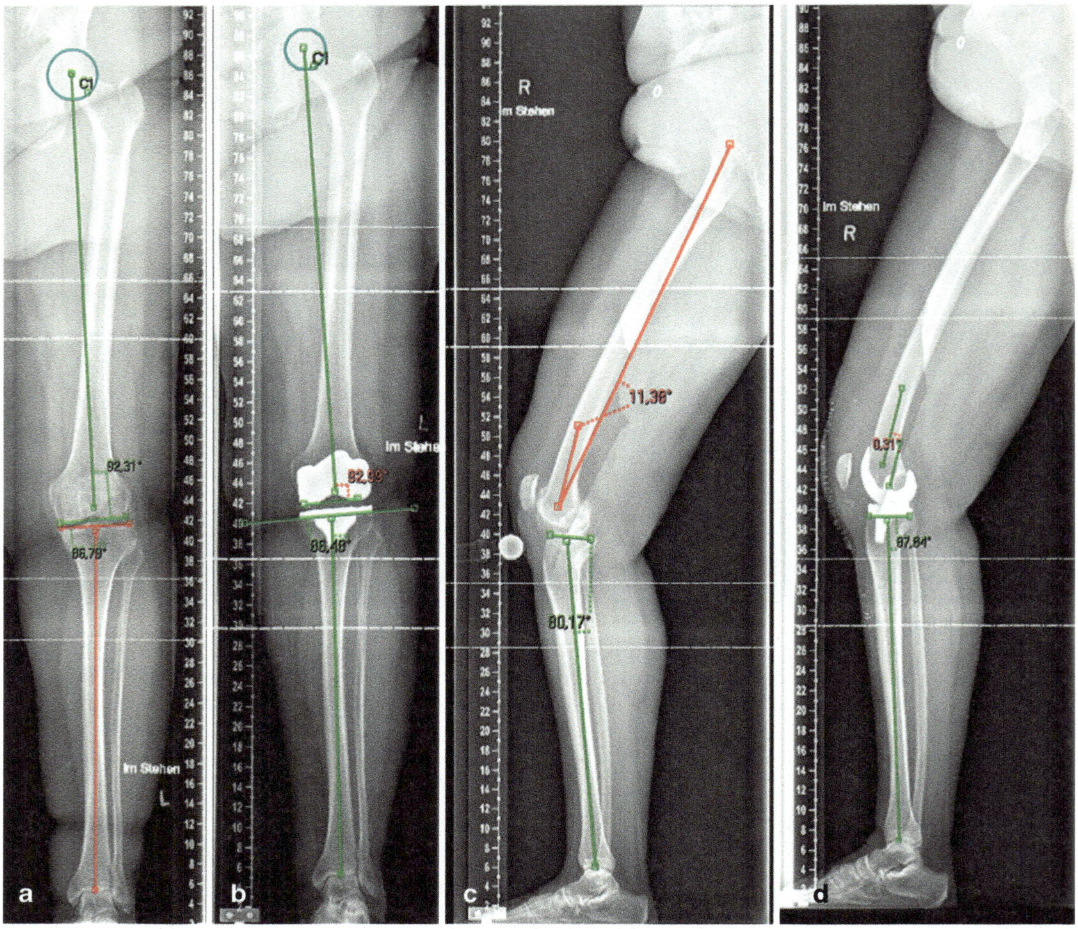

Fig. 3.15 The software simulates the postoperative situation. This individual KA plan lead to 1° of valgus in the femur and 4° of varus in the tibia, leading to a postoperative limb alignment of 3° varus. By conducting this plan, the extension gap was equally balanced, while reconstructing the asymmetric natural flexion gap

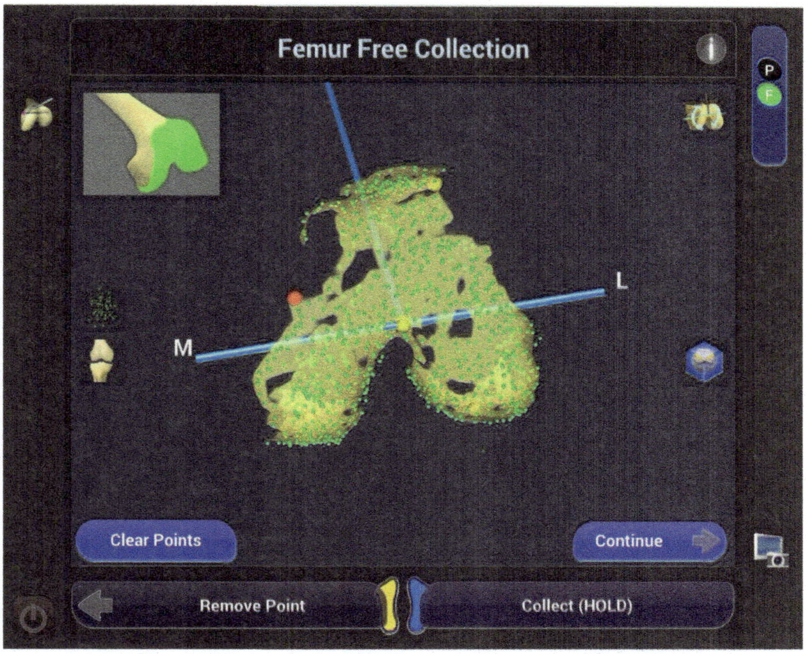

Fig. 3.16 The software calculates an individual 3D reconstruction of the patients knee at the beginning of the surgery

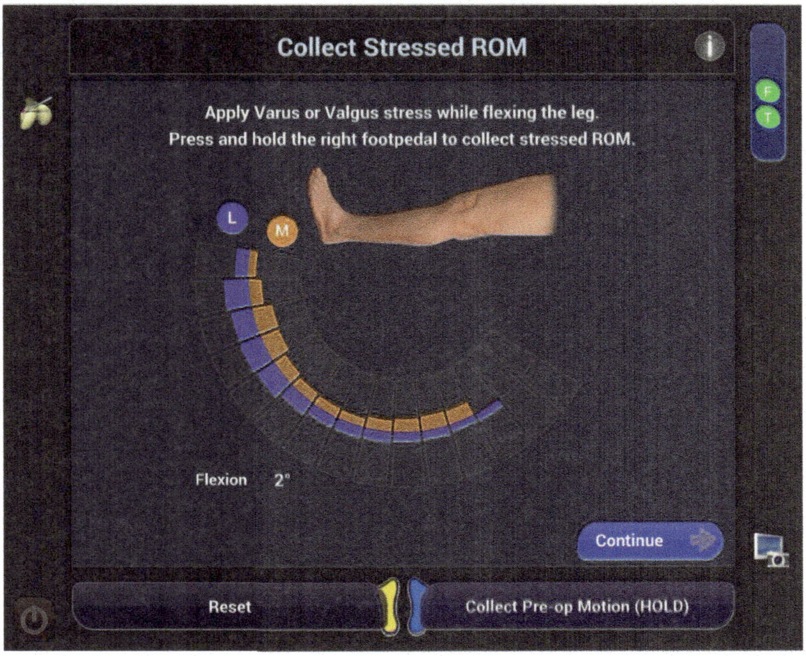

Fig. 3.17 Individual medial and lateral laxity

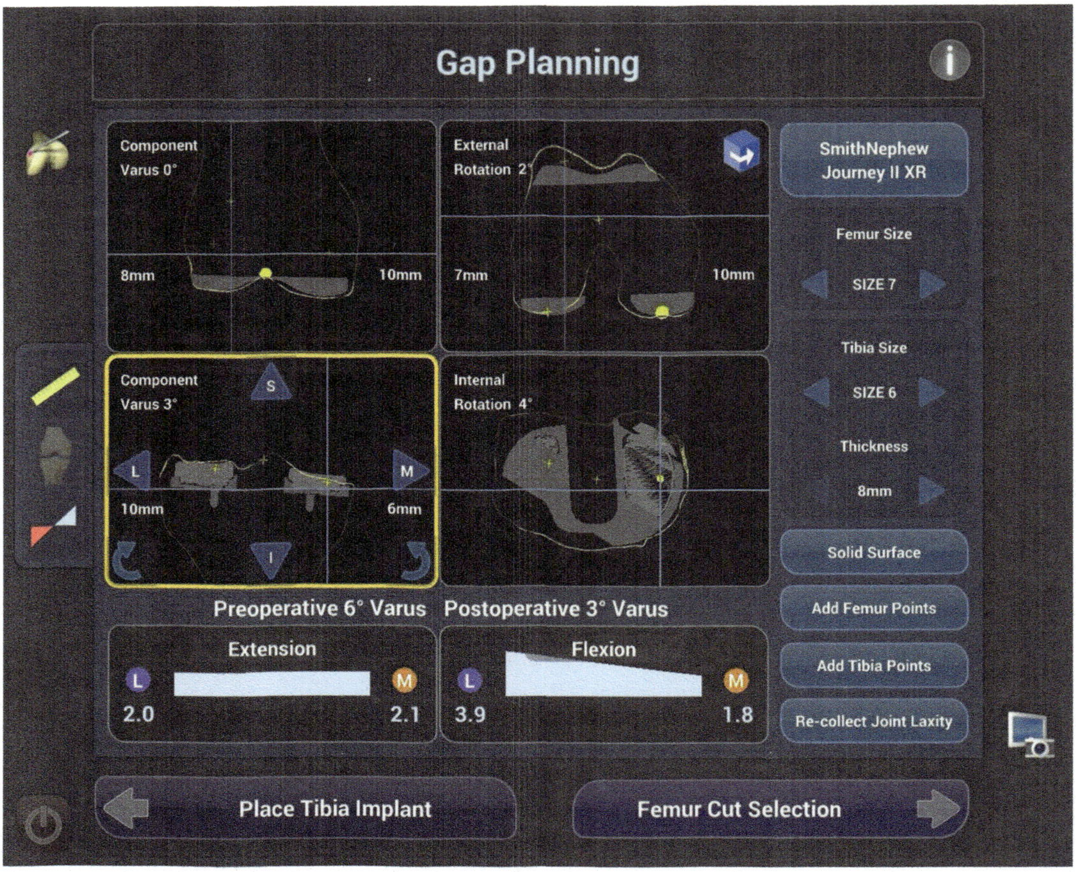

Fig. 3.18 Individual KA plan for a bi-cruciate retaining implant. In contrast to classical CR/PS or medial pivot TKA designs, the gaps have to be more loose

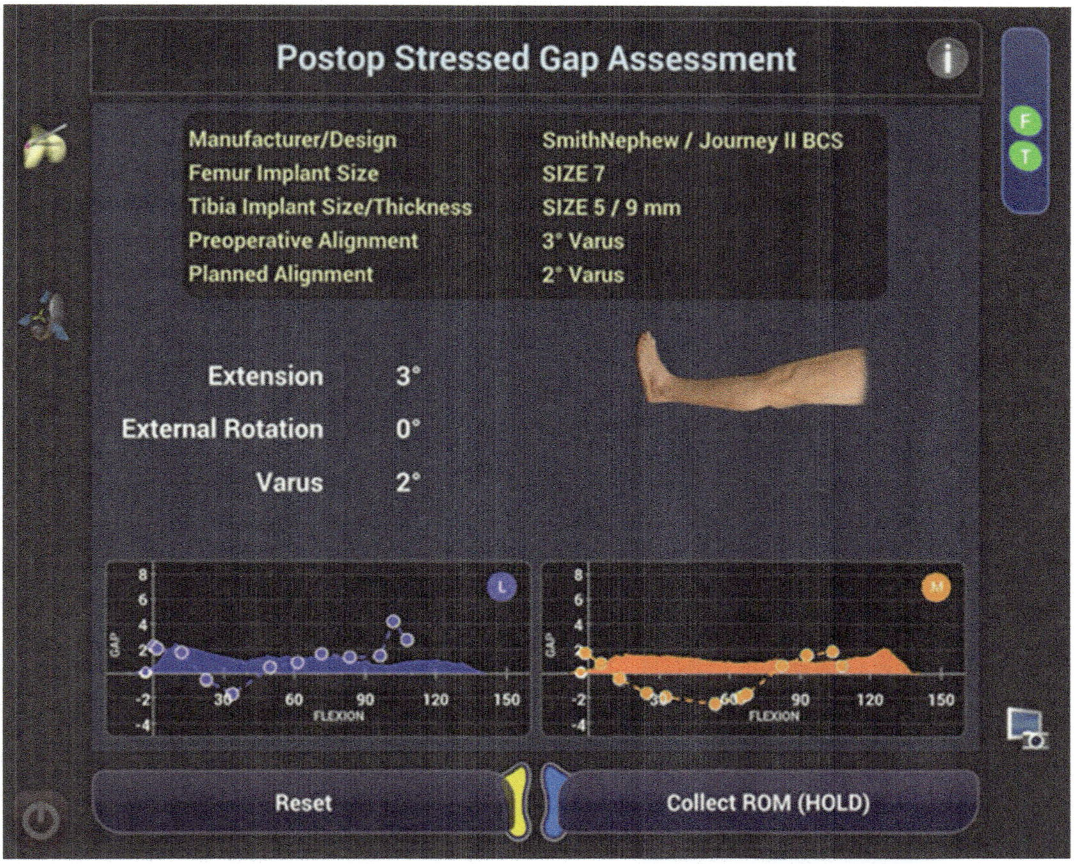

Fig. 3.19 The postoperative balance of the knee throughout the whole range of motion. Figure 3.20 displays the postoperative result

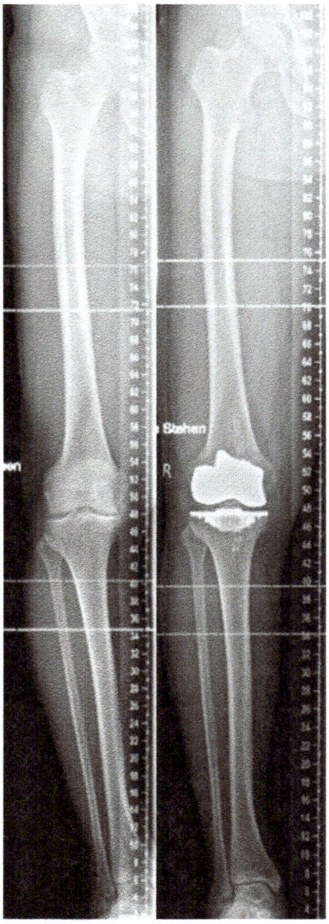

Fig. 3.20 Individual reconstruction of the patient's anatomy using a bi-cruciate retaining implant

References

1. Baker PN, van der Meulen JH, Lewsey J, Gregg PJ, National Joint Registry for E, Wales. The role of pain and function in determining patient satisfaction after total knee replacement. Data from the National Joint Registry for England and Wales. J Bone Joint Surg Br. 2007;89(7):893–900.
2. Bourne RB, Chesworth BM, Davis AM, Mahomed NN, Charron KD. Patient satisfaction after total knee arthroplasty: who is satisfied and who is not? Clin Orthop Relat Res. 2010;468(1):57–63.
3. Bellemans J, Colyn W, Vandenneucker H, Victor J. The Chitranjan Ranawat award: is neutral mechanical alignment normal for all patients? The concept of constitutional varus. Clin Orthop Relat Res. 2012;470(1):45–53.
4. Peters CL, Jimenez C, Erickson J, Anderson MB, Pelt CE. Lessons learned from selective soft-tissue release for gap balancing in primary total knee arthroplasty: an analysis of 1216 consecutive total knee arthroplasties: AAOS exhibit selection. J Bone Joint Surg Am. 2013;95(20):e152.
5. Hollister AM, Jatana S, Singh AK, Sullivan WW, Lupichuk AG. The axes of rotation of the knee. Clin Orthop Relat Res. 1993;(290):259–68.
6. Eckhoff DG, Bach JM, Spitzer VM, Reinig KD, Bagur MM, Baldini TH, et al. Three-dimensional morphology and kinematics of the distal part of the femur viewed in virtual reality. Part II. J Bone Joint Surg Am. 2003;85-A(Suppl 4):97–104.
7. Murakami K, Hamai S, Okazaki K, Ikebe S, Shimoto T, Hara D, et al. In vivo kinematics of healthy male knees during squat and golf swing using image-matching techniques. Knee. 2016;23(2):221–6.
8. Hill PF, Vedi V, Williams A, Iwaki H, Pinskerova V, Freeman MA. Tibiofemoral movement 2: the loaded and unloaded living knee studied by MRI. J Bone Joint Surg Br. 2000;82(8):1196–8.
9. Howell SM, Papadopoulos S, Kuznik KT, Hull ML. Accurate alignment and high function after kinematically aligned TKA performed with generic instruments. Knee Surg Sports Traumatol Arthrosc. 2013;21(10):2271–80.
10. Dossett HG, Swartz GJ, Estrada NA, LeFevre GW, Kwasman BG. Kinematically versus mechanically aligned total knee arthroplasty. Orthopedics. 2012;35(2):e160–9.
11. Young SW, Walker ML, Bayan A, Briant-Evans T, Pavlou P, Farrington B, The Chitranjan S. Ranawat award: no difference in 2-year functional outcomes using kinematic versus mechanical alignment in TKA: a randomized controlled clinical trial. Clin Orthop Relat Res. 2017;475(1):9–20.
12. Jo WL, Lee YK, Ha YC, Park MS, Lyu SH, Koo KH. Frequency, developing time, intensity, duration, and functional score of thigh pain after cementless total hip arthroplasty. J Arthroplast. 2016;31(6):1279–82.
13. Calliess T, Bauer K, Stukenborg-Colsman C, Windhagen H, Budde S, Ettinger M. PSI kinematic versus non-PSI mechanical alignment in total knee arthroplasty: a prospective, randomized study. Knee Surg Sports Traumatol Arthrosc. 2017;25(6):1743–8.
14. Waterson HB, Clement ND, Eyres KS, Mandalia VI, Toms AD. The early outcome of kinematic versus mechanical alignment in total knee arthroplasty: a prospective randomised control trial. Bone Joint J. 2016;98-B(10):1360–8.
15. Dossett HG, Estrada NA, Swartz GJ, LeFevre GW, Kwasman BG. A randomised controlled trial of kinematically and mechanically aligned total knee replacements: two-year clinical results. Bone Joint J. 2014;96-B(7):907–13.
16. Matsumoto T, Takayama K, Ishida K, Hayashi S, Hashimoto S, Kuroda R. Radiological and clinical comparison of kinematically versus mechanically aligned total knee arthroplasty. Bone Joint J. 2017;99-B(5):640–6.
17. Nam D, Lin KM, Howell SM, Hull ML. Femoral bone and cartilage wear is predictable at 0 degrees

and 90 degrees in the osteoarthritic knee treated with total knee arthroplasty. Knee Surg Sports Traumatol Arthrosc. 2014;22(12):2975–81.

18. Williams TG, Holmes AP, Bowes M, Vincent G, Hutchinson CE, Waterton JC, et al. Measurement and visualisation of focal cartilage thickness change by MRI in a study of knee osteoarthritis using a novel image analysis tool. Br J Radiol. 2010;83(995):940–8.
19. Hosseini A, Van de Velde SK, Kozanek M, Gill TJ, Grodzinsky AJ, Rubash HE, et al. In-vivo time-dependent articular cartilage contact behavior of the tibiofemoral joint. Osteoarthr Cartil. 2010;18(7):909–16.
20. Nedopil AJ, Howell SM, Hull ML. What clinical characteristics and radiographic parameters are associated with patellofemoral instability after kinematically aligned total knee arthroplasty? Int Orthop. 2017;41(2):283–91.
21. Ettinger M, Calliess T, Howell SM. Does a positioning rod or a patient-specific guide result in more natural femoral flexion in the concept of kinematically aligned total knee arthroplasty? Arch Orthop Trauma Surg. 2017;137(1):105–10.

4 Medial Opening Wedge High Tibial Osteotomy

Sufian S. Ahmad

The most widely spread and frequently performed osteotomy around the knee joint is the medial opening wedge high tibial osteotomy (mwHTO), a procedure that has managed to occupy a spotlight position as a powerful modality for the treatment of medial compartment gonalgia and degeneration [1–3]. The art is surely not in the technicality aspect of the procedure, but in correct patient selection. Therefore, the procedure would provide an elegant modality for the symptomatic patient with a constitutional metaphyseal varus of the proximal tibia. A few aspects are provided in the following chapter.

The art is with no doubt in patient selection and correct planning of the procedure. A correct analysis of the deformity is necessary to achieve favourable results.

To simplify the matter, it is essential to determine the origin of the varus deformity and the severity of medial compartment degeneration. The clinician should evaluate whether the varus is resultant of joint wasting only as is the case in medial joint degeneration with cartilage loss, or due to the bony morphology of the femur or tibia, or a combination of all, as may be the case in some late presenting cases.

There has been sufficient evidence to prove that correcting the bony pathology whilst respecting the anatomic boundaries, is likely to result in the best outcome [4]. This should mean that allocation of the origin of the deformity is of major importance. An intra-articular varus would best be treated with an intra-articular procedure to build up the joint space and cartilage loss; this may be achieved with a medial compartment resurfacing procedure. A deformity originating from the distal femur should be treated with a distal femur osteotomy and one originating from the proximal tibia with high tibial osteotomy. So it is important to underline that mwHTO should not be the only working horse in the surgical portfolio for the treatment of varus malalignment.

When planning to perform an mwHTO, it is furthermore important to consider and respect anatomic norms. Overcorrection that would result in reverse joint line obliquity is detrimental and would alter the biomechanics negatively due to the introduction of shear stresses that would contribute to progressive degenerative medial compartment change despite valgisation [4, 5]. This is an unwanted phenomenon that should be avoided. Overcorrection also rules out the future option of medial compartment resurfacing, which clinicians should bear in mind. The medial collateral ligament (MCL) is an important structure to consider, given that partial release of the distal fibres has been shown to be associated with optimized effects [6].

S. S. Ahmad (✉)
Department of Reconstructive Surgery & Traumatology, Eberhard Karls University of Tübingen, Tübingen, Germany

M. T. Hirschmann et al. (eds.), *ESSKA Instructional Course Lecture Book*,
https://doi.org/10.1007/978-3-662-61264-4_4

The technical aspects of mwHTO have been revolutionized with modern implants that allow for improved rotational stability. Previous catastrophic failures are no longer a primary matter of concern [7]. However, recognition of hinge fractures remains of major importance and may mandate hinge plating to avoid secondary complications that may constitute loss of correction or a prolonged healing period [8]. After perfect planning, two technical aspects need special consideration when performing the procedure. The first is MCL management and the second is protection of the neurovascular structures. Sharp subperiosteal dissection must be achieved using a periosteal elevator, to allow for controlled release of the MCL fibres, in a fashion to allow for sufficient posterior retraction without comprimising continuity of the ligament. Complete release of the MCL fibres should be avoided. After exposure of the medial aspect of the proximal tibia, it is important to release the insertion of the popliteus muscle with a subperiosteal elevator and insert a retractor between the posterior aspect of the tibia and the popliteus muscle, only then is sufficient protection of the neurovascular structures achieved. Careful consideration of the above mentioned planning and technical aspects should allow for optimized outcome and least complication rates when performing mwHTO.

References

1. Naudie D, Bourne RB, Rorabeck CH, et al. The install award. Survivorship of the high tibial valgus osteotomy. A 10-to-22-year followup study. Clin Orthop Relat Res. 1999;(367):18–27.
2. Fujisawa Y, Masuhara K, Shiomi S. The effect of high tibial osteotomy on osteoarthritis of the knee. An arthroscopic study of 54 knee joints. Orthop Clin North Am. 1979;10:585–608.
3. Floerkemeier S, Staubli AE, Schroeter S, et al. Outcome after high tibial open-wedge osteotomy: a retrospective evaluation of 533 patients. Knee Surg Sports Traumatol Arthrosc. 2013;21:170–80.
4. Nakayama H, Schröter S, Yamamoto C, et al. Large correction in opening wedge high tibial osteotomy with resultant joint-line obliquity induces excessive shear stress on the articular cartilage. Knee Surg Sports Traumatol Arthrosc. 2018;26:1873–8.
5. Brinkman J-M, Lobenhoffer P, Agneskirchner JD, et al. Osteotomies around the knee. J Bone Joint Surg (Br). 2008;90-B:1548–57.
6. Agneskirchner JD, Hurschler C, Wrann CD, et al. The effects of valgus medial opening wedge high tibial osteotomy on articular cartilage pressure of the knee: a biomechanical study. Arthroscopy. 2007;23:852–61.
7. Jackson JP, Waugh W. The technique and complications of upper tibial osteotomy. J Bone Joint Surg (Br). 1974;56-B:236–45.
8. Spahn G. Complications in high tibial (medial opening wedge) osteotomy. Arch Orthop Trauma Surg. 2004;124:649–53.

5 Reverse Arthroplasty Versus Other Options: Case Examples

Pascal Gleyze, Nikos Tzanakakis, and Tina Moraiti

5.1 Introduction

There are certain cases where the indications for shoulder surgery have never been clear. We can describe them as 'cuff arthropathy and other clinical cases with a variable combination of arthropathy and cuff lesions'. This is a description of complex and intercorrelated damages between cuff, cartilage and function which lead to a huge variety of consequences.

Analysis of these multiple causalities of this pathologic state is an important process that we must focus on. We need for that to understand how multiple factors are cumulated to create and make the evolution of (1) anatomical lesion, (2) clinical status and (3) natural evolution.

Before decision-making and proposing a reverse shoulder arthroplasty (RSA) versus other options, we have to check and to take into consideration the pathology for each patient, and we must never forget to estimate the future for each component of the problem: (1) the cuff, (2) the cartilage and (3) the functional demands of the patient.

This process takes time, it demands a lot of thinking and experience, and at the end it may be difficult to take the good decision, especially if we choose a technical solution without quick and spectacular results like the reverse shoulder arthroplasty. We are living in a period of 'limited efforts' from the patient side who are asking for immediate and perfect results. Surgeons are also demanding a great reputation of efficiency, they need to preserve their 'image' by all means, and they often have to forget the influence of industrial and commercial pressure.

Under all these circumstances, we have nowadays an 'over-indication' of reverse shoulder arthroplasty. The significant augmentation of the rate of reverse shoulder arthroplasty is not normal according to the population health evolution (from 15 to 64% in France in less than 10 years).

We do think that all patients should have a period of rehabilitation first (and not immediate RSA) and a cuff repair when possible (and not immediate RSA). In addition, all trauma or degenerative arthropathies with preserved cuff should have anatomical arthroplasty even if a limited cuff repair should be performed (and not immediate systematic RSA) and so on.

This chapter tries to demonstrate through several clinical cases that we need to consume time for a good clinical examination, with special attention to muscle equilibrium of the shoulder, scapula and the 'cervical-to-shoulder zone'. These tasks can help for decision-making, and they serve the opportunity to give clear explanations to the patients about all the different options

P. Gleyze (✉) · N. Tzanakakis
Arthroscopy and Orthopedic Sport Unit, 3 Frontières Saint Louis Hospital, Saint Louis, France

T. Moraiti
Orthopedic and traumatology Unit, Hôpital Nord Franche Comté, Trevenans, France

M. T. Hirschmann et al. (eds.), *ESSKA Instructional Course Lecture Book*,
https://doi.org/10.1007/978-3-662-61264-4_5

that we can propose to them. This sharing time with the patient is precious, especially when the clinical examination and history are not clear with potential hidden problems that could influence our decision, avoiding the error.

5.2 Practical Guideline for Decision-Making and Treatment Options

1. *What has to be checked as fundamental criteria?*
   (a) *Age, activity and psychologic profile* of the patient (active or not): actual and future
   (b) *Muscles*
      - *'Shoulder'*: cuff and deltoid muscles: history (sport, hard workers, …), state at examination and future
      - *'Regional compensation'*: trapezius muscle, para cervical muscles, scapula stabilizers, etc.
   (c) *Cartilages* of gleno–humeral joint but also acromio–clavicular joint
   (d) *Clinical examination*
      - Mechanic/inflammatory pain
      - Active/passive range of motion
      - Handicap
      - Clear clinical conflict (precise painful point in adduction internal rotation test)
      - Analytic muscular testing
2. *What can we propose to the patient according to the combination of anatomical state, age and functional profile?*
   (a) Nothing, if no pain, no functional limitation and no danger for the future
   (b) Rehabilitation and self-rehabilitation exercises with precise, intensive and realistic protocol
   (c) Acromioplasty with or without partial or complete cuff repair
   (d) Patch, graft and spacer techniques
   (e) Surface, anatomical or reverse prosthesis

Without a precise analysis of all of these criteria, if we do not have time to propose and explain to the patient the benefits and risks for each treatment option and if we do not have the possibility to propose to the patient most of the possible techniques, then we have not done a good job. In this situation, proposing a RSA will only be the mask of our deficiency.

RSA for everybody will give satisfaction to all, but the price will be payed later:

- Irreparable cuff with severe arthropathy for patient with limited functional demand is the actual state of the arts as defined by scientific societies and should be followed.
- The biomechanical constrain of the prosthesis design, the definitive sacrifice of residual cuff and the bone capital lost will make it easy to jump from heaven to hell if anything during and/or after the procedure fail and especially if the functional demand of the patient is over the limited biomechanical service given by the implant.

5.3 Clinical Case 1: When We Do Think We Have No Choice…

1. *Presentation of the case*
   (a) *Profile*: Male, 65 years old.
   (b) *Evolution*: 2 years evolution with limited cuff rupture suspected (supraspinatus) and 4 months small trauma and limited post extension of the rupture/pain limited/important handicap/constant score: 30/100. Pseudo paralytic shoulder.
   (c) *Prior treatment*: Rehabilitation 4 months.
   (d) *Clinical examination*
      - Pain: Limited during the day/no pain at night.
      - Handicap: Major handicap.
      - Active range of forward flexion: 70°.
      - Passive range of forward flexion: 170°.
      - Clinical and superior conflict: No.
      - Muscular testing
         - Supraspinatus: OK (deltoid compensation).
         - Infraspinatus: OK.
         - Sub-scap: OK.

(e) *Muscles*
   - *Cuff and deltoid:* Massive rotator cuff tears supra (fatty stage 3) + sup part of infra infraspinatus (fatty stage 2) + sub-scap (fatty stage 2) + no teres minor rupture (but fatty stage 2).
   - *Regional compensation:* Major compensation, trapezius and para cervical: permanent contraction/trumpet sign and pain on the muscular bodies.

(f) *Cartilage*: *No arthropathy*, centred, not medialized/limited superior translation (Visotsky 1A/Hamada 1/Samilson/Sirveaux E0).

(g) *Synthesis of the case*: Pain, limited function, major compensation, no arthrosis. Failure of rehabilitation.

(h) Figure 5.1 *shows arthro-CT scanner.*

2. *Therapeutic options*
   (a) Rehabilitation and intensive self-rehabilitation (2–3 h a day).
   (b) Acromioplasty ± partial repair.
   (c) Reverse shoulder arthroplasty.
3. *Therapeutic decision*
   (a) My first decision: Continuing rehab with the addition of intensive self-rehabilitation/3 months to be certain that we cannot make better: failure of this first option. Absolutely no improvement on pain, handicap, ROM.
   (b) My second decision after 3 months of intensive self-rehab (more than 2 h a day reported on a special following document) and physiotherapy: acromioplasty and partial repair. No partial repair was possible during the procedure. Only

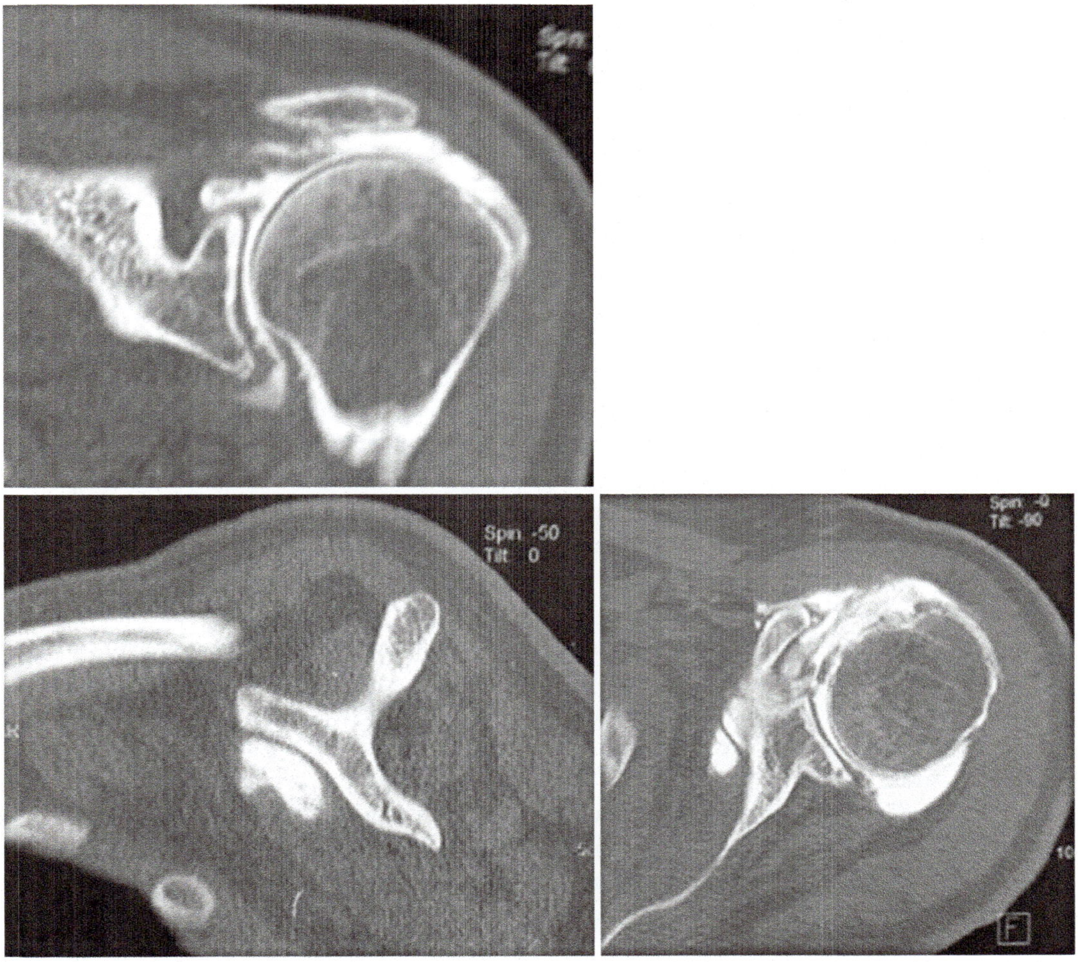

Fig. 5.1 Case 1: Arthro CT scanner

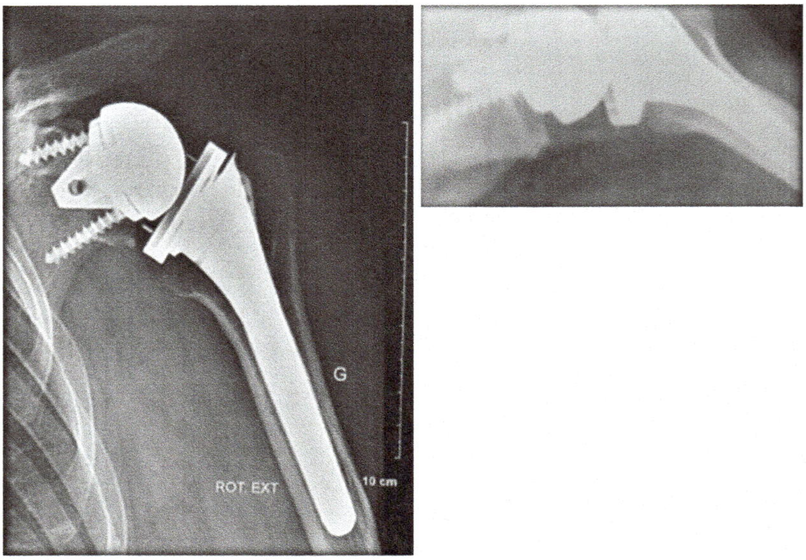

Fig. 5.2 Case 1: Post-op RSA

acromioplasty was performed. Stiff and no pain at 3 months, complete passive range of motion at 6 months, no pain but steel pseudoparalytic shoulder with major trapezius compensation.

(c) My third decision 9 months after acromioplasty: Reversed shoulder prosthesis, no operative difficulty; Fig. 5.2 *shows the post-op control X-rays.*

4. *Final results:* The clinical result was similar at 3 months, 6 months and final revision and it was a bad result. Moderate/no pain night and day with an active ROM below 70° with still a major regional compensation and important handicap. Ten points of constant score improvement. The clinical status was equivalent as it was the first time the patient came.
   (a) Figure 5.3 *shows the final clinical examination in 18 months.*
5. *Analysis*
   (a) The initial clinical state was due to a massive cuff tear with a permanent and major compensation prior to the start of all daily movements. This antalgic reflex position is systematic when shoulder pain is after trauma, recent cuff rupture or other aetiology but should disappear with the use of the shoulder rehabilitation protocols, self-control of the trapezius and time. Sometimes it stays and becomes part of the spontaneous usage of the shoulder as new 'corporeal image'.
   (b) This 'compensation' reflex locks the shoulder and makes a stimulation of the residual cuff muscles and deltoid impossible. Forward flexion and abduction are impossible when trapezius and para cervical muscles are contracted because the shoulder moves into the scapulo–thoracic joint and oblige to spine adaptation. The 'trumpet sign' shows this regional compensation. This clinical sign is a consequence of the massive cuff tear but can also be a causality of the impossible active range of motion when this reflex is maintained by the patient as a systematic antalgic reflex day after day.
      - Figure 5.3 *shows the final examination in 18 months.*
   (c) This explains why the patient was not moving before the prosthesis, and in the same way, it explains why he was not moving better after. It was just because of the persistence of this antalgic reflex.
   (d) We can say that the indication of RSA for this patient was not a good indication because he had no arthropathy, and the handicap and limited function were only due to the 'compensation reflex' and not because of the absence of the cuff. Acromioplasty was not a good indication because he had no clinical conflict and no possibility of any endoscopic reparation during the procedure.

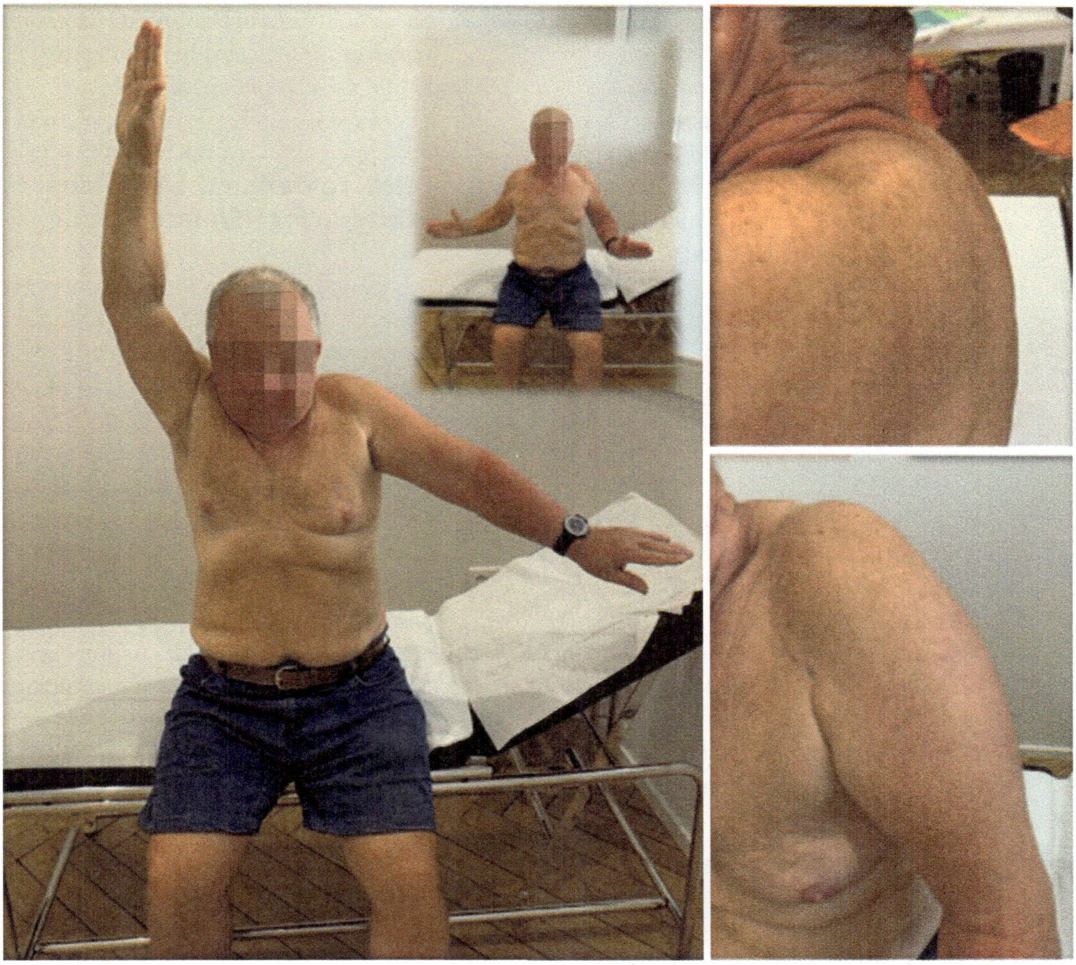

Fig. 5.3 Case 1: Final examination—18 months

(e) What could help to make the decision? The key point is to know the exact potential of the residual cuff and deltoid before decision-making. This can be done with the evaluation of the physiologic age of the patient and muscles. A combination of MRI or CT scan imaging with a precise description of the fatty degeneration of each muscle is vital and specially when it is possible to individualize the state of the superior and inferior part of the infraspinatus and teres minor state. The fatty degeneration of the inferior part of the infraspinatus or teres minor will determine the 'red line frontier'. If it is preserved, the patient should be able to move full ROM specially if he has no significant arthropathy. In this case we observed a fatty degenerescence of infra residual infra and teres minor without rupture, and this could sign the absence of use of these muscles for a long time. On a biomechanical point of view, the preserved inferior part of the infraspinatus in combination with an efficient sub-scapular and a good deltoid is enough to have full range of motion in most of the cases. More posterior extension of the rupture can be accepted as the limit that will give us the decision for RSA.

6. *Conclusion:* No arthropathy with a residual inferior part of the infraspinatus and a good deltoid should be able to give to the patient full range of motion with no pain or limited pain and no handicap or limited handicap.

(a) If a clear clinical conflict sign is present and can explain the pain, acromioplasty with ± partial cuff repair could be proposed.
(b) If there is no pain, the educational control of the compensation should be enough to make this shoulder recover without pain, full range of motion and limited handicap in correlation with limited muscular forces.
(c) Natural evolution of this patient if he has no RSA at this time will be a progressive severe cuff arthropathy. But according to the fact that it is difficult to precisely know and explain to the patient when and how this cuff arthropathy will oblige him to a RSA, the only solution is to control evolution of the shoulder and to propose RSA when the adequate time will come. This can be 10 years after good use of the original shoulder, and this will then be justified by a surgical procedure with an adequate benefit–risk ratio decision. Prevention arthroplasty is not acceptable.
(d) In this specific case as presented, this is not possible for the gleno–humeral joint, with or without arthroplasty, if the corporeal image of the patient is to lock the shoulder before the start of any movement.

5.4 How to Define the 'Red Line Criteria for RSA Índication?

1. *Case 2: Good Result with Rehabilitation*
   (a) Clinical case: Male, 72 years old, active profile. Well-known old cuff tear (SSP) for 4 years. Fall on the shoulder 4 months ago and pseudo-paralytic shoulder, 'trumpet sign' and limited stiffness in forward flexion (130°) and external rotation (20°). On arthro-CT scan, a diagnosis of massive cuff tears with fatty degeneration grade 3 for SS and with a preserved post part of ISS (with fatty grade 2). Eccentric arthropathy, and he had three proposals of RSA. At the time of the first consultation, the patient was not believing anymore in his shoulder (Fig. 5.4 shows standard X rays and CT scan).

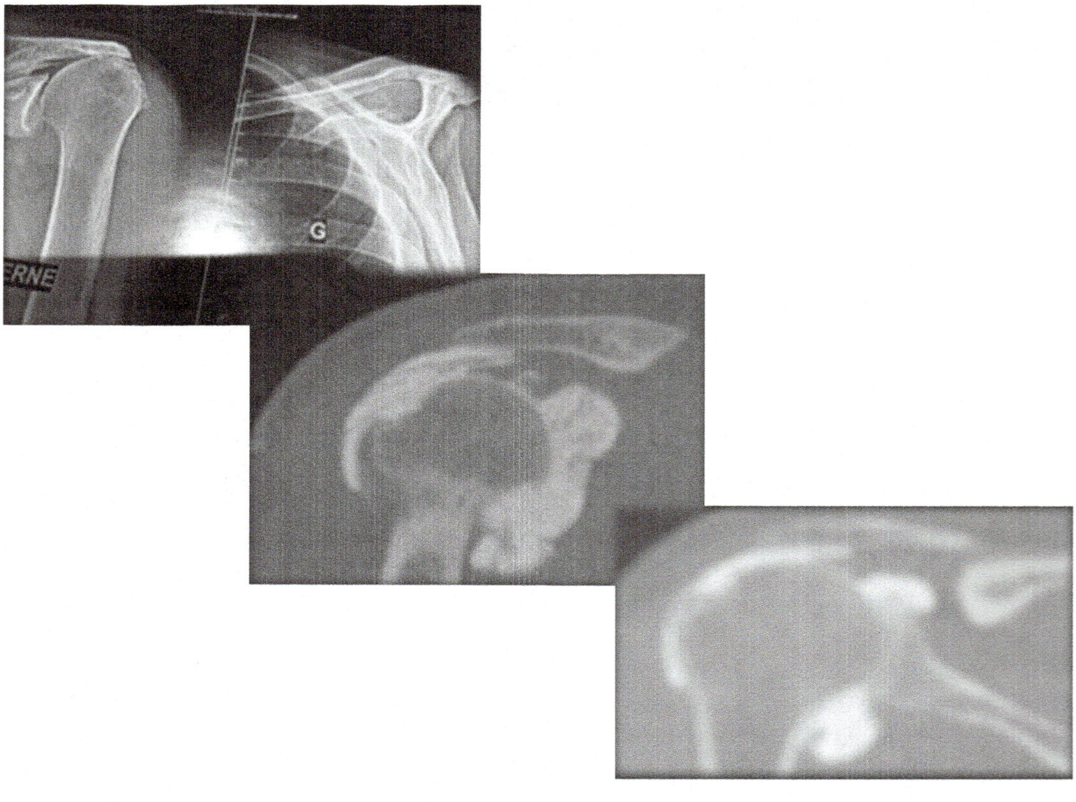

Fig. 5.4 Case 2: State before treatment

(b) Option of intensive rehab and self-stretching over the pain limits. The patient has followed this protocol with more than 2 h per day over the pain limits: Pain-free and complete recover after 3 months with a preserved perfect clinical result and no arthropathy evolution after 5 years. Figure 5.5 *shows the clinical evaluation before treatment simulated at posteriori and after 3 months.*

(c) This clinical case is exactly the same as the prior case except that he has arthropathy and a preserved no fatty degenerescence of the teres minor, but the results are finally very good because the patient moved.

2. *Case 3: Temporally Limited Results Due to Insufficiency of the Rehabilitation and Self-rehabilitation Rxercises*
   (a) Female, 66 years old, not an active profile, no stiffness, limited centred arthropa-

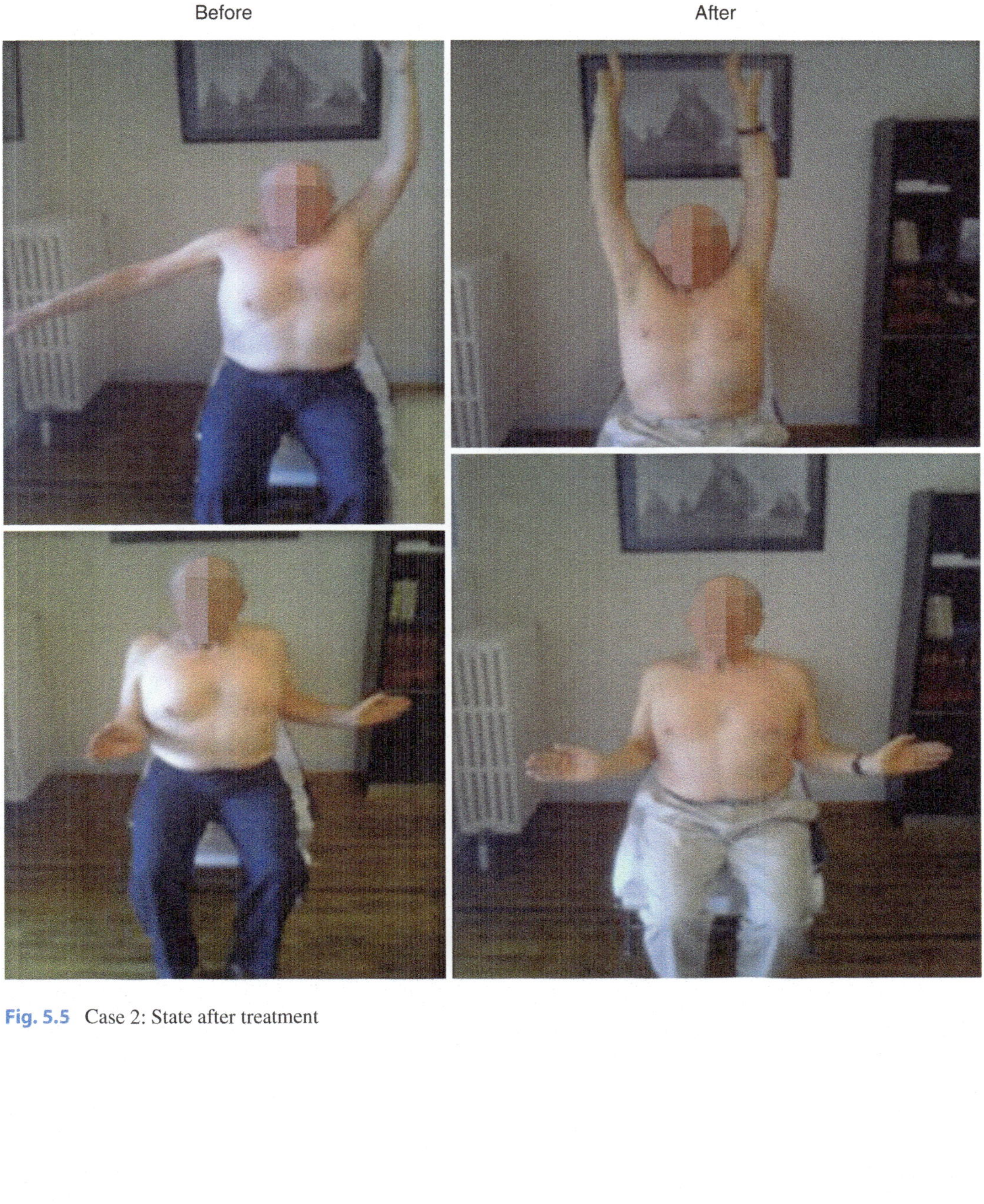

Fig. 5.5 Case 2: State after treatment

thy, pain night and day and importantly handicap. No compensation but no real self-rehab work, bad results after 3 months and still in depressed psychic condition. What to do? We asked her to continue, and we explained her that she was in good progress and that she has now only to pass horizontal angulation. If a patient is able to maintain the arm over horizontally, he or she should be able to make the full active range of motion if he or she works hard on rehabilitation and self-rehabilitation. For this patient, 6 weeks after the examination, she could recover full ROM, no pain night and day. This good clinical result is stable after 2 years.

(b) Figure 5.6 *patient at first following evaluation at 6 weeks without help and then with little help for forward flexion.*

3. *Case 4: No Need of a Doctor, Don't Touch Me*
   (a) Male, 75 years old, very active profile. Massive cuff tear involving post part of the infraspinatus. Eccentric arthropathy. Limited passive ROM. No pain, no handicap (as analysed by the patient). No doctors needed, came for the knee. No treatment and happy active guy.
   (b) Figure 5.7 *shows the photo of the patient with difficult abduction.*
4. *Case 5: Acromioplasty and Partial Repair of Post Part of Infraspinatus*

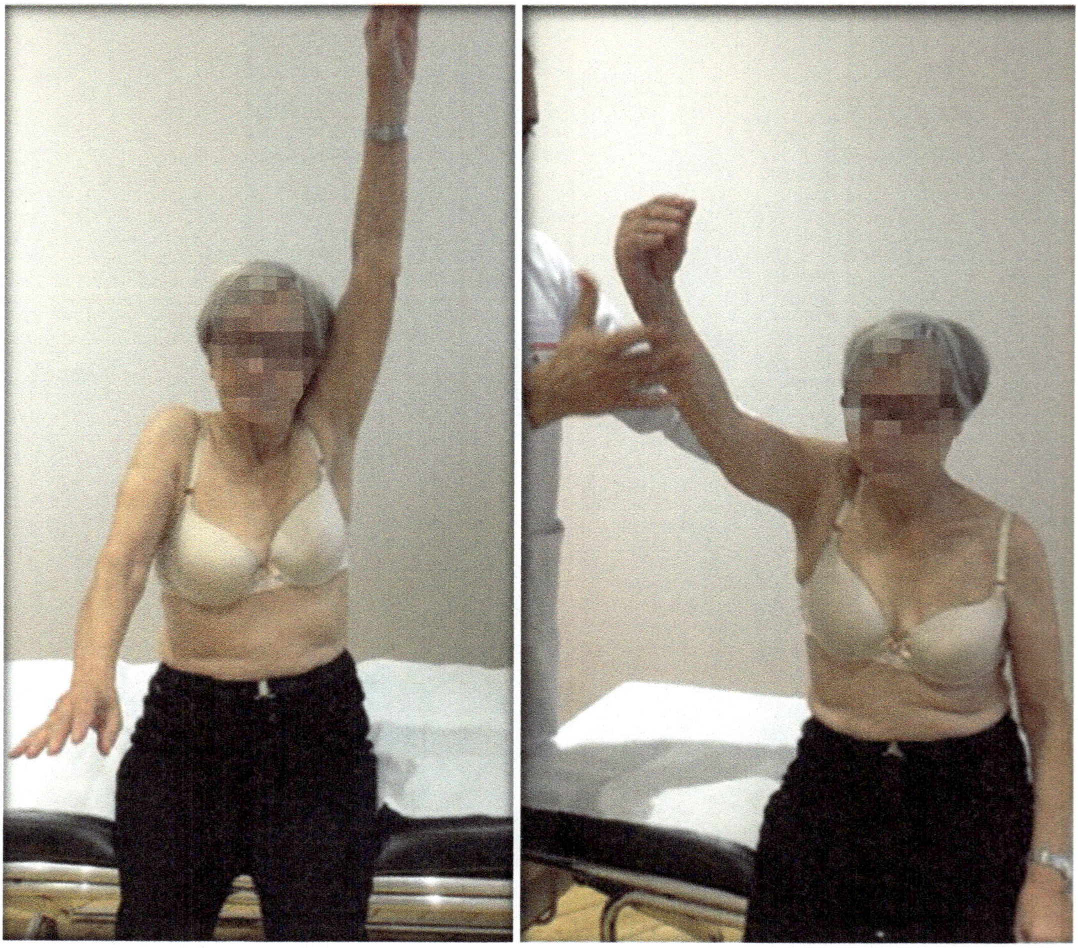

Fig. 5.6 Photo of the patient at first following evaluation at after six weeks physio without help and then with little help for forward flexion

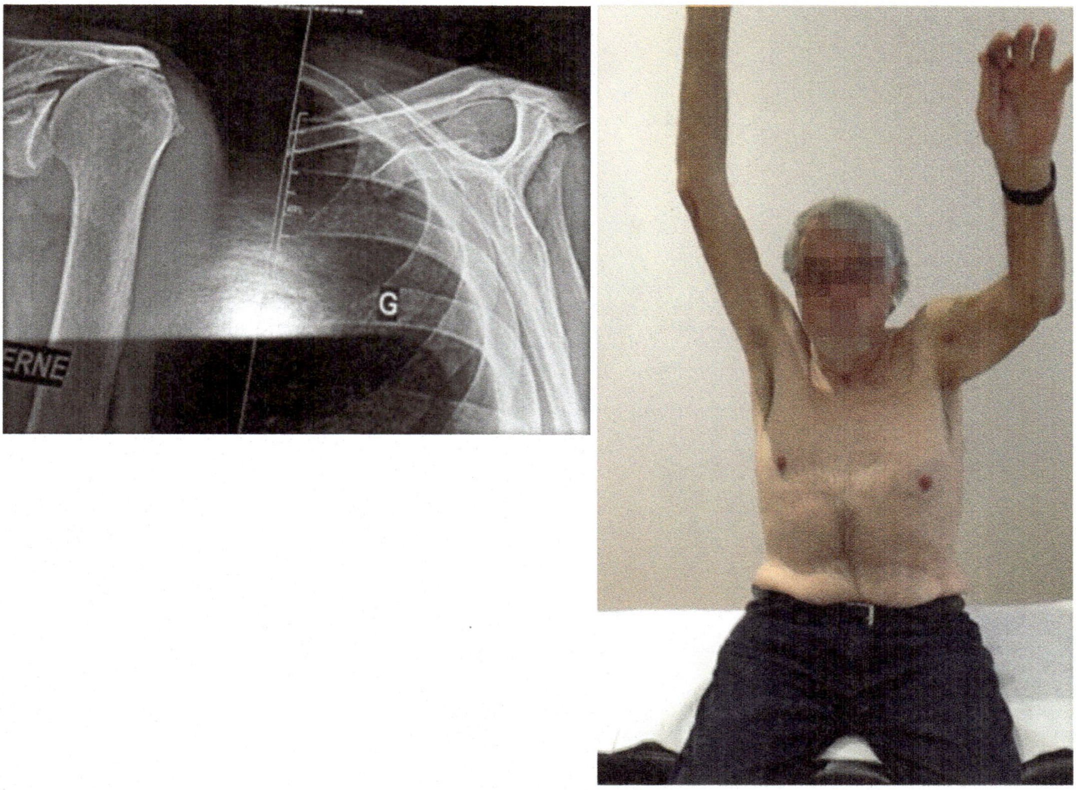

Fig. 5.7 Photo of the patient with difficult abduction

(a) Male, 68 years old, active, rupture of the supraspinatus more than 5 years ago and effort 3 months ago with complete supra and infraspinatus rupture (no fatty degeneration of the infraspinatus). Eccentric arthropathy. Pseudo-paralytic shoulder. Acromioplasty and repair of the infraspinatus, no repair of the supraspinatus.

(b) Clinical result at 3 months, no pain, full ROM and limited force in external rotation.

(c) Figure 5.8 *shows the clinical result 3 months after acromioplasty and partial repair with eccentric arthropathy.*

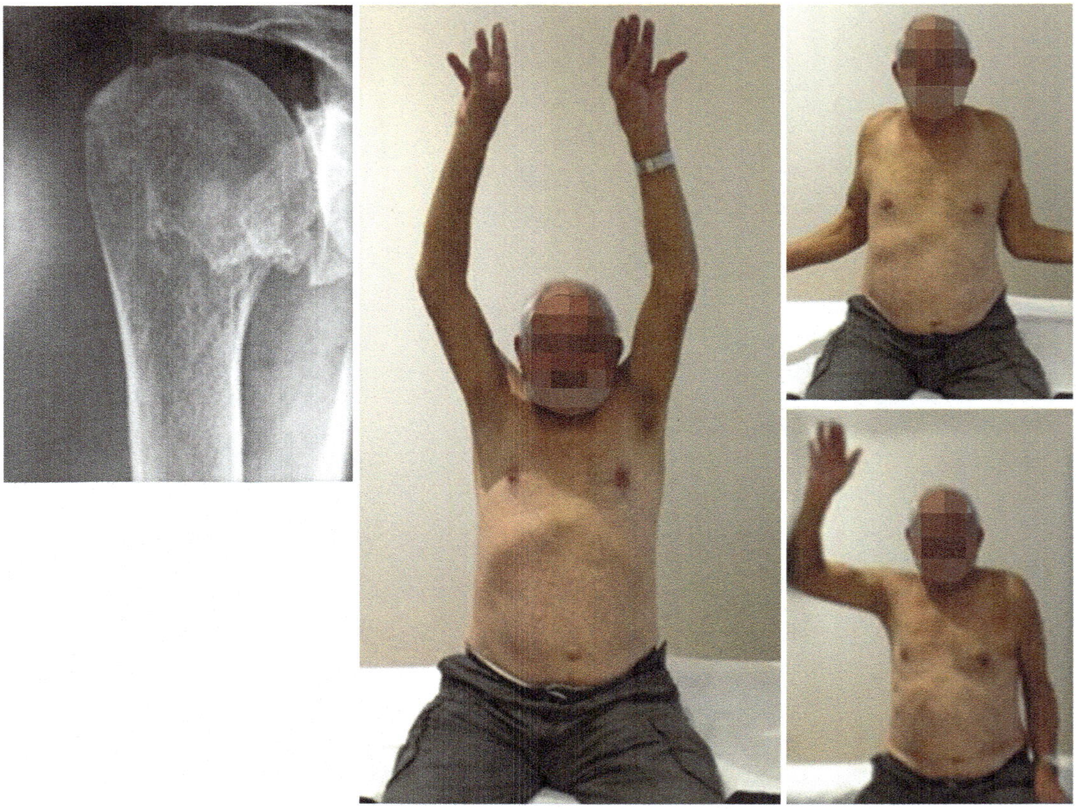

Fig. 5.8 Clinical result 3 months after acromioplasty and partial repair with eccentric arthropathy

5.5 Final Conclusion

We must never propose any surgical solution before we are sure that we have reached the far end of what nature can give. This mean that we have to perform musculation, stretching, self-exercise and physiotherapy on a very intensive way for a minimum of 4 weeks before making the decision to conduct RSA. And we should be very careful in all cases of the compensation reflex which may mask the real potential of the shoulder.

6 How to Avoid Complications in Hip Arthroscopy

Sverre Løken and Olufemi R. Ayeni

Complications in hip arthroscopy are relatively rare, particularly severe complications. In a large review of 36,761 patients, the total complication rate was 3.3%, and there were 0.2% major complications [1]. Complications can be recognised during surgery or after surgery. The consequence of a complication can be transient or permanent. Although the rate of reported complications varies in the literature, higher complication rates are detected when analysing large databases compared with smaller patients series [2]. Higher incidences are also reported in studies where patients are actively asked about specific symptoms after hip arthroscopy [3]. Before surgery it is important to inform the patient about the risk of surgery as well as the possible complications. This overview is limited to surgical complications.

6.1 Breakage of Instruments

Check that all instruments are undamaged and in good shape before surgery. Using instruments of good quality designed for hip arthroscopy is important. Avoid bending or applying unnecessary force to instruments. It is better to make an additional portal if access to the instruments is difficult from an established portal.

6.2 Cartilage and Labral Injuries

These injuries most commonly occur when introducing the instruments at the start of the procedure. The frequency is unknown and probably underreported. To start with the peripheral compartment can help to avoid these injuries. When starting from the central compartment however, an image intensifier is used by most surgeons. Sufficient traction should be applied, possibly with muscle paralysis if needed to achieve joint distraction of 10–15 mm. When introducing the spinal needle into the joint, it should be kept distal, close to the femoral head to avoid the labrum. The needle should be rotated so that the sharp tip of the needle is distal. If too much resistance is felt, this may indicate that the needle is entering the labrum. After having introduced the needle and observed an air arthrogram, saline can be injected through the needle while observing that the needle is directed downwards by the water pressure. This indicates that the needle has avoided the labrum. After that, gentle introduction of the probe is performed, then the probe with cannula and finally the arthroscope. By first introducing the probe and then the

S. Løken (✉)
Oslo University Hospital, Oslo, Norway
e-mail: uxsvlo@ous-hf.no

O. R. Ayeni
McMaster University, Hamilton, ON, Canada
e-mail: ayenif@mcmaster.ca

M. T. Hirschmann et al. (eds.), *ESSKA Instructional Course Lecture Book*,
https://doi.org/10.1007/978-3-662-61264-4_6

probe + cannula, a stepwise dilatation of the capsular opening is achieved. The second portal is introduced under direct visualisation and fluoroscopic control, avoiding the cartilage and labrum. The portals should be enlarged enough to reduce the levering force needed to move the instruments in the joint. Make a capsulotomy sufficient, but be prepared for capsular closure at the completion of surgery. When using a shaver, make sure that the whole aperture of the shaver is visible to avoid injury to tissue that is outside of the visual field. Avoid radiofrequency usage close to the labrum and cartilage. When performing pincer or cam resections, be careful not to over-resect both in depth and area. Make smooth resection surfaces without sharp edges or angles. When placing suture anchors, there is a risk for penetration into the acetabulum with the suture anchor. To avoid this, a distal mid anterior portal is safer. Curved anchor introducers may help direct anchors away from the acetabulum which can also be useful.

6.3 Dislocation/Instability

Avoid scoping dysplastic hips. Treat the capsule carefully by making as small openings as possible and repair the capsule if a capsulotomy has been performed. Dislocation has been reported following iliopsoas tenotomy as well [4], so this procedure should be considered very carefully particularly in dysplastic or unstable hips (connective tissue disorders).

6.4 Nerve Injuries

Pudendal Nerve: The incidence of pudendal nerve injury is reported to be 4.3% with the use of perineal post and 0.5% without. All cases in these series have been resolved within 3 months [5]. Avoid traction time over 90 min and avoid very high traction forces. Some surgeons use instruments to measure the traction force. Another technique to reduce traction force is to angle the table with lowering of the head end—Trendelenburg position [6]. It is also very important to use a large well-padded perineal post to distribute the forces to a large area. Post-free techniques have been developed by placing a material under the patients combined with a Trendelenburg position which prevents the patients from sliding on the table [7]. A post-free technique using duct tape to stabilise the patient has also been described [8].

Lateral Femoral Cutaneous Nerve: This is the most common complication following hip arthroscopy, around 10% still persistent after 1 year [3], but usually without too serious consequences for the patient. The nerve is also vulnerable when not transected. Restricting the use of a scalpel to the skin only and staying as lateral as possible may reduce the risk of injury to this nerve and its branches.

Dorsal Sensory Nerves of the Foot: These nerves may be injured due to the traction by pressure from the traction boot. A well-padded boot should be used to reduce this risk. The boot may also be loosened when traction is released. Keeping the traction time and force down is also important to protect these nerve branches.

Sciatic Nerve: Injury to this nerve is very uncommon during arthroscopy of the hip joint. Some patients may be more vulnerable due to previous injuries, scar tissue, etc. Meticulous preoperative investigations may identify individuals at risk. Newer procedures such as hamstring repair and ischiofemoral impingement work may place this nerve at risk.

Femoral Neck Fracture: A few cases have been reported [9]. The obvious prevention is to avoid over-resection when performing a cam resection. Generally, 30% of the head–neck junction is the maximum limit for resection. Restricted weight bearing following surgery should be considered.

6.5 Infection

Deep infections are very rare following hip arthroscopy [10]. Most surgeons use prophylactic antibiotics. A preoperative injection less than 3 months before surgery has been shown to double the risk of postoperative surgical site infection (including superficial infections) from 1 to 2% [11], so surgery should be delayed by at least 3 months following an injection.

6.6 Heterotopic Ossification

Heterotopic ossification (HO) has become well recognised following hip arthroscopy, being regularly present on post-operative radiographs [12, 13]. It is well documented that NSAIDs reduce the prevalence of radiological HO [14]. Nonetheless, the clinical relevance of radiological HO remains unknown, as most cases are not symptomatic. Although no consensus exists, NSAIDs for 2 weeks are commonly prescribed if there are no contraindications.

6.7 Thromboembolic Complications

The risk of thromboembolic complications is low, and it is debated whether prophylaxis in patients without increased risk factors is justified from a cost–benefit perspective. The use of prophylaxis varies between centres/countries. The indication will also depend on national guidelines and understanding each patient's risk profile [15].

6.8 Conclusion

The safest way to avoid any complication is to avoid surgery; however, this is not always possible with a symptomatic patient. Therefore, there should be good indications for surgery, safe access to joint, detailed approach to addressing surgical lesion and robust post-operative surveillance to address any complications promptly.

References

1. Nakano N, Lisenda L, Jones TL, Loveday DT, Khanduja V. Complications following arthroscopic surgery of the hip: a systematic review of 36 761 cases. Bone Joint J. 2017;99-B(12):1577–83.
2. Truntzer JN, Hoppe DJ, Shapiro LM, Abrams GD, Safran M. Complication rates for hip arthroscopy are underestimated: a population-based study. Arthroscopy. 2017;33(6):1194–201.
3. Dippmann C, Thorborg K, Kraemer O, Winge S, Hölmich P. Symptoms of nerve dysfunction after hip arthroscopy: an under-reported complication? Arthroscopy. 2014;30(2):202–7.
4. Sansone M, Ahldén M, Jónasson P, Swärd L, Eriksson T, Karlsson J. Total dislocation of the hip joint after arthroscopy and iliopsoas tenotomy. Knee Surg Sports Traumatol Arthrosc. 2013;21(2):420–3.
5. Habib A, Haldane CE, Ekhtiari S, de Sa D, Simunovic N, Belzile EL, Ayeni OR. Pudendal nerve injury is a relatively common but transient complication of hip arthroscopy. Knee Surg Sports Traumatol Arthrosc. 2018;26(3):969–75.
6. Lall AC, Saadat AA, Battaglia MR, Maldonado DR, Perets I, Domb BG. Perineal pressure during hip arthroscopy is reduced by use of trendelenburg: a prospective study with randomized order of positioning. Clin Orthop Relat Res. 2019;477(8):1851–7.
7. Kollmorgen RC, Ellis T, Lewis BD, Harris JD. Achieving post-free distraction in hip arthroscopy with a pink pad patient positioning device using standard hip distraction tables. Arthrosc Tech. 2019;8(4):e363–8.
8. Salas AP, Mazek J, Araujo-Reyes D, Gonzalez-Campos M, Castillo-Trevizo A, Garcia JM. The tutankhamun technique in hip arthroscopy. Arthrosc Tech. 2018;7(11):e1167–71.
9. Horner NS, Vikas K, MacDonald AE, Naendrup JH, Simunovic N, Ayeni OR. Femoral neck fractures as a complication of hip arthroscopy: a systematic review. J Hip Preserv Surg. 2017;4(1):9–17.
10. Harris JD, McCormick FM, Abrams GD, Gupta AK, Ellis TJ, Bach BR Jr, Bush-Joseph CA, Nho SJ. Complications and reoperations during and after hip arthroscopy: a systematic review of 92 studies and more than 6,000 patients. Arthroscopy. 2013;29(3):589–95.
11. Wang D, Camp CL, Ranawat AS, Coleman SH, Kelly BT, Werner BC. The timing of hip arthroscopy after intra-articular hip injection affects postoperative infection risk. Arthroscopy. 2017;33(11):1988–94.
12. Randelli F, Pierannunzii L, Banci L, Ragone V, Aliprandi A, Buly R. Heterotopic ossifications after arthroscopic management of femoroacetabular impingement: the role of NSAID prophylaxis. J Orthop Traumatol. 2010;11(4):245–50.
13. Kurz AZ, LeRoux E, Riediger M, Coughlin R, Simunovic N, Duong A, Laskovski JR, Ayeni OR. Heterotopic ossification in hip arthroscopy: an updated review. Curr Rev Musculoskelet Med. 2019;12(2):147–55.
14. Beckmann JT, Wylie JD, Potter MQ, Maak TG, Greene TH, Aoki SK. Effect of naproxen prophylaxis on heterotopic ossification following hip arthroscopy: a double-blind randomized placebo-controlled trial. J Bone Joint Surg Am. 2015;97(24):2032–7.
15. Haldane CE, Ekhtiari S, de Sa D, Simunovic N, Safran M, Randelli F, Duong A, Farrokhyar F, Ayeni OR. Venous thromboembolism events after hip arthroscopy: a systematic review. Arthroscopy. 2018;34(1):321–30.

7 State of the Art in Ankle Ligament Surgery—Repair vs. Reconstruction: How to Choose?

Masato Takao

Surgery for lateral ankle instability has evolved over time from non-anatomical open procedures to anatomical open procedures and more recently to arthroscopic procedures. They can be roughly divided into the ligament repair using a remnant and the ligament reconstruction using a graft, and the choice of a surgical procedure should be done by evaluating the quality of the residual ligament [1, 2]. If the quality of the remnant is sufficient, repair technique to suture the remnant to its attachment to fibula is indicated. Reconstruction technique is chosen if the quality of the remnant is insufficient. But there have been few reports for how to choose repair or reconstruction.

Morvan A et al. compared the result of preoperative MRI including axial T2-weighted image evaluation and the arthroscopic evaluation [3]. The correlation between MRI and arthroscopy was 90.9% in observer 1 and 86.4% in observer 2, and the authors concluded that preoperative MRI of the ATFL is a reliable and valid decisional tool to choose the surgical technique for stabilization of chronic lateral ankle instability.

The quality of the remnant depends on the type of major collagen. Type I collagen consists 90% in normal ligament and is primarily responsible for stiffness of the ligament [4]. We compared the results of type I collagen staining and gene expression of type I collagen by RT-PCR with arthroscopic evaluation of the ATFL remnant. As a result, cases where the remnant was stained with type I collagen staining, gene expression of type I collagen was found in all cases in RT-PCR (Fig. 7.1). Significant correlation was recognized between the staining result of type 1 collagen staining and the arthroscopic evaluation [5] (Fig. 7.2). Accordingly, arthroscopy can be relied as a tool to accurately assess the quality of the remnant. We also compared the results of arthroscopic evaluation with the results of stress radiography, MRI, and stress ultrasonography and found that only stress ultrasonography showed significantly correlation with arthroscopic evaluation (Fig. 7.3).

Accordingly, I recommend repair surgery for cases in which ligament fibers are found and reconstruction for cases in which regiment fibers are not found by preoperative stress ultrasound examination. And the operative procedure is finally determined by intraoperative arthroscopic evaluation.

M. Takao (✉)
Clinical and Research Institute for Foot and Ankle Surgery, Jujo Hospital, Kisarazu, Japan
e-mail: m.takao@carifas.com

M. T. Hirschmann et al. (eds.), *ESSKA Instructional Course Lecture Book*,
https://doi.org/10.1007/978-3-662-61264-4_7

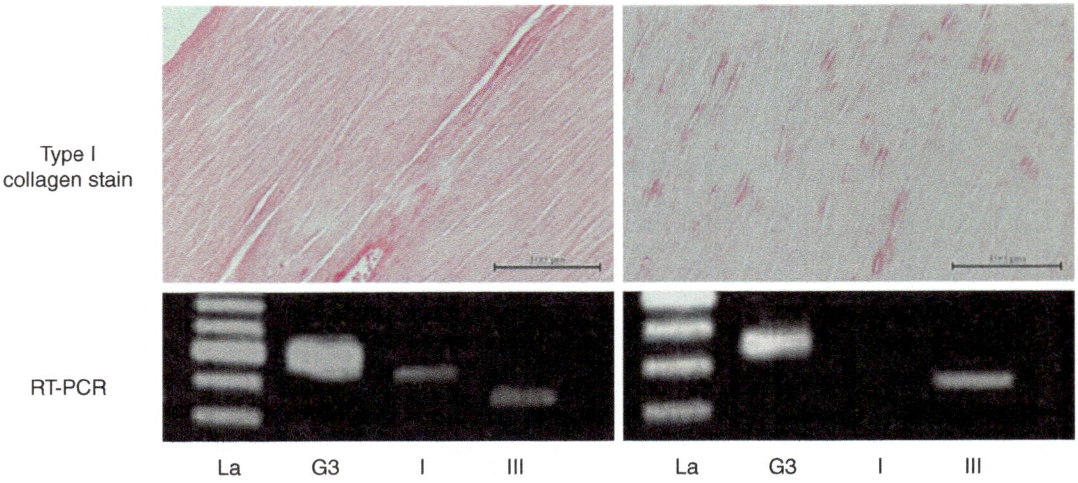

Fig. 7.1 Results of type I collagen stain and the RT-PCR. Left shows that the remnant is stained with type I collagen staining and the gene expression of type I collagen is found in RT-PCR. Right shows that the remnant is not stained with type I collagen staining, and there is no gene expression of type I collagen in RT-PCR. *La* ladder, *G3* G3PDH, *I* type I collagen, *III* type III collagen

Fig. 7.2 Results of the type 1 collagen staining and the arthroscopic evaluation. Left shows that the ligament fibers remain in arthroscopic evaluation (arrow), and the remnant is stained with type I collagen staining. Right shows the scar tissue without ligament fiber in arthroscopic evaluation (arrowhead), and the remnant is not stained with type I collagen staining

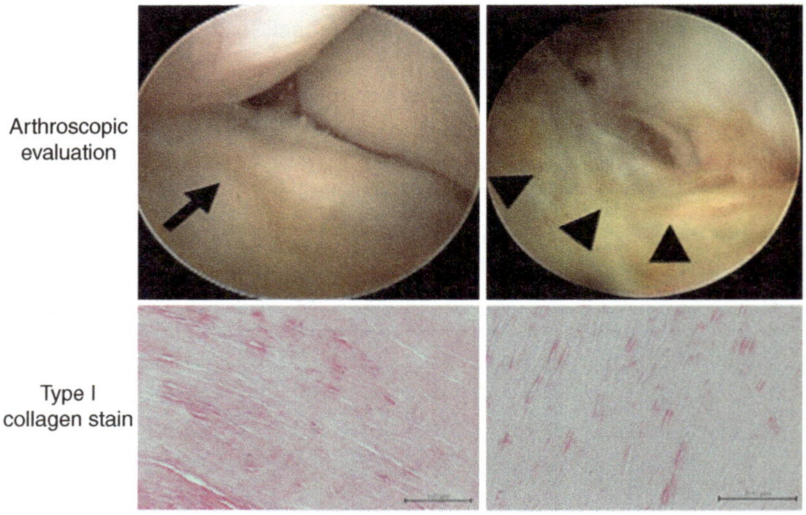

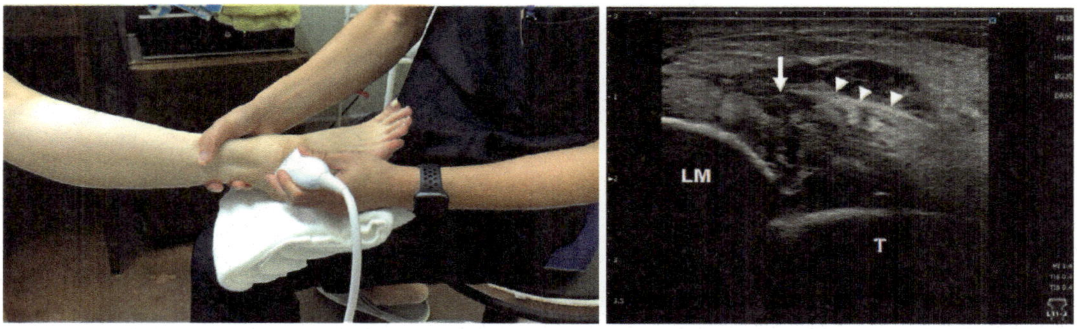

Fig. 7.3 Stress ultrasonography. The patient's heel is placed on the examiner's thigh, and the ATFL is described while applying manual stress in the anterior-posterior direction. *LM* lateral malleolus, *T* talus, *arrowhead* ATFL, *arrow* stump of the ruptured ATFL

References

1. Prisk VR, Imhauser CW, O'Loughlin PF, Kennedy JG. Lateral ligament repair and reconstruction restore neither contact mechanics of the ankle joint nor motion patterns of the hindfoot. J Bone Joint Surg Am. 2010;92(14):2375–86.
2. Karlsson J, Bergsten T, Lansinger O, Peterson L. Reconstruction of the lateral ligaments of the ankle for chronic lateral instability. J Bone Joint Surg Am. 1988;70(4):581–8.
3. Morvan A, Klouche S, Thes A, Hardy P, Bauer T. Reliability and validity of preoperative MRI for surgical decision making in chronic lateral ankle instability. Eur J Orthop Surg Traumatol. 2018;28(4):713–9.
4. Frank C, Amiel D, Woo SL, Akeson W. Normal ligament properties and ligament healing. Clin Orthop Relat Res. 1985;196:15–25.
5. Yasui Y, Takao M. Comparison of arthroscopic and histological evaluation on the injured anterior talofibular ligament. The American Academy of Orthopaedic Surgeons (AAOS) 2013 annual meeting, Chicago, USA.

Mind Your Head: Potential Short- and Long-Term Effects of Concussion in Sport

8

Anna Nordström, N. Feddermann-Demont, and Peter Nordström

8.1 Introduction

Concussions are becoming an important topic in sports research and has gained significant public attention in recent years. What sometimes used to be considered just a bump or a jolt to the head is now clearly considered a true brain injury. Even more concerning, injuries that were previously considered minor can have major impacts on the individual—both short-term and long-term. However, while we may recognize concussions in the acute setting on the playing field, there is limited knowledge about the long-term impact of both concussions and sub-concussive head impacts (e.g., the heading of a football). Despite these knowledge gaps, there appears to be sufficient evidence that current protocols, if properly used, are effective tools in the clinical identification of concussion or more severe brain injury and management of return to training and competition if properly used [1, 2].

In this report, we summarize the most important information about concussions, including their occurrence, symptoms, pathophysiology, and short-term and long-term effects. Our aim is to underscore the importance of following current guidelines and getting expert advice when an athlete has sustained a head injury. Doing so will ensure the best possible outcome and avoid potentially devastating long-term sequelae.

8.2 Seeing and Reporting the Tip of the Iceberg?

Trauma is one of the most common causes of injury to the human brain, with more than ten million people globally suffering a traumatic brain injury (TBI) each year [3]. Most reports of the incidence of TBI have been around 200–300 per 100,000 persons [4], but the actual incidence may be as high as 600 per 100,000 since especially sports-related concussions do not come to medical attention [5, 6]. Therefore, several authors describe TBI as a 'silent epidemic' [7–9].

When it comes to sports-related concussions, these occur most frequently in contact sports

A. Nordström (✉)
Department of Public Health and Clinical Medicine, Section of Sustainable Health, Umeå University, Umeå, Sweden

School of Sport Sciences, UiT Arctic University of Norway, Tromsö, Norway
e-mail: anna.h.nordstrom@umu.se

N. Feddermann-Demont
University Hospital and University of Zurich, Zürich, Switzerland

Swiss Concussion Center, Zürich, Switzerland
e-mail: nina.feddermann@swissconcussion.com

P. Nordström
Department of Community Medicine and Rehabilitation, Unit of Geriatric Medicine, Umeå University, Umeå, Sweden
e-mail: peter.nordstrom@umu.se

M. T. Hirschmann et al. (eds.), *ESSKA Instructional Course Lecture Book*,
https://doi.org/10.1007/978-3-662-61264-4_8

such as American football, hockey, rugby, soccer, and basketball [10]. Among men, most sports-related concussions occur in American football, cycling, and basketball; among women, most occur in cycling and horseback riding. Children and teens are more likely to get a concussion and can take longer to recover than adults.

8.3 Pathophysiology

Given the high incidence of concussion and the risk for short- and long-term sequelae, it is critical to understand the pathophysiology of this condition. While we currently understand the pathophysiology of concussion at a broad level, much is still poorly understood. Most concussions are caused by a direct or indirect linear or rotational force to the head, face, or other area of the body, in which the force is transmitted to the brain. The initial impact is followed by a complex cascade of ionic, metabolic, and physiological events that can adversely affect brain function for several days up to weeks [11]. Progress has been made in the diagnosis of concussions in emergency settings, but there is still much to learn about their multifactorial mechanics and pathophysiology [12]. Such knowledge is needed to improve prevention, diagnosis, and treatment [13].

8.4 Symptoms to Watch Out for

The recognition and management of concussions in sports is an evolving topic for both science and practice. The matter is complicated by the fact that symptoms can come and go at different stages after the initial trauma and include headache, fatigue, sluggishness, difficulty concentrating, dizziness, light sensitivity, memory dysfunction, visual problems, and balance problems. Loss of consciousness is not a requirement for the diagnosis of concussion, and it is reported to occur in less than 5% of cases [14, 15].

The complex picture calls for a comprehensive approach that includes clinical examination, cognitive testing, assessment of balance and vestibular function, and symptom reports. Both national and international guidelines exist for different sports [16–26]. Research shows that concussion assessments need to be repeated, ideally with preseason testing of all athletes to provide a comparison in the case of injury. Useful tools for both baseline and post-injury assessments include SCAT5, Sport Concussion Assessment Tool—5th Edition, the standardized tool for evaluating concussions [27], computerized neuropsychological instruments, which measure reaction time, memory capacity, speed of mental processing and executive functioning [28], and balance test (BESS) at baseline and at follow-ups after trauma [28].

8.5 Short-Term Effects of Concussion

A much-debated topic in treatment of concussion in sports is how and when to decide whether an athlete is fit to return to sport after a head trauma. Despite a growing body research, few evidence-based guidelines are available for determining how long it takes for an athlete to recover after concussion and when it is safe to return to competition.

The changes in brain that occur after a single concussion do not appear to have long-term clinically detectable symptoms. These symptoms usually disappear within 7–10 days, which is often when play is resumed [29, 30]. However, the literature suggests that symptom and cognitive recovery can take anywhere from several hours to several weeks after a sports-related concussion [31–34]. Approximately 85–90% of athletes with a concussion recover from symptoms within 1–2 weeks, and only a small percentage have symptoms lasting weeks to months [30, 35]. However, it is important to keep in mind that most studies on return to sports have been performed in American Football and that in most cases symptom relieve was stated at reduced levels of cognitive and physical load. Moreover, it can be challenging to make an accurate prognosis for return to play since scientific data are limited and because the signs and symptoms of concussions vary considerably. This variability in symptoms is evident in studies investigating short-term recovery periods in the weeks after the impact, where concussion has been associated with subtle cognitive impairments such as impaired attention, executive functioning, and visuospatial skills in computerized tests [36]. These impairments may lead to increased risks of new injuries up to a year later [37–40], perhaps because delayed neural processing can affect the athlete's ability to anticipate changes in external conditions and workloads and to adapt movement accordingly [41]. Since the possible lingering effects may affect an athlete's safety and performance, we need to develop more sensitive tests for field use. As of now, the best recommendation clinical guidelines can give is the use of return-to-sports protocols and computerized cognitive testing, which will ensure a controlled stepwise return to sport and liberal reevaluations [16, 20, 42, 43]. When in doubt sit them out.

8.6 Long-Term Effects of Concussion

Sports and specifically contact sports have received widespread media attention in recent years as being a risk factor for the development of dementia and chronic traumatic encephalopathy (CTE). This attention has sparked fears about the potential long-term effects of head trauma of any severity on cognitive functioning, leading to a public health concern. Evidence has emerged suggesting a connection between contact sports and increased risk of neurodegenerative disease [44, 45]. While the short-term symptoms of concussion are reversible, the evidence suggests that even a single trauma to the head can have severe consequences later in life [46–48]. To date, only a few studies, mostly autopsy studies, have examined whether sports trauma increases the risk of developing dementia or CTE [49–52]. Outside the sports field, the data suggest that the risk of developing dementia is detectable more than 30 years after the trauma and that the risk increases with the severity of the injury [6, 53].

8.7 Summary

Concussion is one of the greatest health challenges in sports today, and there is still a large knowledge gap in regard to its short- and long-term consequences. It is important that athletes with a concussion receive care and be cleared to return to sports by a medical team trained in concussion diagnosis and management. Individuals experiencing a prolonged recovery may have a particular need for knowledgeable and coordinated management of their symptoms.

References

1. Brolinson PG. Management of sport-related concussion: a review. Clin J Sport Med. 2014;24:89–90.
2. Choe MC. The pathophysiology of concussion. Curr Pain Headache Rep. 2016;20:42.
3. Murray CJL, Lopez AD, Organization WH, Bank W, Health HSoP. Global health statistics: a compendium of incidence, prevalence, and mortality estimates for over 200 conditions. Cambridge: Harvard School of Public Health; 1996.
4. Peloso PM, Von Holst H, Borg J. Mild traumatic brain injuries presenting to Swedish hospitals in 1987–2000. J Rehabil Med. 2004;36:22–7.
5. Cassidy JD, Carroll LJ, Peloso PM, et al. Incidence, risk factors and prevention of mild traumatic brain injury: results of the WHO collaborating centre task force on mild traumatic brain injury. J Rehabil Med. 2004;36:28–60.
6. King NS. 'Mild traumatic brain injury' and 'Sport-related concussion': different languages and mixed messages? Brain Inj. 2019;33(12):1156–63.
7. Coburn K. Traumatic brain injury: the silent epidemic. AACN Clin Issues Crit Care Nurs. 1992;3:9–18.
8. Langlois JA, Marr A, Mitchko J, Johnson RL. Tracking the silent epidemic and educating the public: CDC's traumatic brain injury-associated activities under the TBI Act of 1996 and the Children's Health Act of 2000. J Head Trauma Rehabil. 2005;20:196–204.
9. National Center for Injury Prevention and Control. Report to congress on mild traumatic brain injury in the United States: steps to prevent a serious public health problem. Atlanta: Center for Disease Control and Prevention; 2003.
10. Prien A, Grafe A, Rossler R, Junge A, Verhagen E. Epidemiology of head injuries focusing on concussions in team contact sports: a systematic review. Sports Med. 2018;48:953–69.
11. Giza CC, Hovda DA. The new neurometabolic cascade of concussion. Neurosurgery. 2014;75(Suppl 4):S24–33.

12. Satarasinghe P, Hamilton DK, Buchanan RJ, Koltz MT. Unifying pathophysiological explanations for sports-related concussion and concussion protocol management: literature review. J Exp Neurosci. 2019;13:1179069518824125.
13. Laksari K, Kurt M, Babaee H, Kleiven S, Camarillo D. Mechanistic insights into human brain impact dynamics through modal analysis. Phys Rev Lett. 2018;120:138101.
14. Castile L, Collins CL, McIlvain NM, Comstock RD. The epidemiology of new versus recurrent sports concussions among high school athletes, 2005-2010. Br J Sports Med. 2012;46:603–10.
15. Meehan WP 3rd, d'Hemecourt P, Comstock RD. High school concussions in the 2008-2009 academic year: mechanism, symptoms, and management. Am J Sports Med. 2010;38:2405–9.
16. McCrory P, Meeuwisse W, Dvorak J, et al. Consensus statement on concussion in sport-the 5(th) international conference on concussion in sport held in Berlin, October 2016. Br J Sports Med. 2017;51:838–47.
17. Makdissi M, Davis G, McCrory P. Updated guidelines for the management of sports-related concussion in general practice. Aust Fam Physician. 2014;43:94–9.
18. Patricios J, Fuller GW, Ellenbogen R, et al. What are the critical elements of sideline screening that can be used to establish the diagnosis of concussion? A systematic review. Br J Sports Med. 2017;51(11):888–94. https://doi.org/10.1136/bjsports-2016-097441.
19. Summary of evidence-based guideline update: evaluation and management of concussion in sports. 2013. www.aan.com/Guidelines/home/GuidelineDetail/582.
20. Harmon KG, Clugston JR, Dec K, et al. American Medical Society for Sports Medicine position statement on concussion in sport. Br J Sports Med. 2019;53:213–25.
21. Sports-related head injury. www.aans.org/Patients/Neurosurgical-Conditions-and-Treatments/Sports-related-Head-Injury.
22. World rugby concussion management. https://playerwelfare.worldrugby.org/concussion.
23. NFL Head, Neck and spine committee's concussion diagnosis and management protocol. 2017. https://www.playsmartplaysafe.com/wp-content/uploads/2017/06/2017-nfl-concussion-protocol.pdf.
24. Concussion evaluation and management protocol. 2016. http://cdn.agilitycms.com/nhlpacom/2016-17_ConcussionProtocol.pdf.
25. Medical. https://eiha.co.uk/eiha-education-program/medical/.
26. Concussion education & protocols. http://www.waterpolo.ca/concussionprotocol.aspx.
27. Echemendia RJ, Meeuwisse W, McCrory P, et al. The Sport Concussion Assessment Tool 5th Edition (SCAT5): Background and rationale. Br J Sports Med. 2017;51:848–50.
28. Gordon J, Nordstrom A. Trauma and medical emergencies. New York: Thieme Medical Publishers; 2017.
29. Slobounov S, Slobounov E, Sebastianelli W, Cao C, Newell K. Differential rate of recovery in athletes after first and second concussion episodes. Neurosurgery. 2007;61:338–44. discussion 44.
30. McCrea M, Guskiewicz KM, Marshall SW, et al. Acute effects and recovery time following concussion in collegiate football players: the NCAA Concussion Study. JAMA. 2003;290:2556–63.
31. Macciocchi SN, Barth JT, Alves W, Rimel RW, Jane JA. Neuropsychological functioning and recovery after mild head injury in collegiate athletes. Neurosurgery. 1996;39:510–4.
32. McCrea M, Kelly JP, Randolph C, et al. Standardized assessment of concussion (SAC): on-site mental status evaluation of the athlete. J Head Trauma Rehabil. 1998;13:27–35.
33. Collins MW, Grindel SH, Lovell MR, et al. Relationship between concussion and neuropsychological performance in college football players. JAMA. 1999;282:964–70.
34. Echemendia RJ, Putukian M, Mackin RS, Julian L, Shoss N. Neuropsychological test performance prior to and following sports-related mild traumatic brain injury. Clin J Sport Med. 2001;11:23–31.
35. Guskiewicz KM, McCrea M, Marshall SW, et al. Cumulative effects associated with recurrent concussion in collegiate football players: the NCAA Concussion Study. JAMA. 2003;290:2549–55.
36. Belanger HG, Curtiss G, Demery JA, Lebowitz BK, Vanderploeg RD. Factors moderating neuropsychological outcomes following mild traumatic brain injury: a meta-analysis. J Int Neuropsychol Soc. 2005;11:215–27.
37. Nordstrom A, Nordstrom P, Ekstrand J. Sports-related concussion increases the risk of subsequent injury by about 50% in elite male football players. Br J Sports Med. 2014;48:1447–50.
38. Burman E, Lysholm J, Shahim P, Malm C, Tegner Y. Concussed athletes are more prone to injury both before and after their index concussion: a data base analysis of 699 concussed contact sports athletes. BMJ Open Sport Exerc Med. 2016;2:e000092.
39. Cross M, Kemp S, Smith A, Trewartha G, Stokes K. Professional Rugby Union players have a 60% greater risk of time loss injury after concussion: a 2-season prospective study of clinical outcomes. Br J Sports Med. 2016;50:926–31.
40. McPherson AL, Nagai T, Webster KE, Hewett TE. Musculoskeletal injury risk after sport-related concussion: a systematic review and meta-analysis. Am J Sports Med. 2019;47:1754–62.
41. Johnson EW, Kegel NE, Collins MW. Neuropsychological assessment of sport-related concussion. Clin Sports Med. 2011;30:73–88, viii–ix.
42. Ellis MJ, Leddy JJ, Willer B. Physiological, vestibulo-ocular and cervicogenic post-concussion disorders: an evidence-based classification system with directions for treatment. Brain Inj. 2015;29:238–48.

43. Sufrinko A, Charek D, Gillie B. Multimodal concussion assessment. Return to play in football. New York: Springer; 2018. p. 683–98.
44. McKee AC, Daneshvar DH, Alvarez VE, Stein TD. The neuropathology of sport. Acta Neuropathol. 2014;127:29–51.
45. Tagge CA, Fisher AM, Minaeva OV, et al. Concussion, microvascular injury, and early tauopathy in young athletes after impact head injury and an impact concussion mouse model. Brain. 2018;141:422–58.
46. Alexander MP. Mild traumatic brain injury: pathophysiology, natural history, and clinical management. Neurology. 1995;45:1253–60.
47. Traumatic brain injury: hope through research. In: Bethesda MNIoH, ed. Office of Communications and Public Liaison, National Institute of Neurological Disorders and Stroke, National Institutes of Health. NIH publication. 2002;02–158.
48. Holm L, Cassidy JD, Carroll LJ, Borg J. Summary of the WHO collaborating centre for neurotrauma task force on mild traumatic brain injury. J Rehabil Med. 2005;37:137–41.
49. Stewart W, McNamara PH, Lawlor B, Hutchinson S, Farrell M. Chronic traumatic encephalopathy: a potential late and under recognized consequence of rugby union? QJM. 2016;109:11–5.
50. Ling H, Morris HR, Neal JW, et al. Mixed pathologies including chronic traumatic encephalopathy account for dementia in retired association football (soccer) players. Acta Neuropathol. 2017;133:337–52.
51. Omalu BI, Hamilton RL, Kamboh MI, DeKosky ST, Bailes J. Chronic traumatic encephalopathy (CTE) in a National Football League Player: case report and emerging medicolegal practice questions. J Forensic Nurs. 2010;6:40–6.
52. Standring OJ, Friedberg J, Tripodis Y, et al. Contact sport participation and chronic traumatic encephalopathy are associated with altered severity and distribution of cerebral amyloid angiopathy. Acta Neuropathol. 2019;138:401–13.
53. Nordstrom A, Nordstrom P. Traumatic brain injury and the risk of dementia diagnosis: a nationwide cohort study. PLoS Med. 2018;15:e1002496.

All the Secrets of Elbow Instability

9

R. Barco, A. Muller, K. Wegman, A. C. Watts, M. van den Bekerom, D. Eygendaal, and L. A. Pederzini

The goal of the present chapter is to have a comprehensive approach to instabilities of the elbow covering from how to diagnose and how to image them to how to treat them. Acute and chronic instability have different approaches and the presence of associated fractures ("complex instability") influences the decision-making process. Surgical techniques will be reviewed covering with an emphasis on how to repair the lateral and medial ligament complex.

R. Barco · A. Muller
Instituto de Investigación Hospital Universitario La Paz (IdiPAZ), Madrid, Spain

K. Wegman
Department of Orthopaedics and Trauma Surgery, Koeln University, Koeln, Germany
e-mail: kilian.wegmann@uk-koeln.de

A. C. Watts
Wrightington, Wigan and Leigh NHS Foundation Trust, Wigan, UK
e-mail: adam.c.watts@wwl.nhs.uk

M. van den Bekerom · D. Eygendaal
Department of Orthopedics, OLVG, Amsterdam, The Netherlands

L. A. Pederzini (✉)
Orthopeadics and Traumatology Unit, Nuovo Ospedale Civile di Sassuolo, Sassuolo, Italy
e-mail: info@luigipederzini.com

9.1 Diagnosis

The elbow represents the crucial mechanical link between the upper arm and the forearm and therewith to the hand. As the hand is one of the key instruments of the human body, functional integrity of the elbow is mandatory. Besides many pathologies like stiffness or inflammatory processes, elbow instability is a common and challenging issue. As in all pathologies, diagnosing it is the basic step of treatment. However, diagnosis of elbow instability is difficult and poses high demands on the surgeon. The difficulties in the diagnosis of elbow instability begin with the fact that only very little biomechanical data is available, which helps to define elbow stability itself. As individual variability is high, the investigator could be fooled by joint laxity, which is present in every patient as a normal variant. Furthermore, if pathological instability has been identified, it is not clearly defined which amount of instability is worth surgical treatment and which is safely treated conservatively. Recent research will have to tackle this task. Also, the elbow is comprised of three joints functioning together as a biomechanical construct, surrounded by several critical neurovascular bundles, making direct and indirect investigations complex. However, this section shall cover the available and reasonable clinical tests for elbow instability.

As imaging is going to be discussed in the following section, we will focus on signs of

M. T. Hirschmann et al. (eds.), *ESSKA Instructional Course Lecture Book*,
https://doi.org/10.1007/978-3-662-61264-4_9

instability that can be found in patient history and manual clinical tests of elbow instability. For obvious reasons, we concentrate on subtle instability and not gross acute instability, which is usually apparent and easy to find.

9.1.1 Patient History

It is mandatory to take information on prior injuries, surgeries, and also injection therapies from the patients. Subtle signs of elbow instability may be clicking sensations, that is, the patient's report. The clicking can be a consequence of transitional motions of the radial head against the capitulum, especially in posterolateral rotatory instability (PLRI). Due to the shift of the radial head, the posterolateral plica can get impinged and inflamed. These subtle subluxations can cause the clicking sensations reported by the patients. In cases of marked subluxation or even dislocations of the radial head behind the capitulum, the patients may even sensate a "giving way symptom," as known from other joints like the knee. If posterolateral rotatory instability is present, this giving-way would typically happen when the patient is leaning on a table with the affected arm, or poses axial weight-bearing on the arm in another way. Concerning posterolateral instability, when the forearm is externally rotated during this motion, the instability is increased. Some patients will realize this influence and report it when asked. Furthermore, symptoms of patients with lateral instability will be more present in varus loading, while patients with medial instability will suffer distinctively from valgus loading. The typical case would be a thrower, reporting a minor distortion of the joint during exercise or a sudden pain during daily routine practice, with now ongoing pain over the medial joint space, with increasing pain under valgus load. Even closing doors with the affected arm may lead to increased pain, and thus is reported by the patients. Hence, patient's history may offer important leads in the search of elbow instability and should not be neglected.

9.1.2 Manual Clinical Investigations

Palpation is an important part of investigating elbow instability. Tenderness may be found over the tendons and muscles adjacent to the ligaments and the joint space. In case of medial instability, this would be found over the common flexor origin and the pronator mass. Often, the ulnar nerve is also involved and shows signs of inflammation, exhibiting pain on palpation and tapping. Be aware of subluxation of the ulnar nerve out of the sulcus. Laterally, tenderness can be found over the common extensor origin, and also over the posterolateral joint aspect. Typically, manual clinical investigations of joint instability aim to imitate the motion and direction of the suspected instability pattern. In the case of the PLRI test or lateral pivot shift test [1], the elbow should be brought into valgus loading, axial compression, and supination while the patient is in the supine position. When moving from extension to flexion, subluxation may be noted especially between 40 and 20°. This test is difficult to perform in the awake patient, but sensitive if positive. Further testing can be done by the push-up test. With this test, the patient pushes himself up from a sitting position with the arm for example on the arm rest, while the forearm is supinated. Therewith the arm is moved from a supinated flexed position into extension. The test—if positive—will lead to pain over the lateral joint and may lead to clicking, subjective instability, and also apprehension.

Medial instability however is checked via valgus stress testing of the elbow in increasing flexion, starting at 30°. Instability will be noted by gapping medially and pain. Also the moving valgus stress test [2], which is performed with the arm abducted at 90°, where the elbow is extended from a flexed position under valgus loading and therewith shoulder external rotation. Positive would be pain especially between 70 and 120° of flexion. Several other tests have been reported with varying sensitivity and specificity. Imaging and intraoperative tests will be discussed in the following chapters.

9.2 Imaging

When considering imaging for instability we need to consider the following situations: diagnosis of acute traumatic injury, injury grading and prognostic indicators, chronic injury diagnosis, and pre-operative planning.

9.2.1 Acute Traumatic Injury

Plain radiographs are the initial investigation of choice for a patient presenting with a history of trauma and elbow deformity. This will differentiate between a simple elbow dislocation, defined as a dislocation of the ulnohumeral joint without fracture, and an elbow fracture or fracture dislocation. Minor flake avulsion fragments associated with ligament avulsion from the lateral ligament, posterior capitellum, or medial epicondyle may be seen in a simple dislocation, but a coronoid injury however minor in appearance would make this an elbow fracture dislocation, probably of a posteromedial rotatory pattern. Simple dislocations are classified by the direction of dislocation: posteromedial, posterolateral, posterior, anterior, and divergent. The risk of recurrent instability after simple dislocation is dependent on the extent of the soft tissue injury, with a greater degree of instability where the tendons have been avulsed from the epicondyles. Fluoroscopy can be used at the time of closed reduction to assess the degree of instability, and by inference the presence of tendon avulsion, with joint gapping of more than 10° on lateral or medial side associated with an eightfold increase in the risk of recurrent instability. Magnetic resonance imaging (MRI) or ultrasound (US) can also be used to grade the injury.

Elbow fracture and fracture dislocations can be identified from plain radiographs but classification of the pattern of injury is enhanced by the use of computer tomography (CT). There are a number of classification systems in use for coronoid fractures (Regan and Morrey, O'Driscoll), radial head (Mason Johnson, Hotchkiss) and olecranon fracture (Mayo), Monteggia fracture dislocation (Bado, Ring), and transolecranon fracture dislocation (Jupiter). A universal classification system for elbow fracture dislocations including the coronoid, radial head, and olecranon has been developed (Wrightington classification) that guides management of the injury and has been shown to be reproducible, accurate from CT, and, when the suggested treatment algorithms are applied, can result in predictably good outcomes.

Anticipating acute ligament injury in an elbow that is reduced at the time that initial plain radiographs are taken can be challenging, but may be indicated from careful history and examination of the elbow as detailed above. The higher the grade of radial head fracture, the greater the risk of lateral ligament injury, but the clinical significance of these injuries is uncertain. Loss of cortical contact of radial head fragments is predictive of instability as shown by Ring. Plain MRI or US can be used where clinical concern exists. The addition of contrast is not required as the haemarthrosis will typically provide adequate definition of the injury in the acute setting.

9.2.2 Chronic Instability

Chronic instability may occur as a result of ligamentous and neuromuscular incompetence, osseous defect, or a combination of these. Most soft tissue injuries result from traumatic avulsion but attenuation may develop as a result of connective tissue disorders, iatrogenic intervention, or abnormal loading patterns. MRI with intra-articular contrast injection (MR arthrography (MRA)) is the gold standard investigation for the identification of chronic injury to the lateral ligament complex with evidence of contrast between the origin of the radial collateral or lateral ulna collateral ligaments and the humerus or more rarely at the insertion of the ligaments on the ulna. An annular ligament that is not closely opposed to the radial head may be an indication of injury. Avulsion of the posterolateral ligament (Osborne–Cotterill ligament) can be appreciated on sagittal cuts.

Posterior subluxation of the radial head relative to the capitellum on the sagittal images is not a reliable sign of instability as there is such a wide variation in what is normal. The medial ligament can be reliably assessed with US or MRA. US offers the advantage of dynamic assessment and demonstration of functional incompetence if joint gapping is observed. MRA will demonstrate ligament avulsion from the humerus or ulna with the classic "T" sign observed in distal avulsion of the anterior band. Plain CT can be helpful where there is felt to be an osseous element to the instability, but CT arthrography (CTA) is probably more helpful because in most there will be an associated ligament injury. CTA will also identify the presence of cartilage degeneration which may influence the treatment decisions. MRA can also provide adequate assessment of osseoligamentous injuries if 3D rendering is not required.

9.3 Indications

9.3.1 Acute Simple Elbow Instability

After manual reduction of the dislocated elbow this acute instability can often be treated conservatively. It has been shown that immediate mobilization of the elbow does not increase the risk of recurrent instability [2–4]. If the elbow "spontaneously" dislocates at flexion angles more than about 30°, early surgical repair is usually advocated [1]. Routine use of stress radiographs to evaluate acute instability is not indicated. A surgical exploration and repair are indicated if closed reduction is not possible or if the elbow remains grossly unstable following closed reduction. In high-level athletes or manual laborers, ligamentous repair on the lateral and/or medial site can be indicated and often leads to good results. [2].

9.3.2 Chronic Simple Elbow Instability

Recurrent (complete) dislocations are rare, but recurrent subluxations may lead to symptoms as clicking or weakness. Patients with chronic instability are first treated conservatively. When this treatment fails, surgery is indicated. This is more complex than in acute cases because ligaments may be scarred and retracted, so that a direct repair may no longer be possible, and a reconstruction with a graft has to be performed.

Medial instability can occur in overhead athletes because attenuation of the MCL complex can lead to symptomatic but often subtle medial instability. This patients also start with strengthening exercises of the wrist flexors and pronator muscles, and if this treatment fails, ulnar collateral ligament reconstruction can be indicated dependent from future sport ambitions.

9.3.3 Acute Complex Instability

When elbow instability is associated with a fracture, the dislocation is classified as complex. Fractures can include the distal humerus, radial head, proximal ulna, or coronoid process. The coronoid fracture dictates treatment of many of these cases. For understanding the principles of treatment, it can be helpful to differentiate between dislocation and disruption injuries [5]. In general, there are transolecranon fracture dislocations, terrible triad injuries, and the anteromedial coronoid fractures.

9.3.4 Chronic Complex Instability

Most of these cases with symptomatic chronic complex instability have to be treated operatively, and in some cases, this will be a salvage procedure because treatment of this group can be challenging. Most of these patients had an inappropriate initial treatment and have persistent instability, post-traumatic arthritis, stiffness, and pain.

9.4 Non-operative Treatment of Elbow Instability

Elbow instability is often times subject to surgical treatment to correct pain, catching or locking, subjective sensation of instability, and objective episodes of instability. However, there is a role for non-operative treatment.

Conceptually a stable elbow will stay aligned throughout its arc of motion. Failure to maintain this alignment can produce different forms of instability and highlight injury to one or more structures that participate in elbow stability.

We will briefly review the anatomic elements that contribute to stability, injury patterns that can produce elbow instability to understand the basis of non-operative management but will focus on reduced unstable elbows.

The primary stabilizers of the elbow are a congruous distal humerus and proximal ulna and a stable medial and collateral lateral ligament complex. Secondary stabilizers are the radial head, the anterior and posterior capsule and the correct function of muscles around the elbow [1]. Each of the previous structures can be injured to different degrees and can combine in different patterns that make interpretation of instability difficult in certain situations. Most typically, however, they present in a predictable fashion that helps us understand the possible mechanism of injury and will lead to identifying the key injury and possible associated injuries. In reduced unstable elbows, we will find injuries to soft tissues alone (simple instabilities) or associating bony injuries (complex instabilities) in an acute and chronic setting. Anteroposterior and lateral radiographs will typically delineate the associated fractures. To better define existing fractures and joint congruity, CT scans can be helpful. We do not advocate for MRI scanning in these cases as there is a risk of over-treatment although some authors perform scans to screen for high-grade elbow dislocations [2].

The basis for non-operative treatment is to allow for healing of the injuries while keeping an aligned joint. Motion can be started as soon as there is a certain degree of dynamic control over the elbow and within the ranges permitted by the loads applied to injured ligaments and fractures.

Simple elbow dislocations are typically posterolateral, produced by either a PLRI mechanism that can start directly on the lateral side of the elbow and progress medially or start with an initial injury to the MCL and progress laterally.

After initial reduction, placing the elbow though a functional range of motion can assess stability. If there is residual instability, it will typically show at the last degrees of elbow extension or might increase with varus or valgus testing. We avoid using exam under anesthesia as this decreases muscle contribution to elbow stability and does not mimic real-life conditions and might generate over-treatment. If within 30° of extension the elbow is stable, we will follow conservative management.

Non-operative treatment of simple elbow dislocations consist of immobilization with a brachiopalmar plaster cast. We favor a short-term immobilization period of 7–10 days with concentric elbow exercises within the cast followed by progressive advancement in elbow motion as allowed by the patient. Iordens et al. recently showed that early use of the arm when compared to 3 weeks of plaster achieved faster return to activities and sooner regain of range of motion with no increased risk of residual instability, albeit patients should be advised that initially they might have more pain [3].

Some patients will feel very confident and can resume their normal activities very fast, but some will take longer. Gravity-assisted range-of-motion exercise are recommended for the fearful or the more unstable patients as it helps regaining motion while helping reduce the ulnohumeral joint by means of gravity [4]. Avoidance of varus will help protect the lateral ligament complex, but some patients have difficulty grasping the concept of reaching out without loading the elbow into varus [6]. At 6 weeks we will encourage advanced strengthening exercises and will allow normal sporting activities by 3 months.

The use of orthotic devices is controversial. Some patients may feel safer with the use of an orthotic device, but they are difficult to wear correctly. Not infrequently they will slide down the arm altering the center of rotation of the device, which along with the weight of the device can help to subluxate the forearm. Potentially this can be detrimental for adequate healing of the ligaments [4, 5].

In complex elbow instability, the extent of bony injury will influence the stability of the elbow. Of particular interest is the role of coronoid and radial head fractures. Radiocapitellar contact becomes especially important in the setting of a coronoid fracture. If there is integrity of the radial head, coronoid fractures are well tolerated with a specific treatment protocol including 3 weeks of plaster and three additional weeks of sling while starting flexion-extension exercises with the forearm in pronation [7]. It is critical to assess adequate congruity with the use of CT examination.

The degree of involvement of the coronoid in size and location might influence the magnitude and pattern of instability [8–10]. Fracture of the sublime tubercle produces MCL insufficiency and generally requires surgical treatment. Fractures of the lateral coronoid may produce an insufficiency of the annular ligament and may contribute to lateral ligament insufficiency. Tip fractures of up to 50% of coronoid height can be well tolerated, however, with conservative management.

Terrible triad injuries combining a radial head fracture and a coronoid fracture are generally unstable injuries requiring surgical treatment, but small tip coronoid fractures combined with undisplaced radial head fractures can be treated successfully with non-operative treatment in a similar manner as described earlier [11–14].

9.5 Operative Management of Elbow Instability

Elbow instability is a spectrum of injuries. Both the lateral and the medial ligament can be involved as well the radial head and the coronoid. "Terrible Triad" is first described by Hotchkiss in 1996. He described a fracture dislocation of the elbow with a radial head fracture, fractured coronoid, and a dislocation of the elbow joint (Fig. 9.1). This type of elbow injury is notoriously difficult to treat. A careful stepwise approach addressing each of the component of this challenging injury can yield reliable results [15–17].

9.5.1 Surgical Technique for the Terrible Triad

Direct lateral approach is advised as the medial anblel ligament tends to heal naturally, if the ulnohumeral joint is reduced. A grasping stitch is placed through the postero-lateral soft tissues for lateral repair. The coronoid fracture is addressed first; type 1 with sutures (Fig. 9.2). Type 2 with small screws. Second, the radial head is reconstructed, if reconstruction is not anble replacement is indicated as a stable radial head is the key to prevent re-dislocation. After the abovementioned reconstruction, the elbow is assessed for stability. If there is a persistent tendency of the elbow to dislocate in 30 or more degrees of flexion, an additional fixation of the MCL is advised. In exceptional cases, the elbow remains

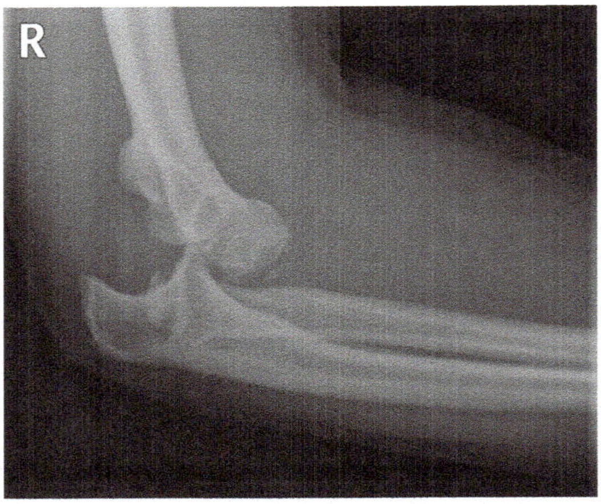

Fig. 9.1 Plain X-ray of terrible triad

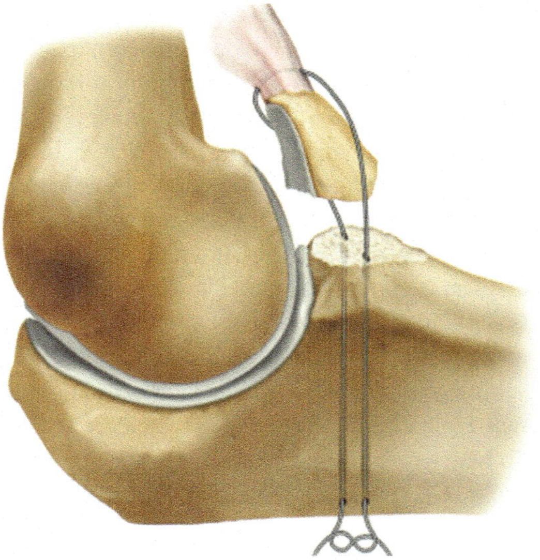

Fig. 9.2 Trans-osseous sutures for type 1 coronoid fractures

unstable after MCL fixation; in those particular cases, an external fixator or transfixation with plaster, as described by David Ring and co-workers, is indicated.

Summary Instability of the elbow encompasses many different injuries that require extensive knowledge of anatomy of the elbow to guide proper physical examination and adequate imaging techniques. Proper physical examination has to be emphasized to gauge the clinical relevance of imaging findings. Simple radiographs remain the first imaging technique to rule out associated fractures. If a fracture is seen or highly suspicious, a CT scan can be helpful to define the magnitude of the fracture and the congruency of the ulnohumeral joint. Rarely, there will be a need for MRI in the acute setting.

The majority of simple elbow dislocations will do well after non-operative management. The addition of associated injuries will add severity to the instability and the need for a surgical intervention greatly increases. The goals of surgery will be to achieve stability and congruity of the joint. Most typically, complex injuries will require a stepwise surgical approach with adequate repair of the LCL complex, the coronoid, and radial head. In selected cases, replacement of the radial head is indicated.

Following these guidelines, a functional elbow will be achieved most of the time.

References

1. O'Driscoll SW, Bell DF, Morrey BF. Posterolateral rotatory instability of the elbow. J Bone Joint Surg Am. 1991;73:440–6.
2. O'Driscoll SW, Lawton RL, Smith AM. The "moving valgus stress test" for medial collateral ligament tears of the elbow. Am J Sports Med. 2005;33(2):231–9. PubMed PMID: 15701609.
3. O'Driscoll SW, Jupiter JB, King GJ, Hotchkiss RN, Morrey BF. The unstable elbow. Instr Course Lect. 2001;50:89–102.
4. Savoie FH III, Trenhaile SW, Roberts J, Field LD, Ramsey JR. Primary repair of ulnar collateral ligament injuries of the elbow in young athletes: a case series of injuries to the proximal and distal ends of the ligament. Am J Sports Med. 2008;36:1066–72.
5. Lordens GI, Van Lieshout EM, Schep NW, et al. Early mobilization versus plaster immobilisation of simple elbow dislocations: results of the FuncSiE multicenter randomised clinical trial. Br J Sports Med. 2017;51(6):531–8.
6. Maripuri SN, Debnath UK, Rao P, Mohanty K. Simple elbow dislocation among adults: a comparative study of two different methods of treatment. Injury. 2007;38:1254–8.
7. Chan K, King GJ, Faber KJ. Treatment of complex elbow fracture-dislocations. Curr Rev Musculoskelet Med. 2016;9(2):185–9.
8. Doornberg J, Ring D, Jupiter JB. Effective treatment of fracture-dislocations of the olecranon requires a stable trochlear notch. Clin Orthop Relat Res. 2004;429:292–300.
9. Karbach LE, Elfar J. Elbow instability: anatomy, biomechanics, diagnostic maneuvers, and testing. J Hand Surg Am. 2017;42(2):118–26.
10. Robinson PM, Griffiths E, Watts AC. Simple elbow dislocation. Shoulder Elbow. 2017;9(3):195–204.
11. Lee AT, Schrumpf MA, Choi D, Meyers KN, Patel R, Wright TM, et al. The influence of gravity on the unstable elbow. J Shoulder Elb Surg. 2013;22(1):81–7.
12. Duckworth AD, Kulijdian A, McKee MD, Ring D. Residual subluxation of the elbow after dislocation or fracture-dislocation: treatment with active elbow exercises and avoidance of varus stress. J Shoulder Elb Surg. 2008;17(2):276–80.
13. Manocha RH, King GJW, Johnson JA. In vitro kinematic assessment of a hinged elbow orthosis following lateral collateral ligament injury. J Hand Surg Am. 2018;43(2):123–32.
14. Foruria AM, Gutierrez B, Cobos J, Haeni DL, Valencia M, Calvo E. Most coronoid fractures and fracture-dislocations with no radial head involvement can be treated nonsurgically with elbow immobilization. J Shoulder Elb Surg. 2019;28(7):1395–405.
15. Mellema JJ, Doornberg JN, Dyer GS, Ring D. Distribution of coronoid fracture lines by specific patterns of traumatic elbow instability. J Hand Surg Am. 2014;39(10):2041–6.
16. Hotchkiss RN. Fractures and dislocations of the elbow. In: Rockwood Jr CA, Green DP, Bucholz RW, Heckman JD, editors. Fractures in adults; 1996. p. P929–1024.
17. Ring D. Posterior dislocation of the elbow with fractures of the radial head and coronoid. J Bone Joint Surg Am. 2002;84-A(4):547–51.

10 Basics of 2D Planning in Total Knee Replacement

Christian Fink and Elisabeth Abermann

10.1 Introduction

Successful outcomes after total knee arthroplasty (TKA) are strongly dependent on accurate component alignment and soft tissue balancing [1]. Postoperative performance can be altered due to inadequate patellofemoral and tibiofemoral kinematics caused by malpositioning of the components [2]. Thorough preoperative planning is critical for optimizing implant position and soft tissue balancing and also minimizes the probability of subsequent TKA failure [3]. Furthermore, it allows for anticipating intraoperative problems, implant choice and size estimation [4, 5].

Planning a TKR (total knee replacement) starts with talking to and examining the patient very closely. Obtaining a thorough history is crucial for patient selection and for the evaluation of potential postoperative complications. Factors that should be considered include preoperative diagnosis, age, characteristics of the knee pain, level of activity, functional limitations, involvement of other joints (e.g., back, hip, and foot), mechanical symptoms and previous treatment [5]. Patients should have good dental health prior to surgery [6], and sources of chronic infection such as urinary tract infections should be eliminated. Morbid obesity, poor nutritional status, anaemia, poorly treated diabetes and heavy smoking raise the risk of infection. Patients with neuromuscular conditions are at high risk of instability following TKA and may benefit from specific implant options (e.g., constrained or hinged components) [7].

10.2 Clinical Examination

The patient's gait should be assessed. In addition to observing the overall knee alignment, the surgeon should look for the presence of thrust and/or hyperextension during walking, which indicates ligamentous laxity. An in-toeing or out-toeing gait may indicate pre-existing rotational deformities [5]. Therefore, hip anteversion and tibial external rotation should be estimated, at least clinically. A hindfoot inspection should also be part of the examination because hindfoot valgus is not uncommon, and it tends to shift the mechanical axis of the lower extremity after TKA [8].

A close look at the preoperative ROM is necessary because the more limited the preoperative ROM, the greater the likelihood that the associated stiffness of the extensor mechanism may contribute to limited flexion after surgery [9].

Preoperative assessment of the collateral and cruciate ligaments is required to guide the

C. Fink (✉) · E. Abermann
Gelenkpunkt—Sports and Joint Surgery, Innsbruck, Austria

Research Unit for Orthopaedic Sport Medicine and Injury Prevention (OSMI), UMIT, Hall in Tirol, Tyrol, Austria
e-mail: c.fink@gelenkpunkt.com

M. T. Hirschmann et al. (eds.), *ESSKA Instructional Course Lecture Book*,
https://doi.org/10.1007/978-3-662-61264-4_10

strategy for soft tissue balancing and the selection of the implant. Any fixed coronal deformity found on physical examination should be noted to allow for planning of an intraoperative correction [5].

10.3 Radiographic Examination

The standard radiographic evaluation in our planning algorithm for patients undergoing primary TKA includes a weight-bearing one-leg AP (anterior-posterior) fixed-flexion view, a lateral view of the knee, a patellofemoral joint view such as a skyline view, a full-length hip-to-ankle AP weight-bearing view, an axial view to assess rotational alignment [10] and an optional Cobey's view of the ankle to assess hindfoot alignment.

The one-leg fixed-flexion AP radiograph is superior to the normal weight-bearing AP X-rays [11–13] and is primarily used to verify the diagnosis and indication as well as to identify medial and lateral osteophytes. In this view, the patient is facing the detector with the foot rotated 10° externally, the toes are touching the detector and the knees are bent until they touch the table. The X-ray beam is angled 10° caudal pointing onto the joint space [11, 14]. As the patient is facing the detector, he/she can hold on to the detector and stand on only the affected limb to further increase the stress [13].

The lateral views are mid-flexion views. The true lateral view can be verified if no overlap is present between the medial and lateral femoral condyles. This view is necessary to detect posterior osteophytes, to assess the vertical position of the patella in relationship to the joint line, to measure the tibial slope and the posterior femoral offset and for size estimation in templating.

The axial view of the patellofemoral joint is performed with the knee in 45° of flexion with the X-ray beam perpendicular to the detector plane [15]. In the axial view the patellar lateralization, the tilt and lateral overhang should be determined for intraoperative planning of lateral facet resection or release of the retinaculum, and the patellar depth should be measured in cases of patella replacement.

The full-length hip to ankle AP weight-bearing view is necessary for the assessment of the load-bearing axis of the lower limb, for estimating coronal laxity, for ruling out extra-articular deformity, for templating in the frontal plane and for planning the bony cuts with respect to the mechanical axis. For this view, the patient stands in front of the detector and is instructed to bear weight on both feet equally. The patella is felt with the index finger and thumb and rotated until it points forward, irrespective of the foot position.

The radiograph confirms the correct position, when it shows the patella centred between the femoral condyles [16].

For the rotation radiograph, the patient sits on a wooden table facing the detector with the lower legs hanging down at neutral rotation. The X-ray beam is directed at a 10° upward angle from behind [10].

In the case of abnormal hindfoot alignment, a weight-bearing modified Cobey's view is taken. This radiograph is obtained with the patient standing on a radiolucent platform, with the radiographic beam angled from behind at an angle of 15° downward from the horizontal plane [17].

All radiographs used for templating should be carried out with a reference ball at the level of the joint to increase the accuracy of size estimation [3, 4].

10.4 Radiologic Assessment

10.4.1 Frontal Plane

10.4.1.1 Alignment

The first step in radiographic templating is to find the mechanical axis in the frontal plane. It is defined as a line drawn from the centre of the femoral head to the centre of the ankle joint [18]. In the case of the neutral mechanical axis, the line passes through the centre of the knee joint. The distance of this line from the centre provides the most accurate measure of coronal alignment. The normal range is 8 ± 8 mm; however, the ideal is 4 ± 4 mm. Malalignment refers to the loss of collinearity of the hip, knee and ankle joints in the frontal plane outside the normal range [19]. To further quantify the deformity, the hip–knee–ankle angle (HKA), formed by the tibial mechanical axis and the femoral mechanical axis, is measured. Frontal plane malalignment can arise from femoral deformity, tibial deformity, knee joint laxity or subluxation and knee joint condylar deformity. To differentiate these, the LDFA (lateral distal femoral angle), the MPTA (medial proximal tibial angle) and the JLCA (joint line convergence angle) are measured [19] (see Figs. 10.1a, 10.2a, and 10.3a). Any extra-articular deformity and the corresponding CORA (centre of rotation of angulation) should be noted. Normal alignment of the knee does not identify malorientation of the hip and ankle. The intramedullary valgus correction angle needs to be defined, and the individual entry point on the distal femur needs to be planned since it depends on the distal femur anatomy [20]. According to the surgeon's alignment philosophy (i.e., mechanical, anatomical, or kinematic; see Fig. 10.1b, c), the necessary correction for the bone cuts can be estimated (see Fig. 10.4a–c). In case of clinical hindfoot malalignment, the modified Cobey's view can objectify the degree of deformity (>180° indicates valgus deformity or <180° indicates varus deformity). As hindfoot deformity tends to persist after correction of the HKA and influences the ground mechanical axis, the hindfoot alignment should be taken into account for over- or under-correction of the HKA [8, 21].

10.4.1.2 Joint Line Height

The distance between a line perpendicular to the mechanical axis of the tibia at the apex of the fibular head and a parallel line to this line at the level of the distal aspect of the lateral femoral condyle is measured [22] (see Fig. 10.5).

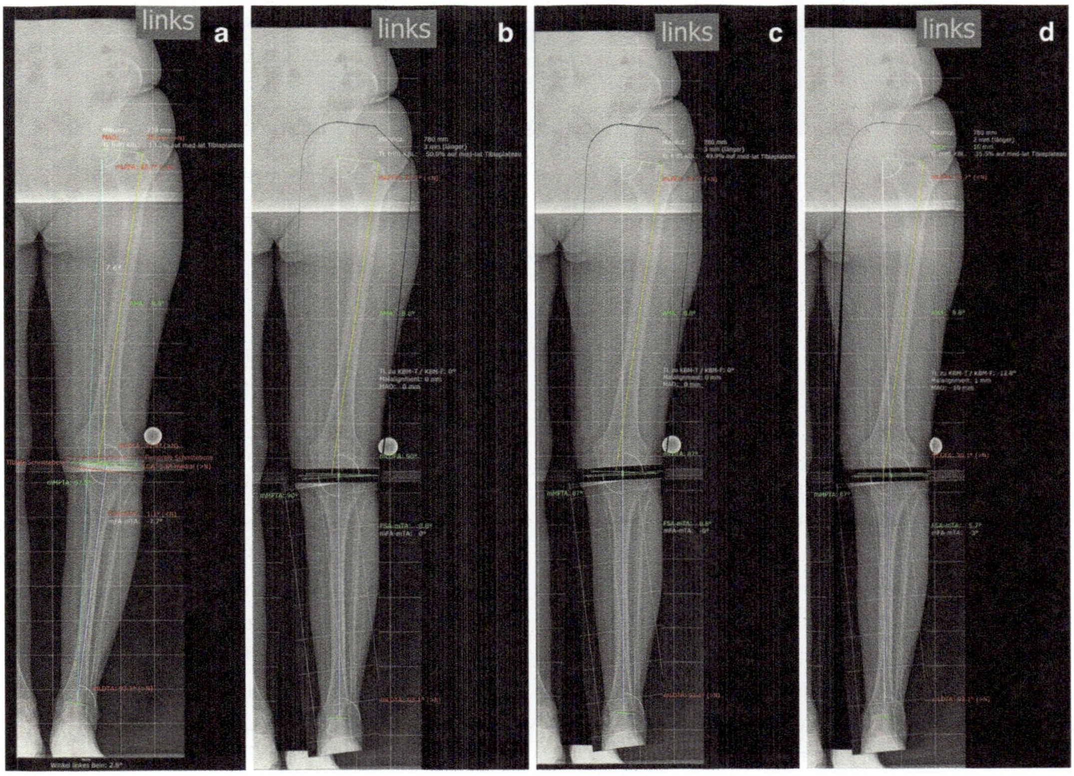

Fig. 10.1 Varus arthritis of a left knee with 8° of varus (LDFA 91.4°, MPTA 87.5°, JLCA 3.8°). (**a**) The preoperative alignment measurements and the intramedullary valgus correction angle using Orthoview Software. (**b**) The correction following mechanical alignment with a neutral HKA angle, (**c**) anatomical alignment again with a neutral HKA and (**d**) kinematic alignment with a persistent varus deformity of 3°

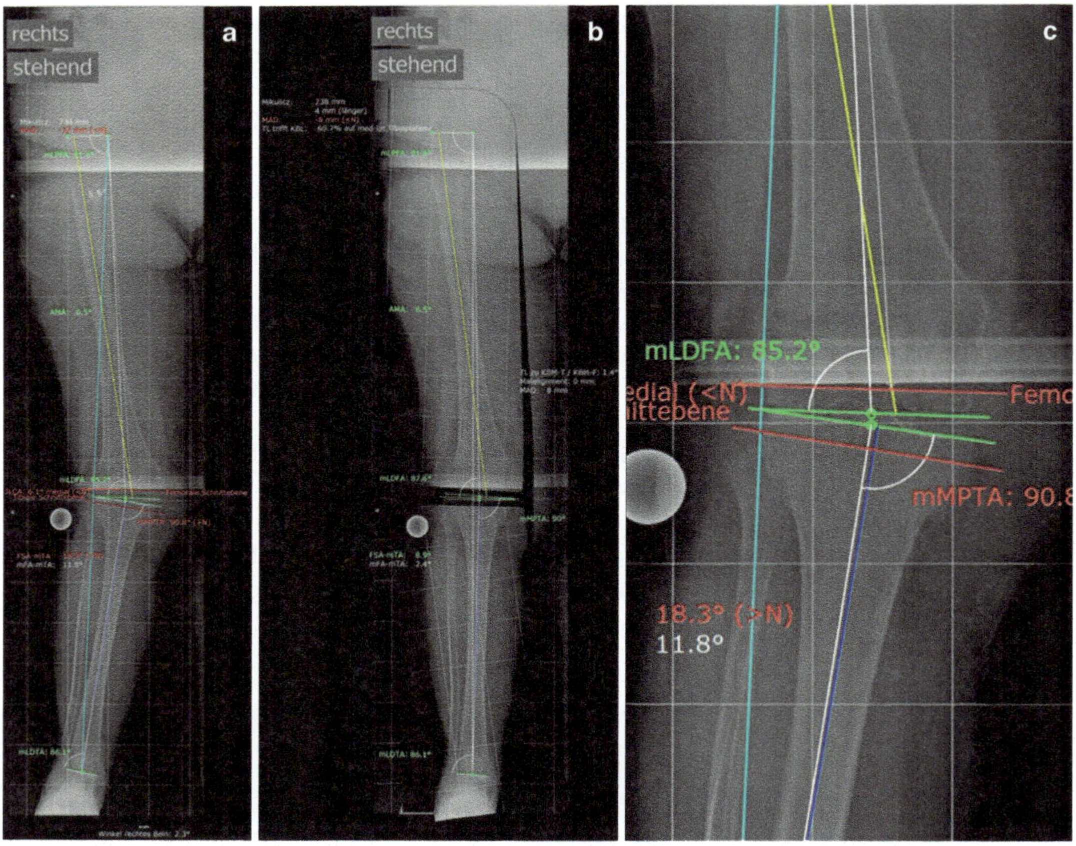

Fig. 10.2 Kinematic alignment in case of severe valgus knee arthritis. (**a**) The preoperative alignment measurements (LDFA 85.2°, MPTA 90.8°, JLCA 6.1° and a HKA angle of 11.8°). (**b**) A correction according to the concept of kinematic alignment is shown. (**c**) A close-up of the correction cuts

Finally, the AP view is used to detect medial and lateral osteophytes influencing soft tissue balancing, and component sizing can be performed in the frontal plane (see Fig. 10.6b).

10.4.2 Sagittal Plane

10.4.2.1 Slope

To measure the slope on a lateral radiograph, consideration of a lateral convex and a medial concave joint line is needed; however, for a medial parapatellar approach, the medial slope is more relevant intraoperatively. Thereafter, the slope between a line tangent to the medial or lateral joint line and the sagittal tibial anatomical line, obtained by connecting the furthest midpoint on the diaphysis visible on the X-ray and a midpoint 10 cm below the joint line, is measured (range 5–11°) [23–25] (see Fig. 10.7a). For the sagittal tibial anatomical axis, several anatomical landmarks are described: the anterior cortical line, the proximal anatomical axis, the central anatomical axis, the posterior cortical line and the fibular shaft axis [26]. The values of the slope change markedly according to the reference axis used but show significant correlations and thus may be used safely if differences with the mechanical axis of the tibia are considered [27].

10.4.2.2 Posterior Condylar Offset

The posterior condylar offset is evaluated on true lateral radiographs by measuring the maximal thickness of the posterior condyle, projected pos-

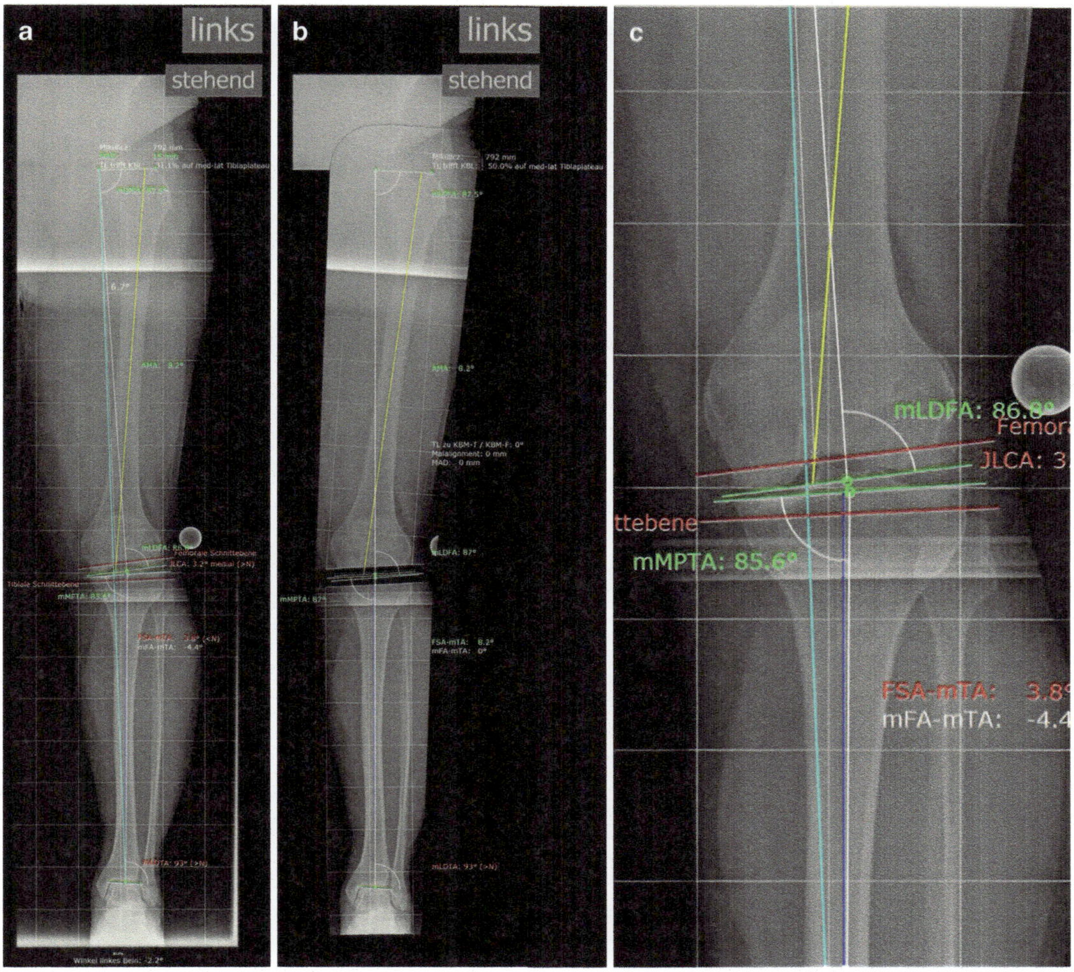

Fig. 10.3 Anatomical alignment in case of slight varus knee arthritis. (**a**) The preoperative alignment measurements (LDFA 85.6°, MPTA 86.8°, JLCA 3.2° and a HKA angle of 4.4°). (**b**) A correction according to the concept of anatomical alignment is shown. (**c**) A close-up of the correction cuts

teriorly to the tangent of the posterior cortex of the femoral shaft [28] (see Fig. 10.7b). The maximal obtainable flexion for PCL-retaining TKAs is determined by impingement of the posterior tibial insert against the femur, which is exaggerated by aberrant kinematics involving anterior sliding of the femur during flexion. For every millimetre lost by posterior condylar offset, the maximal final flexion is reduced by a mean of 6.1°. Therefore, a full restoration of the posterior condylar offset is recommended for PCL-retaining TKAs, since it allows a greater degree of flexion before impingement occurs [28].

10.4.2.3 Patellar Height

Several methods exist to measure patellar height. In the case of TKA, only methods referencing the tibia, such as the Insall-Salvati index [29], the Caton-Deschamps index (see Fig. 10.7c) [30] and the Blackburne-Peel index (see Fig. 10.7d) [31], are useful because they are reproducible after TKA as well. Whereas the Insall-Salvati ratio is good for the identification of a true patella baja or alta, it has inferior interobserver correlation and reproducibility, and its measurements after the operation are misleading if the position of the joint line has

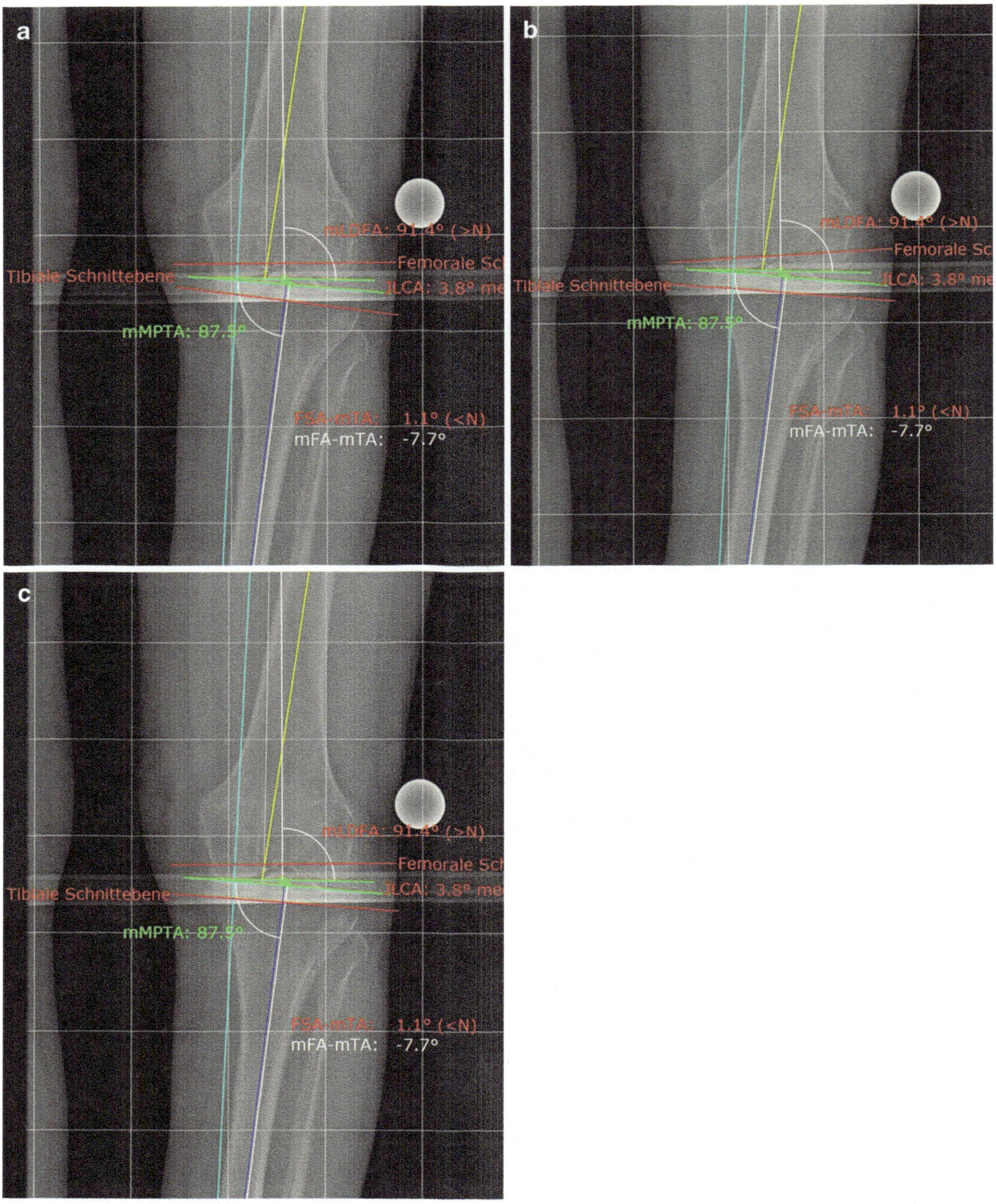

Fig. 10.4 A close-up of the correction cuts of the knee shown in Fig. 10.1. (**a**) The femoral and tibial cuts (red lines) following mechanical alignment, (**b**) the correction cuts following anatomical alignment and (**c**) the ones for kinematic alignment, which seems to be the best fitting option in this case

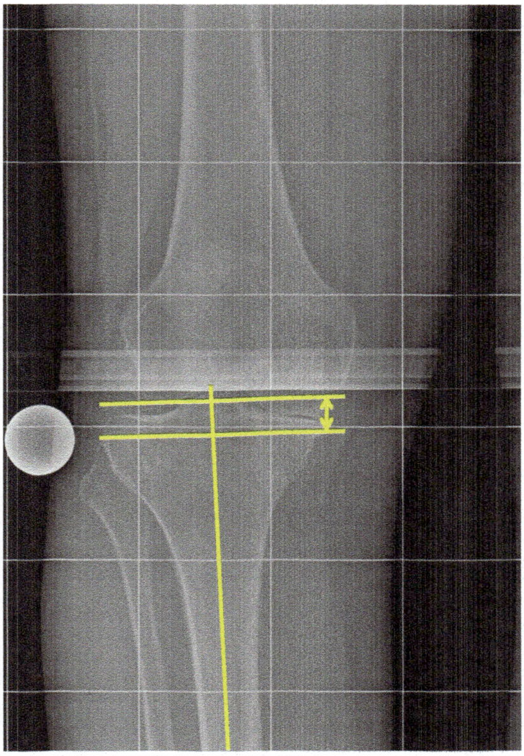

Fig. 10.5 The measuring method of the joint line height. The distance is measured between a line perpendicular to the mechanical axis of the tibia at the apex of the fibular head and a parallel line to the first line at the level of the distal aspect of the lateral femoral condyle

been altered. The Blackburne-Peel and Caton-Deschamps ratios evaluate patellar height relative to the joint surface and will identify a pseudo-patella baja. These methods have superior reliability and interobserver correlation after TKA [32].

Furthermore, anterior and posterior osteophytes, which might cause flexion contracture or limit full flexion, should be identified. As the size of the components is dictated most commonly by the anterior-posterior dimensions of the femur and the tibia, sizing is performed in the lateral view [5]. By templating the size of the components in the frontal and sagittal planes, a possible mismatch might be identified before surgery [33] (see Fig. 10.6a, b).

10.4.3 Axial Plane

10.4.3.1 Axial View of the Patella

Patellofemoral alignment measured according to the American Knee Society Total Knee Arthroplasty Roentgenographic Evaluation and Scoring System takes into account patellar thickness, width, tilt and medial-/lateral displacement [25]. Most important for preoperative planning in cases of patella replacement is the patellar thickness. The patellar thickness refers to the vertical distance from the anterior cortex of the patella to the depth of the femoral sulcus [25]. Multiple studies have confirmed the association between decreased patellar thickness and increased fracture risk [34]. Bone stock preservation is therefore critical. In thin patellae reconstitution of patellar thickness when resurfacing can be problematic. In these cases, an increase in patellar thickness can be accepted without major loss of flexion [34, 35].

10.4.3.2 Rotational Alignment

The angle between the clinical epicondylar axis—a line connecting the medial and lateral femoral prominences—and the posterior condylar axis—a line connecting the posterior margins of the medial and lateral femoral condyles—is measured [10] and kept for intraoperative adjustment of rotation (see Fig. 10.8).

Rotational alignment of the femoral component during TKA has an influence on patellofemoral kinematics [36] and on the balance of the flexion gap, which can affect the femorotibial kinematics [37, 38]. There is no consensus regarding the best method to achieve consistent intraoperative femoral component rotation.

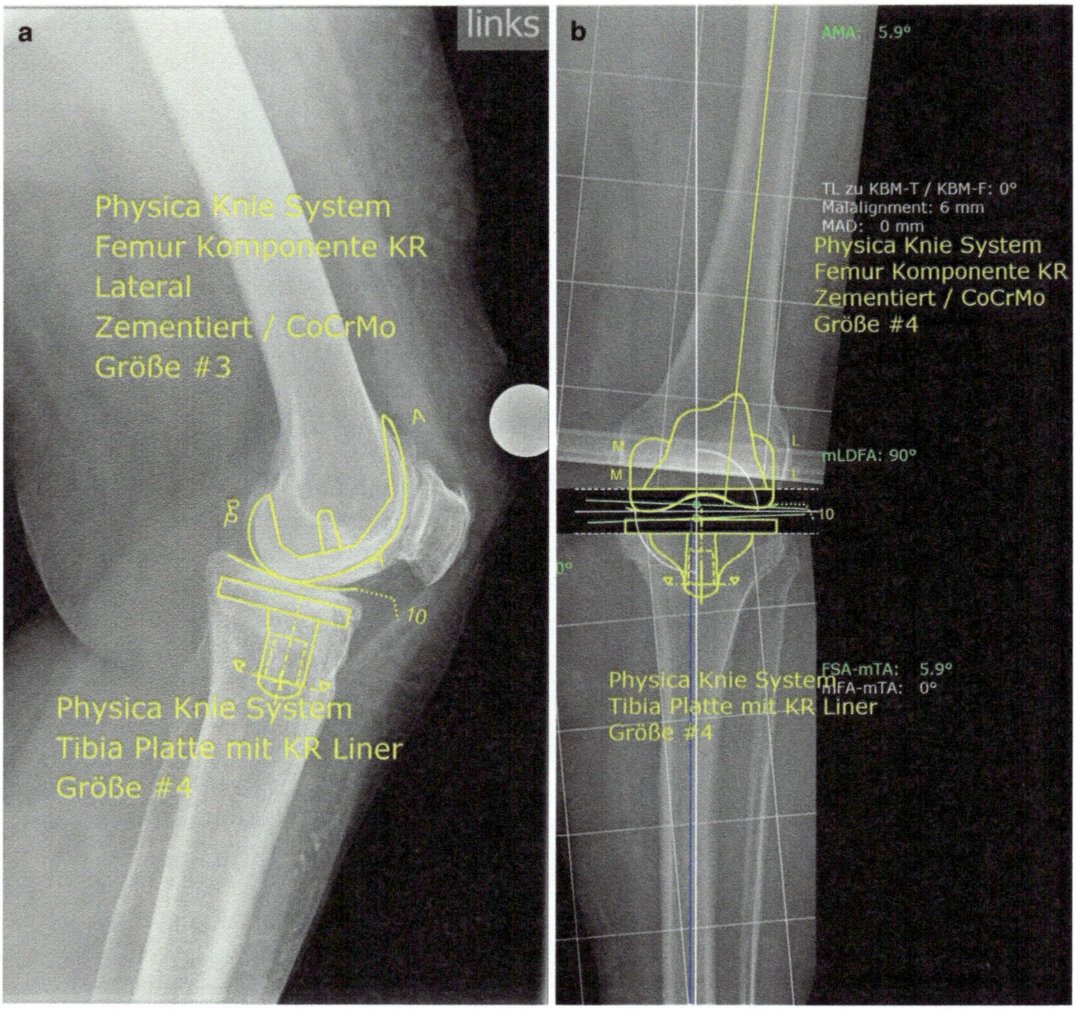

Fig. 10.6 Size templating. It shows the discrepancy of component sizing in the lateral (**a**) and AP view (**b**). However, as the size is most commonly dictated by the anterior-posterior dimensions of femur and tibia, the lateral size estimation is more reliable

Traditionally, two techniques have been used: the gap-balancing technique, in which the femoral component is positioned parallel to the resected proximal tibia with each collateral ligament under equal tension, and the measured resection technique, in which bony landmarks are used as references to set femoral rotation regardless of the ligament tension [39, 40]. At least five distal femoral rotational reference axes are described: the transcondylar axis [41], the posterior condylar axis (PCA) [42, 43], the anatomic and surgical transepicondylar axes (TEAs) [44, 45] and Whiteside's anterior-posterior axis [46]. The surgical TEA is a line connecting the medial epicondylar sulcus with the most prominent point on the lateral epicondyle. It is considered to be the most accurate bony landmark for approximating the flexion axis of the knee [44, 47]. However, whether the TEA is reproducible and accurately identified intraoperatively has been debated in the literature with contradictory reports [44, 47–50]. The PCA, formed by a tangent to the posterior aspect of both femoral condyles, has been used as a surrogate for the TEA. In the case of normal condylar anatomy, the PCA is 3–4° internally rotated in relation to the TEA. Nonetheless,

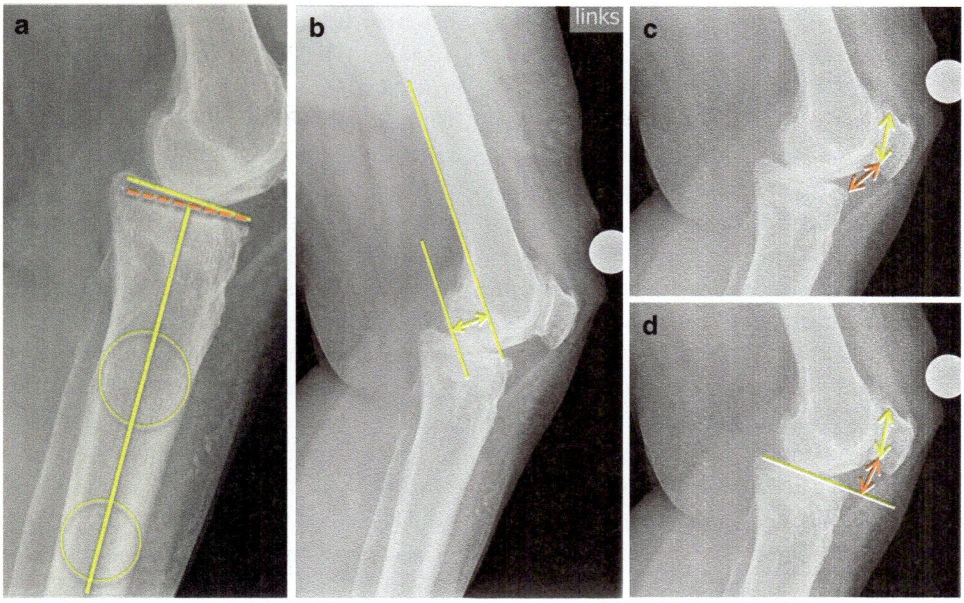

Fig. 10.7 Sagittal plane radiographic evaluations. (**a**) Posterior slope angle is formed by a line perpendicular to the lateral longitudinal axis of the tibia and a line parallel to the medial tibial plateau joint line. Its value is positive when it is under the line and it is negative when it is above. In this case, it is a negative slope of 5°. (**b**) Posterior condylar offset: thickness of the posterior condyle projected posteriorly to the tangent of the posterior cortex of the femoral shaft. (**c**, **d**) Patella height. (**c**) Caton-Deschamps index: The ratio between the distance of the lower edge of the patellar joint surface to the upper edge of the tibial plateau (orange) and the length of the patellar articular surface (yellow). (**d**) Blackburne-Peel index: The ratio between the perpendicular distance from the lower articular margin of the patella and the joint line level (orange) and the length of the articular surface of the patella (yellow)

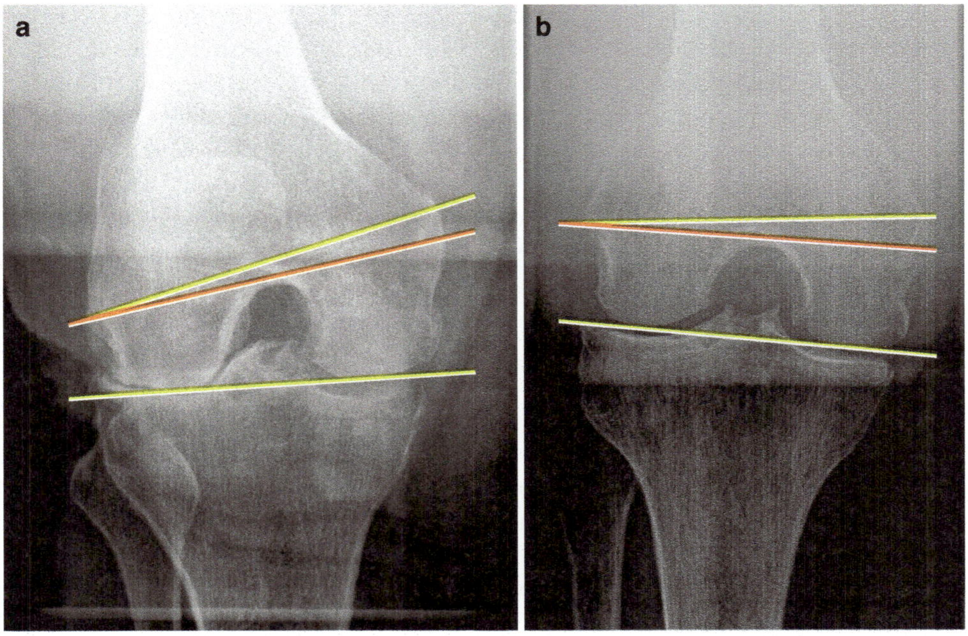

Fig. 10.8 Rotational alignment. The angle between the clinical epicondylar axis—a line connecting the medial and lateral femoral prominences—and the posterior condylar axis—a line connecting the posterior margins of the medial and lateral femoral condyles—is measured (two yellow lines). The TEA is 4° internally rotated relative to the CEA (orange line). (**a**) Valgus knee arthritis with 7° of TEA-PCA angle and (**b**) varus knee arthritis with 2° of TEA-PCA angle

several studies have shown variations regarding the relationship of the PCA to the TEA, potentially leading to component malrotation [47, 51–53]. The anatomic or clinical epicondylar axis (CEA), a line that connects the medial and lateral epicondylar prominences, and the PCA are easily identified in the rotational radiograph [10]. The TEA is 4° internally rotated relative to the CEA, and the angle is constant because the sulcus is the attachment of the medial collateral ligament and should have a fairly constant ratio to the mediolateral length of the femur [53] (orange line, Fig. 10.8). The PCA-CEA angles in the rotational radiograph are comparable to those measured by CT and help interpret the PCA as an intraoperative reference for rotational alignment. Furthermore, the preoperative flexion gap imbalance can be estimated, and soft tissue balancing can be adjusted accordingly [10].

Ng et al. stated that the PCA-TEA strongly correlates with proximal tibial joint line obliquity, indicating a relationship between distal femoral rotational geometry and proximal tibial inclination. These findings could imply that the natural knee in flexion attempts to balance the collateral ligaments towards a rectangular flexion space. A higher tibial varus inclination is matched with a more internally rotated distal femur relative to the TEA [52]. As bony defects due to arthritis mainly occur in the main load carrying areas and not in deep flexion, this could be a hint to estimating the alignment prior to arthritis.

Although not all of these measurements can be verified intraoperatively, they should at least be used for postoperative self-assessment and improving accuracy.

10.5 Alignment Concepts

According to the measurements, one must decide which alignment approach to follow. Historically, the alignment philosophy for TKA was driven by the desire to maximize durability and relieve pain with less regard to restoring normal knee kinematics and function. Michael Freeman introduced the concept of right-angled femoral and tibial bone cuts (mechanical alignment, see Figs. 10.1b and 10.4a) and the idea of parallel and equal flexion and extension spaces [54]. Jeffery et al. popularized the restoration of the mechanical axis to 0° ± 3°, relative to Maquet's line, with the use of long-leg radiographs [55]. This choice of alignment is based on the long-held tenet that postoperative alignment of the lower limb should be within 3° of a neutral mechanical axis [56]. The aim of the mechanical alignment technique for TKA is not to restore the constitutional patient-specific alignment but rather to systematically create a "biomechanically friendly prosthetic knee" [57]. The concept of restoring knee joint line obliquity to a few degrees of varus in total knee arthroplasty using the "anatomic" method was first proposed by Hungerford et al. [42]. Anatomic alignment still aims for a neutral HKA, but the bones are cut 3° oblique to their mechanical axes [54] (see Figs. 10.1c, 10.4b, and 10.3). The rationale supporting this technique is that it promotes a better load distribution on the tibial component and better patella biomechanics as it reduces the risk of lateral retinacular ligament stretching when the knee flexes [57]. In contrast to the classically aligned TKA, the surgical goal of kinematic TKA is not attainment of neutral limb alignment. Instead, the emphasis is placed on the soft tissue and the restoration of alignment to the pre-arthritic state [52] (see Figs. 10.1d, 10.4c, and 10.2). The kinematic alignment technique was first introduced by Stephen Howell in 2006 and is a pure bone procedure with predictable "expected thickness of bone cuts" and intraoperative ability to perform quality assurance checks (calliper measurements) and correct low-quality cuts [57]. The knee kinematics of patients with kinematically aligned TKAs were found to resemble more closely those of normal healthy controls [58], and gait analysis showed a lower knee adduction moment [59]. However, their functional outcome is not necessarily superior to that of mechanically aligned TKAs [60]. Accurate restoration of the distal femoral, posterior femoral and tibial joint lines within ±1 mm is necessary to avoid an increase in tibial compartment forces beyond those of the natural knee, which result in stiffness and limited range of motion [54, 61–63].

As great variability in the lower limb alignment of non-osteoarthritic knees was shown [64–66], an individualized approach is perhaps the best option.

References

1. Insall J, Scott WN, Ranawat CS. The total condylar knee prosthesis. A report of two hundred and twenty cases. J Bone Joint Surg Am. 1979;61(2):173–80.
2. Rienmuller A, Guggi T, Gruber G, Preiss S, Drobny T. The effect of femoral component rotation on the five-year outcome of cemented mobile bearing total knee arthroplasty. Int Orthop. 2012;36(10):2067–72. https://doi.org/10.1007/s00264-012-1628-0.
3. Kniesel B, Konstantinidis L, Hirschmuller A, Sudkamp N, Helwig P. Digital templating in total knee and hip replacement: an analysis of planning accuracy. Int Orthop. 2014;38(4):733–9. https://doi.org/10.1007/s00264-013-2157-1.
4. Peek AC, Bloch B, Auld J. How useful is templating for total knee replacement component sizing? Knee. 2012;19(4):266–9. https://doi.org/10.1016/j.knee.2011.03.010.
5. Tanzer M, Makhdom AM. Preoperative planning in primary total knee arthroplasty. J Am Acad Orthop Surg. 2016;24(4):220–30. https://doi.org/10.5435/JAAOS-D-14-00332.
6. Kotze MJ. Prosthetic joint infection, dental treatment and antibiotic prophylaxis. Orthop Rev (Pavia). 2009;1(1):e7. https://doi.org/10.4081/or.2009.e7.
7. Macaulay W, Geller JA, Brown AR, Cote LJ, Kiernan HA. Total knee arthroplasty and parkinson disease: enhancing outcomes and avoiding complications. J Am Acad Orthop Surg. 2010;18(11):687–94.
8. Mullaji A, Shetty GM. Persistent hindfoot valgus causes lateral deviation of weightbearing axis after total knee arthroplasty. Clin Orthop Relat Res. 2011;469(4):1154–60. https://doi.org/10.1007/s11999-010-1703-z.
9. Gandhi R, de Beer J, Leone J, Petruccelli D, Winemaker M, Adili A. Predictive risk factors for stiff knees in total knee arthroplasty. J Arthroplast. 2006;21(1):46–52. https://doi.org/10.1016/j.arth.2005.06.004.
10. Kanekasu K, Kondo M, Kadoya Y. Axial radiography of the distal femur to assess rotational alignment in total knee arthroplasty. Clin Orthop Relat Res. 2005;434:193–7.
11. Peterfy C, Li J, Zaim S, Duryea J, Lynch J, Miaux Y, Yu W, Genant HK. Comparison of fixed-flexion positioning with fluoroscopic semi-flexed positioning for quantifying radiographic joint-space width in the knee: test-retest reproducibility. Skelet Radiol. 2003;32(3):128–32. https://doi.org/10.1007/s00256-002-0603-z.
12. Kan H, Arai Y, Kobayashi M, Nakagawa S, Inoue H, Hino M, Komaki S, Ikoma K, Ueshima K, Fujiwara H, Yokota I, Kubo T. Fixed-flexion view X-ray of the knee superior in detection and follow-up of knee osteoarthritis. Medicine (Baltimore). 2017;96(49):e9126. https://doi.org/10.1097/MD.0000000000009126.
13. Pinsornsak P, Naratrikun K, Kanitnate S, Sangkomkamhang T. The one-leg standing radiograph: an improved technique to evaluate the severity of knee osteoarthritis. Bone Joint Res. 2016;5(9):436–41. https://doi.org/10.1302/2046-3758.59.BJR-2016-0049.R1.
14. Kan H, Arai Y, Kobayashi M, Nakagawa S, Inoue H, Hino M, Komaki S, Ikoma K, Ueshima K, Fujiwara H, Kubo T. Radiographic measurement of joint space width using the fixed flexion view in 1,102 knees of Japanese patients with osteoarthritis in comparison with the standing extended view. Knee Surg Relat Res. 2017;29(1):63–8. https://doi.org/10.5792/ksrr.16.046.
15. Merchant AC. Patellofemoral imaging. Clin Orthop Relat Res. 2001;389:15–21. https://doi.org/10.1097/00003086-200108000-00004.
16. Paley D. Principles of deformity correction. Berlin: Springer; 2003.
17. Cobey JC, Sella E. Standardizing methods of measurement of foot shape by including the effects of subtalar rotation. Foot Ankle. 1981;2(1):30–6.
18. Maquet P. Biomechanics of gonarthrosis. Acta Orthop Belg. 1972;38(Suppl 1):33–54.
19. Paley D. What is alignment and malalignment? In: Thienpont E, editor. Improving accuracy in knee arthroplasty, vol. 1. New Delhi: Jaypee Brothers Medical Publishers (P) Ltd; 2012.
20. Pietsch M, Hofmann S. Value of radiographic examination of the knee joint for the orthopedic surgeon. Radiologe. 2006;46(1):55–64. https://doi.org/10.1007/s00117-005-1292-0.
21. Yoshimoto K, Noguchi M, Yamada A, Nasu Y. Compensatory function of the subtalar joint for lower extremity malalignment. Adv Orthop. 2019;2019:7656878. https://doi.org/10.1155/2019/7656878.
22. Song SJ, Bae DK, Kim KI, Jeong HY. Changes in femoral posterior condylar offset, tibial posterior slope angle, and joint line height after cruciate-retaining total knee arthroplasty. Knee Surg Relat Res. 2016;28(1):27–33. https://doi.org/10.5792/ksrr.2016.28.1.27.
23. Maestro A, Harwin SF, Sandoval MG, Vaquero DH, Murcia A. Influence of intramedullary versus extramedullary alignment guides on final total knee arthroplasty component position: a radiographic analysis. J Arthroplast. 1998;13(5):552–8.
24. Denis K, Van Ham G, Bellemans J, Labey L, Sloten JV, Van Audekercke R, Van der Perre G, De Schutter J. How correctly does an intramedullary rod represent the longitudinal tibial axes? Clin

Orthop Relat Res. 2002;397:424–33. https://doi.org/10.1097/00003086-200204000-00050.
25. Baldini A, Traverso F. Alignment? How do we measure it? In: Thienpont E, editor. Improving accuracy in knee arthroplasty, vol. 1. New Delhi: Jaypee Brothers Medical Publishers (P) Ltd; 2012.
26. Yoo JH, Chang CB, Shin KS, Seong SC, Kim TK. Anatomical references to assess the posterior tibial slope in total knee arthroplasty: a comparison of 5 anatomical axes. J Arthroplast. 2008;23(4):586–92. https://doi.org/10.1016/j.arth.2007.05.006.
27. Han HS, Chang CB, Seong SC, Lee S, Lee MC. Evaluation of anatomic references for tibial sagittal alignment in total knee arthroplasty. Knee Surg Sports Traumatol Arthrosc. 2008;16(4):373–7. https://doi.org/10.1007/s00167-008-0486-1.
28. Bellemans J, Banks S, Victor J, Vandenneucker H, Moemans A. Fluoroscopic analysis of the kinematics of deep flexion in total knee arthroplasty. Influence of posterior condylar offset. J Bone Joint Surg Br. 2002;84(1):50–3.
29. Insall J, Salvati E. Patella position in the normal knee joint. Radiology. 1971;101(1):101–4. https://doi.org/10.1148/101.1.101.
30. Caton J, Deschamps G, Chambat P, Lerat JL, Dejour H. Patella infera. Apropos of 128 cases. Revue de chirurgie orthopedique et reparatrice de l'appareil moteur. 1982;68(5):317–25.
31. Blackburne JS, Peel TE. A new method of measuring patellar height. J Bone Joint Surg Br. 1977;59(2):241–2.
32. Rogers BA, Thornton-Bott P, Cannon SR, Briggs TW. Interobserver variation in the measurement of patellar height after total knee arthroplasty. J Bone Joint Surg Br. 2006;88(4):484–8. https://doi.org/10.1302/0301-620X.88B4.16407.
33. Hofmann S, Djahani O, Pietsch M. Frontal and sagittal alignment in knee arthroplasty. In: Thienpont E, editor. Improving accuracy in knee arthroplasty, vol. 1. New Delhi: Jaypee Brothers Medical Publishers (P) Ltd; 2012.
34. Pierce TP, Jauregui JJ, Cherian JJ, Elmallah RK, Harwin SF, Mont MA. Is there an ideal patellar thickness following total knee arthroplasty? Orthopedics. 2016;39(1):e187–92. https://doi.org/10.3928/01477447-20151222-03.
35. Bengs BC, Scott RD. The effect of patellar thickness on intraoperative knee flexion and patellar tracking in total knee arthroplasty. J Arthroplast. 2006;21(5):650–5. https://doi.org/10.1016/j.arth.2005.07.020.
36. Akagi M, Matsusue Y, Mata T, Asada Y, Horiguchi M, Iida H, Nakamura T. Effect of rotational alignment on patellar tracking in total knee arthroplasty. Clin Orthop Relat Res. 1999;366:155–63. https://doi.org/10.1097/00003086-199909000-00019.
37. Puloski SK, McCalden RW, MacDonald SJ, Rorabeck CH, Bourne RB. Tibial post wear in posterior stabilized total knee arthroplasty. An unrecognized source of polyethylene debris. J Bone Joint Surg Am. 2001;83(3):390–7. https://doi.org/10.2106/00004623-200103000-00011.
38. Berger RA, Crossett LS, Jacobs JJ, Rubash HE. Malrotation causing patellofemoral complications after total knee arthroplasty. Clin Orthop Relat Res. 1998;356:144–53. https://doi.org/10.1097/00003086-199811000-00021.
39. Heesterbeek PJ, Jacobs WC, Wymenga AB. Effects of the balanced gap technique on femoral component rotation in TKA. Clin Orthop Relat Res. 2009;467(4):1015–22. https://doi.org/10.1007/s11999-008-0539-2.
40. Dennis DA, Komistek RD, Kim RH, Sharma A. Gap balancing versus measured resection technique for total knee arthroplasty. Clin Orthop Relat Res. 2010;468(1):102–7. https://doi.org/10.1007/s11999-009-1112-3.
41. Iranpour F, Merican AM, Dandachli W, Amis AA, Cobb JP. The geometry of the trochlear groove. Clin Orthop Relat Res. 2010;468(3):782–8. https://doi.org/10.1007/s11999-009-1156-4.
42. Hungerford DS, Kenna RV, Krackow KA. The porous-coated anatomic total knee. Orthop Clin North Am. 1982;13(1):103–22.
43. Laskin RS. Flexion space configuration in total knee arthroplasty. J Arthroplast. 1995;10(5):657–60.
44. Berger RA, Rubash HE, Seel MJ, Thompson WH, Crossett LS. Determining the rotational alignment of the femoral component in total knee arthroplasty using the epicondylar axis. Clin Orthop Relat Res. 1993;286:40–7.
45. Griffin FM, Insall JN, Scuderi GR. The posterior condylar angle in osteoarthritic knees. J Arthroplast. 1998;13(7):812–5.
46. Whiteside LA, Arima J. The anteroposterior axis for femoral rotational alignment in valgus total knee arthroplasty. Clin Orthop Relat Res. 1995;321:168–72.
47. Olcott CW, Scott RD. A comparison of 4 intraoperative methods to determine femoral component rotation during total knee arthroplasty. J Arthroplast. 2000;15(1):22–6.
48. Jenny JY, Boeri C. Low reproducibility of the intra-operative measurement of the transepicondylar axis during total knee replacement. Acta Orthop Scand. 2004;75(1):74–7. https://doi.org/10.1080/00016470410001708150.
49. Kinzel V, Ledger M, Shakespeare D. Can the epicondylar axis be defined accurately in total knee arthroplasty? Knee. 2005;12(4):293–6. https://doi.org/10.1016/j.knee.2004.09.003.
50. Franceschini V, Nodzo SR, Gonzalez Della Valle A. Femoral component rotation in total knee arthroplasty: a comparison between transepicondylar axis and posterior condylar line referencing. J Arthroplast. 2016;31(12):2917–21. https://doi.org/10.1016/j.arth.2016.05.032.
51. Patel AR, Talati RK, Yaffe MA, McCoy BW, Stulberg SD. Femoral component rotation in total knee arthroplasty: an MRI-based evaluation of our options.

J Arthroplast. 2014;29(8):1666–70. https://doi.org/10.1016/j.arth.2014.02.033.

52. Ng CK, Chen JY, Yeh JZY, Ho JPY, Merican AM, Yeo SJ. Distal femoral rotation correlates with proximal tibial joint line obliquity: a consideration for kinematic total knee arthroplasty. J Arthroplast. 2018;33(6):1936–44. https://doi.org/10.1016/j.arth.2017.12.025.
53. Matsui Y, Kadoya Y, Uehara K, Kobayashi A, Takaoka K. Rotational deformity in varus osteoarthritis of the knee: analysis with computed tomography. Clin Orthop Relat Res. 2005;433:147–51. https://doi.org/10.1097/01.blo.0000150465.29883.83.
54. Hirschmann MT, Becker R, Tandogan R, Vendittoli PA, Howell S. Alignment in TKA: what has been clear is not anymore! Knee Surg Sports Traumatol Arthrosc. 2019;27(7):2037–9. https://doi.org/10.1007/s00167-019-05558-4.
55. Jeffery RS, Morris RW, Denham RA. Coronal alignment after total knee replacement. J Bone Joint Surg Br. 1991;73(5):709–14.
56. Abdel MP, Oussedik S, Parratte S, Lustig S, Haddad FS. Coronal alignment in total knee replacement: historical review, contemporary analysis, and future direction. Bone Joint J. 2014;96-B(7):857–62. https://doi.org/10.1302/0301-620X.96B7.33946.
57. Riviere C, Iranpour F, Auvinet E, Howell S, Vendittoli PA, Cobb J, Parratte S. Alignment options for total knee arthroplasty: a systematic review. Orthop Traumatol Surg Res. 2017;103(7):1047–56. https://doi.org/10.1016/j.otsr.2017.07.010.
58. Blakeney W, Clement J, Desmeules F, Hagemeister N, Riviere C, Vendittoli PA. Kinematic alignment in total knee arthroplasty better reproduces normal gait than mechanical alignment. Knee Surg Sports Traumatol Arthrosc. 2019;27(5):1410–7. https://doi.org/10.1007/s00167-018-5174-1.
59. Niki Y, Nagura T, Nagai K, Kobayashi S, Harato K. Kinematically aligned total knee arthroplasty reduces knee adduction moment more than mechanically aligned total knee arthroplasty. Knee Surg Sports Traumatol Arthrosc. 2018;26(6):1629–35. https://doi.org/10.1007/s00167-017-4788-z.
60. Luo Z, Zhou K, Peng L, Shang Q, Pei F, Zhou Z. Similar results with kinematic and mechanical alignment applied in total knee arthroplasty. Knee Surg Sports Traumatol Arthrosc. 2019. https://doi.org/10.1007/s00167-019-05584-2.
61. Riley J, Roth JD, Howell SM, Hull ML. Increases in tibial force imbalance but not changes in tibiofemoral laxities are caused by varus-valgus malalignment of the femoral component in kinematically aligned TKA. Knee Surg Sports Traumatol Arthrosc. 2018;26(11):3238–48. https://doi.org/10.1007/s00167-018-4841-6.
62. Riley J, Roth JD, Howell SM, Hull ML. Internal-external malalignment of the femoral component in kinematically aligned total knee arthroplasty increases tibial force imbalance but does not change laxities of the tibiofemoral joint. Knee Surg Sports Traumatol Arthrosc. 2018;26(6):1618–28. https://doi.org/10.1007/s00167-017-4776-3.
63. Shelton TJ, Howell SM, Hull ML. A total knee arthroplasty is stiffer when the intraoperative tibial force is greater than the native knee. J Knee Surg. 2019;32(10):1008–14. https://doi.org/10.1055/s-0038-1675421.
64. Hirschmann MT, Hess S, Behrend H, Amsler F, Leclercq V, Moser LB. Phenotyping of hip-knee-ankle angle in young non-osteoarthritic knees provides better understanding of native alignment variability. Knee Surg Sports Traumatol Arthrosc. 2019;27(5):1378–84. https://doi.org/10.1007/s00167-019-05507-1.
65. Moser LB, Hess S, Amsler F, Behrend H, Hirschmann MT. Native non-osteoarthritic knees have a highly variable coronal alignment: a systematic review. Knee Surg Sports Traumatol Arthrosc. 2019;27(5):1359–67. https://doi.org/10.1007/s00167-019-05417-2.
66. Hirschmann MT, Moser LB, Amsler F, Behrend H, Leclercq V, Hess S. Phenotyping the knee in young non-osteoarthritic knees shows a wide distribution of femoral and tibial coronal alignment. Knee Surg Sports Traumatol Arthrosc. 2019;27(5):1385–93. https://doi.org/10.1007/s00167-019-05508-0.

Minimally Invasive Osteotomies Around the Knee

11

Kristian Kley

11.1 Introduction/Historical Background

Osteoarthritis is a very common cause of knee pain. It affects high percentages of patients above 60 years of age [1] but is also seen in younger patients as a result of different etiologies including rheumatoid arthritis, a genetic predisposition, poor cartilage quality, or obesity.

In addition, mechanical malalignment is widely accepted as a major source of osteoarthritis. Numerous studies have shown that at least 30% of the male population and almost 20% of the female population have a lower limb malalignment of more than 3° [1–3]. Regardless of the underlying cause of this malalignment, it then secondarily leads to high pressure loads and peak load areas resulting in mechanical abrasion. The patient then enters a vicious circle of progressive cartilage loss and worsening malalignment [4–7].

It is widely accepted that the best way realigning and treating malalignment is with an osteotomy performed around the knee. Depending on the malalignment in the coronal plane, varus or valgus corrections can be achieved by open or closed wedge osteotomies which can be carried out laterally or medially at femur or tibia.

Regardless of the type of osteotomy, the aim is to correct the malalignment by changing the weight-bearing line and shift the peak load areas [8]. Recently more attention was paid to the orientation of the joint line in relation to Mikulicz line to restore the kinematic alignment profile [1, 9, 10]. To avoid creating a new deformity and malalignment of the joint line orientation, proper analysis is mandatory [11–13]. Having carried out the deformity analysis, it is not uncommon to find that there is a degree of deformity in both the distal femur and proximal tibia. And it is the experience of our unit and other centers [10] that the best results can be achieved by making the corrective realignment procedure at the level of the osteotomy. That in many cases is in both, the distal femur and proximal tibia with a double osteotomy. Though newer techniques of high tibial osteotomies (HTO) led to superior results, HTO and distal femoral osteotomy (DFO) are still considered to be difficult procedures with high potential risk in terms of complications [14, 15]. In the case of HTO, the number of recent outcome papers is low and mostly based on historical techniques with relatively poor long-term outcome [16, 17]. Again in DFO surgery, the procedure is considered technically challenging with higher complication rates, although meta-analysis could not find evidence [18].

It is now widely accepted that there is at least a 20% dissatisfaction rate with total knee replacement (TKR) surgery. There are also limitations of

K. Kley (✉)
Orthoprofis Hannover, Luisenstrasse 10/11, Hannover 30159, Germany

M. T. Hirschmann et al. (eds.), *ESSKA Instructional Course Lecture Book*,
https://doi.org/10.1007/978-3-662-61264-4_11

what can be achieved with a TKR, and we always need to have a plan "B" in the event of failure and think about the next procedure in an ever-aging population with high demands. Adversely, that does not affect the rising figures of these procedures [19]. The dilemma is that osteotomy shows excellent results [15, 20, 21]; however, the number of osteotomies carried out is decreasing. This could be explained by the feeling that these procedures are considered to be difficult and high risk. Furthermore, the shift to joint replacement surgeries over the last decades has been encouraged by the industry, and at the same time, we have seen a relatively few centers of excellence and training initiatives in osteotomy surgery.

Taking that into consideration, there has been a need to adopt the recent major advantages of osteotomies around the knee and simplify the procedures to make them more reproducible and less traumatic.

11.2 State-of-the-Art Treatment/ Biomechanical Problems: HTO and DFO

One of the problems in a review of the literature of osteotomy surgery is the vast number of heterogeneous treatments and techniques that have been reported. As a result, there is a strong need to define a surgical standard that needs to be reproducible in terms of indication, planning, execution and teaching. At the moment, the only standardized teaching and techniques to meet these criteria for osteotomy is that recommended by the Joint Preservation Expert Group of AO (JPEG).

Correcting the tibia is achieved by medial open or closed wedge technique for valgus or varus deformity. The more reproducible and accurate approach for high tibial osteotomy surgery is to carry out a medial opening wedge procedure to the proximal tibia. Unlike the lateral closing wedge technique, where there is a risk of common peroneal nerve injury, there is a need to perform a fibula osteotomy and more soft tissue dissection to the lateral compartment, the medial approach involves minimal soft tissue dissection, significantly less risk of neurovascular damage, and the open wedge approach allows "fine tuning" of the osteotomy [22, 23].

For femoral malalignments, routinely closed wedge osteotomies, either medially or laterally, are performed to correct coronal plane deformities. The distal femur shows different biomechanics than the proximal tibia. The surface at the level of osteotomy is smaller on the femoral side. There is no natural "hinge-preserver" such as the fibers of the proximal tibio-fibular joint in the area of the safe zone [24, 25], and the lever arm of the DFO is longer. As a result, DFO is inherently more unstable. To help with this problem of potential instability, we recommend as a routine that a proximal biplane second cut is made to provide more stability and also to help with the healing process [26, 27] (Figs. 11.1 and 11.2).

The biplanar technique for DFO and HTO shows numerous advantages. Geometrically the volume of the osteotomy is reduced, the osteotomy

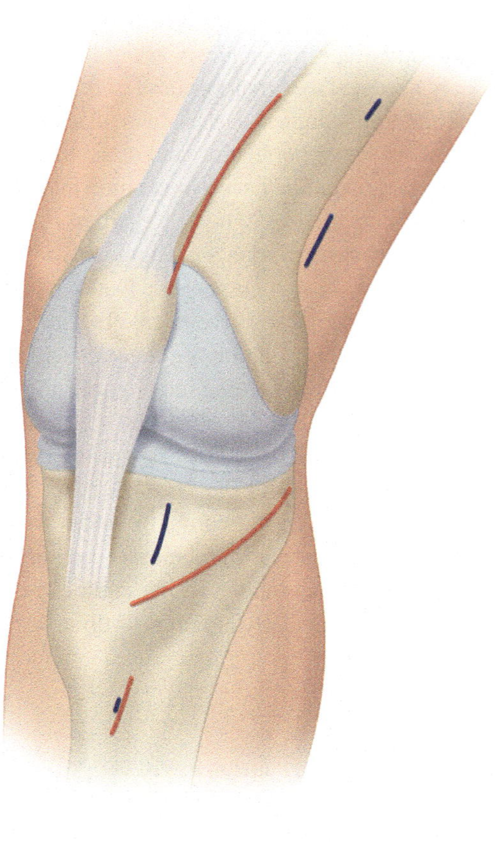

Fig. 11.1 Incisions for conventional (red) and MIS (blue) technique

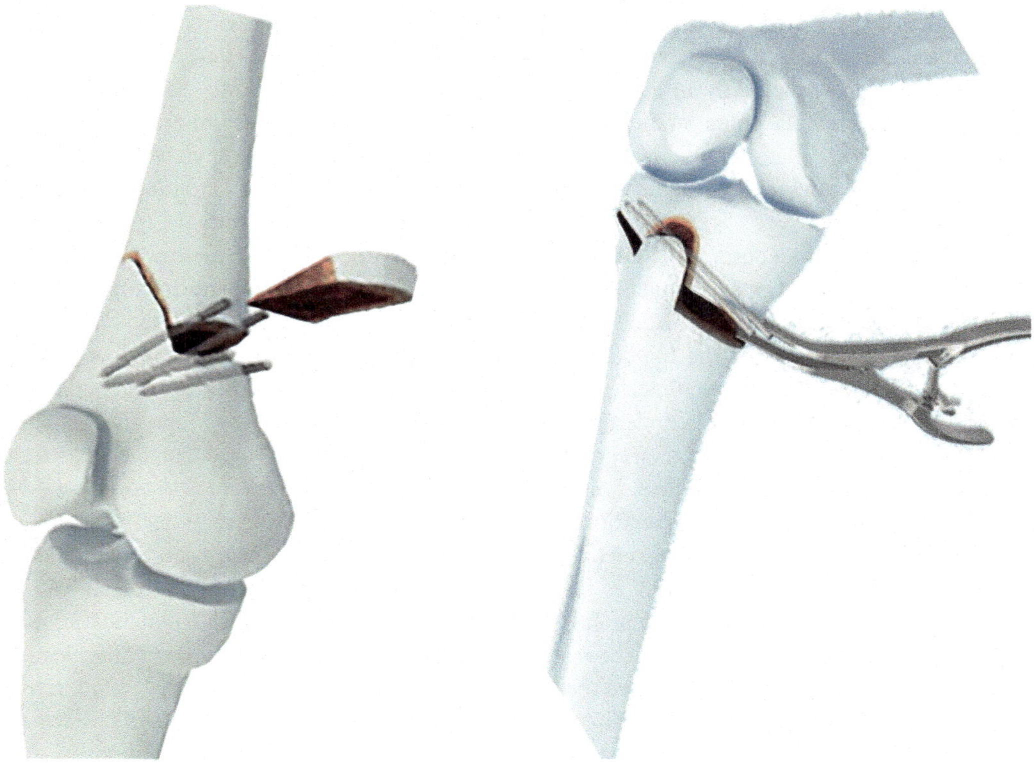

Fig. 11.2 Biplanar osteotomy at distal femur (DFO) and proximal tibia (HTO)

can be performed closer to the metaphysis with better bone-healing, and there is an inherent higher axial stability, protection against the potential issue of malrotation, and an option for reduction in case of a hinge-fracture [23, 26, 27].

These biplanar techniques along with angle stable plate fixators reproducibly showed excellent midterm results and patient satisfaction [15, 28, 29]. A further technical advancement has been the introduction of a minimally invasive (MIS) approach to both the proximal tibia and distal femur, which has been the standard in our department for the last 2 years.

11.3 MIS Technique/Future Options

The MIS biplanar technique that we have developed is less invasive but still allows the procedures to be carried out safely in experienced hands. The key is to make the incision in the optimal location to allow good visualization. This incision allows a window to be created, and like any MIS technique, this window is moved as is required. With increasing surgical experience in osteotomy surgery, it is possible to bring down the incisions to less than 4 cm for DFO and HTO. We do not advocate this technique for less experienced osteotomy surgeons at the start of their learning curve and would suggest a stepwise progression toward the MIS technique as the surgeon gains experience and confidence.

MIS in medial open wedge HTO is linked to the incision length. As there is no critical structure in the approach up to the MCL, MIS does not help to reduce the surgical trauma. But taking into consideration that osteotomy patients undergo revision surgery, the surgical pathways need to be planned thoughtfully. The skin-bridge between two proximal tibial incisions should at least be 5 cm [30]. An incision shorter than that can be considered non-critical. Substantial change with the MIS approach is the direction of the incision, which at the distal end is medial to the tibial tubercle and goes slightly obliquely to the level of joint line and no longer to the posteromedial corner. The two osteotomy cuts need to be performed sequentially in a window shift technique, so as the placement of the drill sleeves being used for the plate fixator in the proximal part. The shaft screws are placed through a single stab-incision.

For the DFO procedure, the MIS approach moved significantly from a long median incision to a medial or lateral 4 cm incision some 4 cm above the epicondyles. At the medial side, the fascia of vastus medialis is then incised and longitudinally split. Blunt dissection around the muscle is performed to the dorsal circumference. At the lateral aspect, the upper border of the iliotibial band needs to be identified and divided in a longitudinal way. Care is to be taken at the distal parts around the vastus lateralis as branches of the lateral ascending genicular artery penetrate the intermuscular septum. These either need to be ligated or coagulated. From there it is possible to lift the vastus medialis or lateralis to gain access to the medial or lateral intermuscular septum, which is then incised close to the femur. The key is to dissect the posterior aspect of the femur that has to be revealed, and this can be done minimally invasively without lifting the whole muscles at each side. By doing this, there is minimal compromise to the vascularity of the area. It has been shown with conventional plating vs. MIPO (minimal invasive plate osteosynthesis) causes and limitations for periosteal and bone marrow perfusion, leading to compromised osteotomy consolidation [31–33]. Performing the osteotomy and applying the plate like in HTO is achieved by window-shifting. The placement of the shaft screws is also done by stab incision. To establish a safe portal with limited damage to the muscle, a cannula is placed in the stab incision. Following these MIS principles in our hands, surgical trauma has been reduced. Following deformity analysis, we have found significant numbers of varus patients with femoral deformity and now correct up to 20% of our varus deformity with lateral closing wedge DFO surgery. In conclusion, femoral osteotomy procedures are currently not carried out in sufficient numbers. Where appropriate, osteotomy needs to be performed in the femur and not always carried out in the tibia for varus deformity. The same is true in valgus deformity, where a significant number of patients have deformity in the tibia as opposed to the femur, and it is here therefore where the osteotomy should be carried out, to prevent the surgery creating joint line obliquity and a new deformity. In recent times, attention has been payed to the orientation of the joint-line, along with the postoperative correction of the weight-bearing line [1, 10, 34]. From the dynamic perspective, the knee medializes during gait. That leads to a horizontal joint-line orientation, when the joint-line is medially inclined in stance. As a consequence, altering the MPTA to abnormal values to correct the weight-bearing line might lead to disturbed kinematics. Though at present there is no scientific evidence, our threshold for a postoperative MPTA is 93°. It is important to understand, that the femur decides on the joint-line orientation. If the desired correction cannot be achieved within reasonable values for mLDFA and/or MPTA, we tend to plan a DLO (double-level osteotomy).

11.4 Take Home Message

Biplanar osteotomy with angle-stable plate fixators produces excellent results when carried out for the right indications. As our understanding of malalignment, planning and execution of osteotomy surgery has evolved, the vast majority of the technical challenges of the past have been largely solved. Having said that this field will continue to develop and improve with time. These interesting new concepts of correction philosophies have led to controversial discussion over the last years and led to promising concepts such as the MIS technique and focus on joint-line orientation. The big challenge of the next decades will be to bring osteotomy back to a broader surgical society and establish these working concepts as standard treatment pathways.

References

1. Victor JMK, Bassens D, Bellemans J, Gürsu S, Dhollander AAM, Verdonk PCM. Constitutional varus does not affect joint line orientation in

the coronal plane knee. Clin Orthop Relat Res. 2014;472(1):98–104.
2. Bellemans J, Colyn W, Vandenneucker H, Victor J. The Chitranjan Ranawat award: is neutral mechanical alignment normal for all patients? The concept of constitutional varus. Clin Orthop Relat Res. 2012;470(1):45–53.
3. Cooke TD, Scudamore RA, Bryant JT, Sorbie C, Siu D, Fisher B. A quantitative approach to radiography of the lower limb. Principles and applications. J Bone Joint Surg Br. 1991;73(5):715–20.
4. Sharma L, Song J, Dunlop D, Felson D, Lewis CE, Segal N, et al. Varus and valgus alignment and incident and progressive knee osteoarthritis. Ann Rheum Dis. 2010;69(11):1940–5.
5. Jordan JM, Kington RS, Lane NE, Nevitt MC, Zhang Y, Sowers MF. Systemic risk factors for osteoarthritis. In Felson DT. Osteoarthritis: new insights. Part 1: The disease and its risk factors. Ann Intern Med. 2000; 133:637–9.
6. Felson DT, Naimark A, Anderson J, Kazis L, Castelli W, Meenan RF. The prevalence of knee osteoarthritis in the elderly. The framingham osteoarthritis study. Arthritis Rheum. 1987;30(8):914–8.
7. Brouwer RW, Jakma TSC, Bierma-Zeinstra SM A, Verhagen A P, Verhaar J, et al. Osteotomy for treating knee osteoarthritis. Cochrane database Syst Rev. 2005;(1):CD004019.
8. Agneskirchner JD, Hurschler C, Wrann CD, Lobenhoffer P. The effects of valgus medial opening wedge high tibial osteotomy on articular cartilage pressure of the knee: a biomechanical study. Arthroscopy. 2007;23(8):852–61.
9. Cooke T, Pichora D, Siu D, Scudamore R, Bryant J. Surgical implications of varus deformity of the knee with obliquity of joint surfaces. Bone Joint J. 1989;71–B(4):560–5.
10. Babis GC, An K-N, Chao EYS, Rand JA, Sim FH. Double level osteotomy of the knee: a method to retain joint-line obliquity. Clinical results. J Bone Joint Surg Am. 2002;84–A(8):1380–8.
11. Cooke TDV, Sled EA, Scudamore RA. Frontal plane knee alignment: a call for standardized measurement. J Rheumatol. 2007;34(9):1796–801.
12. Paley D. Malalignment and malorientation in the frontal plane. In: Principles of deformity correction. Berlin: Springer; 2002. p. 19–30.
13. Paley D. Normal lower limb alignment and joint orientation. In: Principles of deformity correction. Berlin: Springer; 2002. p. 1–18.
14. Saithna A, Kundra R, Modi CS, Getgood A, Spalding T. Distal femoral varus osteotomy for lateral compartment osteoarthritis in the valgus knee. A systematic review of the literature. Open Orthop J. 2012;6:313–9.
15. Rosso F, Margheritini F. Distal femoral osteotomy. Curr Rev Musculoskelet Med. 2014;7(4):302–11.
16. Felson DT, Niu J, Gross KD, Englund M, Sharma L, Cooke TDV, et al. Valgus malalignment is a risk factor for lateral knee osteoarthritis incidence and progression: findings from the multicenter osteoarthritis study and the osteoarthritis initiative. Arthritis Rheum. 2013;65(2):355–62.
17. Nelissen EM, van Langelaan EJ, Nelissen RGHH. Stability of medial opening wedge high tibial osteotomy: a failure analysis. Int Orthop. 2010;34(2):217–23.
18. Chahla J, Mitchell JJ, Liechti DJ, Moatshe G, Menge TJ, Dean CS, et al. Opening- and closing-wedge distal femoral osteotomy: a systematic review of outcomes for isolated lateral compartment osteoarthritis. Orthop J Sport Med. 2016;4(6):2325967116649901.
19. W-Dahl A, Robertsson O, Lidgren L. Surgery for knee osteoarthritis in younger patients. Acta Orthop. 2010;81(2):161–4.
20. Spahn G, Hofmann GO, von Engelhardt LV, Li M, Neubauer H, Klinger HM. The impact of a high tibial valgus osteotomy and unicondylar medial arthroplasty on the treatment for knee osteoarthritis: a meta-analysis. Knee Surg Sports Traumatol Arthrosc. 2013;21(1):96–112.
21. Floerkemeier S, Staubli AE, Schroeter S, Goldhahn S, Lobenhoffer P. Outcome after high tibial openwedge osteotomy: a retrospective evaluation of 533 patients. Knee Surg Sports Traumatol Arthrosc. 2013;21(1):170–80.
22. Lobenhoffer P, Agneskirchner J, Zoch W. Die öffnende valgisierende Osteotomie der proximalen Tibia mit Fixation durch einen medialen Plattenfixateur. Orthopäde. 2004;33:153–60.
23. Brinkman J-M, Lobenhoffer P, Agneskirchner JD, Staubli AE, Wymenga AB, van Heerwaarden RJ. Osteotomies around the knee: patient selection, stability of fixation and bone healing in high tibial osteotomies. J Bone Joint Surg Br. 2008;90–B(12):1548–57.
24. Han SB, Lee DH, Shetty GM, Chae DJ, Song JG, Nha KW. A “safe zone” in medial open-wedge high tibia osteotomy to prevent lateral cortex fracture. Knee Surg Sports Traumatol Arthrosc. 2013;21(1):90–5.
25. Vanadurongwan B, Siripisitsak T, Sudjai N, Harnroongroj T. The anatomical safe zone for medial opening oblique wedge high tibial osteotomy. Singapore Med J. 2013;54(2):102–4.
26. van Heerwaarden R, Najfeld M, Brinkman M, Seil R, Madry H, Pape D. Wedge volume and osteotomy surface depend on surgical technique for distal femoral osteotomy. Knee Surg Sports Traumatol Arthrosc. 2013;21(1):206–12.
27. Brinkman J-M, Hurschler C, Agneskirchner JD, Freiling D, van Heerwaarden RJ. Axial and torsional stability of supracondylar femur osteotomies: biomechanical comparison of the stability of five different plate and osteotomy configurations. Knee Surg Sports Traumatol Arthrosc. 2011;19(4):579–87.
28. Hofmann S, Lobenhoffer P, Staubli A, Van Heerwaarden R. Osteotomien am Kniegelenk bei

Monokompartmentarthrose. Orthopade. 2009;38(8): 755–70.
29. Bonasia DE, Governale G, Spolaore S, Rossi R, Amendola A. High tibial osteotomy. Curr Rev Musculoskelet Med. 2014;7:292–301.
30. Sanna M, Sanna C, Caputo F, Piu G, Salvi M. Surgical approaches in total knee arthroplasty. Joints. 2013;1(2):34–44.
31. Farouk O, Krettek C, Miclau T, Schandelmaier P, Guy P, Tscherne H. Minimally invasive plate osteosynthesis and vascularity: preliminary results of a cadaver injection study. Injury. 1997;28:A7–12.
32. Farouk O, Krettek C, Miclau T, Schandelmaier P, Tscherne H. The topography of the perforating vessels of the deep femoral artery. Clin Orthop Relat Res. 1999;368:255–9.
33. Farouk O, Krettek C, Miclau T, Schandelmaier P, Tscherne H. Effects of percutaneous and conventional plating techniques on the blood supply to the femur. Arch Orthop Trauma Surg. 1998;117(8):438–41.
34. Amis AA. Biomechanics of high tibial osteotomy. Knee Surg Sports Traumatol Arthrosc. 2013; 21(1):197–205.

12 ACL Reconstruction Using a Flat Quadriceps Tendon Graft Without Bone Block

Christian Fink, Elisabeth Abermann, Robert Smigielski, Rainer Siebold, and Mirco Herbort

12.1 Introduction

The selection of a graft for reconstructing the anterior–cruciate ligament (ACL) continues to be a controversial issue. While the patellar tendon was long considered the "gold standard" for ACL reconstructions, it was surpassed gradually in popularity by the semitendinosus and gracilis tendons, and more recently quadriceps tendon got increased attention [1–3].

Clinical studies have documented similar excellent results with less donor site morbidity than patellar tendon BTB grafts [4]. Clinical results are also comparable to the more commonly used hamstring graft, but QT was found to be associated with a lower re-rupture rate [1, 5].

C. Fink (✉) · E. Abermann
Gelenkpunkt—Sports and Joint Surgery, Innsbruck, Austria

Research Unit for Orthopaedic Sport Medicine and Injury Prevention (OSMI), UMIT, Hall, Austria
e-mail: c.fink@gelenkpunkt.com

R. Smigielski
Mirai Institute, Warsaw, Poland

R. Siebold
ATOS Clinic, Heidelberg, Germany
e-mail: rainer.siebold@atos.de

M. Herbort
Research Unit for Orthopaedic Sport Medicine and Injury Prevention (OSMI), UMIT, Hall, Austria

OCM Clinic München, Munich, Germany
e-mail: mirco.herbort@ocm-muenchen.de

While many knee surgeons currently accept QT as an ideal revision graft, to date it has not been widely utilized as a standard graft for primary ACL reconstructions [6]. One reason might be that QT graft harvesting is more technically demanding. This downside may be overcome by using a standardized minimal invasive technique that makes QT harvest saver and yields to more favorable cosmetic results [7].

Recent evidence has suggested that broad flat QT soft tissue grafts may more closely mimic native ACL "ribbon-like" morphology than hamstring tendon grafts (Fig. 12.1).

Neither a QT graft nor a patellar tendon graft is inherently round [8–10]. Only the reaming technique necessitates to harvest a graft that would fit snugly in a classic bone tunnel.

These considerations led us to develop a technique for creating rectangular bone tunnels (Karl Storz, Tuttlingen) that conform to graft shape. In vitro, this modification has been shown to have a biomechanical advantage with respect to rotational laxity [10, 11].

As a further advancement of these technique, an even flatter and wider femoral tunnel can be created on the femur, and instead of a squared tunnel on the tibia, a C-shaped tunnel, even more closely resembling the natural anatomy, can be created using newly developed instrumentation (MARS; Medacta, Lugano).

A soft tissue QT graft is suitable for both techniques.

M. T. Hirschmann et al. (eds.), *ESSKA Instructional Course Lecture Book*,
https://doi.org/10.1007/978-3-662-61264-4_12

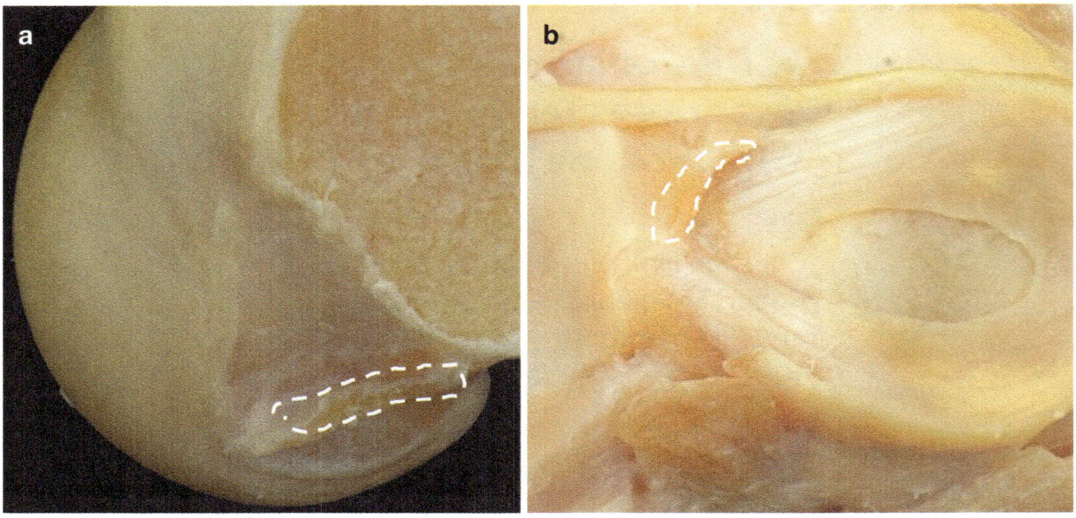

Fig. 12.1 Femoral (**a**) and tibial (**b**) attachments of the ACL

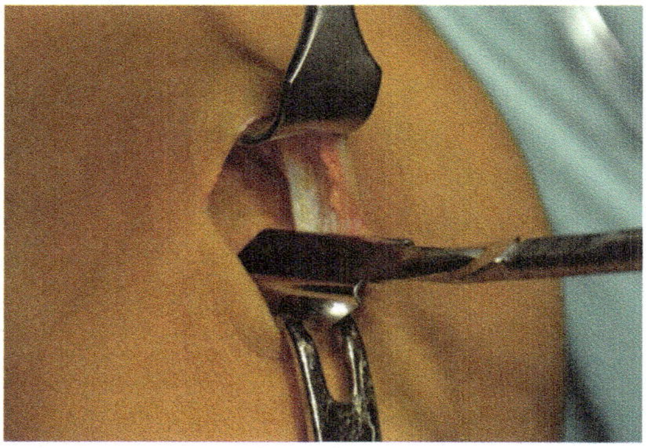

Fig. 12.2 Subcutaneous advancement of the tendon knife. The cutting edges are spaced at the desired graft width (Karl Storz, Tuttlingen)

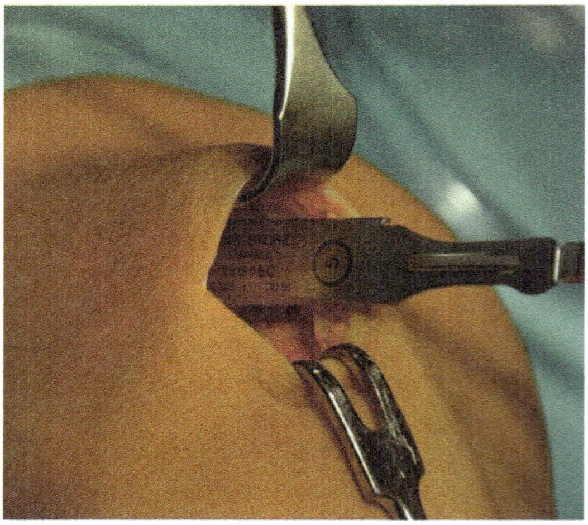

Fig. 12.3 Insertion and advancement of the 5-mm tendon separator (Karl Storz, Tuttlingen)

12.2 Operative Technique

12.2.1 Graft Harvest and Preparation

A transverse skin incision approximately 3 cm long is made over the superior border of the patella. The bursal layer is then dissected aside to expose the QT, and a long Langenbeck retractor is introduced. Next a tendon knife with two parallel blades (10 mm width) (Karl Storz, Tuttlingen) is advanced to 7 cm (Fig. 12.2).

The thickness of the graft is then defined with the tendon separator (Karl Storz, Tuttlingen), which is set to a depth of 5 mm and is also advanced to the 7-cm mark (Fig. 12.3).

Finally, graft length is determined with the quadriceps tendon cutter (Karl Storz, Tuttlingen), a punch-action instrument that is introduced 1–2 cm proximal to the superior–patellar border. It is advanced to the desired length and activated to free the proximal end of the graft. The graft is now reflected distally, and the distal end of the graft is outlined with a scalpel, cutting down to the patella (Fig. 12.4) [7].

A periosteal strip equal to the graft width and 1.5–2 cm long can be dissected from the anterior–patellar surface (Fig. 12.5a). The strip is then folded over (Fig. 12.5b) and whipstitched with two nonabsorbable No. 2 sutures (Fig. 12.5c). This yields a rounded end that will facilitate later graft passage. The sutures are passed through the central holes of a FlippTack® fixation button (Karl Storz, Tuttlingen). Finally, the free end of the tendon is whipstitched with two nonabsorbable Nr. 2 lead sutures (e.g. Fibre Wire®, Arthrex Naples FL) and passed through an Endotack® (Karl Storz, Tuttlingen) or a Tibial button (PSP®, Medacta Lugano), respectively (Fig. 12.5d).

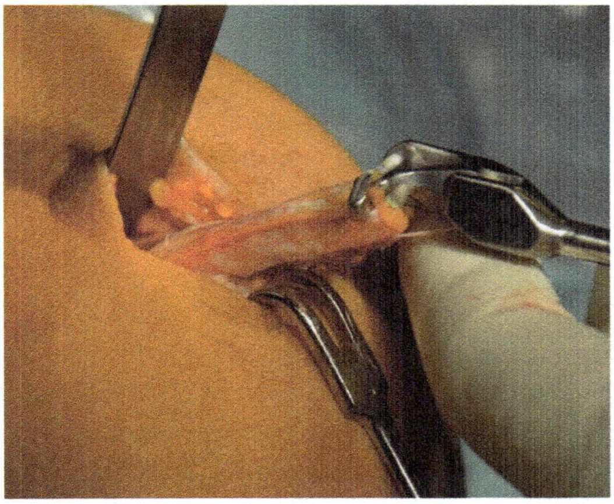

Fig. 12.4 Subcutaneous advancement of the quadriceps tendon cutter (Karl Storz, Tuttlingen) and retrieving the graft

12.2.2 Femoral Bone Tunnel

A standard arthroscope portal is placed just lateral to the patellar tendon at the level of the patellar apex. A low medial portal is then placed under vision, using a trial needle to determine the portal site. The cruciate ligament remnants are resected, leaving a tibial stump.

With the knee flexed 90°, the anatomic femoral insertion site of the ACL is marked with a microfracture awl. The position of this point is checked by viewing through the medial arthroscope portal (Fig. 12.6).

A 2.4-mm guide wire is now introduced through the medial portal using a femoral drill guide. The guide wire is advanced to a 1 cm laser mark (Fig. 12.7a). Then the length of the tunnel is measured with a special depth gauge (Karl Storz, Tuttlingen) (Fig. 12.7b, c).

When the correct position of the guide wire has been confirmed, it is overdrilled with a 4.5-mm drill bit. Then a 10 mm rasp is passed through the medial portal. With the knee flexed 115°, the rasp is aligned parallel to the tibial plateau (Fig. 12.8). The smooth surface of the rasp is fac-

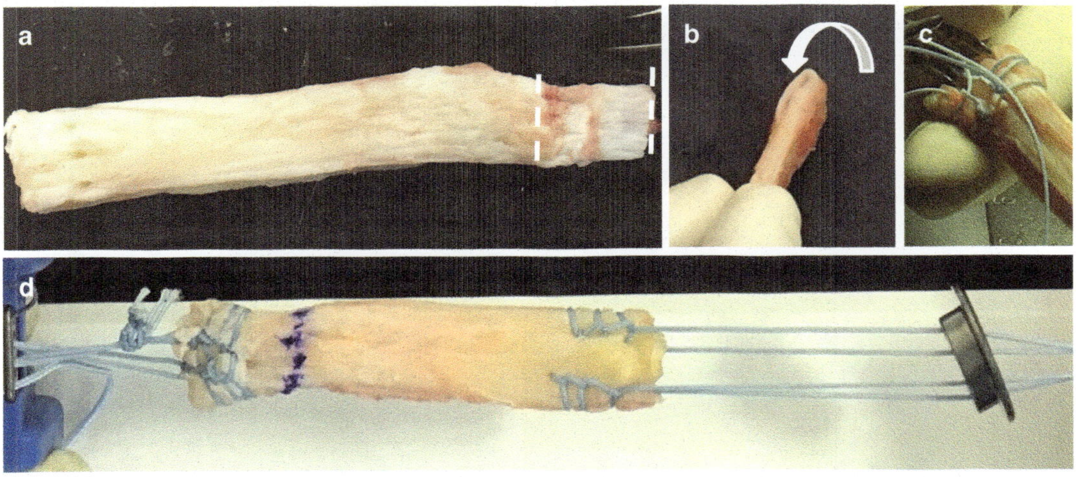

Fig. 12.5 (a) Harvesting a QT graft with a 2-cm-long periosteal strip conforming to the graft width. (b) The periosteal strip is folded over and (c) whipstitched with two nonabsorbable No. 2 sutures. (d) The final graft proximally tied to a flip button and distally instrumented with a special suture button (PSP® Medact Lugano)

ing the posterior cruciate ligament to protect that structure from injury. A socket is formed by driving the rasp in slowly to a depth of approximately 25–30 mm. The rasp is then tapped back out.

Alternatively, the MARS femoral guide (Medacta, Lugano) is slided over the central guide wire and two more 2.4-mm guide wires are placed at the femoral insertion (Fig. 12.9). The guide wires are over-reamed by a 4.5-mm cannulated reamer, and then the tunnel is finalized using a dilatator of the appropriate graft size (small, medium, or large) (Fig. 12.10).

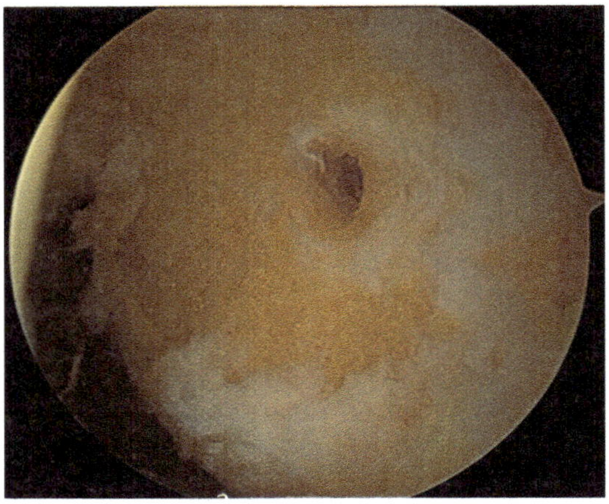

Fig. 12.6 Arthroscopic view from the medial portal controlling the position of the marking for the femoral tunnel

12.2.3 Tibial Bone Tunnel

12.2.3.1 Rectangular Bone Tunnel

The tibial drill guide is introduced through the medial arthroscope portal. Then a vertical skin incision approximately 1.5 cm long is made medial to the tibial tuberosity. The first guide wire is now drilled in through the center of the drill sleeve, and its relation to the roof of the intercondylar notch is evaluated by extending the knee. The guide sleeve is removed and a cannulated 10-mm (or 12-mm) drill bit is advanced over the wire. It is predrilled to a depth of 0.5–1 cm to create a countersunk bed for the later placement of an EndoTack® (Karl Storz, Germany). Now the drill sleeve is reintroduced and fixed securely in the predrilled hole. A second guide wire is drilled in parallel to the first at a slightly more anterior position (Fig. 12.11).

Each wire is overdrilled with a 5-mm drill bit. Both the wires are removed, and any bony bridges that remain between the drill holes are disrupted with a shaver. Now a guide wire is inserted for orientation purposes, and a 10 mm rasp is carefully driven into the tunnel. Finally a tibial dilator of the appropriate size is carefully tapped into place to complete the tibial tunnel (Fig. 12.12).

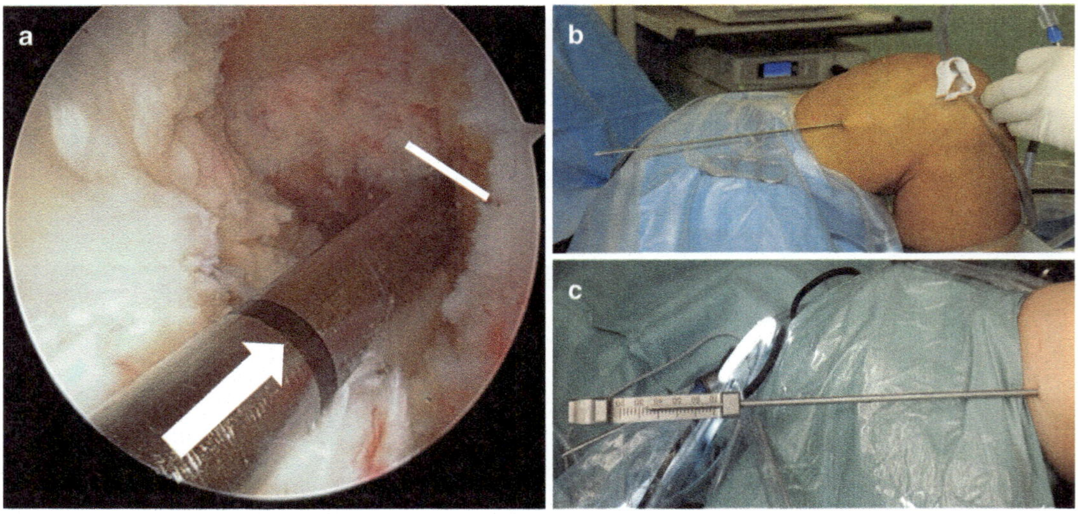

Fig. 12.7 The 2.4-mm guide wire is advanced to a 1 cm laser mark (**a**). Then the length of the tunnel is measured with a special depth gauge (Karl Storz, Tuttlingen) (**b** and **c**)

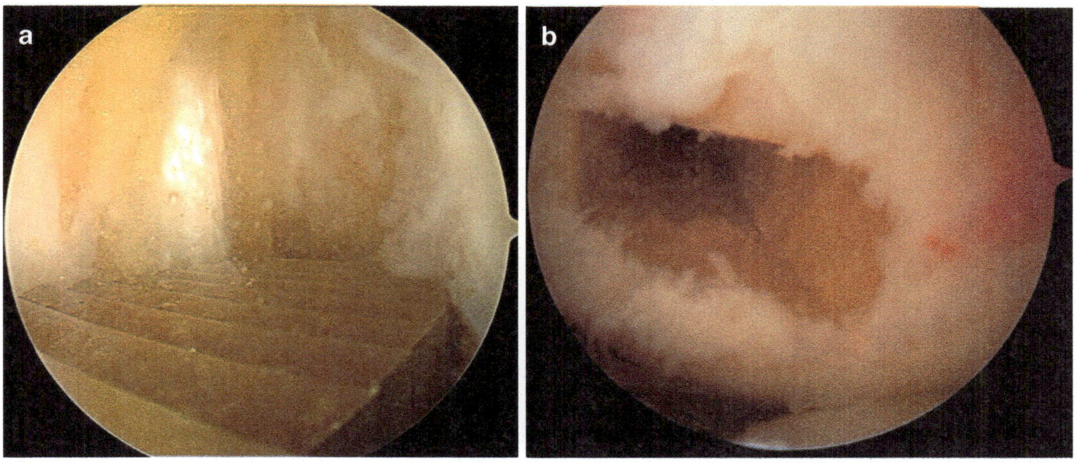

Fig. 12.8 (**a**) A rasp (8 or 10 × 5 mm) (Karl Storz, Tuttlingen) is driven into the bone tunnel with the knee flexed approximately 115°. (**b**) Final appearance of the squared femoral bone tunnel through a medial arthroscopic portal

Fig. 12.9 Using the MARS femoral drill guide (Medacta, Lugano) to place three 2.4 mm K-wires in the femoral ACL footprint (schematic drawing and arthroscopic visualization)

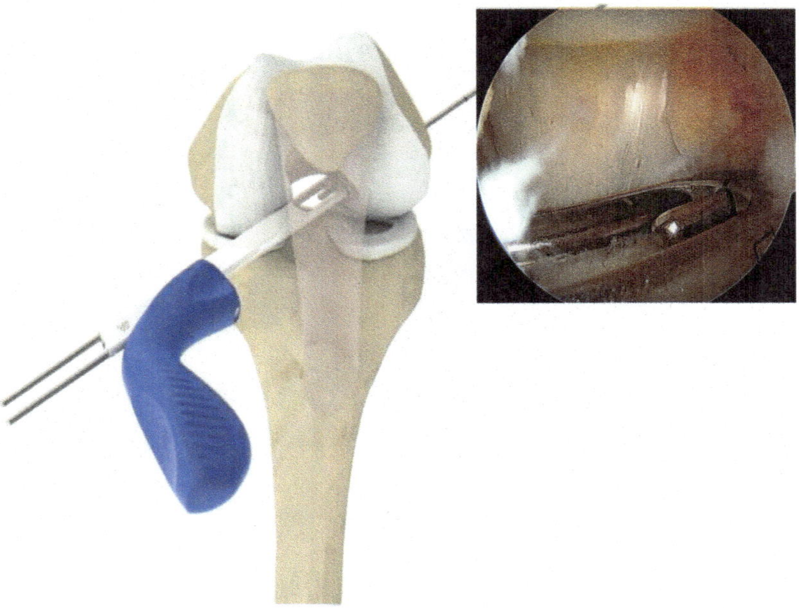

12.2.3.2 C-Shaped Bone Tunnel

The MARS tibial aimer (Medacta, Lugano) is inserted through the medial portal with the knee in 90° of flexion again and placed around the anterior horn of the lateral meniscus and with reference to the ACL remnant. The guide wire is drilled into the center of the ACL footprint (Fig. 12.13).

Now two 4.5-mm drill bits are drilled anterior and posterior to the guide pin. Finally, the tibial aimer is removed and a cannulated 4.5-mm drill bit is used to over drill the guide wire.

The tibial tunnel is finalized using a C-shaped dilatator of the appropriate graft size (small, medium, or large) (Fig. 12.14).

12.2.3.3 Graft Passage (Fig. 12.15)

The suture loop from the free suture ends from the tendon end of the graft to the button are now tied off to equal the measured length of the femoral tunnel.

Correct graft rotation is an important consideration during graft [8, 9] passage. It is easier to

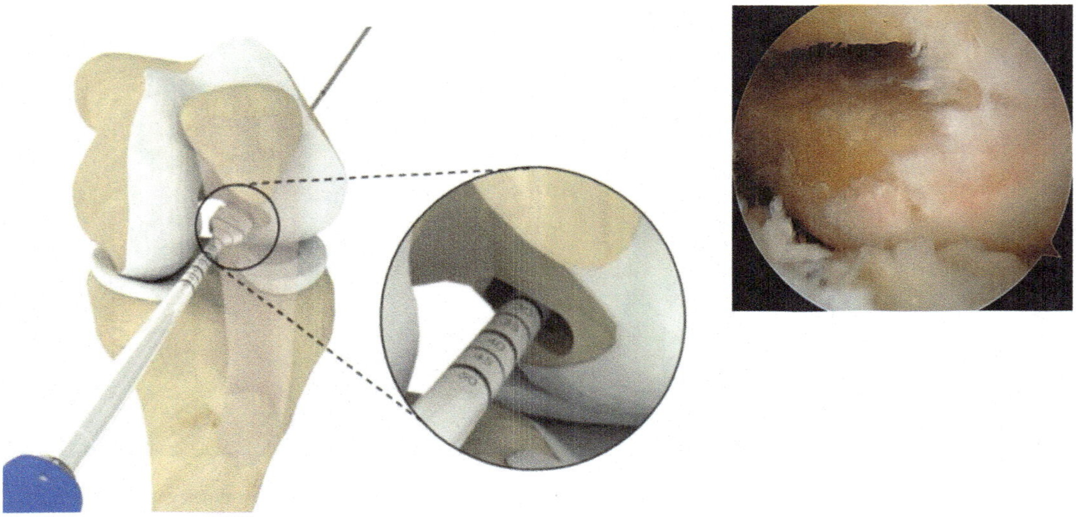

Fig. 12.10 Dilating the femoral tunnel in the appropriate size equal to graft dimensions (schematic drawing and arthroscopic visualization)

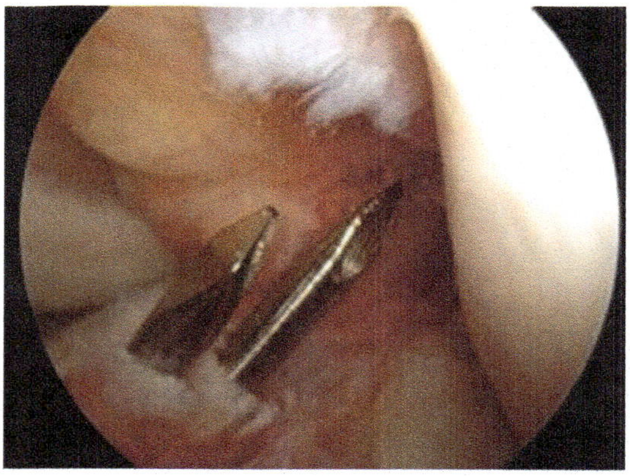

Fig. 12.11 Two K-wires are placed parallel in the tibial footprint with a special tibial aimer (Karl Storz, Tuttlingen)

achieve correct graft rotation with the knee slightly extended. When it is confirmed that the fixation button has been flipped, the graft is pulled back through the tibial tunnel to seat the button securely against the femoral cortex. Now the knee joint is taken through ten cycles of flexion extension while traction is maintained on the distal leads. Then, with the knee flexed approximately 20°, the tibial end of the graft is fixed with an 8 × 28 mm absorbable interference screw inserted on the lateral side of the graft. Additionally, the sutures are tied over an EndoTack® (Karl Storz, Germany) - rectangular tibial tunnel.

For the C-shaped tibial tunnel, the distal sutures are tied over a special tibial fixation button (PSP®; Medacta, Lugano) (Fig. 12.16).

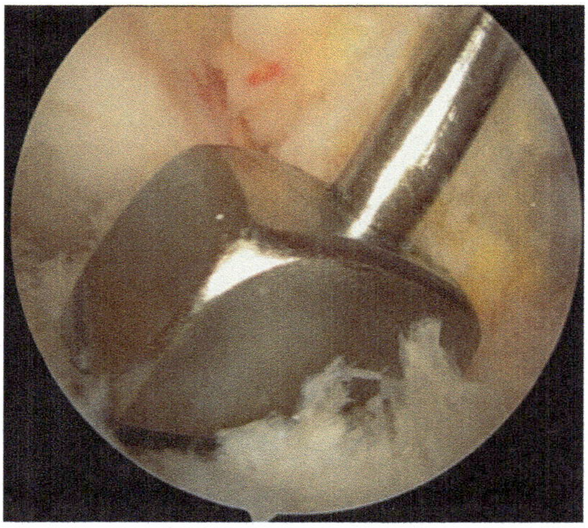

Fig. 12.12 A tibial dilator of the appropriate size (Karl Storz, Tuttlingen) is carefully driven into place

Finally the QT tendon graft is inspected, and ACL remnants that might impinge in full extension are carefully removed using a shaver (Fig. 12.17).

12.3 Postoperative Care

While still in the operating room, the knee is positioned in an extension brace following application of the wound dressing and a Cryo cuff.

If the patient is hospitalized, drains are removed and radiographs are obtained on the first postoperative day. A 0–0–90° knee brace is

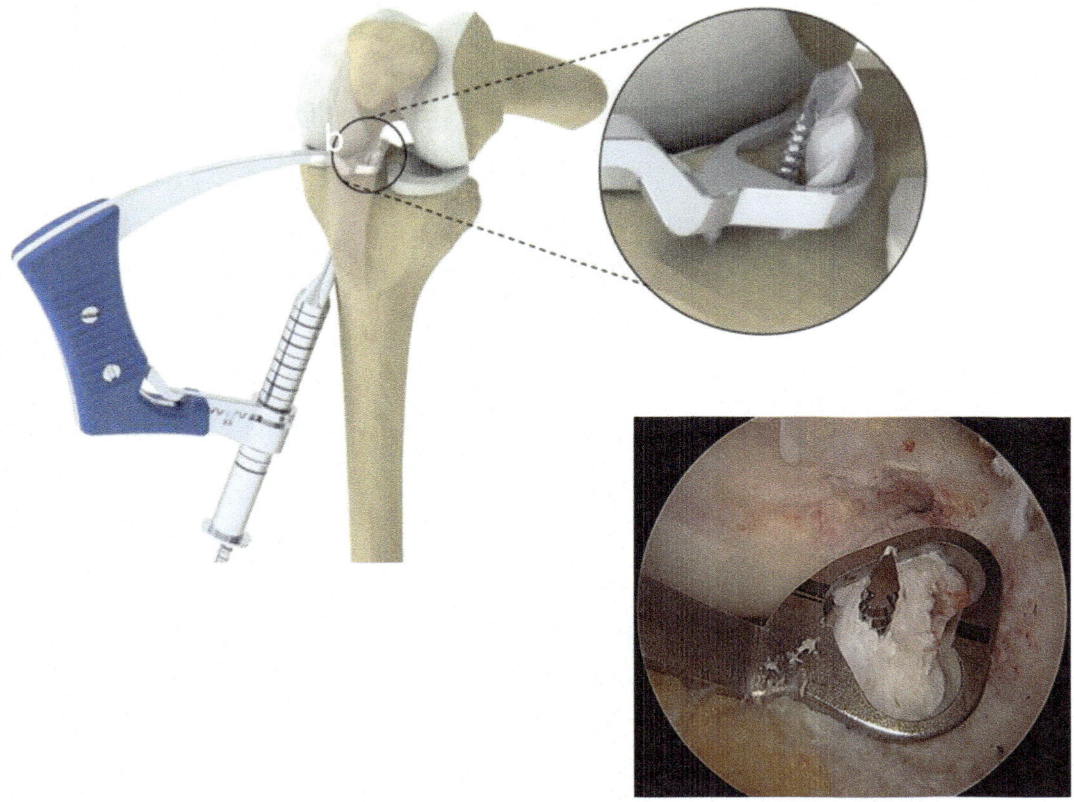

Fig. 12.13 The MARS tibial aimer (Medacta, Lugano) is inserted through the medial portal with the knee in 90° of flexion again and placed around the anterior horn of the lateral meniscus and with reference to the ACL remnant. The guide wire is drilled into the center of the ACL footprint (schematic drawing and arthroscopic visualization)

Fig. 12.14 The tibial tunnel is finalized using a C-shaped dilatator of the appropriate graft size

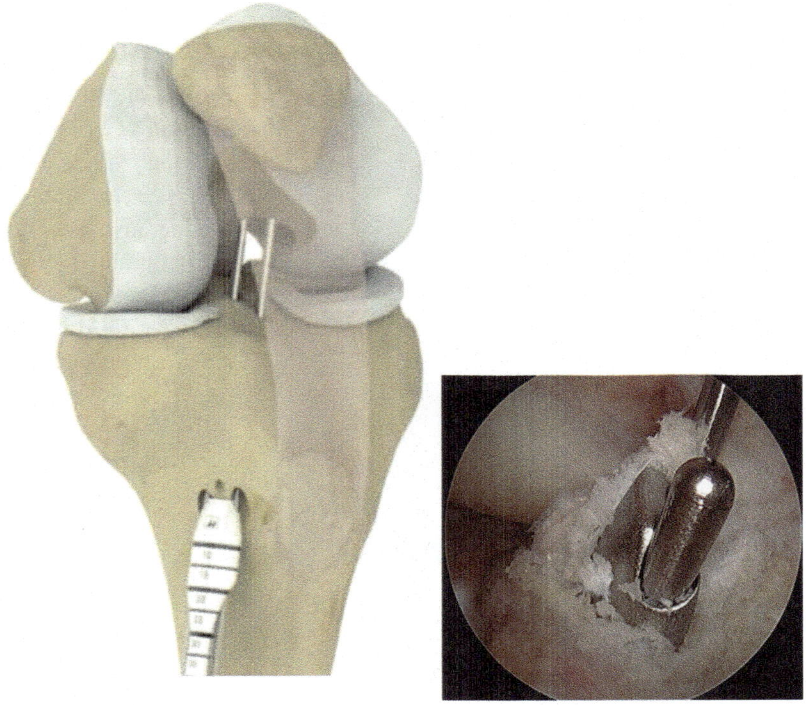

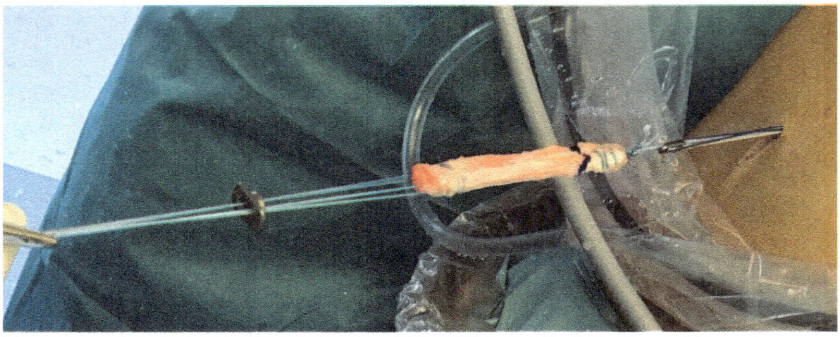

Fig. 12.15 Insertion of the graft through the tibial tunnel

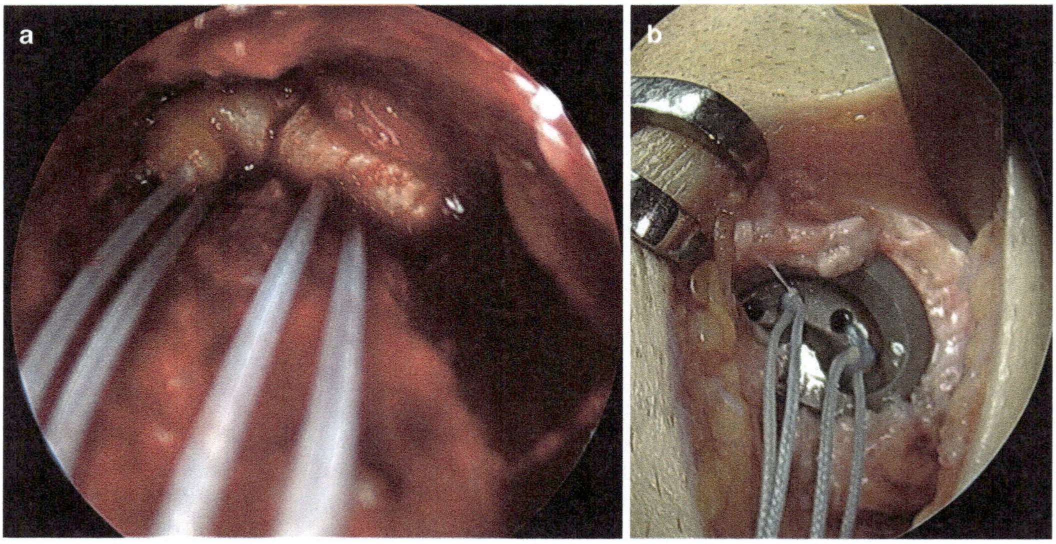

Fig. 12.16 (**a**) Endoscopic view of the graft in the C-shaped tibial tunnel. (**b**) Fixation through tying the knots over a special tibial suture button (PSP®; Medacta, Lugano)

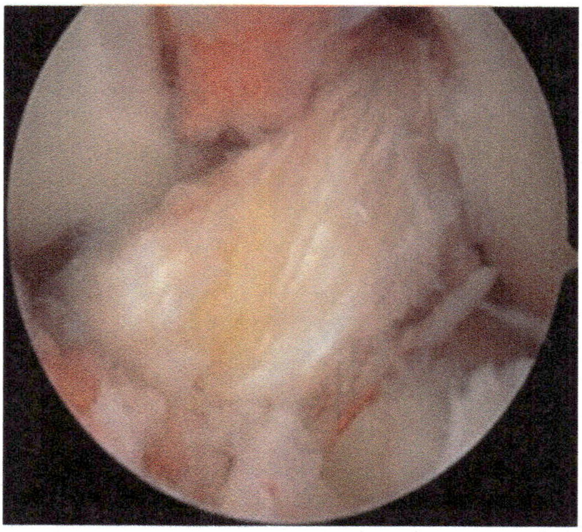

Fig. 12.17 Final arthroscopic appearance of a flat QT graft

applied, and the patient is mobilized under the direction of a physical therapist.

Partial weight-bearing at approximately 20–30 kg should be maintained for the first two postoperative weeks. The brace and crutches can be discontinued by the third postoperative week. In most cases, the patient is discharged on the second or third postoperative day and continues outpatient physical therapy 2 or 3 times per week for at least 6 weeks.

12.4 Discussion

A soft tissue QT graft allows for new, more anatomic ACL reconstruction techniques. Commonly used ACL reconstruction techniques use drills to create bone tunnels for graft insertion. However, this seems to be the only explanation for them being round, because neither the femoral nor the tibial insertion sites are round. On the femoral side, the rectangular or flat tunnel mimics the native insertion better than a round tunnel, and the tibia a rectangular or C-shaped tunnel potentially reduces the risk for laceration of the anterior horn of the lateral meniscus. Additionally, the increased graft bone contact area of a flat ACL graft compared to a round graft with similar cross-sectional area may provide a biological advantage leading to accelerated ingrowth and probably less central graft necrosis.

12.5 Take Home Message

The quality of the QT is often underestimated in cruciate ligament surgery. The tendon is very flexible in its dimensions. QT harvest without a bone block is technically easier (e.g., no risk of patellar fracture), and the addition of a periosteum flap facilitates its insertion and is potentially beneficial for graft to bone healing.

Because neither the bony attachments nor the mid-substance of the native ACL is round, the use of round tunnels and tubular hamstring tendon (HT) grafts as the optimum reconstruction technique has been questioned. Anatomically oriented rectangular femoral tunnels and rectangular or C-shaped tibial tunnels may more closely replicate the native anatomy, allowing graft rotation during knee flexion that is similar to the biomechanics of the native ACL [11].

References

1. Chen CH, Chuang TY, Wang KC, Chen WJ, Shih CH. Arthroscopic anterior cruciate ligament reconstruction with quadriceps tendon autograft: clinical outcome in 4–7 years. Knee Surg Sports Traumatol Arthrosc. 2006;14(11):1077–85.
2. Geib TM, Shelton WR, Phelps RA, Clark L. Anterior cruciate ligament reconstruction using quadriceps tendon autograft: intermediate-term outcome. Arthroscopy. 2009;25(12):1408–14.
3. Slone HS, Romine SE, Premkumar A, Xerogeanes JW. Quadriceps tendon autograft for anterior cruciate ligament reconstruction: a comprehensive review of current literature and systematic review of clinical results. Arthroscopy. 2015;31(3):541–54.
4. Lund B, Nielsen T, Fauno P, Christiansen SE, Lind M. Is quadriceps tendon a better graft choice than patellar tendon? A prospective randomized study. Arthroscopy. 2014;30(5):593–8.
5. Hoeher J, Balke M, Albers M. Anterior cruciate ligament (ACL) reconstruction using a quadriceps tendon autograft and press-fit fixation has equivalent results compared to a standard technique using semitendinosus graft: a prospective matched-pair analysis after 1 year. Knee Surg Sports Traumatol Arthrosc. 2012;20:147.
6. Stäubli HU, Schatzmann L, Brunner P, Rincon L, Nolte LP. Mechanical tensile properties of the quadriceps tendon and patellar ligament in young adults. Am J Sports Med. 1999;27(1):27–34.
7. Fink C, Herbort M, Abermann E, Hoser C. Minimally invasive harvest of a quadriceps tendon graft with or without a bone block. Arthrosc Tech. 2014;3(4):e509–13.
8. Fink C, Hoser C. Einzelbündeltechnik: quadrizepssehne in portaltechnik. Arthroskopie. 2013;26(1):35–41.
9. Fink C, Lawton R, Förschner F, Gföller P, Herbort M, Hoser C. Minimally invasive quadriceps tendon single-bundle, arthroscopic, anatomic anterior cruciate ligament reconstruction with rectangular bone tunnels. Arthrosc Tech. 2018;24(7):e1045–56.
10. Shino K, Nakata K, Nakamura N, Toritsuka Y, Horibe S, Nakagawa S, Suzuki T. Rectangular tunnel double-bundle anterior cruciate ligament reconstruction with bone-patellar tendon-bone graft to mimic natural fiber arrangement. Arthroscopy. 2008;24(10):1178–83.
11. Herbort M, Tecklenburg K, Zantop T, Raschke MJ, Hoser C, Schulze M, Petersen W, Fink C. Single-bundle anterior cruciate ligament reconstruction: a biomechanical cadaveric study of a rectangular quadriceps and bone—patellar tendon—bone graft configuration versus a round hamstring graft. Arthroscopy. 2013;29(12):1981–90.

Void Filler in Opening Wedge Osteotomies Around the Knee

13

Asif Parkar, Philip Pastides, Raghbir S. Khakha, and Matt Dawson

Opening wedge osteotomy around the knee is a safe, effective and satisfactory surgical technique used in active patients in order to restore coronal and sometimes sagittal alignment in the management of osteoarthritis and other conditions.

An opening wedge osteotomy relies on the natural healing processes of the bone to consolidate the gap and unite. Recognised risks and complications of these procedures include malunion, delayed union or even non-union, with or without an associated loss of the deformity correction. The advent of angle stable plates and recent advances in technique have been shown to increase the stability across the osteotomy site. This allows early weight bearing, which thus stimulates the mechanical environment and accelerates osseous healing. In fact, locking plates compared to non-locking plates appear to have a more favourable outcome in terms of stability at the osteotomy site, with or without the addition of void filler [1, 2].

Despite this finding, some surgeons advocate the use of void fillers to enhance bone healing and increase initial mechanical stability. Furthermore, in vitro studies have shown that use of void filler increases initial axial and rotational stability compared to leaving the osteotomy gap empty [3]. Options to fill the osteotomy gap include autografts (such as those derived from the iliac crest graft), allograft (such as femoral head wedges), cement blocks or synthetic grafts (in wedges or powder form).

An autograft is tissue that is harvested from and transplanted to another part in the same individual. Based on the anatomical location of the donor site, this can be cortical, cancellous, corticocancellous, vascularised graft or bone marrow. Autograft is generally regarded as the gold standard because it is the only graft option that has the potential of providing mechanical stability as well as the patient's own osteogenic cells to promote bone healing. The exemplar for an autograft that gives excellent structural support and osteogenic cells is tricortical iliac crest bone graft. This provides structural support as well as living cells with growth factors having excellent osteogenic and osteoinductive properties. This facilitates rapid incorporation at the recipient site without the risk of disease transmission or immunogenic complications and at no extra cost for material or tissue. The disadvantages of autograft are donor-site morbidity such as pain, haematoma, infection, scar, increased operative time and also limited supply.

A. Parkar
Locum Consultant Trauma & Orthopaedics, Queens Hospital, London, UK

P. Pastides · R. S. Khakha
Guys and St Thomas Hospital, London, UK
e-mail: raghbir.khakka@nhs.net

M. Dawson (✉)
North Cumbria University Hospital, Cumbria, UK
e-mail: matt.dawson@ncuh.nhs.uk

M. T. Hirschmann et al. (eds.), *ESSKA Instructional Course Lecture Book*,
https://doi.org/10.1007/978-3-662-61264-4_13

An allograft is a graft that is harvested from one individual and implanted into another of the same species. This can be cortical, cancellous or corticocancellous, and based on the processing method, it can be fresh, frozen, freeze-dried and demineralised. The greatest advantage of allograft is that there is no donor site morbidity. Large amounts of graft can be made available and hence making it more suitable for bigger defects. Important disadvantages, however, are that structural properties as well as the biological potential of the allograft may be adversely affected by the processing techniques employed. Disease transmission remains a concern when using allografts, and thorough screening is mandatory when supplying allografts. Bone banks screen the graft for hepatitis B, hepatitis C, HIV, syphilis and rhesus status. Other exclusion criteria include malignancy, inflammatory arthritis, autoimmune disease, prolonged steroid use and diseases such as Alzheimer's, multiple sclerosis and Creutzfeldt–Jakob disease. The reported risk of infection with allograft for HIV is one in 1.6 million, and hepatitis C is one in 150,000. Other disadvantages of allograft are the risk of immunogenic reaction and the cost.

Xenograft is when a graft is harvested from one species and implanted into a different species. This method is not readily used as of yet, but studies have shown encouraging results.

Synthetic or artificial grafts are also an option. These have neither donor site morbidity nor risk of cross infection, as compared to autograft and allograft, respectively. However, their unique biological and biomechanical properties need to be carefully considered.

The aim of this chapter is to discuss the various options to use if void filler is desired and also summarise the evidence for each option.

13.1 In Vitro Evidence

13.1.1 Simulation Testing

Large osteotomy gaps (>10 mm) have been shown to be associated with a high risk of lateral cortex fracture [4, 5]. Using saw bone tibiae, Belsey et al. [6, 7] performed two laboratory studies looking at the effect of void fillers for larger osteotomy gaps.

In the study published earlier this year, Belsey et al. [6] performed 12 mm biplanar MOWHTOs in ten medium-sized tibiae. Five of the gaps were filled with an allograft wedge whilst the other five were left empty. The osteotomies were fixed using a Tomofix plate (Synthes GmbH, Oberdorf, Switzerland) on the medial side, in the standard fashion. Both groups underwent static compression testing and cyclical fatigue testing until failure of the osteotomy. Peak force, valgus malrotation, number of cycles, displacement and stiffness around the tibial head were analysed. Intraoperative hinge fractures occurred in all specimens. Under static compression, the allograft group withstood higher peak forces (6.01 kN) compared with the control group (5.12 kN). Valgus malrotation was lower, and stiffness was higher, in the allograft group. During cyclical fatigue testing, results within the allograft group were more consistent than within the control group.

The second paper by Belsey et al. looked at three groups of five artificial tibiae that underwent 10 mm biplanar MOWHTO [7]. In two groups, the gaps were filled with either an Osferion wedge (OSferion60, Olympus Terumo Biomaterials, Tokyo, Japan) or an allograft bone wedge, and the third group left empty. Fixation was achieved using an Activmotion plate (NewClip Technics, Haute-Goulaine, France) on the medial side. Static compression was applied axially to each specimen until failure of the osteotomy. Ultimate load, horizontal and vertical displacements were measured and used to calculate construct stiffness and valgus malrotation of the tibial head. The synthetic group failed at 6.3 kN, followed by the allograft group (6 kN) and the control group (4.5 kN). The most valgus malrotation of the tibial head was observed in the allograft group (2.6°). The synthetic group showed the highest stiffness at the medial side of the tibial head (9.54 kN mm^{-1}), but the lowest stiffness at the lateral side (1.59 kN mm^{-1}). The allograft group showed high stiffness on the medial side of the tibial head (7.54 kN mm^{-1}) as well as the highest stiffness on the lateral side (2.18 kN mm^{-1}).

13.2 In Vivo Evidence

13.2.1 Autografts

13.2.1.1 Iliac Crest Autograft

Between 2005 and 2009, Fucentese et al. [8] randomised patients undergoing a medial open wedge high tibial osteotomy (MOWHTO) with a medial angular stable locking plate (Surfix-Integra, France), to receive either cancellous bone graft from ipsilateral iliac crest (group A, 15 patients) or no void filler (group B, 25 patients). At 3 and 12 months postoperatively, the healing of the osteotomy gap was measured using a 40 slice CT scan. The reconstruction was performed in axial, coronal and sagittal planes with slice thickness of 2 mm at an increment of 0.5 mm. The osteotomy was divided into anteromedial, anterolateral, posteromedial and posterolateral quadrants. They used the mean value of the four quadrants as the percentage of bone healing. This quantitative CT measurement was performed twice by a blinded musculoskeletal radiologist and a blinded orthopaedic knee surgeon. Functional assessment was carried out using pre- and postoperative KSS and WOMAC scores. The groups were similar in age, sex ratio, knee varus deformity, body mass index and smoking status. Group A and B had similar preoperative varus (6.9° vs. 7.6°) and postoperative valgus (2.2° vs. 3.0°). Compared with the control, group A had a significantly greater degree of osseous gap healing after 3 months (40.1% vs. 10.8%, $p = 0.045$) and 12 months (91.5% vs. 59.1%, $p \leq 0.001$). Multiple linear regression analysis found that bone grafting was an independent promoting factor for gap healing, whilst increased preoperative varus and older age were independent retardant factors. They noted that iliac crest autograft significantly increased healing of the osteotomy gap. However, no functional advantage was found at 3 or 12 months postoperatively.

Another similarly designed prospective randomised controlled study looked at the clinical and radiological results of 46 OWHTO using Puddu locking plate. Twenty-three patients were randomised to having iliac crest autograft in the osteotomy gap and 23 were randomised to no graft [9]. They harvested cancellous bone graft from opposite iliac crest in all patients including the group where it was not used. The authors have expressed their view that with modern locking plate structural allograft is not necessary. Bone union was assessed by two blinded investigators using Apley and Solomon's criteria which were originally described for fracture union. As per these criteria, union occurs when there is no pain on local palpation, absence of swelling in the limb, painless walking without crutches, and presence of bridging callus on plain radiographs. This assessment was carried out every 2 weeks until both investigators agreed with osteotomy union. They found comparable mean time to radiological bone union in both groups, the autograft group at 12.35 weeks and the no void filler group at 13.65 weeks. This study reported higher incidence of haematoma in no void filler group involving four patients (17.4%) compared to two patients (8.7%) in autograft group.

13.2.1.2 Autologous Osteophytes

Akiyama et al. [10] described a technique of arthroscopically harvesting osteophytes to then use as a void filler from the affected knee in patients undergoing OWHTO. Their theory for using these as autografts is that development of osteophytes is associated with the process of endochondral bone formation and expression of various growth factors such as transforming growth factor β, insulin-like growth factor 1, bone morphogenetic proteins and cartilage-derived morphogenetic proteins and therefore have osteoinductive properties. In their published single surgeon series of 11 patients, the bone-healing process was evaluated with computed tomography. The average age of the patients was 60.6 years. As a result, bone healing was observed at 5.3 weeks postoperatively on average. Subsequent follow-up CT images showed favourable union rates. They compared this technique to a single patient who had undergone a MOWHTO with autologous osteophyte grafting in one knee and without bone grafting in the other knee. They noted that bone healing at the site of osteotomy was accelerated for the knee treated with autologous osteophyte grafting than that for the knee without bone grafting.

13.2.1.3 Reamer Irrigator Aspirator Autograft

Seagrave et al. [11] published a novel technique of using reamer irrigator aspirator (RIA) autograft as a void filler. The autograft was taken via a retrograde femoral technique during the MOWHTO. Although a very small case series of three patients, all patients went on to union and had no sequelae due to the collection method. They did not comment on the type of plate used for their fixation method. The aforementioned study is the only published article found using this technique. Whilst this technique provides excellent quality and volume of cancellous autograft, it is associated with significant risks [12]. The senior author has personally used this technique on two occasions and perceives that on balance, the risk of comorbidity using this technique outweighs the potential benefit.

13.3 Synthetic Fillers

13.3.1 Cement

Bone cement has been used with great success in multiple areas throughout orthopaedics. In part due to its excellent compressive properties, bone cement has also been described as void filler during OWHTO procedures.

In a series of 245 OWHTO in 197 patients, Hernigou et al. [13] used a wedge-shaped fashioned cement block, placed within the posteromedial part of the osteotomy, to fill the void and maintain the height of the wedge. The size of the block was predetermined according to preoperative planning based on the degree of correction required. An anteromedial placed plate (non-locking) was used to provide a stable fixation. Patients were kept non-weight-bearing for 45 days on average.

They noted four postoperative infections; two in the early phase treated with a replacement of the cement block with an antibiotic impregnated equivalent. They noted two late infections at 2 and 3 years, which resolved with the removal of the metalwork. Union was assessed on radiographs. They defined delayed union as a period of more than 45 days, of which they had three cases. Only one required further intervention in the form of a revision with the removal of the cement wedge and replacement with iliac crest bone grafting. Complete filling of the osteotomy was noted at 3 months in all other cases. The authors report that this technique eliminates the morbidity associated with iliac crest harvest and avoids the potential risk of infection linked to allograft used.

13.3.2 Tricalcium Phosphate

A lot of research has been done looking at the use of tricalcium phosphate (TCP) as a void filler in either granular or wedge form. It has osteoconductive properties and allows osteoblasts to adhere to it, deposit bony tissue on its surface and thus act as a scaffold to fill in the osteotomy site [14]. The degree of porosity of this synthetic filler has shown to be related to its mechanical and bioabsorptive properties. Krall et al. [15] showed that complete resolution of 30% microporosity rigid b-TCP wedges did not take place up to 8 years postoperatively. Tanaka et al. [16] have shown traditional b-TCP with 75% porosity is unsuitable for weight-bearing until integration and resorption have occurred. As a result, they developed a b-TCP block with 60% porosity, which is approximately seven times greater in terms of compressive strength compared to a similar block of 75% porosity. In 25 patients who underwent OWHTO, they used two different blocks of b-TCP to fill the osteotomy site, using a Puddu plate (Arthrex) plate for fixation. They inserted a block of 75% porosity b-TCP laterally and another block of 60% porosity medially (at the cortex). In the longer term follow-up period, they had no cases of delayed or non-union and no cases of correction loss. Complete or near complete resorption of the b-TCP was obtained within 3.5 years. Furthermore they were able to take biopsies from the medial wedge (60% porosity) in 13 cases to assess the degree of resorption and incorporation. Within the specimens taken, they found lamellar bone formation with a mean percentage of residual b-TCP/lamellar bone ratio of 6.7% (range 0.3–14.5%).

The clinical relevance and importance of the porosity of the b-TCP wedge was also shown by Lim et al. [17] in their study using porcine models. They performed OWHTO in 12 porcine specimens. Six procedures were augmented with a 70% porosity b-TCP wedge whilst the rest were left empty. Follow-up both radiographically and with CT scan showed complete union in both groups by 6 months with no significant difference in healing times between the two groups. However, the cohort that also had the void filler did show evidence of a statistically significant higher bone mineral density.

In contrast to the above findings, Ferner et al. [18] reported a significantly higher delayed union and non-union rate with the use of tricalcium phosphate bone graft. In their prospective non-randomised study of MOWHTO, they initially treated 19 osteotomies (group A) with a TCP void filler (Actifuse granules, Apatech Limited, United Kingdom). Based on their experience of delayed union and non-union in these 19 patients, they stopped using TCP void filler. Remaining 30 patients (group B) in this study who had surgery at a later date, did not have any void filler in their osteotomies. The same locking plate (Tomofix) was used in all cases. Bone healing was assessed clinically and radiologically using radiographs at 6 and 12 months after surgery. CT scan was used only in cases with loss of correction or patients who required revision surgery. Unfortunately, authors made no differentiation between non-union and delayed union. Also, time to bony consolidation with or without synthetic augmentation was not measured. It was noted that patients with TCP augmentation had larger corrections with opening angles (6–18°) compared to patients who did not have any void filler (4–15°). Another finding was 13 out of 19 patients (68%) in group A with TCP graft required sagittal plane correction compared to 16 out of 30 patients (53%) in group B without any void filler. Their results showed that TCP void filler group showed a 26% non-union rate (five out of 19 patients required revision surgery) compared to a 3.3% non-union rate (one out of 30 patients required revision surgery) in the later technique of not utilising any form of void filler.

13.4 Comparative Studies

13.4.1 B-TCP vs. HA Wedge

Onodera et al. [19] compared the use of b-TCP and hydroxyapatite wedges in 38 OWHTO (19 in each group). They noted that b-TCP had statistically significant greater osteoconductive and absorbability properties compared to HA using a modified van Hermert score. However, this did not translate in any significant differences in complications or clinical outcomes at 18 months.

Lind-Hansen TB et al. [20] compared injectable calcium phosphate cement with local bone autograft or iliac crest autograft, in a randomised controlled trial using 45 patients (3 groups of 15 patients). Osteotomy was secured with titanium spacer plate and non-locking titanium screws (Dynafix VS Osteotomy system, Biomet, Warsaw, IN) in all patients. Stability of the bony healing was evaluated with radiostereometric analysis (RSA) up to 24 months postoperatively. Clinical outcome was evaluated with the knee injury and osteoarthritis outcome score (KOOS). RSA revealed translations and rotations close to zero regardless of bone grafting material, with no statistically significant differences between the groups. Clinically, the group with the injectable calcium phosphate cement had lower quality of life KOOS sub-score at 2 years follow-up. This was statistically significant ($p = 0.047$). Authors have proposed that this might be due to the inflammatory response in the soft tissue from calcium phosphate cement injection. Their study therefore concluded that with a stable implant and 6 weeks of partial weight-bearing, local autografting is sufficient to achieve solid bone consolidation following MOWHTO.

13.4.2 B-TCP vs. No Void Filler vs. Autologous Bone Graft and b-TCP

Jung et al. [21] compared the radiological bone union rate after MOWHTO in three patient groups. Osteotomy gaps were filled with β-tricalcium phosphate (β-TCP) (group A), left unfilled (group B) or autologous bone graft and β-TCP (group C). In all cases, a TomoFix™ plate (Synthes, Oberdorf, Switzerland) was used to stabilise the osteotomy. The mean time for radiological bone union was 8.3 ± 3.1 months in group A, 7.2 ± 3.2 in group B and 3.4 ± 1.5 in group C ($p = 0.001$). There was statistically significant faster bone union in group C. If the opening distance was more than 10 mm, group A united in 8.6 ± 3.6 months, group B in 8.8 ± 3.4 and group C in 3.5 ± 1.7 ($p = 0.001$). IKDC and Lysholm knee scores improved significantly ($p = 0.004$ for IKDC and 0.001 for Lysholm knee scores) in group C when compared to groups A and B at 6-month follow-up. At final follow-up, there was no difference in IKDC and Lysholm knee scores. Less delayed union occurred in group C.

13.4.3 Xenograft vs. bTCP

Maffulli et al. [22] undertook a prospective cohort study using a Puddu plate for MOWHTO, using either bovine xenograft or bTCP. All patients were followed up at 6 weeks and at 3, 6, 12 and 24 months postoperatively. Clinical outcomes were assessed preoperatively and at 24 months postoperatively. They found that all clinical scores improved significantly in both groups after surgery, without any significant difference between the two groups. Immediately after surgery, the HKA angle went from 9.1 ± 5.2° in varus to 3.1 ± 4.8° in valgus ($P = 0.01$) in the xenograft group and from 8.5 ± 5.9° in varus to 3.4 ± 4.2° in valgus ($P = 0.01$) in the tricalcium phosphate group. At the last follow-up, the tricalcium phosphate group showed a significant loss of correction ($P = 0.03$).

13.5 Systematic Reviews and Meta-analyses

Lash et al. [23] performed a systematic review to research this question. Their initial review included 56 peer-reviewed articles and 3033 cases of MOWHTO with a mean patient age of 50 years and mean follow-up period of 42 months. Of the 56 studies included, only 17 reported on time to union of the osteotomy site. The types of fillers used were autograft bone (29.5%), allograft bone (25.9%), tricalcium phosphate (12.6%), calcium phosphate (7.2%), HA/tricalcium phosphate (3.4%), bioglass (1.7%), combined fillers (0.9%), coralline wedge (0.9%) and no filler (17.3%).

Autograft was associated with the shortest mean time to union (3.1 months), followed by allograft bone (3.8 months). Calcium phosphate, tricalcium phosphate and no filler had mean union times of 25 months, 10.6 months and 9 months, respectively. Bioglass was only used in two cases with a mean union time of 4 months.

There was a combined delayed union rate of 2% (60 cases) and 1.4% non-union (43 cases). Delayed/non-union rates were 1.4%, 2.6%, 4.6% and 4.5% for the no filler group, autologous bone graft, allograft bone graft and synthetic bone substitutes, respectively. They concluded that in terms of union timing and overall healing rates, the use of autograft shown statistically significant superiority compared to allograft use. Similarly, the use of allograft showed a statistically significant benefit compared to not using a void filler at all. Comparative rates using autograft or no filler showed no statistically significant benefit.

In terms of loss of correction, interestingly the cases that reported this outcome all used HA/tricalcium phosphate filler and were associated with a mean loss of 4 degrees of correction. This review also noted that the use of locking plates had a mean loss of correction of 2.3° compared to non-locking plates that had a mean loss of 0.5°. However, all cases that used HA/tricalcium phosphate filler were included in the locking plate analysis and thus might be a confounding factor.

Finally HA/tricalcium phosphate use appeared to be associated with a superficial wound infection rate of 6.2% compared to 0.6% with other fillers. However, caution should be noted in analysing this finding as all cases came from a single study.

Han et al. [24] performed a meta-analysis to compare the radiological outcomes of MOWHTO with bone graft (autograft, allograft and synthetic bone) and those without bone graft. The hypotheses were that the use of bone graft would produce superior radiological outcomes. This included 25 studies and 1841 patients who underwent MOWHTO using four different void fillers. Out of 1841 patients, 352 had autograft, 547 had allograft, 541 had synthetic graft and 401 had no void filler. Overall, they reported comparable results in all four void filler options with regard to delayed union, non-union and loss of correction. However, based on their observation, they reported union time of about 3 months for autograft, synthetic graft and no void filler group whereas longer union time over 5 months with allografts. A hinge fracture was found to be a significantly negative prognostic factor to failure of the procedure. With this in mind, one may consider whether a procedure that undergoes a larger correction should be supplemented with a void filler. The authors attempted to extrapolate the data based on osteotomy gap size. They concluded that a void filler of any type is not recommended if the osteotomy is smaller than 14 mm as long as it has been stabilised with a rigid fixation using a locking system.

Another systematic review was performed by Slevin et al. [25]. Of the 1421 MOWHTO included from the 22 studies, 647 underwent MOWHTO using allografts, 367 using synthetic material (β-TCP, hydroxyapatite or combination of both), in 208 no bone void filler and in 199 iliac crest autograft was used. With a mean follow-up of 41 months (range 6 months to 9 years) and mean gap of 9.9 mm, they demonstrated similar results in terms of union rates and loss of correction with or without the use of gap filler. This was irrespective of the type of filler used. They made an important observation that the gap size had direct correlation with the healing time. For gaps less than 9 mm, 90% of the osteotomies had healed within 12 weeks. Based on this observation, they recommended that standard osteotomies with gap around 10 mm can be safely performed without the use of any void filler. They also recommended the use of autograft for osteotomy gaps larger than 10 mm. They observed that when bone grafting was needed, autograft bone provides higher rates of clinical and radiographic union. They also analysed the deep infection and non-union rates. The infection rate was lowest 0.3% in the allograft group, 0.4% in the no filler group followed by 1.1% in both autograft and synthetic group. Non-union rate was lowest 0.4% in the no filler group followed by 0.5% in both autograft and allograft. It was highest 1.1% in the synthetic group. Based on these observations, the authors recommended that the standard MOWTHO procedure, with gaps smaller than 10 mm and a locking plate fixation, should be performed without bone grafting. Furthermore they concluded that the use of synthetic void filler cannot be recommended in opening wedge high tibial osteotomy.

13.6 Discussion

Surgeons demonstrate a wide range of practice with regard to gap filling in open wedge osteotomy. In some European countries, there is constraint around material costs, and in others, the decision depends solely on the surgeon's preference. There is also often great variation between surgeons within the same nation. Behind this sometimes random situation is the lack of strong scientific evidence which would provide the backbone for consensus. Much of the available evidence is based on low numbers in studies which often have a flawed methodology. There are often too many variables in terms of plate design, surgical technique and postoperative rehabilitation running alongside the investigation of void fillers for any clear conclusions to be drawn. There is also an absence of a consistent and reliable standard for the investigation of bone union. What we have, therefore, is a clear requirement for robust level one evidence from larger well-planned studies. Results should yield the evidence for a properly structured guidance document to instruct upon best practice.

As evidenced from a number of papers discussed above, the role of synthetic fillers has been scrutinised, and in the systematic review of Slevin et al. [25] there is clear advice against their use. This should not deter investigators from attempts to discover solutions involving biocomposites, but it is important to recognise the relative value of currently available products and place these in the context of other available alternatives.

When investigating the relative worth of the different gap fillers or indeed the choice to leave the gap empty, it is crucial that we both produce accurate outcome data and importantly that we interpret these data in a clinically relevant fashion. In one study [8], whilst one methodology proved to have a faster bone healing time, the slower healing group had comparatively no adverse outcome. Is it therefore justifiable to promote a technique with a demonstrably quicker healing time even if there is no clinical benefit?

As the practice of osteotomy has advanced over the last two decades in both technology and technique, different questions have started to surface.

- Larger corrections, revision surgery and osteotomies to change the tibial slope as well as in the frontal plane produce a more demanding situation for the surgeon. Hinge fractures which may follow bigger corrections both intraoperatively and postoperatively are now much better understood. Laboratory evidence [6, 7] supports the use of structural support in the osteotomy gap in situations such as these where the mechanical environment may otherwise be suboptimal for good bone healing.
- There is greater interest in osteotomy surgery in older active patients including postmenopausal women which together with other risk factors such as obesity, diabetes and smoking presents the likelihood that bone strength and healing will not always match the ideal standard of a fit 45-year-old male. The requirement therefore exists to investigate the potential for augmenting the healing response to avoid complications such as infection, nonunion or loss of correction.
- Early recovery from osteotomy including the control of pain and swelling [9] is the subject of enquiry regarding the effect of gap filling. The additional benefits of accelerated rehabilitation in single leg correction and even same-sitting bilateral surgery have now become important to explore.

13.7 Conclusion and Considerations for Gap Filling

A large, multicentred randomised controlled trial dedicated to answering specific questions around this subject is now overdue. The opinions of high volume surgeons around Europe do vary significantly but based on limited scientific evidence and current ‘perceived wisdom’, we are led to make the following recommendations for medial opening wedge high tibial osteotomy.

13.8 Our Recommendations

Based on the above-mentioned literature and current expert practice, there is good evidence to suggest that the use of a graft filler for medial opening high tibial osteotomy is appropriate in the following categories.

1. Revision surgery. This can be a result of nonunion of the osteotomy or loss of correction. Commonest causes of loss of correction are either fixation failure or significant breach of the lateral cortex. Autograft remains the filler of choice in the revision scenario for its properties mentioned above.
2. In high-risk patients (high BMI, smokers, diabetics on insulin, steroid use and poor bone quality).
3. Severe deformity needing large correction. The role of a void filler here is twofold. One is to minimise the risk of delayed union and

healing time and second is to maintain structural support to avoid collapse of the lateral cortex. Other coexisting factors will affect decision-making, but gaps of 10 mm and above are appropriate for primary bone grafting.

4. In case of significant disruption of lateral cortex. In such a scenario, this should be identified and addressed intraoperatively with the combination of a use of a filler and augmented fixation.
5. In bilateral opening wedge surgery to augment healing and enable more rapid rehabilitation.
6. In double osteotomy surgery where a closing wedge may provide a suitable graft to transplant to a recipient opening wedge site.
7. In tibial slope changing surgery where a bespoke allograft may safely and robustly support the multiplanar correction until the angle stable plate fixation has been achieved. It may also offer subsequent mechanical support in addition to the plate in such a situation when the hinge has necessarily been destabilised.
8. In patients older than 60 years.

References

1. Brosset T, PAsquier G, Migaud H, Gougeon F. Opening wedge high tibial osteotomy performed without filling the defect but with locking plate fixation (TomofixTM) and early weight bearing: prospective evaluation of bone union, precision and maintenance of correction in 51 cases. Orthop Traumatol Surg Res. 2011;97(7):705–11.
2. Martinez de Albornoz P, Meyes M, Forriol F, Del Buono A, Maffulli N. Opening wedge high tibial osteotomy: plate position and biomechanics of the medial tibial plateau. Knee Surg Sports Traumatol Arthrosc. 2014;22(11):2641–7.
3. Takeuchi R, Bito H, Akamatsu Y, Shiraishi T, Morishita S, Koshino T, Saito T. In vitro stability of open wedge high tibial osteotomy with synthetic bone graft. Knee. 2010;17(3):217–20.
4. Miller BS, Downie B, McDonough EB, Wojtys EM. Complications after medial opening wedge high tibial osteotomy. Arthroscopy. 2009;25(6):639–46.
5. Spahn G. Complications in high tibial (medial opening wedge) osteotomy. Arch Orthop Trauma Surg. 2004;124(10):649–53.
6. Belsey J, Diffo Kaze A, Jobson S, Faulkner J, Maas S, Khakha R, Pape D, Wilson AJ. The biomechanical effects of allograft wedges used for large corrections during medial opening wedge high tibial osteotomy. PLoS One. 2019;14(5):e0216660. https://doi.org/10.1371/journal.pone.0216660.
7. Belsey J, Kaze AD, Jobson S, Faulkner J, Maas S, Khakha R, Wilson AJ, Pape D. Graft materials provide greater static strength to medial opening wedge high tibial osteotomy than when no graft is included. J Exp Orthop. 2019;6:13.
8. Fucentese SF, Tscholl PM, Sutter R, Brucker PU, Meyer DC, Koch PP. Bone autografting in medial open wedge high tibial osteotomy results in improved osseous gap healing on computed tomography, but no functional advantage: a prospective, randomised, controlled trial. Knee Surg Sports Traumatol Arthrosc. 2019;27(9):2951–7. https://doi.org/10.1007/s00167-018-5285-8. {Epub ahead of publication}.
9. Zorzi A, Da Silva H, Muszkat C, Marques L, Cliquet A Jr, Batista de Miranda J. Opening-wedge high tibial osteotomy with and without bone graft. Artif Organs. 2010;35(3):301–7.
10. Akiyama T, Okazaki K, Mawatari T, Ikemura S, Nakamura S. Autologous osteophyte grafting for open wedge high tibial osteotomy. Arthrosc Tech. 2016;5(5):989–95.
11. Seagrave RA, Sojka J, Goodyear A, Munns SW. Utilising reamer irrigator aspirator autograft for opening wedge high tibial osteotomy: a new surgical technique and report of three cases. Int J Surg Case Rep. 2014;5(1):37–42.
12. Marchand LS, Rothberg DL, Kubiak EN, Higgins TF. Is this autograft worth it? The blood loss and transfusion rates associated with reamer irrigator aspirator bone graft harvest. J Orthop Trauma. 2017;31(4):205–9.
13. Hernigou P, Ma W. Open wedge tibial osteotomy with acrylic bone cement as bone substitute. Knee. 2001;8(2):103–10.
14. Roesgen M. Knöcherne Regeneration und Calciumphosphatkeramiken. In: Weller S, Hierholzer G, editors. Traumatologie aktuell. 4th ed. Stuttgart: Thieme; 1997.
15. Kraal T, Mullender M, de Bruine JH, Reinhard R, de Gast A, Kuik DJ, van Roen BJ. Resorbability of rigid beta-tricalcium phosphate wedges in open-wedge high tibial osteotomy: a retrospective radiological study. Knee. 2008;15(3):201–5.
16. Tanaka T, Kumagae Y, Saito M, Chazono M, Komaki H, Kikuchi T, Kitasato S, Marumo K. Bone formation and resorption in patients after implantation of beta-tricalcium phosphate blocks with 60% and 75% porosity in opening-wedge high tibial osteotomy. J Biomed Mater Res B Appl Biomater. 2008;86(2):453–9.
17. Lim HC, Bae JH, Song HR, Teoh SH, Kim HK, Kum DH. High tibial osteotomy using polycaprolactone-tricalcium phosphate polymer wedge in a micro pig model. J Bone Joint Surg Br. 2011;93(1):120–5.

18. Ferner F, Dickschas J, Ostertag H, Poske U, Schwitulla J, HArrer J, Strcker W. Is a synthetic augmentation in medial open wedge high tibial osteotomies superior to no augmentation in terms of bone-healing? Knee. 2016;23(1):2–7.
19. Onodera J, Kondo E, Omizu N, Ueda D, Yagi T, Yasuda K. Beta-tricalcium phosphate shows superior absorption rate and osteoconductivity compared to hydroxyapatite in open-wedge high tibial osteotomy. Knee Surg Sports Traumatol Arthrosc. 2014;22(11):2763–70.
20. Lind-Harsen TB, Lind MC, Nielsen PT, Laursen MB. Open-wedge high tibial osteotomy: RCT 2 years RSA follow-up. J Knee Surg. 2016;29(8):664–72.
21. Jung W, Takeuchi R, Kim D, et al. Faster union rate and better clinical outcomes using autologous bone graft after medial opening wedge high tibial osteotomy. Knee Surg Sports Traumatol Arthrosc. 2019. https://doi.org/10.1007/s00167-019-05463-w.
22. Maffulli N, Loppini M, Longo UG, Denaro V, Olivia F. Bovine xenograft locking Puddu plate versus tricalcium phosphate spacer non-locking plate in opening-wedge high tibial osteotomy: a prospective double-cohort study. Int Orthop. 2013;37(5):819–26.
23. Lash NJ, Feller JA, Batty LM, Wasiak J, Richmond AK. Bone grafts and bone substitutes for opening-wedge osteotomies of the knee: a systematic review. Arthroscopy. 2015;31(4):720–30.
24. Han JH, Kim HJ, Song JG, Yang JH, Bhandare NN, Fernandez AR, Park HJ, Nha KW. Is bone grafting necessary in opening wedge high tibial osteotomy? A meta-analysis of radiological outcomes. Knee Surg Relat Res. 2015;27(4):207–20.
25. Slevin O, Ayeni OR, Hinetrwimmer S, Tischer T, Feucht MJ, Hirschmann MT. The role of bone void fillers in medial opening wedge high tibial osteotomy: a systematic review. Knee Surg Sports Traumatol Arthrosc. 2016;24(11):3584–98.

14 Mobile-Bearing Unis

M. Clarius and L. M. Clarius

14.1 Introduction

Unicompartmental knee arthroplasty (UKA) has many advantages over total knee arthroplasty (TKA) [1–3] including better function, a better feel, better range of motion, higher patient satisfaction, less blood loss, lower infection rate, lower morbidity and even lower mortality [4–6]. Therefore, for many surgeons, UKA is option number one in the treatment of unicompartmental medial or lateral knee arthritis [7].

14.2 Unicompartmental Knee Designs: Fixed- or Mobile-Bearing

When the decision is made for a UKA, surgeons have basically two options of implant designs they can use.

Fixed-bearing designs are more or less anatomical designs consisting of an anatomically shaped metal femoral component in combination with an all-polyethylene tibial component or a metal-backed tibial component with a polyethylene insert.

Mobile-bearing uni knees combine a metal femoral with a metal tibial component. Between them lies an unconstrained mobile bearing made out of polyethylene. The mobile bearing is driven by the femoral component throughout the range of motion and has to move unrestrictedly concerning anterior–posterior translation and rotation inside the knee to work successfully.

For both uni knee designs, a careful patient selection is recommended [8]. The classical indication for UKA is the isolated medial or lateral bone on bone arthritis of the knee with intact medial and lateral collateral ligaments as well as an intact cruciate ligament complex. Ligament deficiency, inflammatory disease and previous high tibial or distal femoral osteotomy are considered as contraindications.

14.3 Fixed- or Mobile-Bearing: Comparative Studies and Meta-analysis

A lot of studies have been undertaken to investigate the difference between the results of mobile-bearing and fixed-bearing UKAs in the literature.

In summary, no significant differences have been found between the two design options concerning quality of life [9], muscle activity and gait [10], survival rate, clinical result [11, 12] or complication rate [13, 14] even in the long term after 15 years [15] and in obese patients [16].

M. Clarius (✉) · L. M. Clarius
Department of Orthopaedic and Trauma Surgery, Vulpius Klinik GmbH, Bad Rappenau, Germany
e-mail: Michael.clarius@vulpiusklinik.de

M. T. Hirschmann et al. (eds.), *ESSKA Instructional Course Lecture Book*,
https://doi.org/10.1007/978-3-662-61264-4_14

Meta-analysis found out that both the designs have similar results and that no essential differences were observed [17, 18]. However, the failure mode between the two designs is different [13]. Polyethylene wear and instability were more common in fixed-bearing implants, whereas pain and bearing dislocation [13] were more common in mobile-bearing implants [19]. Bonutti et al. concluded that the keys to long-term survival of both fixed and mobile-bearing designs in unicompartmental knee arthroplasty are patient selection, surgical technique and surgical experience [20].

14.4 Design of Mobile-Bearing Unis

There are several designs of mobile-bearing uni knees on the market. The first and probably the clinically best documented mobile-bearing uni knee was developed in 1974 by John Goodfellow and John O'Connor in England and is known as the Oxford Uni Knee.

At that time, wear was the main problem of a fixed-bearing uni knee. The anatomical, non-congruent, shape of the femoral component articulating on a flat tibia with a minimum of polyethylene results in high contact stress, and therefore, wear of the polyethylene was inevitable. Both the designers, an orthopaedic surgeon and an engineer, wanted to address this problem "wear" with a spherical femoral component articulating with a mobile, fully congruent meniscal bearing with a flat tibial surface moving on a flat tibial metal component. Despite some significant changes in this implant system, these design features have not changed over the last 45 years. The meniscofemoral interface behaves like "a ball in a socket" and allows the angular movements of flexion-extension, the meniscotibial interface (flat on flat) allows translational movements, and axial rotation is allowed by a combination of translation and spinning movements at both interfaces [21]. In other words, in all positions of knee flexion and knee rotation a fully congruent meniscal bearing transfers the load and shear forces via tibial and femoral component into bone and therefore wear of the mobile bearing is reduced to a minimum.

All other mobile-bearing uni designs use polyradial, more anatomical, femoral components in combination with a flat or slightly curved tibia. In such implants, the concavity on the upper surface of the meniscal bearing must have a radius of a curvature large enough to accommodate the largest radius of the femoral condyle offered in extension and therefore too large to match the smaller radii in flexion. This may result in higher contact stress and consecutive in wear in flexion, because compression forces are greater in flexion.

Moreover, due to limited congruency, rotational forces may lead to impingement and may increase the risk of dislocation.

In most unicompartmental knee systems, the same design is used for the medial and lateral compartment. The Oxford Group reported good clinical and functional results with the Oxford Uni Knee in the lateral compartment; however, with a flat tibia design, the dislocation rate was reported to be 10%. That was the reason to change to a domed tibial plateau shape and a biconcave meniscal bearing in combination with the traditional femoral spherical design to reduce the dislocation rate.

14.5 Clinical Results of Medial Mobile-Bearing UKA

Excellent long-term survival of mobile-bearing UKA have been described in the literature. Bontemps et al. found 96% survival of a polycentric femoral component mobile-bearing UKA after 10 years [22]. The Oxford Group published excellent long-term data with 93% survival in more than 1000 patients operated by 90 surgeons after 10 years and 96% survival in 1000 patients operated by two surgeons after 15 years [23, 24]. While these data came from designer centres and may be judged carefully, several other authors have confirmed the excellent survival in experienced hands. Lim et al. described a 94% survival

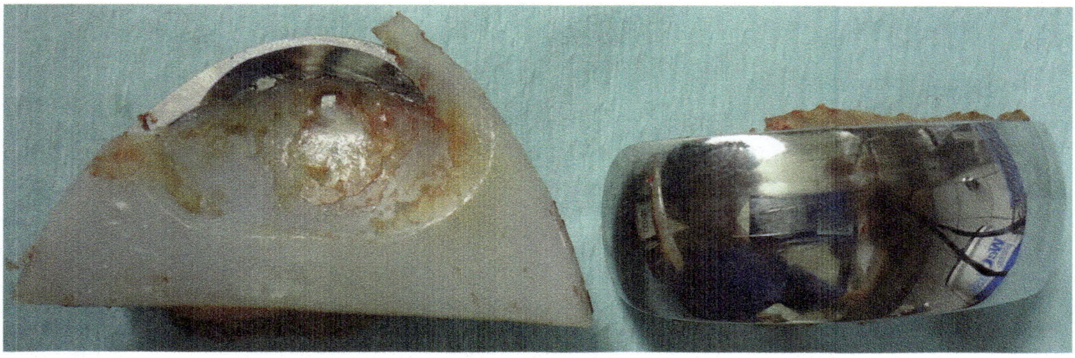

Fig. 14.1 Fixed-bearing UKA components with wear of the polyethylene and metallosis due to the contact of the metal femur and the metal tibial plate

after 10 years [25], Yoshida found 95% survival in 1279 patients after 10 years [26], and Faour-Martin et al. published 95% survival in 416 patients after 10 years [27]. The most impressing data come from Sweden, where Ulf Svard reported a long-term survival of 91% in 683 patients after 20 years [28].

However, registered data from several countries have shown that in general higher revision rates are documented, suggesting that the clinical and surgical experience of the surgeon is key for the success of a UKA.

14.6 Failure Modes

Common reasons for a revision of a uni knee are infection, progression of arthritis, loosening of one of the components, periprosthetic tibial fractures and persistent pain.

Fixed-bearing and mobile-bearing uni knees have different, specific failure modes.

14.7 Wear as a Major Mode of Failure in Fixed-Bearing Designs

Due to the anatomical shape of the fixed-bearing implants, high contact stress is applied on a limited area on the tibia especially in flexion, where the radius of the femoral component is smaller and contact area is limited. This in combination with a thin polyethylene layer on the tibia leads to wear and finally to revision (Fig. 14.1).

Mobile-bearing unis especially the Oxford Uni with the spherical femoral component design and full congruency with the mobile-bearing theoretically should have solved the problem of wear despite the fact that there are two interfaces between the meniscal bearing and the femur and the tibia. Several studies have shown that the theoretical expectation of limited wear has been fulfilled in practice. The wear rate of retrieved bearings of failed Oxford Unis 1–9 years from the implantation was 0.03 mm/year on average [29]. A second study confirmed this data with 0.036 mm/year, 1–13 years on average from the implantation [30].

If unrestricted movement of the meniscal bearing is secured, a wear rate in vivo of 0.01 mm/year was found [31]. However, in case of restricted movement of the meniscal bearing because of bone or cement impingement, wear of the meniscal bearing can be excessive [31, 32].

14.8 Dislocation as a Mode of Failure in Mobile-Bearing Unis

Dislocation of the bearing can only occur in mobile-bearing unis. The incidence of bearing dislocation in the medial side is relatively low,

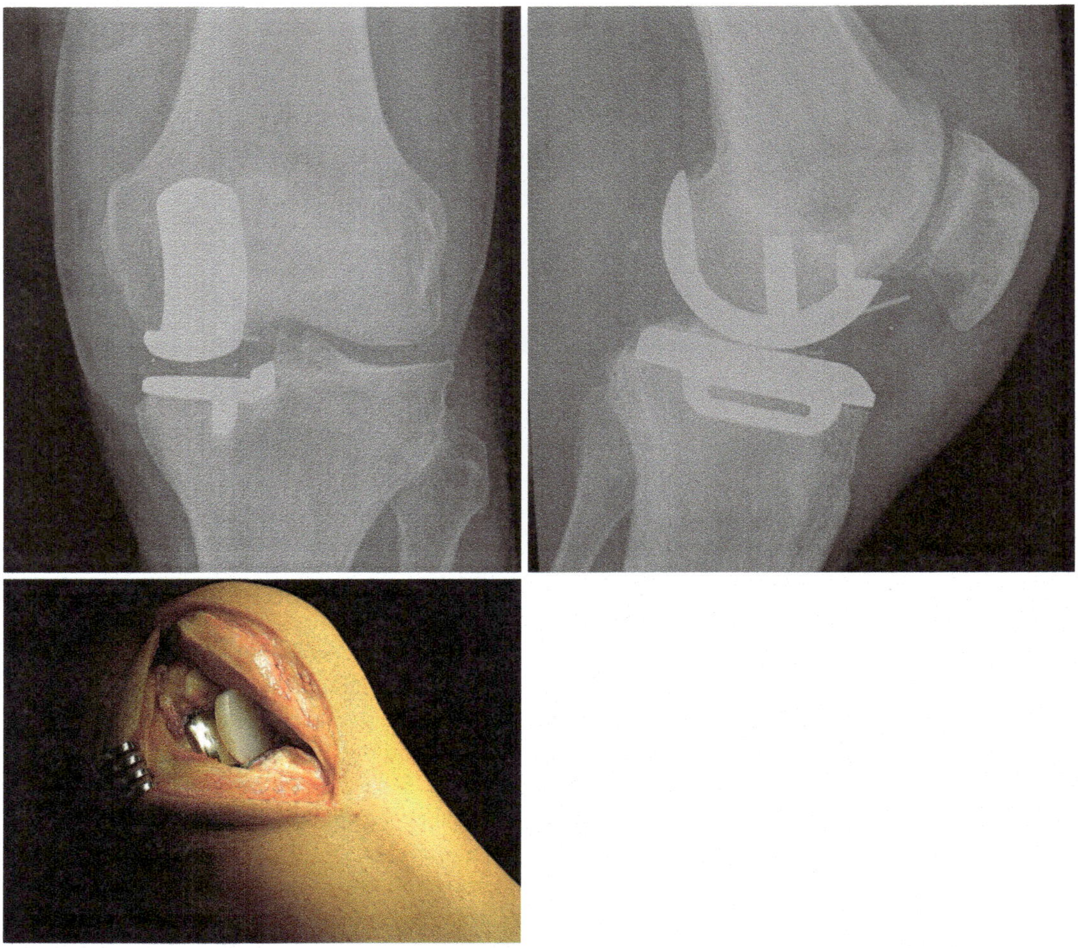

Fig. 14.2 X-ray and intraoperative view of an anterior dislocation of a mobile bearing in medial compartment

but clearly dependant on the experience of the surgeon, because most dislocations are related to technical errors during surgery such as component malposition, gap imbalance [33] and impingement of the bearing [21]. The mobile bearing passively follows the track of the femoral component as it moves anterioposteriorly and mediolaterally relative to the plateau. The limits of the movement are set by the length of the ligaments, and within these limits, the freedom of the bearing to translate in all directions should be unrestricted [21]. Then tensile forces and loads can be transmitted into bone. If the bearing movement is resisted by impingement against bone, cement or the lateral wall of the tibial component, shear stresses develop at the femoral and/or tibial interface and can lead to loosening, dislocation of the bearing and persistent pain [21]. Therefore, a careful surgical technique can prevent this failure mode to a minimum in the medial side. In large series in experienced hands, the rate of bearing dislocation is 0.58 [34, 35]–1% even in the long term [28]. However, higher incidences up to 3.6% are described in the literature [33] (Fig. 14.2).

While the pathology of dislocation of a mobile bearing in the medial side is mostly understood and can therefore be prevented, dislocation of a mobile bearing on the lateral side remains to be a challenge [36] (Fig. 14.3). In combination with

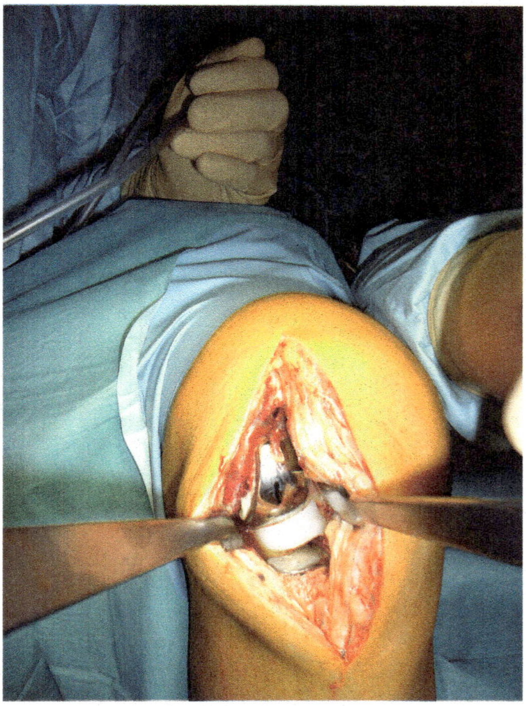

Fig. 14.3 Dislocation of a mobile bearing in the lateral knee. The bearing slipped up the medial wall

the flat tibia medial Oxford UKA design implanted on the lateral side, high dislocation rates of 10% after years have been reported in the literature [37]. The reason is a more complex motion in the lateral compartment in flexion with a very individual amount of internal rotation relative to the femur and that the lateral collateral ligament can be very loose in flexion. A domed tibia design in combination with a biconcave mobile bearing was developed to address the problem of dislocation, and the first published short-term results were encouraging because the reported dislocation rate was minimised compared to the flat tibia design with excellent clinical outcome [37–40]. However, the problem of dislocation was not solved. Dislocations occurred also in the longer term. A multicentre study of 363 consecutive patients who underwent lateral UKA showed a high revision rate of 15% at 5 years with dislocation of the bearing (8.5% after 5 years) as a main reason for implant failure with the domed design. The authors concluded that despite the observed good functional and clinical results and the high patient satisfaction rate in this series, they decided to discontinue to use the domed mobile-bearing UKA instead of a fixed bearing component [41].

14.9 Progression of Patellofemoral Arthrosis as a Mode of Failure in Fixed-Bearing Unis

Fixed-bearing unis aim to reconstruct the anatomical shape of the femoral condyle. A perfect surgical technique should place the metal component in line with the intact cartilage of the condyle. An overhang must be avoided to prevent an impingement of the femoral component with the patella in flexion. Impingement can happen when the femoral component is placed in flexion or prominent due to anterior placement [42]. But patellar impingement can also occur due to degeneration of the femoral cartilage as a matter of time in fixed-bearing uni knees and can cause clinical problems and pain and can lead to revision. In a study by Berger et al., patellar impingement and development of a patellofemoral arthrosis were the main reasons for revision in a 15-year follow-up after a fixed-bearing uni [43]. The authors observed a progression of the patellofemoral arthrosis with time. After a 10-year period of time, 1.6% of the patients showed clinical signs and 6% showed radiological changes of patellofemoral arthrosis, whereas after 15 years 10% of the patients were clinically symptomatic and showed 26% radiological signs of arthrosis. In the series of Hernigou, 29% of the patients showed patellofemoral arthrosis after 14 years [42] (Fig. 14.4).

To our knowledge, progressive arthrosis in the patellofemoral joint has not been described in patients who underwent mobile-bearing UKA as a major problem. Because the spherical femoral component usually ends up in an underhang and leaves a gap that is filled with fibrous tissue [21], patellar impingement and consecutive patellofemoral arthrosis do not seem to be a problem in mobile-bearing UKA.

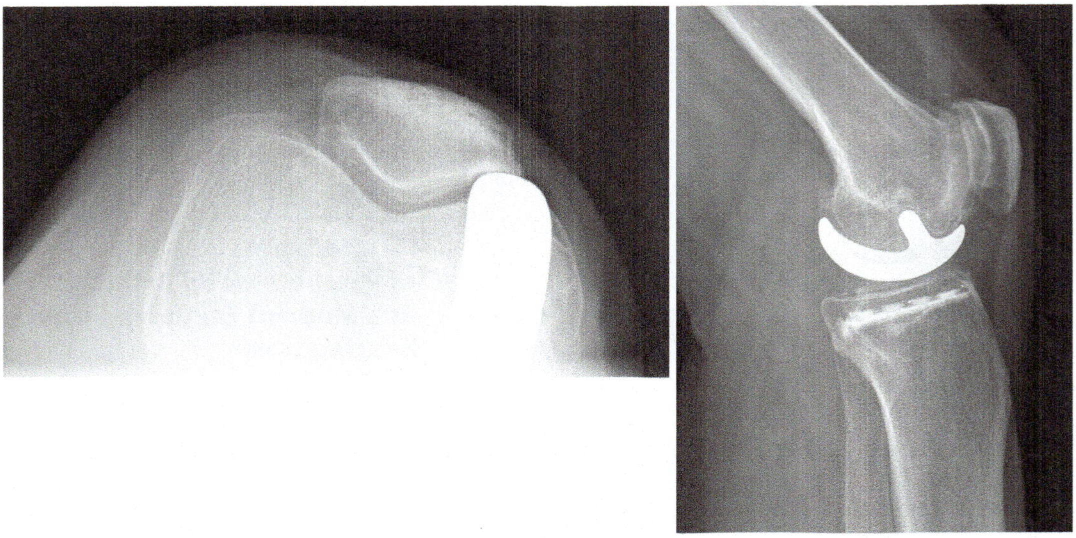

Fig. 14.4 A significant bone defect of the patella due to patellofemoral impingement of a fixed-bearing UKA

14.10 Summary

- Both fixed- and mobile-bearing uni knees have excellent clinical long-term survival in experienced hands.
- Wear is inevitable in fixed-bearing unis due to a small contact area of the anatomical shape of the femur and high contact stress on a thin polyethylene tibia.
- Wear is not a problem in mobile-bearing unis as long as unrestricted movement of the bearing is secured.
- Dislocation of the meniscal bearing can be a problem of mobile-bearing unis and can be prevented by a proper surgical technique.
- Progressive patellofemoral arthrosis is a problem in the second decade after fixed-bearing unis and a common reason for revision, but not after mobile-bearing unis.

References

1. Beard DJ, Davies LJ, Cook JA, MacLennan G, Price A, Kent S, et al. The clinical and cost-effectiveness of total versus partial knee replacement in patients with medial compartment osteoarthritis (TOPKAT): 5-year outcomes of a randomised controlled trial. Lancet. 2019;394:746–56.
2. Murray DW, Liddle AD, Dodd CA, Pandit H. Unicompartmental knee arthroplasty: is the glass half full or half empty? Bone Joint J. 2015;97-B:3–8.
3. Walker T, Gotterbarm T, Bruckner T, Merle C, Streit MR. Total versus unicompartmental knee replacement for isolated lateral osteoarthritis: a matched-pairs study. Int Orthop. 2014;38:2259–64.
4. Liddle AD, Judge A, Pandit H, Murray DW. Adverse outcomes after total and unicompartmental knee replacement in 101,330 matched patients: a study of data from the National Joint Registry for England and Wales. Lancet. 2014;384:1437–45.
5. Liddle AD, Pandit H, Judge A, Murray DW. Optimal usage of unicompartmental knee arthroplasty: a study of 41,986 cases from the National Joint Registry for England and Wales. Bone Joint J. 2015;97-B:1506–11.
6. Liddle AD, Pandit H, Judge A, Murray DW. Patient-reported outcomes after total and unicompartmental knee arthroplasty: a study of 14,076 matched patients from the National Joint Registry for England and Wales. Bone Joint J. 2015;97-B:793–801.
7. Aldinger PR, Clarius M, Murray DW, Goodfellow JW, Breusch SJ. Medial unicompartmental knee replacement using the "Oxford Uni" meniscal bearing knee. Orthopade. 2004;33:1277–83.
8. Berend KR, Berend ME, Dalury DF, Argenson JN, Dodd CA, Scott RD. Consensus statement on indications and contraindications for medial unicompartmental knee arthroplasty. J Surg Orthop Adv. 2015;24:252–6.
9. Biau DJ, Greidanus NV, Garbuz DS, Masri BA. No difference in quality-of-life outcomes after mobile and fixed-bearing medial unicompartmental knee replacement. J Arthroplast. 2013;28:220–226.e221.
10. Catani F, Benedetti MG, Bianchi L, Marchionni V, Giannini S, Leardini A. Muscle activity around

the knee and gait performance in unicompartmental knee arthroplasty patients: a comparative study on fixed- and mobile-bearing designs. Knee Surg Sports Traumatol Arthrosc. 2012;20:1042–8.
11. Neufeld ME, Albers A, Greidanus NV, Garbuz DS, Masri BA. A comparison of mobile and fixed-bearing unicompartmental knee arthroplasty at a minimum 10-year follow-up. J Arthroplast. 2018;33:1713–8.
12. Whittaker JP, Naudie DD, McAuley JP, McCalden RW, MacDonald SJ, Bourne RB. Does bearing design influence midterm survivorship of unicompartmental arthroplasty? Clin Orthop Relat Res. 2010;468:73–81.
13. Ko YB, Gujarathi MR, Oh KJ. Outcome of unicompartmental knee arthroplasty: a systematic review of comparative studies between fixed and mobile bearings focusing on complications. Knee Surg Relat Res. 2015;27:141–8.
14. Smith TO, Hing CB, Davies L, Donell ST. Fixed versus mobile bearing unicompartmental knee replacement: a meta-analysis. Orthop Traumatol Surg Res. 2009;95:599–605.
15. Parratte S, Pauly V, Aubaniac JM, Argenson JN. No long-term difference between fixed and mobile medial unicompartmental arthroplasty. Clin Orthop Relat Res. 2012;470:61–8.
16. Kuyucu E, Bulbul AM, Kara A, Say F, Erdil M. Which unicondylar prosthesis is better in the mid-term in obese patients: fixed or mobile? Acta Orthop Belg. 2018;84:257–61.
17. Cao Z, Niu C, Gong C, Sun Y, Xie J, Song Y. Comparison of fixed-bearing and mobile-bearing unicompartmental knee arthroplasty: a systematic review and meta-analysis. J Arthroplasty. 2019;34(12):3114–3123.e3. https://doi.org/10.1016/j.arth.2019.07.005.
18. Peersman G, Stuyts B, Vandenlangenbergh T, Cartier P, Fennema P. Fixed-versus mobile-bearing UKA: a systematic review and meta-analysis. Knee Surg Sports Traumatol Arthrosc. 2015;23:3296–305.
19. Cheng T, Chen D, Zhu C, Pan X, Mao X, Guo Y, et al. Fixed-versus mobile-bearing unicondylar knee arthroplasty: are failure modes different? Knee Surg Sports Traumatol Arthrosc. 2013;21:2433–41.
20. Bonutti PM, Dethmers DA. Contemporary unicompartmental knee arthroplasty: fixed vs mobile bearing. J Arthroplast. 2008;23:24–7.
21. Goodfellow J, O'Connor J, Dodd C, Murray DW, editors. Unicompartmental knee arthroplasty with the Oxford knee. Oxford: Oxford University Press; 2006.
22. Schlueter-Brust K, Kugland K, Stein G, Henckel J, Christ H, Eysel P, et al. Ten year survivorship after cemented and uncemented medial Uniglide(R) unicompartmental knee arthroplasties. Knee. 2014;21:964–70.
23. Bottomley N, Jones LD, Rout R, Alvand A, Rombach I, Evans T, et al. A survival analysis of 1084 knees of the Oxford unicompartmental knee arthroplasty: a comparison between consultant and trainee surgeons. Bone Joint J. 2016;98-B:22–7.
24. Pandit H, Hamilton TW, Jenkins C, Mellon SJ, Dodd CA, Murray DW. The clinical outcome of minimally invasive phase 3 Oxford unicompartmental knee arthroplasty: a 15-year follow-up of 1000 UKAs. Bone Joint J. 2015;97-B:1493–500.
25. Lim HC, Bae JH, Song SH, Kim SJ. Oxford phase 3 unicompartmental knee replacement in Korean patients. J Bone Joint Surg Br. 2012;94:1071–6.
26. Yoshida K, Tada M, Yoshida H, Takei S, Fukuoka S, Nakamura H. Oxford phase 3 unicompartmental knee arthroplasty in Japan—clinical results in greater than one thousand cases over ten years. J Arthroplast. 2013;28:168–71.
27. Faour-Martin O, Valverde-Garcia JA, Martin-Ferrero MA, Vega-Castrillo A, de la Red Gallego MA, Suarez de Puga CC, et al. Oxford phase 3 unicondylar knee arthroplasty through a minimally invasive approach: long-term results. Int Orthop. 2013;37:833–8.
28. Price AJ, Svard U. A second decade lifetable survival analysis of the Oxford unicompartmental knee arthroplasty. Clin Orthop Relat Res. 2011;469:174–9.
29. Argenson JN, O'Connor JJ. Polyethylene wear in meniscal knee replacement. A one to nine-year retrieval analysis of the Oxford knee. J Bone Joint Surg Br. 1992;74:228–32.
30. Psychoyios V, Crawford RW, O'Connor JJ, Murray DW. Wear of congruent meniscal bearings in unicompartmental knee arthroplasty: a retrieval study of 16 specimens. J Bone Joint Surg Br. 1998;80:976–82.
31. Price AJ. Medial meniscal bearing unicompartmental arthroplasty: wear, mechanics and clinical outcome. DPhil Thesis, University of Oxford; 2003.
32. Price AJ, Short A, Kellett C, Beard D, Gill H, Pandit H, et al. Ten-year in vivo wear measurement of a fully congruent mobile bearing unicompartmental knee arthroplasty. J Bone Joint Surg Br. 2005;87:1493–7.
33. Bae JH, Kim JG, Lee SY, Lim HC, In Y, Group MS. Epidemiology of bearing dislocations after mobile-bearing unicompartmental knee arthroplasty: multicenter analysis of 67 bearing dislocations. J Arthroplasty. 2020;35(1):265–71. https://doi.org/10.1016/j.arth.2019.08.004.
34. Mohammad HR, Strickland L, Hamilton TW, Murray DW. Long-term outcomes of over 8,000 medial Oxford phase 3 unicompartmental knees-a systematic review. Acta Orthop. 2018;89:101–7.
35. Pandit H, Jenkins C, Gill HS, Barker K, Dodd CA, Murray DW. Minimally invasive Oxford phase 3 unicompartmental knee replacement: results of 1000 cases. J Bone Joint Surg Br. 2011;93:198–204.
36. Walker T, Aldinger PR, Streit MR, Gotterbarm T. Lateral unicompartmental knee arthroplasty—a challenge. Oper Orthop Traumatol. 2017;29:17–30.
37. Weston-Simons JS, Kendrick BJ, Mentink MJ, Pandit H, Gill HS, Murray DW. An analysis of dislocation of the domed Oxford lateral unicompartmental knee replacement. Knee. 2014;21:304–9.
38. Streit MR, Walker T, Bruckner T, Merle C, Kretzer JP, Clarius M, et al. Mobile-bearing lateral unicompartmental knee replacement with the Oxford domed tibial component: an independent series. J Bone Joint Surg Br. 2012;94:1356–61.

39. Weston-Simons JS, Pandit H, Gill HS, Jackson WF, Price AJ, Dodd CA, et al. The management of mobile bearing dislocation in the Oxford lateral unicompartmental knee replacement. Knee Surg Sports Traumatol Arthrosc. 2011;19:2023–6.
40. Weston-Simons JS, Pandit H, Kendrick BJ, Jenkins C, Barker K, Dodd CA, et al. The mid-term outcomes of the Oxford domed lateral unicompartmental knee replacement. Bone Joint J. 2014;96-B:59–64.
41. Walker T, Zahn N, Bruckner T, Streit MR, Mohr G, Aldinger PR, et al. Mid-term results of lateral unicondylar mobile bearing knee arthroplasty: a multicentre study of 363 cases. Bone Joint J. 2018;100-B:42–9.
42. Hernigou P, Deschamps G. Patellar impingement following unicompartmental arthroplasty. J Bone Joint Surg Am. 2002;84:1132–7.
43. Berger RA, Meneghini RM, Sheinkop MB, Della Valle CJ, Jacobs JJ, Rosenberg AG, et al. (2004) The progression of patellofemoral arthrosis after medial unicompartmental replacement: results at 11 to 15 years. Clin Orthop Relat Res; https://doi.org/10.1097/01.blo.0000147700.89433.a592-99.

Reconstructions with Tibial Slings. When and How?

15

Pablo E. Gelber

15.1 Introduction

Several surgical techniques have been described to treat posterolateral corner (PLC) injuries. These include advancement of the osseous attachment of the arquate ligament complex [1], proximal advancement of the posterolateral complex [2], biceps tenodesis [3], and tibial sling procedures [4]. More recently, in an attempt to address these injuries with a more anatomic perspective, other techniques have been described. Currently, the two more common groups of PLC reconstructions are considered those involving tunnels in the fibular head [5–7], and those combining this transfibular tunnel with a tibial sling [8, 9].

PLC reconstructions with only with tibial slings have shown similar results comparing to those with isolated transfibular tunnels in order to restore rotational stability at both 30 and 90° of knee flexion [10]. In this study, there was a trend of the fibular-based technique to show slightly more residual rotatory laxity from an objective point of view. Thus, a tibial sling is at least as efficient as a transfibular tunnel to address rotational instability in PLC injuries. The tibial sling can then be performed alone, or concomitantly with a transfibular tunnel technique.

P. E. Gelber (✉)
Department of Orthopaedic Surgery, Hospital de la Santa Creu I Sant Pau, Universitat Autònoma de Barcelona, Barcelona, Spain

Department of Orthopedic Surgery and Traumatology, ICATME-Hospital Universitari Dexeus, Universitat Autònoma de Barcelona, Barcelona, Spain
e-mail: personal@drgelber.com

15.2 Anatomic and Biomechanics Aspects

The static stability of the PLC is mainly provided by the fibular collateral ligament (FCL) and the popliteus muscle–tendon complex [11]. This popliteus complex provides not only static, but also dynamic stability to the knee primarily in response to external tibial rotation [11]. The popliteus complex comprises basically the popliteus muscle and the popliteofibular ligament (PFL). The popliteus muscle originates from the posteromedial aspect of the proximal tibia. The muscle gives rise to the popliteus tendon in the PLC. The popliteus tendon averages 55 mm. It continues proximally through the popliteal hiatus at which point became intra-articular to insert onto the lateral femoral condyle. The insertion is found at the most anterior 1/5 of the popliteus sulcus of the femur; 18.5 mm anterior-inferior from the femoral insertion of the FCL [12]. As the tendon courses into the popliteal hiatus (also known as the bare area of the lateral meniscus), it attaches to the lateral meniscus mainly via the anteroinferior and the posterosuperior popliteomeniscal fascicles, as described by Stäubli and

M. T. Hirschmann et al. (eds.), *ESSKA Instructional Course Lecture Book*,
https://doi.org/10.1007/978-3-662-61264-4_15

Birrer [13]. They are important in providing dynamic stability to the lateral meniscus and preventing medial entrapment of the lateral meniscus with functional varus forces to the knee [11]. The PFL, on the other side, originates at the popliteus musculo-tendinous junction of the popliteus muscle, just distal to the popliteomeniscal fascicles. It courses distally and laterally to attach to the medial edge of the fibular head, 1.6 mm distal to the tip of its fibular styloid process [12] The PFL is a static stabilizer resisting varus, external rotation and posterior tibial translation. It is relatively isometric and can remain functional through a full range of motion [12]. In contrast, the area from the posterolateral corner of the tibia (region of attachment for popliteus tibial sling techniques) to the lateral femoral epicondyle is only tensioned near full extension. In a normal situation, an intact popliteus muscle belly tensions this portion of the PT. This explains why it is so important to include tissue in the position of the PFL when reconstructing the PLC.

15.3 When? Indications

A tibial sling procedure is a more aggressive, demanding, and time-consuming technique comparing to an only fibular-based technique. Therefore, a tibial sling should only be performed for the following indications:

- Grade C Fanelli PLC injuries [14]. These are the most severe cases of PLC injuries. It involves not only the popliteus complex and FCL, but also both cruciate ligaments and the posterolateral capsule. It could also include avulsions of the biceps tendon and other soft tissue or bony injuries. Leaving most of the rotational stability in such tremendous injuries to a single graft within the fibular tunnel might not be enough in most cases. It can lead not only to persistent or recurrent instability, but also to fibular head fractures. Then, it is recommended a stronger construction where the graft introduced in the fibular head is backed up by a tibial sling. The Laprade technique [8] anatomically reconstructs the FCL and also adds a tibial sling graft to fix the PFL as well as the reconstructed popliteus tendon. Similarly, the Lee technique [9] also use tibial and fibular tunnels. However, it reconstructs the popliteus complex more anatomically. While in the Laprade technique the PFL reconstruction is in fact a tibiofibular ligament, the Lee technique uses a split Achilles tendon to independently reconstruct the PFL and the popliteus tendon.
- In primary cases with fibular head fractures or iatrogenic intraoperative fracture of the fibular head. In order to independently address the fibular head fixation and the soft-tissue reconstruction. As commented before, this isolated tibial sling has shown to achieve similar objective results than a fibular-based technique in terms of restoring the rotational stability to the knee [10].
- PLC revision surgeries where a fibular-based technique has already failed. In these cases, a transfibular tunnel can be performed again. But it seems more reasonable to perform a tibial sling, instead. This can be done alone or in combination with another fibular tunnel.
- In those cases with disruption of the proximal tibiofibular joint in grade B Fanelli's PCL injuries [14].

15.4 How? Surgical Pearls

A well-padded tourniquet on the proximal thigh of the operative extremity, although not essential, is recommended. The patient is placed in the supine position on the operating room table. A high lateral post is used to stabilize the lower extremity. The injured knee is flexed approximately 60° and maintained with a foot bump.

Although mini-open techniques or arthroscopically assisted techniques for PLC reconstructions have been described [15], these are not the most appropriate for techniques including a tibial sling.

Initial lateral exposure is made through a gentle hockey stick incision extending from the midlateral aspect of the distal thigh over the lateral femoral epicondyle. This is done parallel to the posterior aspect of the iliotibial band. Distally, it goes either toward Gerdy's tubercle if an isolated tibial sling technique is being performed, or midway between the Gerdy's tubercle and the fibular head, if concomitant transtibial and transfibular tunnels are going to be performed.

Following the most popular surgical approach to PLC of the knee described by Terry and LaPrade [16], a first fascial incision posterior to the biceps tendon is performed. In all this cases, exposing the common peroneal nerve is recommended. It can be just left exposed or, better yet, it can be marked and protected by a rubber patch during the surgical procedure. In those technique where only a fibular tunnel is drilled, the fascial incision can be done anterior to the biceps tendon. Then, the peroneal nerve does not have to be specifically dissected, because the biceps tendon already protects it from being injured.

Next, an incision through the fascia of the lateral head of the gastrocnemius muscle allows to open a window to the posterior aspect of the lateral tibial plateau.

A thin membrane exists between the FCL and the biceps tendon. It is sometimes difficult to reach the area and the fibular head might challenge a correct positioning of the tibial guide. The tunnel should exit the posterior tibia 15 mm below the joint line coming through the lateral tibia from a point just medial to the Gerdy's tubercle (Figs. 15.1 and 15.2). Although there are already some specific guides for this tibial drilling, an ACL tibial guide can also be used (Fig. 15.3). After the guide pin is introduced, a cannulated reamer of proper diameter is advanced. Subsequently, a suture is passed with the help of a suture shuttle though the tunnel to facilitate graft passage. Once the soft-tissue graft has been introduced from posterior to anterior following the specific surgical technique, it is finally fixed with an interference screw. Alternatively, a staple or button in the anterolateral tibia can also be used.

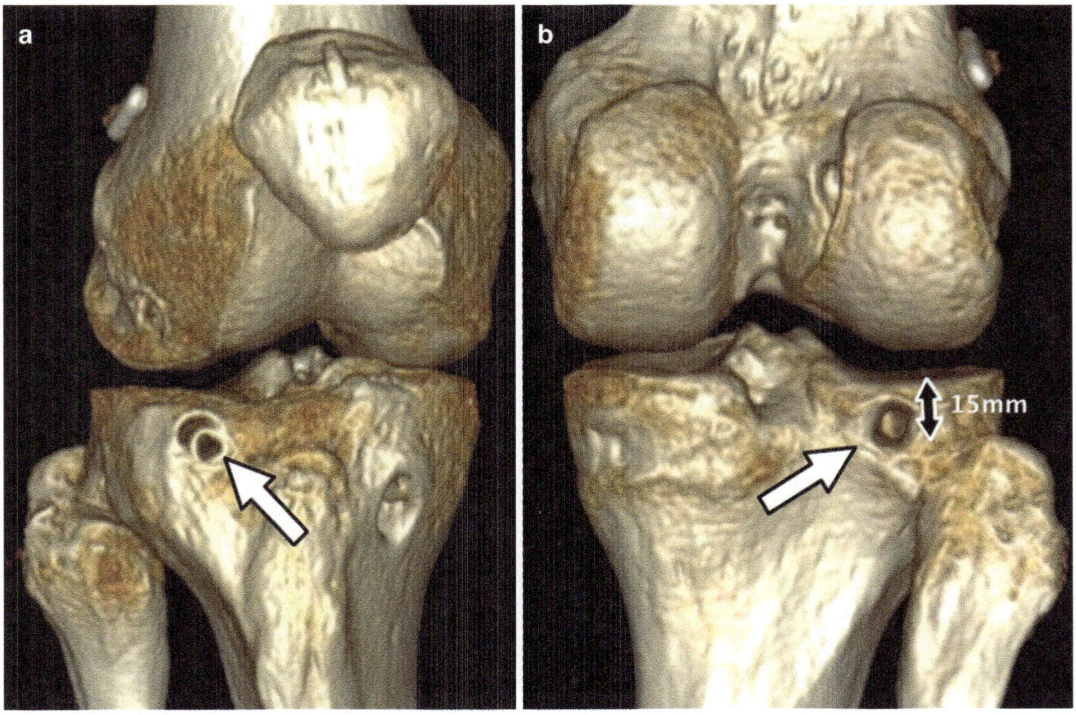

Fig. 15.1 Postoperative 3D CT scan of a right knee. (**a**) anterior view; the entry point of the tibial tunnel (arrow) is seen right medial to Gerdy's tubercle. (**b**) posterior view; the exit of the tibial tunnel (white arrow) is medial to the fibular head and 15 mm distal to the joint line (black arrow)

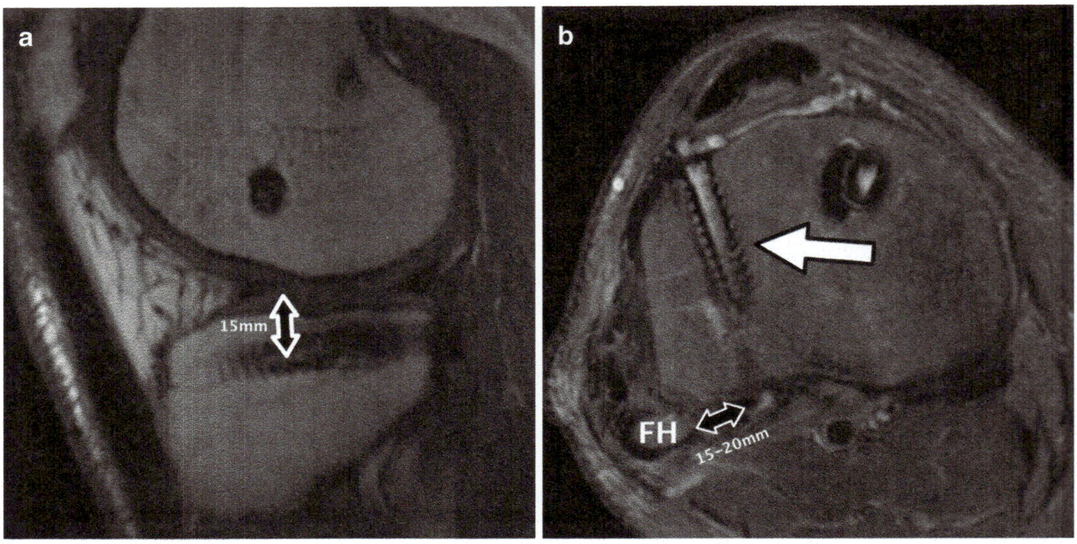

Fig. 15.2 MRI of a right knee after a PLC including a tibial sling. (**a**) sagittal view; the graft and interference screw are seen in the antero-posterior tibial tunnel 15 mm distal to the joint line (arrow). (**b**) axial view; The interference screw fixing the soft-tissue graft within the tibial tunnel is seen; The tunnel is aiming 15–20 mm medial (black arrow) to the posteromedial border of the fibular head (FH)

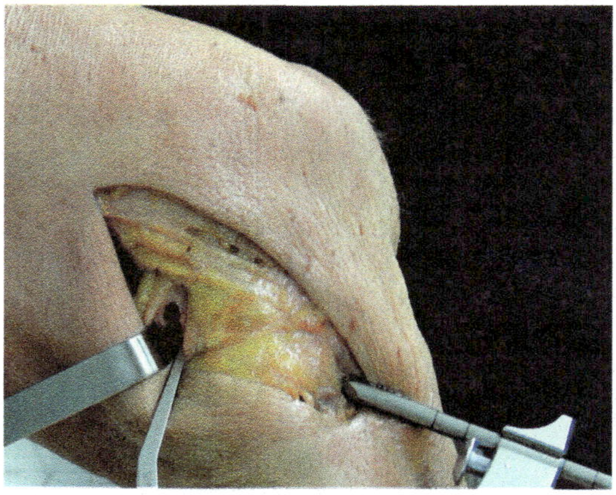

Fig. 15.3 Right knee in a cadaveric specimen. The tibial tunnel can be easily performed with the help of a standard ACL tibial guide. The entry point has to be placed medially to Gerdy's tubercle in the anterolateral aspect of the proximal tibia. The exit point has to be located 15 mm medial to the fibular head y 15 mm distal to the joint line in the posterolateral aspect of the proximal tibia

15.5 Conclusions

A reconstruction of the PLC with techniques including tibial tunnels, restore at least as efficiently the rotational stability as those which are exclusively fibular based. Among the several techniques than have been described to addressed PLC injuries, those including a tibial sling find a crucial role when drilling a tunnel in the fibular head might be a challenge (isolated tibial sling), in revision cases (isolated or combined with a fibular tunnel), and in the most severe injuries (Fanelli Grade C, combined with a fibular tunnel).

References

1. Hughston JC, Jacobson KE. Chronic posterolateral rotatory instability of the knee. J Bone Joint Surg Am. 1985;67:351–9.
2. Noyes FR, Barber-Westin SD. Surgical restoration to treat chronic deficiency of the posterolateral complex and cruciate ligaments of the knee joint. Am J Sports Med. 1996;24:415–26.
3. Fanelli GC, Giannotti BF, Edson CJ. Arthroscopically assisted combined posterior cruciate ligament/posterior lateral complex reconstruction. Arthroscopy. 1996;12:521–30.
4. Albright JP, Brown AW. Management of chronic posterolateral rotatory instability of the knee: surgical technique for the posterolateral corner sling procedure. Instr Course Lect. 1998;47:369–78.
5. Arciero RA. Anatomic posterolateral corner reconstruction. Arthroscopy. 2005;21:1147.
6. Zhang H, Feng H, Hong L, Wang X, Zhang J. Popliteofibular ligament reconstruction for

posterolateral external rotation instability of the knee. Knee Surg Traumatol Arthrosc. 2009;17:1070–7.
7. Larson RV. Isometry of the lateral collateral and popliteofibular ligaments and techniques for reconstruction using a free semitendinosus tendon graft. Op Techniques for Sport Med. 2001;9:84–90.
8. LaPrade RF, Johansen S, Wentorf FA, Engebretsen L, Esterberg JL, Tso A. An analysis of an anatomical posterolateral knee reconstruction: an in vitro biomechanical study and development of a surgical technique. Am J Sports Med. 2004;32:1405–14.
9. Lee MC, Park YK, Lee SH, Jo H, Seong SC. Posterolateral reconstruction using split Achilles tendon allograft. Arthroscopy. 2003;19:1043–9.
10. Jung YB, Jung HJ, Kim SJ, Park SJ, Song KS, Lee YS, Lee SH. Posterolateral corner reconstruction for posterolateral rotatory instability combined with posterior cruciate ligament injuries: comparison between fibular tunnel and tibial tunnel techniques. Knee Surg Sports Traumatol Arthrosc. 2008;16:239–48.
11. Sanchez AR 2nd, Sugalski MT, LaPrade RF. Anatomy and biomechanics of the lateral side of the knee. Sports Med Arthrosc Rev. 2006;14:2–11.
12. LaPrade RF, Ly TV, Wentorf FA, Engenretsen L. The posterolateral attachments of the knee: a qualitative and quantitative morphologic analysis of the fibular collateral ligament, popliteus tendon, popliteofibular ligament, and lateral gastrocnemius tendon. Am J Sports Med. 2003;31:854–60.
13. Staubli HU, Birrer S. The popliteus tendon and its fascicles at the popliteal hiatus: gross anatomy and functional arthroscopic evaluation with and without anterior cruciate ligament deficiency. Arthroscopy. 1990;6:209–20.
14. Fanelli GC, Larson RV. Practical management of posterolateral instability of the knee. Arthroscopy. 2002;18:1–8.
15. Li Y, Zhang H, Zhang J, Li X, Zheng T, Zhang Z, Feng H. The clinical outcome of arthroscopic versus open popliteal tendon reconstruction combined with posterior cruciate ligament reconstruction in patients with type a posterolateral rotational instability. Arthroscopy. 2019;35:2402–9.
16. Terry GC, LaPrade RF. The posterolateral aspect of the knee. Anatomy and surgical approach. Am J Sports Med. 1996;24:732–9.

Arthroscopic Capsulolabral Repair 16

Francesc Soler

The glenohumeral stability is the result of the cooperation of multiple anatomical structures: capsule, ligaments, tendons, bone morphology, and labrum. Each of these contributes in preventing joint dislocation in a sophisticated biomechanical system which allows the shoulder to be the most mobile joint of the human body.

The advent of arthroscopy helped to better understand the normal anatomy, the non-pathological variations and the pathological conditions of these structures.

The labrum is a fibrous structure strongly attached around the glenoid edge (Fig. 16.1) that increases the contact surface between the glenoid itself and the humeral head. The total surface of the head is about four times larger than the glenoid.

The glenoid labrum consists mainly of fibrous cartilage, and some studies showed that is composed of dense fibrous colagen's tissue [1, 2].

The glenoid labrum has multiple effects on the shoulder instability [3]:

- "Chock-block" for limiting translation of the humeral head
- Increase of the "concavity-compression" effect
- Contribute to long head of the biceps anchor stability
- Strength of the inferior glenohumeral ligament.

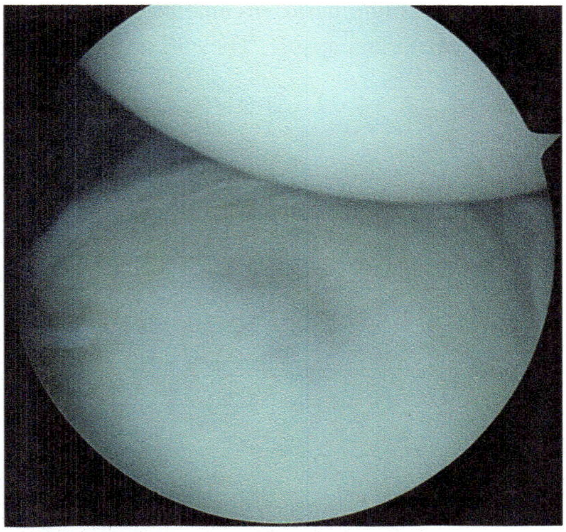

Fig. 16.1 Image from anterosuperior portal. Labrum around the glenoid rim

In order to correctly recognize pathological conditions of the labrum it requires a good knowledge of the normal aspect and also the awareness of the several anatomical variations that may disguise the surgeon:

- Superior meniscoid labrum: The aspect of the superior labrum is somewhat similar to a knee

Electronic supplementary material The online version of this chapter (https://doi.org/10.1007/978-3-662-61264-4_16) contains supplementary material, which is available to authorized users.

F. Soler (✉)
Traumadvance, Terrassa, Barcelona, Spain
e-mail: fsoler@traumadvance.es

M. T. Hirschmann et al. (eds.), *ESSKA Instructional Course Lecture Book*,
https://doi.org/10.1007/978-3-662-61264-4_16

meniscus with triangular cross section and loose edge toward the joint (Fig. 16.2). The glenoid surface is covered by cartilage.

- Anterior sub-labral hole: The glenoid rim has at its anterior part a small notch. The labrum looks detached from the bone without signs of lesion (Fig. 16.3).
- Buford complex: It is a cord-like middle glenohumeral ligament blended with the anteror superior labrum while no labrum is present on the anterior superior glenoid from 12 to 3 o'clock (Fig. 16.4).

There are three distinct thickenings, called anterior glenohumeral ligaments, within the anterior shoulder capsule. They all originate from the anterior and inferior surface of the humeral head and insert on the anterior glenoid.

The function of glenohumeral ligaments has been elucidated in several classic studies [4, 5], which have demonstrated that the stability provided by the ligaments is specific to the position of the arm at the time stress is applied. With the arm in full overhead position with greater abduction and external rotation, the anterior band and axillary pouch of inferior glenohumeral ligament become the most important stabilizers of glenohumeral stability.

The Bankart lesion is the attachment rupture of the anterior band of glenohumeral ligament to the glenoid (Fig. 16.5), allowing the anteroinferior

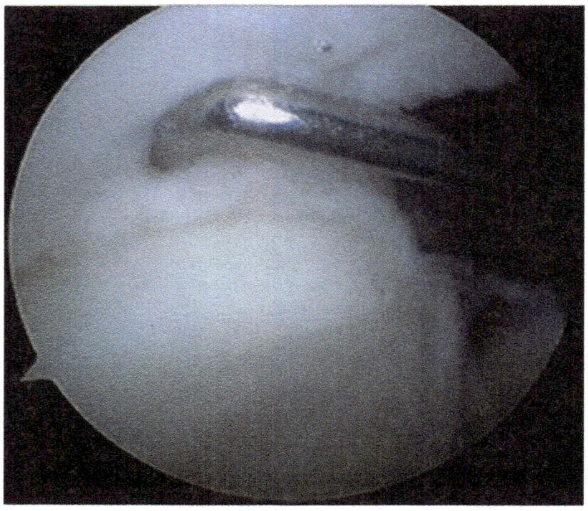

Fig. 16.2 Superior meniscoid labrum

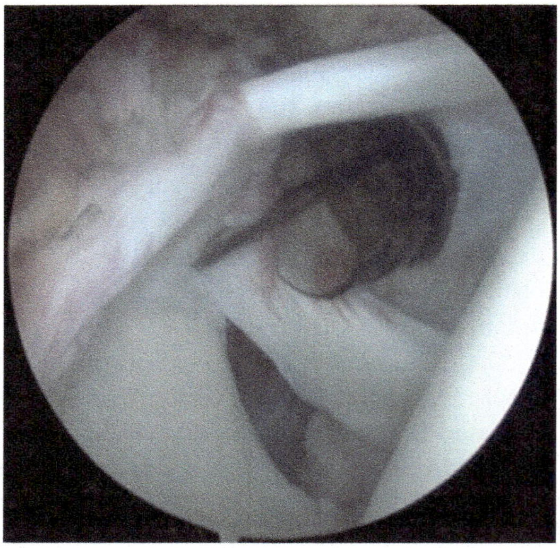

Fig. 16.4 Buford complex

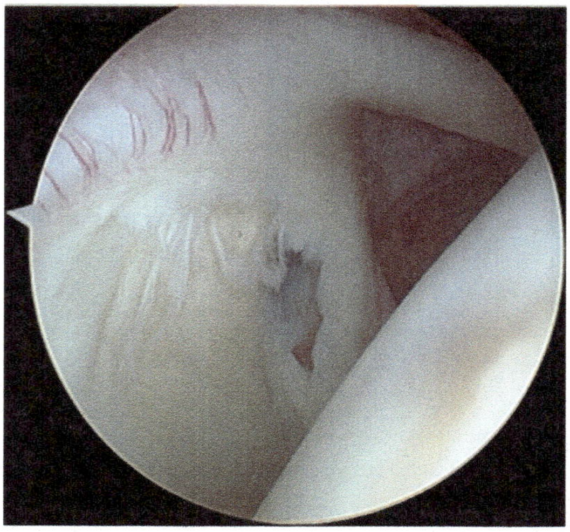

Fig. 16.3 Anterior sub-labral hole

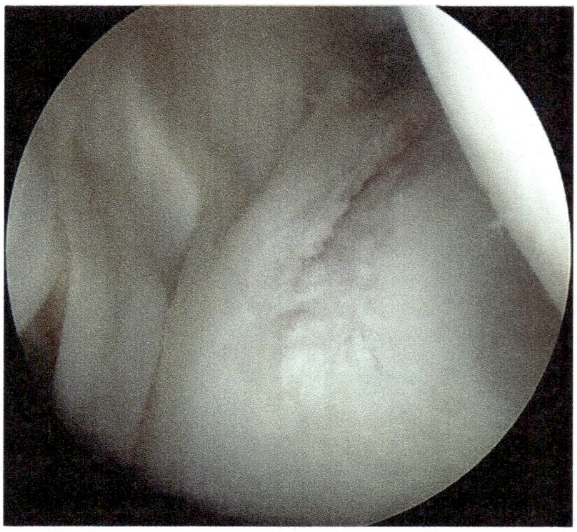

Fig. 16.5 Bankart lesion

displacement of the humeral head, and the glenohumeral joint dislocation. This is the main lesion of the post-traumatic shoulder instability, and it would be necessary to repair it in order to restore the correct glenohumeral stabillity.

16.1 Arthroscopic Surgical Technique

We can perform the arthroscopic procedure with the patient placed in lateral decubitus or beach chair position, depending on the surgeon's preferences.

Following the steps described by Snyder [6], we start de procedure establishing a posterior mid-glenoid portal and introducing the scope, in order to have a first glenohumeral articular view. After, we perform an anterior portar placed in the triangle between the humeral head, the biceps, and the subscapularis tendons. Through this portal, and with the arthroscopic hook, we check all the articular anatomical structures (superior-antero-inferior and posterior labrum, glenoid cartilage, biceps tendon, supraspinatus tendon attachment, and subscapularis tendon). We can identify the Bankart lesion, and define its size.

Afterwards, we perform an anterosuperior portal close to the biceps tendon, and switch the scope from the posterior portal to the anterosuperior portal. The view we obtain form this portal allows us to control the anterior, inferior, and posterior labrum, and also the posterior part of the humeral head. From this portal we can check more accurately the extension of the Bankart lesion, and also have a better control when we separate the labrum from its wrong atachment (Fig. 16.6).

This maneuver has to be very accurate, in order to not damage the labrum. The detachment finishes when we are able to see the subscapularis muscle fibers through it (Fig. 16.7), and put again the labrum at its original place.

Through the anterior portal, we introduce the drill guide in order to make the hole where we'll put the first implant. The first implant will be placed 5 mm superiorly regarding where we'll pass the suture through the labrum and capsule, in order to obtain a capsular plication and a volume reduction of the axillary pouch [7] (Fig. 16.8).

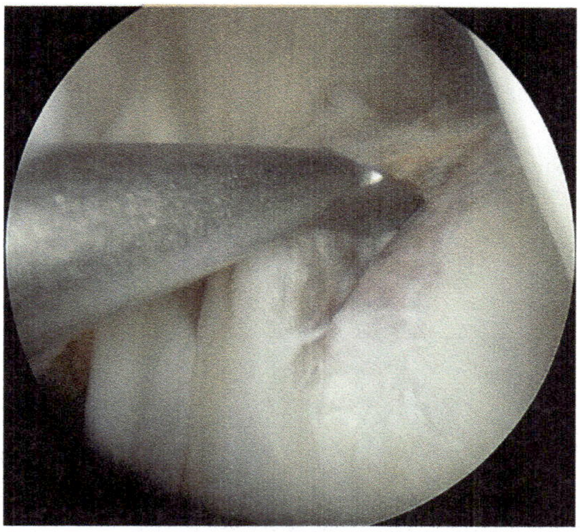

Fig. 16.6 Bankart lesion detachment

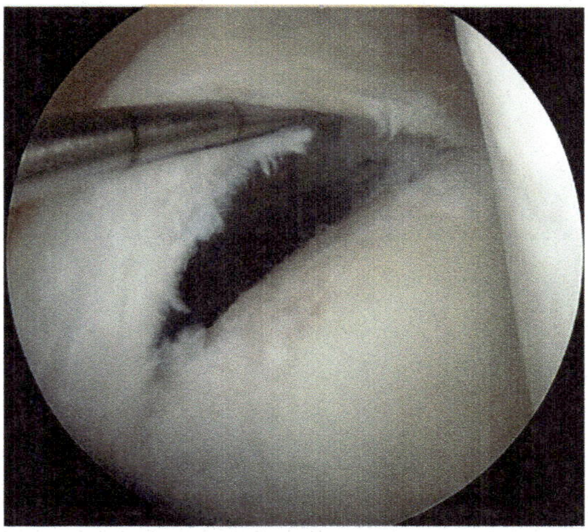

Fig. 16.7 Complet detachment of Bankart lesion

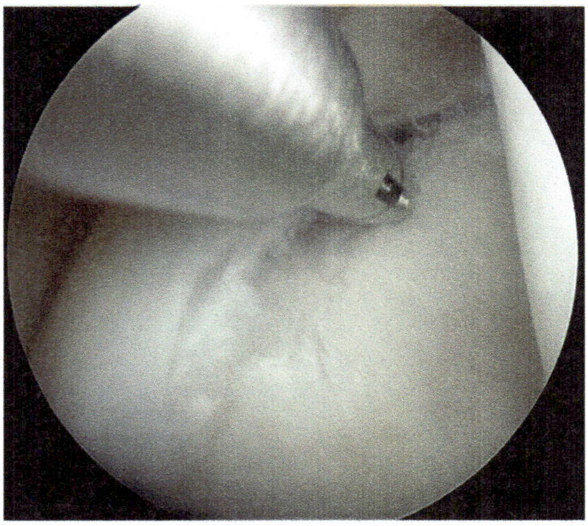

Fig. 16.8 Position of guide-drill first implant

To pass the suture through the capsule and labrum, we can use different devices, holding the suture in a direct or indirect systems (Fig. 16.9a, b).

Finally, we tie the knot, cut the rest of the suture, and check the suture tension (Fig. 16.10).

We'll repeat the same procedure for every implant we place, usually in number of 2–4 for the anteroinferior labrum.

If the posteroinferior labrum is torn, and need to be repaired, we'll perform the same steps, but instead of working from the anterior portal, we create a new portal called "7 o'clock portal", through whom we introduce the implant and the device to perform the sutures (Fig. 16.11).

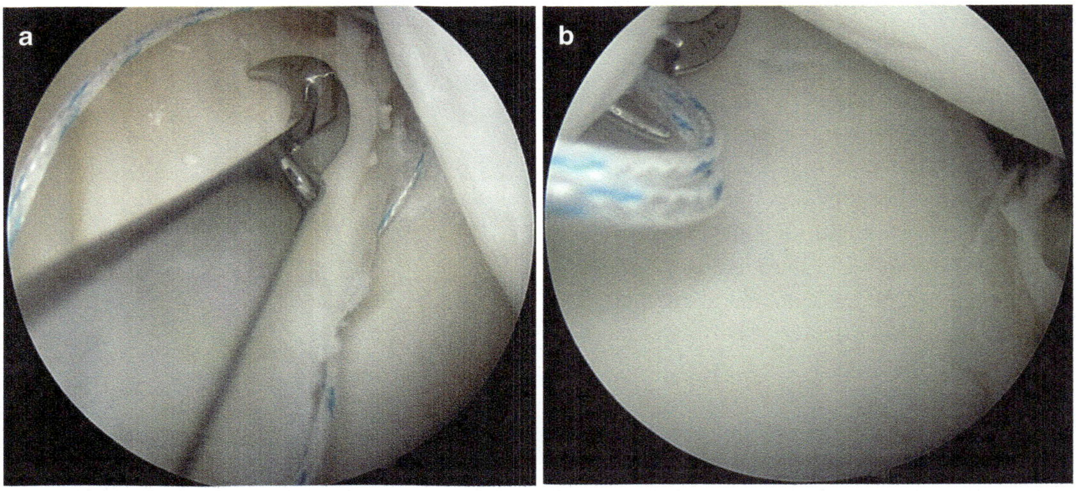

Fig. 16.9 (**a**, **b**) A direct system device

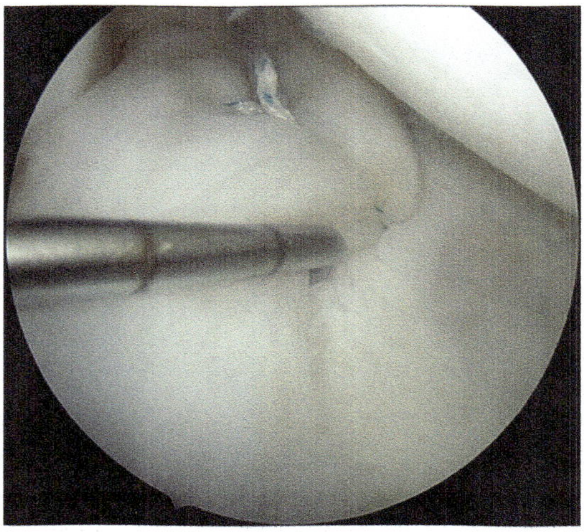

Fig. 16.10 Checking the suture

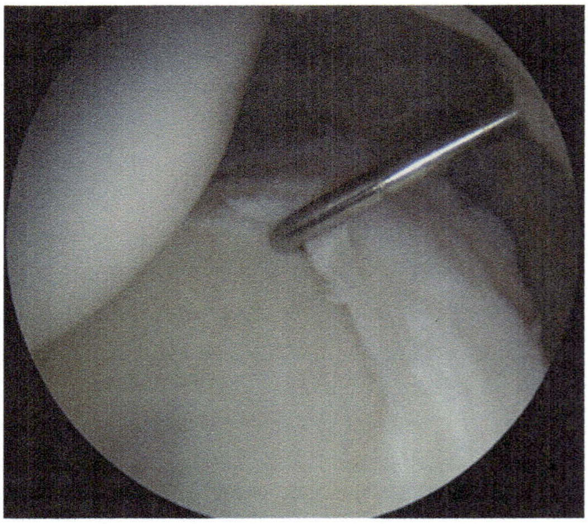

Fig. 16.11 Posteroinferior labrum. 7 o'clock portal

References

1. Cooper D, Arnoczky SP, O'Brien SJ, Warren R, Di Carlo E, Allen A. Anatomy, histology and vascularuty of the glenoid labrum: an anatomical study. J Bone Joint Surg Am. 1992;74A:46–52.
2. Moseley HF, Overgaard B. The anterior capsular mechanism in recurrent anterior dislocation of the shoulder. Morphological and clinical studies with special reference to the glenoid labrum and gleno-humeral ligaments. J Bone Joint Surg. 1962;44B(4):913–27.
3. Matsen FA, Harryman DT, Sidles JA. Mechanics of glenohumeral instability. Clin Sports Med. 1983;2:247–54.
4. Turkel SJ, Panio MW, Marshall JL, et al. Stabilizing mechanisms prevention preventing anterior dislocation of the glenohumeral joint. J Bone Joint Surg Am. 1981;63:1208–13.
5. O'Brien SJ, Neve S, Arnoczky SP. Anatomy and histology od the inferior glenohumeral complex of the shoulder. Am J Sports Med. 1990;18:449–56.
6. Snyder SJ. Shoulder arthroscopy. 2nd ed. Philadelphia: Lippincot Williams & Wilkins; 2003.
7. Boileau P, Chuinard C. Arhtroscopic stabilization of the shoulder: trips and tricks. In: Shoulder artrhoscopy and artrhoplasty. Current concepts. Nice: Saurants Medical; 2006.

17 Managing Cam FAI: Intermediate Hip Arthroscopy

Karadi H. Sunil Kumar, Z. H. Khokher, and Vikas Khanduja

17.1 FAI: Pathology and Assessment

Femoroacetabular impingement (FAI) is a clinical condition characterised by abnormal contact between the femoral head-neck junction and the acetabular rim. The pathology is defined by the consequential rise in stresses across both articulating surfaces, which may eventually lead to labral damage and articular cartilage injury [1]. Other ramifications of this atypical association include osteoarthritis, which has been described by Ganz and colleagues in 2003 to be an eventuality of FAI syndrome based upon the repetitive pathological motion of the hip joint [2]. In the last two decades, several interventions have been developed focused on treating FAI in order to prevent or stop this progression to osteoarthritis, with severe cases often requiring open surgical procedures. There are three major types of FAI that have been described depending on the nature of the deformity; (1) Cam impingement affecting the femoral head-neck junction arising because of an asphericity of the femoral head, defined as an alpha angle of >55°, (2) Pincer impingement, owing to an overcoverage or retroversion of the acetabulum and (3) Mixed involving features of both cam and pincer type impingement [2].

Patients typically present with groin pain or lateral hip pain, with sporadic radiation towards the thigh. The classical presentation involves gripping of the affected hip with the ipsilateral hand, clinically described as the 'C' sign [3]. On physical examination, pain may be exhibited on flexion, adduction and internal rotation of the affected hip (FADIR) [3]. The combination of discomfort in these three planes of movement is otherwise known as the 'Impingement test' which has a high sensitivity but a low specificity, thus can only be used for screening of FAI rather than guiding clinical diagnosis and treatment [4]. Accurate diagnosis of FAI is achieved by incorporation of plain radiographs, CT scans (with 3D reconstruction analysis to assess bony abnormalities), and MRI scanning to assess the condition of the articular cartilage and adjoining acetabular labrum [5].

Successful surgical intervention for FAI can be achieved through both arthroscopic and open procedures [6, 7]. However, in order to attain an outcome identifying with the patient's best interests, thorough clinical assessment of the subject and extensive preoperative investigations are imperative in guiding whether the decision should be made to proceed to surgical intervention. Radiological investigations for example are a practical form of preoperative considerations in assessing the extent of chondral damage and

K. H. Sunil Kumar · Z. H. Khokher · V. Khanduja (✉)
Young Adult Hip Service, Addenbrooke's—Cambridge University Hospital, Cambridge, UK
e-mail: zhk24@cam.ac.uk; vk279@cam.ac.uk

M. T. Hirschmann et al. (eds.), *ESSKA Instructional Course Lecture Book*,
https://doi.org/10.1007/978-3-662-61264-4_17

intra-articular pathology [8]. In the event that early arthritis is evident through imaging, this must be further evaluated as arthroscopic surgery has a limited ability in preventing progression of disease in this cohort of patients.

Cam type deformities frequently lead to labral tears and delamination of the acetabular cartilage due to the increased shear stresses across both the femoral head-neck junction and the acetabular rim. This may result in differences in thickness of acetabular subchondral sclerosis, a key hallmark of osteoarthritis, as a result of the transverse nature of the contact force caused by the dynamic association. An MRI study conducted by Bieri and colleagues described the differences in thickness of subchondral sclerosis between hip joints of young Swiss Army recruits, with and without cam deformities, demonstrating that the subchondral sclerosis in cam type deformities was 0.66 mm thicker compared to those without cam deformities [9]. Mechanical stress in the antero-superior part of the hip joint was thought to increase with cam deformity and it's consequential impingement, resulting in increased subchondral sclerosis in addition to concomitant cartilage damage observed in these same areas, possibly as a repercussion of the hypertrophic bone. This further reinforces the perceived association of cam type deformities with osteoarthritis.

17.2 Assessment of a Patient with FAI

The key to a satisfactory outcome following management of FAI depends on the accurate diagnosis of the deformity, as well as the status of the articular cartilage and labrum. In the case of moderate to severe chondral damage, simple arthroscopic procedures may be insufficient. Aside from standard interventions such as arthroscopic debridement, articular cartilage chondroplasty, and labral repair, cartilage regenerative procedures as well as various biological therapies have been described to be of use in the literature [5].

Table 17.1 Tonnis grading of OA in the hip joint

Tonnis grade	Signs
0	No signs of arthritis
1	Increased sclerosis Slight narrowing of the joint space No or slight loss of head sphericity
2	Small cysts Moderate narrowing of the joint space Moderate loss of head sphericity
3	Large cysts Severe narrowing or obliteration of the joint space Severe deformity of the femoral head

Classification of the hip joint based upon the Tonnis grading system, (see Table 17.1) serves as an additional tool to help guide management [10]. Tonnis Grade 0 and 1 are amenable to hip preservation procedures whereas Tonnis grade 3 hips are beyond preservation surgery and may be in need of arthroplasty. However, there has been no clear guideline for Tonnis grade 2 hips with variable results from hip preservation surgery.

Uemura et al. [8] evaluated 10 different radiographic views commonly performed for evaluation of femoroacetabular impingement, and concluded that each view could identify cam lesions in varying clockface positions at the head-neck junction [11]. Any increase or decrease in femoral anteversion changed the clockwise representation of the cam deformity [11]. Therefore, it is advisable to perform three-dimensional analysis, for instance, a CT scan with 3D reconstruction to evaluate the CAM deformity thoroughly prior to undertaking FAI surgery. However, the 3D CT may still not represent the true impingement, which is a dynamic situation as the hip moves through its range of movement. Furthermore 3D motion analysis of the hip joint with the help of specialised computer software e.g. Clinical Graphics may provide further information into impingement and guide the surgeon to adequately perform targeted osteoplasty of the deformity. Navigated hip arthroscopy or robotics may be used routinely in the future to guide treatment of the cam deformity [12].

17.3 Management Options for FAI

Nonoperative management of FAI includes rest, analgesia with nonsteroidal anti-inflammatory drugs (NSAIDs), activity modification, and focused physiotherapy to strengthen muscles around the hip. Corrective surgical interventions comprise different approaches to reshape the femoral head-neck junction and acetabulum in order to eliminate the impingement [13]. Surgery can be broadly classified into open surgical dislocation, hip arthroscopy, and mini-open procedures. Advantage of the open procedure is that it can correct both intra-articular and extra-articular deformities at the same sitting. However, the procedure carries significantly increased risk, necessitating a high level of expertise by the operating surgeon and involving a steep learning curve for this procedure [14].

Patients younger than 25 years and those with Carlson comorbidity index of <2 had a markedly increased rate of bilateral FAI requiring surgery compared to other patients of age greater than 25 years [15]. In their entire cohort, 15.3% (109 of 694) of patients underwent bilateral hip arthroscopy, with radiographic imaging being unable to successfully anticipate the occurrence of bilateral involvement.

Kaldau and colleagues [16] investigated the conversion rate following hip arthroscopy to total hip arthroplasty (THA), in their series of 84 patients they reported a 18% conversion rate [16]. They identified that high-grade cartilage lesions and age over 40 years were notable risk factors for conversion to THA. Therefore, early identification of cam and pincer type lesions is crucial in order that hip preservation interventions may be performed to stop or delay the conversion to THA.

Utsunomiya et al. [17] from their large single surgeon series of 2396 hip arthroscopies, concluded that older age predisposed towards severe cartilage damage (Outerbridge grade III or IV) for both the femoral head and the acetabulum [17]. In addition, a lower centre-edge angle and larger Tonnis angle inclined patients towards severe cartilage damage for the femoral head; and severe acetabular cartilage damage correlated with male sex, increased body mass index, increased alpha angle, as well as decreased joint space [17].

Table 17.2 Radiological assessment of a patient with FAI

Investigation	Useful assessment
Plain radiographs	Centre-edge angle Tonnis angle Alpha angle Joint space
CT scan	3D view of the Cam deformity 3D view of the Pincer deformity Acetabular version Femoral version Joint space
MRI scan	Extent of chondral injury Labral pathology Joint space

Acetabular retroversion is another important factor to be considered during preoperative evaluation, especially if surgical osteoplasty is planned [18]. Vahedi et al. [18] reported a very high failure rate of 13.7% among the acetabular retroversion group (N = 51) undergoing mini-open femoroacetabular osteoplasty when compared to those patients without any acetabular retroversion (N = 550) [18].

Assessment of comorbidities is crucial, prior to commitment to surgical management, alongside imaging to evaluate the extent of the lesion. Plain radiographs assess the articulating angles involving the hip joint, CT scans provide information regarding the type of deformity and joint space, whilst MRI scanning ascertains the extent and severity of the cartilage and labral lesion. Some of the important parameters assessed with standard radiological investigations are mentioned in Table 17.2.

17.4 Results of Surgery for Cam Deformity

Cam deformity can be treated with three different surgical approaches: (1) hip arthroscopic surgery with osteoplasty, (2) mini-open surgery, and (3) complete surgical dislocation of the hip. Following a multi-criteria decision analysis, Diaz-Ledezma and Parvizi [19] concluded that a mini-open approach was preferred due to a typical association with lower costs [19]. However, Rego et al. [20] in their series of 198 patients with cam FAI did not find any significant functional difference between those treated with either hip arthroscopy or open surgical hip dislocation [20].

Landsdown and colleagues [21] evaluated 707 patients who underwent surgery involving hip arthroscopy, concluding that measurement of the extent of the cam lesion was the strongest predictor of outcome following surgery [21]. The preoperative false profile alpha angle, AP alpha angle and postoperative false profile alpha angle were concluded to be independent predictors of clinical outcome [21].

Reporting on early outcomes of hip arthroscopy in the athletic adolescent population, Philippon et al. [22] determined that postoperatively there was a 35 point increase of modified Harris Hip Score to 90 points [22]. Furthermore, these patients had high levels of satisfaction in the short term as well as exceptional increases in functionality reflected by a mean increase in Hip Outcome Score (HOS) activities-of-daily-living by 54 points. These 16 patients had a combination of lesions: cam (2), pincer, (5) and mixed type (9).

Tran et al. [23] reported that arthroscopic surgery to treat cam type impingement in the adolescent population resulted in a high level of satisfaction, return to sport and significant improvement in postoperative hip scores (modified Harris Hip Score and Non-arthroplasty Hip Score) [23]. In their case series of 34 patients, 88% were satisfied with their operation with 78% of patients returning to full sporting activities [23].

Recently, there have been publications of two large multicentre randomised controlled trials in the UK reporting the outcome of FAI surgery: FAIT and UK FASHIoN, both of which have suggested that hip arthroscopy resulted in significant improvements in outcome in the short term compared with physiotherapy.

FAIT was a multicentre randomised controlled trial on treatment of FAI comparing outcome of arthroscopic surgery versus nonoperative management, involving physiotherapy and activity modification [24]. The trial randomised 222 patients into the two arms equally. The trial determined that patients with symptomatic FAI showed better outcomes with arthroscopic surgery in comparison to physiotherapy. After 8 months of follow up, the mean HOS activities-of-daily-living was ten points greater in the arthroscopic hip surgery group when compared to the physiotherapy program group, showing a statistically significant increase [24]. The minimum clinically important difference (MCID) between the two groups was decided to be nine points [24]. There were no complications noted in either of the groups.

The UK FASHIoN trial, another multicentre, assessor blinded, randomised controlled trial, involved 348 patients and evaluated outcomes of hip arthroscopy versus physiotherapy for FAI [25]. There were a minimum of 170 patients in each arm. Hip arthroscopy once again manifested in a clinically significant improvement in outcome scores when compared to physiotherapy [25].

Currently another ongoing trial, the Femoroacetabular Impingement RandomiSed controlled Trial (FIRST), is looking at the outcome following arthroscopic osteochondroplasty with or without labral repair versus sole arthroscopic lavage of the hip joint. A total of 220 patients are due to be recruited into the study [26].

Summary Our understanding of FAI has improved tremedously since the concept was introduced by Ganz in the 1990s, and as such the forms of intervention too have progressively matured. The management of cam type FAI must be practiced with considerate prior clinical and radiological assessment of the patient to successfully guide treatment. Nonoperative measures should not be disregarded, with physiotherapy, NSAIDs and activity modification being a suitable choice for many patients. However, recent results from two large scale multicentre RCTs—FAIT and UK FASHIoN, have suggested that hip arthroscopy has resulted in significant improvement in the short term and may be of preference over conservative measures. Future large-scale, long-term RCTs are pivotal in assessing the long-term outcomes of patients who decide to undergo such procedures, and whether this improvement is sustained.

References

1. Audenaert EA, Peeters I, Van Onsem S, et al. Can we predict the natural course of femoroacetabular impingement? Acta Orthop Belg. 2011;77(2):188–96.
2. Ganz R, Parvizi J, Beck M, Leunig M, Notzli H, Siebenrock KA. Femoroacetabular impingement: a cause for osteoarthritis of the hip. Clin Orthop Relat Res. 2003;417:112–20.
3. Byrd JW. Evaluation of the hip: history and physical examination. N Am J Sports Phys Ther. 2007;2(4):231–40.
4. Ayeni OR, Belzile EL, Musahl V, et al. Results of the PeRception of femOroaCetabular impingEment by Surgeons Survey (PROCESS). Knee Surg Sports Traumatol Arthrosc. 2014;22(4):906–10.
5. Nakano N, Gohal C, Duong A, et al. Outcomes of cartilage repair techniques for chondral injury in the hip—a systematic review. Int Orthop. 2018;42:2309–22.
6. Khanduja V, Villar RN. The arthroscopic management of femoro-acetabular impingement. Knee Surg Sports Traumatol Arthrosc. 2007;15(8):1035–40.
7. Imam S, Khanduja V. Current concepts in the diagnosis and management of femoroacetabular impingement. Int Orthop. 2011;35(10):1427–35.
8. Uemura K, Atkins PR, Anderson AE, et al. Do your routine radiographs to diagnose cam femoroacetabular impingement visualize the region of the femoral head-neck junction you intended? Arthroscopy. 2019 Jun;35(6):1796–806.
9. Bieri M, Beck M, Limacher A, et al. Increased subchondral bone thickness in hips with cam-type femoroacetabular impingement. Hip Int. 2019;29(4):430–7.
10. Byrd JWT, Jones KS, Bardowski EA. Influence of Tonnis grade on outcomes of arthroscopy for FAI in athletes: a comparative analysis. J Hip Preserv Surg. 2018;5(2):162–5.
11. Uemura K, Atkins PR, Anderson AE, et al. Do your routine radiographs to diagnose cam femoroacetabular impingement visualize the region of the femoral head-neck junction you intended. Arthroscopy. 2019;35(6):1796–806.
12. Nakano N, Audenaert E, Ranawat A, et al. Review: current concepts in computer-assisted hip arthroscopy. Int J Med Robot. 2018;14(6):e1929.
13. Wall PD, Fernandez M, Griffin DR, et al. Nonoperative treatment for femoroacetabular impingement: a systematic review of the literature. PM R. 2013;5(5):418–26.
14. Ganz R, Gill TJ, Gautier E, et al. Surgical dislocation of the adult hip: a technique with full access to the femoral head and acetabulum without the risk of avascular necrosis. J Bone Joint Surg Br. 2001;83:1119–2.
15. Leong NL, Neal W, Alter T, et al. Risk factors for bilateral femoroacetabular impingement syndrome requiring surgery. J Am Acad Orthop Surg Glob Res Rev. 2018;2(11):e070.
16. Kaldau NC, Brorson S, Hölmich P, et al. Good midterm results of hip arthroscopy for femoroacetabular impingement. Dan Med J. 2018;65(6):A5483.
17. Utsunomiya H, Briggs KK, Dornan GJ, et al. Predicting severe cartilage damage in the hip: a model using patient-specific data from 2,396 hip arthroscopies. Arthroscopy. 2019;35(7):2051–2060.e13. https://doi.org/10.1016/j.arthro.2019.02.033. pii: S0749–8063(19)30191–4. [Epub ahead of print].
18. Vahedi H, Aalirezaie A, Schlitt PK, et al. Acetabular retroversion is a risk factor for less optimal outcome after femoroacetabular impingement surgery. J Arthroplasty. 2019;34(7):1342–6. https://doi.org/10.1016/j.arth.2019.02.050. Epub 2019 Feb 25.
19. Diaz-Ledezma C, Parvizi J. Surgical approaches for cam femoroacetabular impingement: the use of multicriteria decision analysis. Clin Orthop Relat Res. 2013;471(8):2509–16.
20. Rego PA, Mascarenhas V, Oliveira FS, et al. Arthroscopic versus open treatment of cam-type femoro-acetabular impingement: retrospective cohort clinical study. Int Orthop. 2018;42(4):791–7.
21. Lansdown DA, Kunze K, Ukwuani G, et al. The importance of comprehensive cam correction: radiographic parameters are predictive of patient-reported outcome measures at 2 years after hip arthroscopy. Am J Sports Med. 2018;46(9):2072–8.
22. Philippon MJ, Yen YM, Briggs KK, et al. Early outcomes after hip arthroscopy for femoroacetabular impingement in the athletic adolescent patient: a preliminary report. J Pediatr Orthop. 2008;28(7):705–10.
23. Tran P, Pritchard M, O'Donnell J. Outcome of arthroscopic treatment for cam type femoroacetabular impingement in adolescents. ANZ J Surg. 2013;83(5):382–6.
24. Palmer AJR, Ayyar Gupta V, Fernquest S, et al. Arthroscopic hip surgery compared with physiotherapy and activity modification for the treatment of symptomatic femoroacetabular impingement: multicentre randomised controlled trial. BMJ. 2019;364:l185. https://doi.org/10.1136/bmj.l185.
25. Griffin DR, Dickenson EJ, Wall PDH, et al. Hip arthroscopy versus best conservative care for the treatment of femoroacetabular impingement syndrome (UK FASHIoN): a multicentre randomised controlled trial. Lancet. 2018;391(10136):2225–35. https://doi.org/10.1016/S0140-6736(18)31202-9. Epub 2018 Jun 1.
26. FIRST Investigators. A multi-centre randomized controlled trial comparing arthroscopic osteochondroplasty and lavage with arthroscopic lavage alone on patient important outcomes and quality of life in the treatment of young adult (18–50) Femoroacetabular impingement. BMC Musculoskelet Disord. 2015;16:64.

18 An Update on Ankle Arthroscopy: Current Evidence and Practical Recommendations for 2020

Daniël Haverkamp

18.1 Introduction

When talking about innovations and progress in the field of arthroscopy, we have to focus on indications and technological improvement. The basic principle of looking in the joint did not change over the year, but technical innovations makes it possible to visualize more and to perform more specific procedures. The synergy with the industry makes that equipment can be invented to perform many surgical procedures which were impossible to do before. Off course being able to get a tool does not automatically mean that it is wise to use it, and we should always remain critical.

Due to many innovations more and more procedures can be done arthroscopically, also in the ankle joint. However, we have to focus on the fact whether it is really an improvement to perform that specific procedure (arthro)scopically compared to the classical open technique. If a successful open procedure can be done scopically it does not automatically mean that it is superior to do so. For the early ages the switch from open to arthroscopic was immense, for instance meniscal removal with large incisions to the option now to perform an arthroscopic repair. For many procedures however it remains to be proven that arthroscopic treatment indeed is better than open.

18.2 Cartilage Repair

Specifically for the ankle we see that there is more focus on cartilage repair arthroscopically. The treatment of osteochondral lesions of the talus (OLT) is one that still can be improved with results reaching 85% in the smaller defects [1]. We see a change going from the classical debridement and bone marrow stimulation to techniques (preferably arthroscopic) to restore the cartilage as much as possible. In the literature, we see an immense increase of interest in biological additions to enhance the healing of talar osteochondral defect in the ankle [2].

The Amsterdam Foot and Ankle group posed the technique of Lift, Drill, Fill, and Fix (LDFF) to preserve the original cartilage and reported their initial results to be good [3, 4]. This technique can be performed all arthroscopically.

Adding PRP or BMAC during the arthroscopic procedures to enhance healing potential of the debrided OLT, literature regarding PRP is not conclusive [5]. Perhaps since many differences in PRP exists [6]. BMAC have been extensively studied in animal models, showing to be promising [7, 8]. Studies report on adding BMAC to

D. Haverkamp (✉)
Xpert Orthopedics, Amsterdam, The Netherlands
e-mail: D.Haverkamp@xpertorthopedie.nl

M. T. Hirschmann et al. (eds.), *ESSKA Instructional Course Lecture Book*,
https://doi.org/10.1007/978-3-662-61264-4_18

debridement and curettage improves the outcome [9, 10]. However comparing BMAC tot MACI, the latter shows to be perhaps a better option as shown by the Rizolli group [11].

Several types of scaffolds are available now, all having limited available evidence [12]. The matrix-induced autologous chondrocyte transplantation (MACT) is a second generation ACI technique using a collagen type I/III bilayer membrane seeded with cultured autologous chondrocytes. The disadvantage of this system is that it is a two-stage procedure. Bone marrow derived cell transplantation (BMDCT) is a one-step system in which concentrated bone marrow aspirate is secured with a hyaluronic based scaffold. Autologous matrix-induced chondrogeneis (AMIC) is a one-stage procedure in which BMS with porcine collagen type I/III scaffold is used. This technique can be done completely arthroscopic as described by Baumfeld reporting on the results of an all arthroscopic AMIC procedure showing it to be a reliable and reproducible procedure [13] (Fig. 18.1).

Most important for the coming years is that we start to perform multicenter studies comparing these different options. For now, there are options on the markets for which no publication exists for OLT, yet they are used in the field.

18.3 Ankle Instability

Another upcoming area in ankle surgery is the arthroscopic treatment of ankle instability. Many publications occurred regarding the surgical options to restore the ankle ligaments arthroscopically in which the ESSKA-AFAS Ankle Instability Group played a major role [14–18]. Most important after reporting on publishing many technical and anatomical studies and 'how to do it' consensus strategies [15, 19–23] also the results are being published [24–27] in which especially the French Arthroscopic Society should be praised for the effort of publishing the outcome of a national prospective series of arthroscopic ligament reconstruction in the ankle [25].

The next challenge will be to prove the superiority of the arthroscopic reconstruction, despite the fact that as arthroscopic surgeons we are convinced that it is a better option, we still have to define it is better. Especially since the arthroscopic surgeries are often more costly as more specialized equipment is needed. A recent systematic review from Song comparing the reported outcome of arthroscopic lateral ankle ligament reconstruction to the golden standard being the well-documented open procedure showed no significant difference in outcome

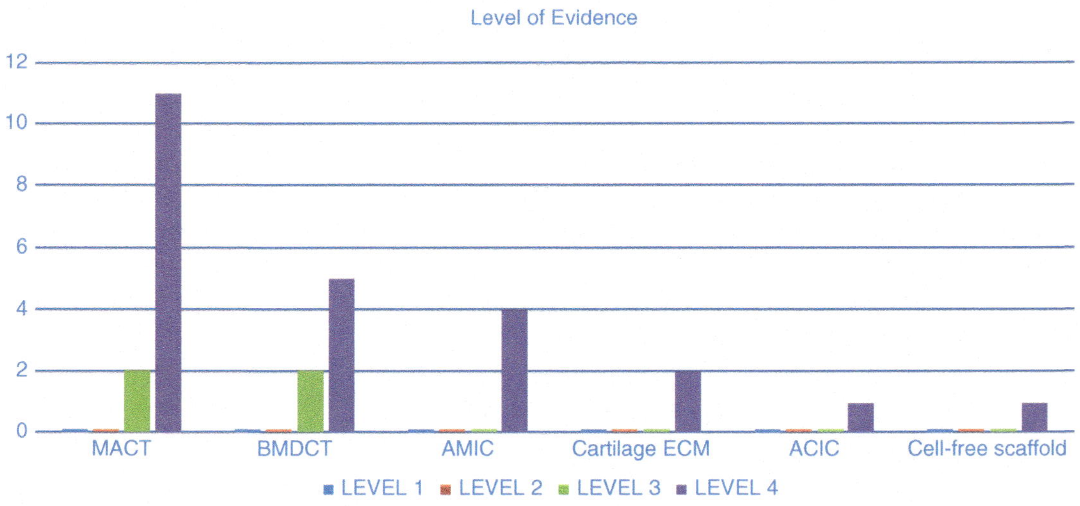

Fig. 18.1 Number of publications and evidence on scaffold bases OCD treatment of the ankle

between these procedures in early outcomes [28]. However, only one level 1 study could be found, and the total of studies included was 4 with only 207 surgical repairs. A previous Systematic review of Guelfi used different criteria including more studies and did not show a difference between open and arthroscopic repair of the ankle ligaments [29]. The most recent publication of Li also did not show superiority of the arthroscopic procedure over the open option [30]. We as surgeons have to define how we will measure and prove that one option is better than the other.

18.4 Arthroscopic Assisted Fracture Care

An upcoming field seems to be the use of arthroscopic assistance during the surgical treatment of ankle fractures. Chen et al. reported on the findings of arthroscopy during ORIF of the ankle fractures finding up to 92% of loose bodies in supination type fractures which would otherwise have been unnoted [31]. However, retrospective descriptive series like these provide valuable information on the amount and type of concomitant injuries in ankle fractures, it remains unclear whether the patients benefit of adding arthroscopy to the ORIF and whether the extra effort is cost-effective.

A large database study from the United States comparing over 32,000 ORIF procedures with or without arthroscopic assistance on reoperation rate and reported complications [32]. As with many database studies we have no clue what really happened to these patients and what the real outcome is. Even not the reason why only 0.8% of these 32,000 had arthroscopic-assisted ORIF. The conclusion of the authors that arthroscopy does not add to the outcome of ORIF cannot be made on the presented data, but the proof that it does have a positive effect is also lacking from literature.

Arthroscopic assistance in fracture care might be beneficial, but still needs to be proven.

18.5 Needle Arthroscopy in Outpatient Setting

Needle arthroscopy which can be performed in the outpatient setting is one of the recent advances which is a major topic of discussion, now mainly for the knee but the same discussion could be held for the ankle joint. Should we go back to invasive diagnostics now that we are in an era where the quality of imaging is enormously improved and still expected to improve. Some authors really advocate going back to invasive, justifying it by degrading the amount of invasiveness [33], Amin justifies the use by doing a cost-effectiveness analyses with a Markov model trying to prove that the use of a needle arthroscopy is justified [34]. Chapman et al. stated it to be a benefit that now a diagnostic arthroscopy is not necessary [35]. However, after the needle arthroscopy is performed and shows a problem, still regular arthroscopy is needed [35]. Gill showed that needle arthroscopy shows more detailed information than MRI, other authors confirmed this [36–38].

However finding details not found on MRI may not automatically mean that they need surgery and result in a better outcome. This is yet to be investigated. Besides that, we have to realize the role of the industry trying to bring this product to the market, and most of the pro studies are indeed sponsored studies. Although the discussion now focusses mainly on knee and shoulder we have to realize that for the ankle the same discussion exists. Especially since for several indications in the ankle, diagnostic arthroscopy is still considered the gold standard [21, 39].

Also, there is more focus on the anatomical structures we can reach with ankle arthroscopy and the correlation of arthroscopic interpretation to anatomical dissection. Dalmau-Pastor showed in an anatomical study for instance that medial and lateral ankle ligaments can be well identified and reached with the dorsiflexion non-distraction anterior ankle arthroscopy [40]. Besides that, we need to redefine what is normal and not normal, since we do not want to address non-pathological variations thinking they are abnormal. Research projects like Lubberts et al. are becoming more important by helping us to define when an arthroscopic finding is relevant [39]. In this study they developed an algorithm defining how to classify a syndesmosis as stable or unstable during arthroscopic investigation.

18.6 Discussion

In the orthopedic field, more and more traditional (arthroscopic) procedures which have been basic treatment options are now questioned whether they really are more efficient than nonoperative treatment. For instance, arthroscopic treatment of the degenerative knee or subacromial decompression are now considered to be non-superior to conservative care after well-conducted multicenter randomized clinical trials.

The main practical recommendation is that we have to prove how successful our (arthroscopic) surgery is by documenting all procedures, preferably by joining forces and conducting large multicenter randomized clinical trials.

We have to keep in mind that with the right tools we can do almost anything, but we should always be aware if the procedures we perform really benefit the patient.

References

1. Zengerink M, van Dijk CN. Complications in ankle arthroscopy. Knee Surg Sports Traumatol Arthrosc. 2012;20(8):1420–31. https://doi.org/10.1007/s00167-012-2063-x. Epub 2012 Jun 5. PubMed PMID: 22669362; PubMed Central PMCID: PMC3402678.
2. McGoldrick NP, Murphy EP, Kearns SR. Osteochondral lesions of the ankle: the current evidence supporting scaffold-based techniques and biological adjuncts. Foot Ankle Surg. 2018;24(2):86–91. https://doi.org/10.1016/j.fas.2017.01.003. Epub 2017 Jan 20. Review. PubMed PMID: 29409225.
3. Reilingh ML, Lambers KTA, Dahmen J, Opdam KTM, Kerkhoffs GMMJ. The subchondral bone healing after fixation of an osteochondral talar defect is superior in comparison with microfracture. Knee Surg Sports Traumatol Arthrosc. 2018;26(7):2177–82. https://doi.org/10.1007/s00167-017-4654-z. Epub 2017 Jul 27. PubMed PMID: 28752185; PubMed Central PMCID: PMC6061443.
4. Kerkhoffs GM, Reilingh ML, Gerards RM, de Leeuw PA. Lift, drill, fill and fix (LDFF): a new arthroscopic treatment for talar osteochondral defects. Knee Surg Sports Traumatol Arthrosc. 2016;24(4):1265–71. https://doi.org/10.1007/s00167-014-3057-7. Epub 2014 May 20. PubMed PMID: 24841940.
5. van Bergen CJ, Kerkhoffs GM, Özdemir M, Korstjens CM, Everts V, van Ruijven LJ, van Dijk CN, Blankevoort L. Demineralized bone matrix and platelet-rich plasma do not improve healing of osteochondral defects of the talus: an experimental goat study. Osteoarthr Cartil. 2013;21(11):1746–54. https://doi.org/10.1016/j.joca.2013.07.014. Epub 2013 Jul 27. PubMed PMID: 23896314.
6. Oudelaar BW, Peerbooms JC, Huis In 't Veld R, Vochteloo AJH. Concentrations of blood components in commercial platelet-rich plasma separation systems: a review of the literature. Am J Sports Med. 2019;47(2):479–87. https://doi.org/10.1177/0363546517746112. Epub 2018 Jan 16. PubMed PMID: 29337592.
7. Fortier LA, Potter HG, Rickey EJ, Schnabel LV, Foo LF, Chong LR, Stokol T, Cheetham J, Nixon AJ. Concentrated bone marrow aspirate improves full-thickness cartilage repair compared with microfracture in the equine model. J Bone Joint Surg Am. 2010;92(10):1927–37. https://doi.org/10.2106/JBJS.I.01284. PubMed PMID: 20720135.
8. Saw KY, Hussin P, Loke SC, Azam M, Chen HC, Tay YG, Low S, Wallin KL, Ragavanaidu K. Articular cartilage regeneration with autologous marrow aspirate and hyaluronic acid: an experimental study in a goat model. Arthroscopy. 2009;25(12):1391–400. https://doi.org/10.1016/j.arthro.2009.07.011. Epub 2009 Sep 17. PubMed PMID: 19962065.
9. Smyth NA, Murawski CD, Haleem AM, Hannon CP, Savage-Elliott I, Kennedy JG. Establishing proof of concept: platelet-rich plasma and bone marrow aspirate concentrate may improve cartilage repair following surgical treatment for osteochondral lesions of the talus. World J Orthop. 2012;3(7):101–8. https://doi.org/10.5312/wjo.v3.i7.101. PubMed PMID: 22816065; PubMed Central PMCID: PMC3399015.
10. Vannini F, Cavallo M, Ramponi L, Castagnini F, Massimi S, Giannini S, Buda RE. Return to sports after bone marrow-derived cell transplantation for osteochondral lesions of the talus. Cartilage. 2017;8(1):80–7. Epub 2016 Apr 12. PubMed PMID: 27994723; PubMed Central PMCID: PMC5154421.
11. Desando G, Bartolotti I, Vannini F, Cavallo C, Castagnini F, Buda R, Giannini S, Mosca M, Mariani E, Grigolo B. Repair potential of matrix-induced bone marrow aspirate concentrate and matrix-induced autologous chondrocyte implantation for talar osteochondral repair: patterns of some catabolic, inflammatory, and pain mediators. Cartilage. 2017;8(1):50–60.

Epub 2016 Apr 13. PubMed PMID: 27994720; PubMed Central PMCID: PMC5154420.
12. Shimozono Y, Yasui Y, Ross AW, Miyamoto W, Kennedy JG. Scaffolds based therapy for osteochondral lesions of the talus: a systematic review. World J Orthop. 2017;8(10):798–808. https://doi.org/10.5312/wjo.v8.i10.798. eCollection 2017 Oct 18. PubMed PMID: 29094011; PubMed Central PMCID: PMC5656496.
13. Baumfeld T, Baumfeld D, Prado M, Nery C. All-arthroscopic AMIC(®) (AT-AMIC) for the treatment of talar osteochondral defects: a short follow-up case series. Foot (Edinb). 2018;37:23–7. https://doi.org/10.1016/j.foot.2018.07.006. Epub 2018 Jul 25. PubMed PMID: 30321855.
14. Nery C, Fonseca L, Raduan F, Moreno M, Baumfeld D, ESSKA AFAS Ankle Instability Group. Prospective study of the "inside-out" arthroscopic ankle ligament technique: preliminary result. Foot Ankle Surg. 2018;24(4):320–5. https://doi.org/10.1016/j.fas.2017.03.002. Epub 2017 Mar 22. PubMed PMID: 29409246.
15. Michels F, Pereira H, Calder J, Matricali G, Glazebrook M, Guillo S, Karlsson J, ESSKA-AFAS Ankle Instability Group, Acevedo J, Batista J, Bauer T, Calder J, Carreira D, Choi W, Corte-Real N, Glazebrook M, Ghorbani A, Giza E, Guillo S, Hunt K, Karlsson J, Kong SW, Lee JW, Michels F, Molloy A, Mangone P, Matsui K, Nery C, Ozeki S, Pearce C, Pereira H, Perera A, Pijnenburg B, Raduan F, Stone J, Takao M, Tourné Y, Vega J. Searching for consensus in the approach to patients with chronic lateral ankle instability: ask the expert. Knee Surg Sports Traumatol Arthrosc. 2018;26(7):2095–102. https://doi.org/10.1007/s00167-017-4556-0. Epub 2017 Apr 25. PubMed PMID: 28439639.
16. Matsui K, Oliva XM, Takao M, Pereira BS, Gomes TM, Lozano JM, ESSKA AFAS Ankle Instability Group, Glazebrook M. Bony landmarks available for minimally invasive lateral ankle stabilization surgery: a cadaveric anatomical study. Knee Surg Sports Traumatol Arthrosc. 2017;25(6):1916–24. https://doi.org/10.1007/s00167-016-4218-7. Epub 2016 Jun 28. PubMed PMID: 27351549.
17. Glazebrook M, Stone J, Matsui K, Guillo S, Takao M, ESSKA AFAS Ankle Instability Group. Percutaneous ankle reconstruction of lateral ligaments (Perc-anti RoLL). Foot Ankle Int. 2016;37(6):659–64. https://doi.org/10.1177/1071100716633648. Epub 2016 Feb 22. PubMed PMID: 26903001.
18. Matsui K, Burgesson B, Takao M, Stone J, Guillo S, Glazebrook M, ESSKA AFAS Ankle Instability Group. Minimally invasive surgical treatment for chronic ankle instability: a systematic review. Knee Surg Sports Traumatol Arthrosc. 2016;24(4):1040–8. https://doi.org/10.1007/s00167-016-4041-1. Epub 2016 Feb 11. Review. PubMed PMID: 26869032.
19. Michels F, Matricali G, Guillo S, Vanrietvelde F, Pottel H, Stockmans F. An oblique fibular tunnel is recommended when reconstructing the ATFL and CFL. Knee Surg Sports Traumatol Arthrosc. 2019;28:124. https://doi.org/10.1007/s00167-019-05583-3. [Epub ahead of print]. PubMed PMID: 31240379.
20. Teixeira J, Guillo S. Arthroscopic treatment of ankle instability—allograft/autograft reconstruction. Foot Ankle Clin. 2018;23(4):571–9. https://doi.org/10.1016/j.fcl.2018.07.004. Review. PubMed PMID: 30414653.
21. Elkaïm M, Thès A, Lopes R, Andrieu M, Cordier G, Molinier F, Benoist J, Colin F, Boniface O, Guillo S, Bauer T, French Arthroscopic Society. Agreement between arthroscopic and imaging study findings in chronic anterior talo-fibular ligament injuries. Orthop Traumatol Surg Res. 2018;104(8S):S213–8. https://doi.org/10.1016/j.otsr.2018.09.008. Epub 2018 Sep 27. PubMed PMID: 30268650.
22. Thès A, Odagiri H, Elkaïm M, Lopes R, Andrieu M, Cordier G, Molinier F, Benoist J, Colin F, Boniface O, Guillo S, Bauer T, French Arthroscopic Society. Arthroscopic classification of chronic anterior talo-fibular ligament lesions in chronic ankle instability. Orthop Traumatol Surg Res. 2018;104(8S):S207–11. https://doi.org/10.1016/j.otsr.2018.09.004. Epub 2018 Sep 20. PubMed PMID: 30243676.
23. Takao M, Glazebrook M, Stone J, Guillo S. Ankle arthroscopic reconstruction of lateral ligaments (ankle anti-ROLL). Arthrosc Tech. 2015;4(5):e595–600. https://doi.org/10.1016/j.eats.2015.06.008. eCollection 2015 Oct. PubMed PMID: 26900560; PubMed Central PMCID: PMC4722511.
24. Crombé A, Borghol S, Guillo S, Pesquer L, Dallaudiere B. Arthroscopic reconstruction of the lateral ankle ligaments: radiological evaluation and short-term clinical outcome. Diagn Interv Imaging. 2019;100(2):117–25. https://doi.org/10.1016/j.diii.2018.09.002. Epub 2018 Nov 13. PubMed PMID: 30446413.
25. Lopes R, Andrieu M, Cordier G, Molinier F, Benoist J, Colin F, Thès A, Elkaïm M, Boniface O, Guillo S, Bauer T, French Arthroscopic Society. Arthroscopic treatment of chronic ankle instability: prospective study of outcomes in 286 patients. Orthop Traumatol Surg Res. 2018;104(8S):S199–205. https://doi.org/10.1016/j.otsr.2018.09.005. Epub 2018 Sep 21. PubMed PMID: 30245066.
26. Cordier G, Lebecque J, Vega J, Dalmau-Pastor M. Arthroscopic ankle lateral ligament repair with biological augmentation gives excellent results in case of chronic ankle instability. Knee Surg Sports Traumatol Arthrosc. 2019;28:108. https://doi.org/10.1007/s00167-019-05650-9. [Epub ahead of print]. PubMed PMID: 31388694.
27. Li H, Hua Y, Li H, Chen S. Anterior talofibular ligament (ATFL) repair using two suture anchors produced better functional outcomes than using one suture anchor for the treatment of chronic lateral ankle instability. Knee Surg Sports Traumatol Arthrosc. 2019;28:221. https://doi.org/10.1007/s00167-019-05550-y. [Epub ahead of print]. PubMed PMID: 31165905.

28. Song YJ, Hua YH. Similar outcomes at early term after arthroscopic or open repair of chronic ankle instability: a systematic review and meta-analysis. J Foot Ankle Surg. 2019;58(2):312–9. https://doi.org/10.1053/j.jfas.2018.08.026. PubMed PMID: 30850101.
29. Guelfi M, Zamperetti M, Pantalone A, Usuelli FG, Salini V, Oliva XM. Open and arthroscopic lateral ligament repair for treatment of chronic ankle instability: a systematic review. Foot Ankle Surg. 2018;24(1):11–8. https://doi.org/10.1016/j.fas.2016.05.315. Epub 2016 May 12. Review. PubMed PMID: 29413768.
30. Li H, Hua Y, Li H, Ma K, Li S, Chen S. Activity level and function 2 years after anterior talofibular ligament repair: a comparison between arthroscopic repair and open repair procedures. Am J Sports Med. 2017;45(9):2044–51. https://doi.org/10.1177/0363546517698675. Epub 2017 Apr 10. PubMed PMID: 28394631.
31. Chen XZ, Chen Y, Zhu QZ, Wang LQ, Xu XD, Lin P. Prevalence and associated factors of intra-articular lesions in acute ankle fractures evaluated by arthroscopy and clinical outcomes with minimum 24-month follow-up. Chin Med J (Engl). 2019;132(15):1802–6. https://doi.org/10.1097/CM9.0000000000000342. PubMed PMID: 31335476.
32. Yasui Y, Shimozono Y, Hung CW, Marangon A, Wollstein A, Gianakos AL, Murawski CD, Kennedy JG. Postoperative reoperations and complications in 32,307 ankle fractures with and without concurrent ankle arthroscopic procedures in a 5-year period based on a large U.S. healthcare database. J Foot Ankle Surg. 2019;58(1):6–9. https://doi.org/10.1053/j.jfas.2018.03.030. Epub 2018 Sep 19. PubMed PMID: 30243789.
33. Crall TS. Editorial commentary: Morton forks a knee: magnetic resonance imaging versus needles arthroscopy for knee meniscus tears. Arthroscopy. 2019;35(2):563–5. https://doi.org/10.1016/j.arthro.2018.11.021. PubMed PMID: 30712632.
34. Amin N, McIntyre L, Carter T, Xerogeanes J, Voigt J. Cost-effectiveness analysis of needle arthroscopy versus magnetic resonance imaging in the diagnosis and treatment of meniscal tears of the knee. Arthroscopy. 2019;35(2):554–562.e13. https://doi.org/10.1016/j.arthro.2018.09.030. PubMed PMID: 30712631.
35. Chapman GL, Amin NH. The benefits of an in-office arthroscopy in the diagnosis of unresolved knee pain. Case Rep Orthop. 2018;2018:6125676. https://doi.org/10.1155/2018/6125676. eCollection 2018. PubMed PMID: 29992071; PubMed Central PMCID: PMC5827882.
36. Gill TJ, Safran M, Mandelbaum B, Huber B, Gambardella R, Xerogeanes J. A prospective, blinded, multicenter clinical trial to compare the efficacy, accuracy, and safety of in-office diagnostic arthroscopy with magnetic resonance imaging and surgical diagnostic arthroscopy. Arthroscopy. 2018;34(8):2429–35. https://doi.org/10.1016/j.arthro.2018.03.010. Epub 2018 May 24. PubMed PMID: 29804955.
37. Deirmengian CA, Dines JS, Vernace JV, Schwartz MS, Creighton RA, Gladstone JN. Use of a small-bore needle arthroscope to diagnose intra-articular knee pathology: comparison with magnetic resonance imaging. Am J Orthop (Belle Mead NJ). 2018;47(2). https://doi.org/10.12788/ajo.2018.0007. PubMed PMID: 29494711.
38. Cooper DE. Editorial commentary: the desire to take a look: surgeons and patients must weigh the benefits and costs of in-office needle arthroscopy versus magnetic resonance imaging. Arthroscopy. 2018;34(8):2436–7. https://doi.org/10.1016/j.arthro.2018.06.002. PubMed PMID: 30077266.
39. Lubberts B, Guss D, Vopat BG, Johnson AH, van Dijk CN, Lee H, DiGiovanni CW. The arthroscopic syndesmotic assessment tool can differentiate between stable and unstable ankle syndesmoses. Knee Surg Sports Traumatol Arthrosc. 2018;28:193. https://doi.org/10.1007/s00167-018-5229-3. [Epub ahead of print]. PubMed PMID: 30367196.
40. Dalmau-Pastor M, Malagelada F, Kerkhoffs GM, Karlsson J, Guelfi M, Vega J. Redefining anterior ankle arthroscopic anatomy: medial and lateral ankle collateral ligaments are visible through dorsiflexion and non-distraction anterior ankle arthroscopy. Knee Surg Sports Traumatol Arthrosc. 2019;28:18. https://doi.org/10.1007/s00167-019-05603-2. [Epub ahead of print]. PubMed PMID: 31292688.

19 ACL Injury: Where Are We Now? Is Prevention the Key for All Sports?

Gilbert Moatshe and Lars Engebretsen

19.1 ACL Update in 2020

19.1.1 Introduction

Anterior cruciate ligament (ACL) injuries are one of the most common injuries of the knee, with an estimated incidence of 200,000 per year in the United States [1, 2]. Treatment of ACL injuries remains one of the most prevalent musculoskeletal procedures performed, affecting 1 in 3000 among the general population of the United States. In Norway, there is an annual population incidence of primary anterior cruciate ligament reconstruction surgeries of 34 per 100,000 citizens (85 per 100,000 citizens in the main at-risk age group of 16–39 years) [3]. ACL injuries in the pediatric and adolescent population has trended much higher in current literature, increasing by 147.8% over the 10-year span from 2005 to 2015, reaching an overall annual rate of 6.79 per 100,000 in patients aged 5–14 [4, 5].

G. Moatshe · L. Engebretsen (✉)
Oslo University Hospital Orthopedic Clinic, Oslo, Norway

Oslo Sports Trauma Research Center, Norwegian School of Sports Sciences, Oslo, Norway
e-mail: lars.engebretsen@medisin.uio.no

19.1.2 ACL Injuries and Risk Factors

Variable factors have been recently identified and reinforced which can be attributed to the recent increase in ACL injury and subsequent treatment, including increased participation in sports, earlier sports specialization in adolescents, and improved diagnosis protocols [6].

Increased sagittal slope of the tibial plateau has recently been suggested in the literature as a significant contributor to ACL *reinjury*. This is attributed to the seemingly synonymous increase in anterior tibial translation that occurs from increases in posterior tibial slope (PTS), which is correlated by an ensuing increased occurrence of noncontact ACL injuries in patients with significantly greater PTS, 9.39° ± 2.58°, relative to control subjects, 8.50° ± 2.67° (P = 0.003) [7]. Measuring PTS by the longitudinal axis method has exhibited significant success in inter-rater (0.898) and intra-rater reliability (0.928), for use as a predictor for noncontact ACL injury [8]. Activities involving large compression forces significantly contribute to ACL failure when combined with greater PTS, with both active and passive models displaying substantial increases in anterior tibial translation and ACL forces upon increased PTS. [9]

New studies have recently surfaced showing significant correlations between ACL injuries and increased PTS. Using a hamstring tendon-based ACL reconstruction (ACLR) procedure with

M. T. Hirschmann et al. (eds.), *ESSKA Instructional Course Lecture Book*,
https://doi.org/10.1007/978-3-662-61264-4_19

interference screw fixation, Salmon et al. [10] found adolescent patients (<18 years) to experience significantly greater ligamentous laxity and ACL graft rupture relative to the adult cohort. A PTS of >12° was found to be a significant predictor of secondary ACL injury as well, with ACL graft rupture and contralateral ACL injury 11 times and 7 times, respectively, more likely to occur in adolescents with PTS of >12° relative to adults with PTS <12° [10]. Within the adult cohort, greater than 12° of PTS made a contralateral knee ACL injury 7 times more likely [10].

Risk factors associated with ACL injuries are not only important for avoiding the initial ACL rupture, potential graft failure, and reinjury concerns, but also due to the implications it may have on the potential development of osteoarthritis (OA) [11]. In a meta-analysis of 4108 patients, Cinque et al. found the likelihood of developing post-traumatic OA (PTOA) following ACLR as 11.3% at 5 years, 20.6% at 10 years, and 51.6% at 20 years, postoperatively [12]. The most significant risk factors associated with this probability of PTOA development were an increased preoperative interval between the ACL tear and ACLR, and increased age at the time of surgery. A study similar in follow-up length was conducted by Risberg et al. except comparing incidence of OA in isolated ACL injuries relative to combined ACL injuries in concomitance of others. Results showed a significant rise in the incidence of tibiofemoral and patellofemoral OA between follow-up of 15 and 20 years (increasing by 13% and 8%), reaching a total incidence of 42% and 21% [13]. Furthermore, patients sustaining ACL injuries with other combined injuries relative to isolated ACL injuries had significantly higher prevalence of tibiofemoral OA [13].

19.1.3 Treatment of ACL Injuries

Anterior cruciate ligament (ACL) rupture is a common knee ligament injury and the treatment can be either surgical or nonsurgical in nature [2]. Regardless of treatment strategy, patients with ACL injuries, especially those with a meniscal injury, have an increased risk of knee osteoarthritis (OA) [1, 14, 15] and decreased knee-related quality of life [16, 17] as compared with the general population [14].

Recent high-quality comparative studies using midterm follow-up have largely failed to show any clear advantage of surgical or nonsurgical treatment on knee OA development and patient-reported outcome measures (PROMs) [18, 19]. Prior systematic reviews with long-term follow-up also lack evidence to support either surgical or nonsurgical treatment [1, 20, 21]. However, a major problem with these comparative studies is the considerable number of patients who initially received nonsurgical treatment but later opted for surgical treatment and thereby make the consequences of the initial treatment harder to track [18, 22, 23]. Another shortcoming of the existing comparative studies is selection bias, since patients with worse injuries (e.g., concomitant ligament, cartilage, and meniscal injuries) are generally the ones initially being treated with surgery.

19.1.4 ACL Injury and Post-traumatic Osteoarthritis

Patients receiving concomitant meniscectomy procedures with ACLR previously have been reported to have a 3.54 elevated probability of OA development [24]. In addition, a recent study by the Mars Group reported a 17-fold increase in the progression of articular cartilage damage in the lateral compartment when >33% of the lateral meniscus was resected at the time of ACLR [25]. This increased risk was not reproduced in similar loss of meniscus in the medial compartment, which may be reflected by the difference in concavity of each compartment and variable function of the meniscus in each respective compartment [25]. This group also found the use of allograft for primary ACLRs resulted in a 15-fold elevated risk of OA in the patellofemoral compartment [25].

Advancement in identifying the risk factors for reinjury and OA progression is vital not only in refining the approach for ACLR procedures but also in developing preventative programs [26, 27]. It is also important to avoid the assumption of direct clinical application from promising biomechanical studies that have yet to show outcome significance. For instance, improved biomechanical graft properties have been observed from the double-bundle ACLR approach compared to single-bundle, [28] but upon analysis of revision rates, recent literature has shown a lack of influence contingent on the single- or double-bundle approach [29]. In fact, the use of bone-patellar tendon-bone grafts were observed to have a lower frequency of revision opposed to double-bundle hamstring tendon grafts [29]. What has been established by current studies is that focus should be attentive toward the means of reducing the interval between injury to surgery by earlier responsive diagnosis and prompt surgical treatment in knees needing early surgery, and of anatomic specific features respective of each patient; more specifically regarding increased PTS and medial/lateral menisci integrity. Preventative programs could partially lessen the increased occurrence of ACL injuries seen in adolescents due to the elevated training programs and increased sports specialization of today's sports culture, with simple decisions having profound impacts upon risk of reinjury [30, 31]. These findings have potential to improve the treatment of patients affected by ACL injuries, and ultimately prevent further damage that frequently occurs following this procedure.

19.1.5 Nonoperative Management

Treatment strategies for anterior cruciate ligament (ACL) injuries continue to evolve. The best practice guidelines for the *surgical* management of ACL injury are often based on studies of low-quality and low-levels of evidence.

Both operative and nonoperative treatment of ACL injury continue to evolve. Improved understanding of the structure and function of the native ACL has supported the development and adoption of anatomic ACLR [32]. Increased recognition of the adaptability of the neuromuscular system to achieve dynamic knee stability despite ACL deficiency has concurrently supported nonoperative treatment as a viable strategy in some patients [32, 33].

Successful outcomes following both operative and nonoperative treatments necessitate progressive rehabilitation in which impairments are addressed, functional stability is achieved, and the readiness to safely return to sport is confirmed [34]. The acute phase after the injury or surgery focuses on the elimination of residual symptoms (effusion, pain) and impairments (range of motion, quadriceps activation, and strength). Subsequently, neuromuscular training with additional perturbation training is implemented to improve knee stabilization strategies [35, 36]. The last phase aims to further enhance muscular strength, return to pre-injury sports level through sport-specific exercises, and assess mental readiness for the return to sport. Any discussion of nonoperative treatment herein implies the completion of a progressive, staged rehabilitation protocol.

Similarly, any discussion of operative treatment implies anatomic ACL reconstruction, which intends to restore the ACL to its native dimensions, collagen orientation, and insertion sites. Anatomic ACLR includes both single- and double-bundle techniques, followed by a progressive rehabilitation program that considers the natural healing cascade and ligamentization of the graft [37]. Both operative and nonoperative treatment aim to restore knee stability and thereby prevent further damage to the meniscus and cartilage, which could contribute to post-traumatic osteoarthritis. Functional bracing, intended to reduce the risk of ACL injury by decreasing peak ligament strain, has not yet been conclusively shown to achieve this goal [38, 39].

There is still uncertainty as to which patient should undergo immediate surgery and which patient may be successfully treated nonoperatively. Regardless, the treatment approach should be determined through a shared decision-making process between the patient and the provider [40]. In particular, the physician should share information on the evidence-based treatment options while also considering the patient's expectations and goals. While the patient and provider are the primary stakeholders in the shared decision-making process, the potential influence of secondary stakeholders, such as family and coaches, may be anticipated so as to minimize interests potentially conflicting with the health of the patient.

19.1.6 Future Directions

There is a need for larger randomized trials with longer-term follow-up in which initial surgery (followed by rehabilitation) is compared with a strategy of initial rehabilitation and delayed surgery. Data from randomized trials are lacking to guide treatment when there are concomitant meniscal and collateral ligament injuries. Data on long-term clinical outcome are needed to better understand the interrelationships of treatment of ACL injuries, subsequent injuries to meniscus and cartilage, and the development of osteoarthritis.

Take Home Message
Anterior cruciate ligament injuries are one of the most common knee injuries in the young and active population. Several patient-related factors and sports types have been demonstrated to increase the risk of ACL injury. Both operative and nonoperative approaches are viable treatment options for ACL injuries and continue to evolve. One of the major challenges is determining which patient with ACL injury will benefit from operation and who will benefit from nonsurgical treatment. Irrespective of the treatment chosen, proper and adequate rehabilitation is important to regain knee function after injury. Furthermore, it is important to implement ACL prevention strategies because ACL injuries have been demonstrated to affect the knee-related quality of life and increase the risk of developing OA.

References

1. Oiestad BE, Engebretsen L, Storheim K, Risberg MA. Knee osteoarthritis after anterior cruciate ligament injury: a systematic review. Am J Sports Med. 2009;37:1434–43.
2. Rahr-Wagner L, Lind M. The Danish knee ligament reconstruction registry. Clin Epidemiol. 2016;8:531–5.
3. Granan LP, Bahr R, Steindal K, Furnes O, Engebretsen L. Development of a national cruciate ligament surgery registry: the Norwegian National Knee Ligament Registry. Am J Sports Med. 2008;36:308–15.
4. Shaw L, Finch CF. Trends in pediatric and adolescent anterior cruciate ligament injuries in Victoria, Australia 2005-2015. Int J Environ Res Public Health. 2017;14.
5. Werner BC, Yang S, Looney AM, Gwathmey FW Jr. Trends in pediatric and adolescent anterior cruciate ligament injury and reconstruction. J Pediatr Orthop. 2016;36:447–52.
6. Frank JS, Gambacorta PL. Anterior cruciate ligament injuries in the skeletally immature athlete: diagnosis and management. J Am Acad Orthop Surg. 2013;21:78–87.
7. Todd MS, Lalliss S, Garcia E, DeBerardino TM, Cameron KL. The relationship between posterior tibial slope and anterior cruciate ligament injuries. Am J Sports Med. 2010;38:63–7.
8. Zeng C, Yang T, Wu S, Gao SG, Li H, Deng ZH, Zhang Y, Lei GH. Is posterior tibial slope associated with noncontact anterior cruciate ligament injury? Knee Surg Sports Traumatol Arthrosc. 2016;24:830–7.
9. Marouane H, Shirazi-Adl A, Adouni M, Hashemi J. Steeper posterior tibial slope markedly increases ACL force in both active gait and passive knee joint under compression. J Biomech. 2014;47:1353–9.
10. Salmon LJ, Heath E, Akrawi H, Roe JP, Linklater J, Pinczewski LA. 20-year outcomes of anterior cruciate ligament reconstruction with hamstring tendon autograft: the catastrophic effect of age and posterior tibial slope. Am J Sports Med. 2018;46:531–43.
11. Grindem H, Eitzen I, Engebretsen L, Snyder-Mackler L, Risberg MA. Nonsurgical or surgical treatment of ACL injuries: knee function, sports participation, and knee reinjury: the Delaware-Oslo ACL cohort study. J Bone Joint Surg Am. 2014;96:1233–41.
12. Cinque ME, Dornan GJ, Chahla J, Moatshe G, LaPrade RF. High rates of osteoarthritis develop after anterior cruciate ligament surgery: an analysis of 4108 patients. Am J Sports Med. 2018;46:2011–9.
13. Risberg MA, Oiestad BE, Gunderson R, Aune AK, Engebretsen L, Culvenor A, Holm I. Changes in knee osteoarthritis, symptoms, and function after anterior cruciate ligament reconstruction: a 20-year prospective follow-up study. Am J Sports Med. 2016;44:1215–24.
14. Ajuied A, Wong F, Smith C, Norris M, Earnshaw P, Back D, Davies A. Anterior cruciate ligament injury and radiologic progression of knee osteoarthritis: a systematic review and meta-analysis. Am J Sports Med. 2014;42:2242–52.
15. van Meer BL, Meuffels DE, van Eijsden WA, Verhaar JA, Bierma-Zeinstra SM, Reijman M. Which determinants predict tibiofemoral and patellofemoral osteo-

arthritis after anterior cruciate ligament injury? A systematic review. Br J Sports Med. 2015;49:975–83.
16. Filbay SR, Ackerman IN, Russell TG, Macri EM, Crossley KM. Health-related quality of life after anterior cruciate ligament reconstruction: a systematic review. Am J Sports Med. 2014;42:1247–55.
17. Filbay SR, Culvenor AG, Ackerman IN, Russell TG, Crossley KM. Quality of life in anterior cruciate ligament-deficient individuals: a systematic review and meta-analysis. Br J Sports Med. 2015;49:1033–41.
18. Frobell RB, Roos HP, Roos EM, Roemer FW, Ranstam J, Lohmander LS. Treatment for acute anterior cruciate ligament tear: five year outcome of randomised trial. BMJ. 2013;346:f232.
19. Wellsandt E, Failla MJ, Axe MJ, Snyder-Mackler L. Does anterior cruciate ligament reconstruction improve functional and radiographic outcomes over nonoperative management 5 years after injury? Am J Sports Med. 2018;46:2103–12.
20. Chalmers PN, Mall NA, Moric M, Sherman SL, Paletta GP, Cole BJ, Bach BR Jr. Does ACL reconstruction alter natural history?: a systematic literature review of long-term outcomes. J Bone Joint Surg Am. 2014;96:292–300.
21. Smith TO, Postle K, Penny F, McNamara I, Mann CJ. Is reconstruction the best management strategy for anterior cruciate ligament rupture? A systematic review and meta-analysis comparing anterior cruciate ligament reconstruction versus non-operative treatment. Knee. 2014;21:462–70.
22. Kessler MA, Behrend H, Henz S, Stutz G, Rukavina A, Kuster MS. Function, osteoarthritis and activity after ACL-rupture: 11 years follow-up results of conservative versus reconstructive treatment. Knee Surg Sports Traumatol Arthrosc. 2008;16:442–8.
23. Streich NA, Zimmermann D, Bode G, Schmitt H. Reconstructive versus non-reconstructive treatment of anterior cruciate ligament insufficiency. A retrospective matched-pair long-term follow-up. Int Orthop. 2011;35:607–13.
24. Claes S, Hermie L, Verdonk R, Bellemans J, Verdonk P. Is osteoarthritis an inevitable consequence of anterior cruciate ligament reconstruction? A meta-analysis. Knee Surg Sports Traumatol Arthrosc. 2013;21:1967–76.
25. Magnussen RA, Borchers JR, Pedroza AD, Huston LJ, Haas AK, Spindler KP, Wright RW, Kaeding CC, Allen CR, Anderson AF, Cooper DE, DeBerardino TM, Dunn WR, Lantz BA, Mann B, Stuart MJ, Albright JP, Amendola A, Andrish JT, Annunziata CC, Arciero RA, Bach BR Jr, Baker CL 3rd, Bartolozzi AR, Baumgarten KM, Bechler JR, Berg JH, Bernas GA, Brockmeier SF, Brophy RH, Bush-Joseph CA, Butler JB, Campbell JD, Carey JL, Carpenter JE, Cole BJ, Cooper JM, Cox CL, Creighton RA, Dahm DL, David TS, Flanigan DC, Frederick RW, Ganley TJ, Garofoli EA, Gatt CJ Jr, Gecha SR, Giffin JR, Hame SL, Hannafin JA, Harner CD, Harris NL Jr, Hechtman KS, Hershman EB, Hoellrich RG, Hosea TM, Johnson DC, Johnson TS, Jones MH, Kamath GV, Klootwyk TE, Levy BA, Ma CB, Maiers GP 2nd, Marx RG, Matava MJ, Mathien GM, McAllister DR, McCarty EC, McCormack RG, Miller BS, Nissen CW, O'Neill DF, Owens BD, Parker RD, Purnell ML, Ramappa AJ, Rauh MA, Rettig AC, Sekiya JK, Shea KG, Sherman OH, Slauterbeck JR, Smith MV, Spang JT, Svoboda SJ, Taft TN, Tenuta JJ, Tingstad EM, Vidal AF, Viskontas DG, White RA, Williams JS Jr, Wolcott ML, Wolf BR, York JJ. Risk factors and predictors of significant chondral surface change from primary to revision anterior cruciate ligament reconstruction: a MOON and MARS cohort study. Am J Sports Med. 2018;46:557–64.
26. Persson A, Fjeldsgaard K, Gjertsen JE, Kjellsen AB, Engebretsen L, Hole RM, Fevang JM. Increased risk of revision with hamstring tendon grafts compared with patellar tendon grafts after anterior cruciate ligament reconstruction: a study of 12,643 patients from the Norwegian cruciate ligament registry, 2004-2012. Am J Sports Med. 2014;42:285–91.
27. Persson A, Gifstad T, Lind M, Engebretsen L, Fjeldsgaard K, Drogset JO, Forssblad M, Espehaug B, Kjellsen AB, Fevang JM. Graft fixation influences revision risk after ACL reconstruction with hamstring tendon autografts. Acta Orthop. 2018;89:204–10.
28. Lehmann AK, Osada N, Zantop T, Raschke MJ, Petersen W. Femoral bridge stability in double-bundle ACL reconstruction: impact of bridge width and different fixation techniques on the structural properties of the graft/femur complex. Arch Orthop Trauma Surg. 2009;129:1127–32.
29. Aga C, Kartus JT, Lind M, Lygre SHL, Granan LP, Engebretsen L. Risk of revision was not reduced by a double-bundle ACL reconstruction technique: results from the Scandinavian registers. Clin Orthop Relat Res. 2017;475:2503–12.
30. Grindem H, Snyder-Mackler L, Moksnes H, Engebretsen L, Risberg MA. Simple decision rules can reduce reinjury risk by 84% after ACL reconstruction: the Delaware-Oslo ACL cohort study. Br J Sports Med. 2016;50:804–8.
31. Risberg MA, Grindem H, Oiestad BE. We need to implement current evidence in early rehabilitation programs to improve long-term outcome after anterior cruciate ligament injury. J Orthop Sports Phys Ther. 2016;46:710–3.
32. Fu FH, van Eck CF, Tashman S, Irrgang JJ, Moreland MS. Anatomic anterior cruciate ligament reconstruction: a changing paradigm. Knee Surg Sports Traumatol Arthrosc. 2015;23:640–8.
33. Eitzen I, Moksnes H, Snyder-Mackler L, Risberg MA. A progressive 5-week exercise therapy program leads to significant improvement in knee function early after anterior cruciate ligament injury. J Orthop Sports Phys Ther. 2010;40:705–21.
34. Paterno MV. Non-operative care of the patient with an ACL-deficient knee. Curr Rev Musculoskelet Med. 2017;10:322–7.
35. Chmielewski TL, Hurd WJ, Rudolph KS, Axe MJ, Snyder-Mackler L. Perturbation training improves

knee kinematics and reduces muscle co-contraction after complete unilateral anterior cruciate ligament rupture. Phys Ther. 2005;85:740–9; discussion 750–754.
36. Fitzgerald GK, Axe MJ, Snyder-Mackler L. The efficacy of perturbation training in nonoperative anterior cruciate ligament rehabilitation programs for physical active individuals. Phys Ther. 2000;80:128–40.
37. Pauzenberger L, Syre S, Schurz M. "Ligamentization" in hamstring tendon grafts after anterior cruciate ligament reconstruction: a systematic review of the literature and a glimpse into the future. Arthroscopy. 2013;29:1712–21.
38. Hangalur G, Brenneman E, Nicholls M, Bakker R, Laing A, Chandrashekar N. Can a knee brace reduce the strain in the anterior cruciate ligament? A study using combined in vivo/in vitro method. Prosthet Orthot Int. 2016;40:394–9.
39. Sitler M, Ryan J, Hopkinson W, Wheeler J, Santomier J, Kolb R, Polley D. The efficacy of a prophylactic knee brace to reduce knee injuries in football. A prospective, randomized study at west point. Am J Sports Med. 1990;18:310–5.
40. Charles C, Gafni A, Whelan T. Shared decision-making in the medical encounter: what does it mean? (or it takes at least two to tango). Soc Sci Med. 1997;44:681–92.

20 Cell Soluble Factors and Matrix in Allograft Integration

Laura de Girolamo

20.1 Introduction

In orthopaedic procedures, allografts play a crucial role due to decreased operative times and donor site morbidity associated with autograft harvesting [1]. Similar to autografts, allograft transplantation has a very high success rate, as shown for meniscal treatments with only 5% drawback in a timeframe up to 5 years [2]. Likewise, only a 2.4% complication rate was reported for osteochondral allograft [3] and revision rates after cruciate ligament reconstruction showed an encouraging success (93%) 24 months after surgery [4]. Very little is known about the basic science of integration, remodelling and healing of allografts. Ideally, a graft should recreate the biomechanical and anatomical features of the native tissues, ensuring a quick biological integration, efficient recovery and reduced donor site morbidity. Since each tissue behave uniquely due to their cellular and mechanical properties, not all allograft tissues are alike.

L. de Girolamo (✉)
Orthopaedic Biotechnology Laboratory, IRCCS Orthopaedic Institute Galeazzi, Milan, Italy
e-mail: laura.degirolamo@grupposandonato.it

20.2 Meniscal Allograft

When the tear is in the outer third of the meniscus, the chances of healing are high. In the cases reduced tissue is left, meniscus transplantation is to be preferred [5]. Mandatory for transplant success, the new meniscus has to perform optimal mechanical and biological functions to stabilize and support the knee. In this view, viable donor cells readily sustain the graft extracellular matrix [6]. Therefore, meniscus procurement should take place no longer than 12 h after donor's death [7]. Nevertheless, after implantation, donor cells are either no longer or in small amounts detectable with respect to host cells. For example, in goats, donor cells did not survive longer than 4 weeks [8]. Despite this, in a rabbit model, graft neo-vascularization and cell repopulation took place at 12 and 26 weeks [9]. This repopulation of cells from the host to the allograft is associated with an increase in the expression of type I and III procollagen mRNAs, especially near the region of the synovial capsule. Intriguingly, at 26 weeks, type I procollagen mRNA expression became prominent with only a small amount of type III procollagen, indicating active cell metabolism [9]. Consistently, in dogs, cells originated from the adjacent synovium were able to populate implanted menisci, being able to migrate over the surface of the meniscus to invade the deeper layers of the tissue [10]. Supporting these in vivo results, in humans, after 12 months, 95%

M. T. Hirschmann et al. (eds.), *ESSKA Instructional Course Lecture Book*,
https://doi.org/10.1007/978-3-662-61264-4_20

of the DNA meniscal allograft was identical to the recipient [11]. These data demonstrated that the implanted graft is almost entirely repopulated by host cells derived from the synovial membrane.

Although graft cells are important for first steps of engraftment even if they disappear quickly, a major issue after transplantation is recipient's immune response [12], since fresh meniscal allografts express class I and II histocompatibility antigens [13]. Consistently, in rats, evidence of rejection was noted [14]. To reduce graft immunogenicity and allow long storage periods, a popular method is deepfreezing, where donor cells are destroyed together with denaturation of histocompatibility antigens [15]. Lyophilisation also preserves the tissue, although it may produce changes in the size of allografts [15]. Finally, gamma irradiation, often used to minimize the risk of disease transmission, may also compromise the mechanical properties of the graft [15]. Thus, to date, fresh-frozen grafts are among the most widely used in clinical practice, and a meta-analysis on 2853 allografts clearly showed no significant difference in allograft survival between frozen and lyophilized/irradiated grafts [16].

20.3 Osteochondral Allograft

The difficulty to reconstruct articular cartilage lesions is mainly due to a lack of vascularisation that could provide regenerative progenitor cells to sites of damage. Osteochondral defects may become naturally filled with a blood clot originating from microfracturing the subchondral bone marrow, that stimulates the mobilization and osteochondro-differentiation of marrow progenitor cells (MSC) [17]. However, the repair tissue is of fibrocartilaginous nature, containing type I collagen without the re-establishment of an arcade-like organization of the fibrillar extracellular matrix (ECM) [17]. Therefore, despite the availability of options to stimulate bone marrow or deliver chondrocytes/MSC, osteochondral allograft transplantation, especially for large defects, remains the most preferred option with long lasting results [18, 19]. For this approach, the initial presence of viable chondrocytes is crucial to maintain tissue composition, structure, and function [20]. Currently, the preferred protocol for storage is preservation at 4 °C [21], able to maintain chondrocyte viability higher than 90% up to 8 days [22]. As an alternative when prolonged storage is required, freezing procedure is selected, despite reduced viability even under addition of cryoprotectants (approximately 15% of initial viability) [23]. Alternatively, physiological temperature of 37 °C has also been proposed with >70% chondrocyte viability for at least 8 weeks [24]. To date, independently from the storage approach, the average time from procurement to implantation of an osteochondral allograft is 24 days [21].

The most important issue remains the integration of implanted osteochondral allograft with host osseous and cartilage tissues. In this view, technical procedures and supplemental treatment options resulted to be crucial. As an example, an aggressive approach to insert the graft may cause cell death and apoptosis leading to matrix degradation and eventual graft failure [25]. To improve viability, the addition of platelet rich plasma (PRP) or bone marrow aspirate concentrate (BMC) to help repopulate the osseous portion of an osteochondral allograft was suggested, bringing stem cells and growth factors to the site of injury [26]. Supporting this notion, in dogs, BMC and PRP provided a superior osseous integration due to release of osteoinductive proteins such as osteoprotegerin, increase of bone mineral density and bone volume, as well as production of bone morphogenetic protein 2, known to stimulate osteogenesis. The paradigm of supporting viable cells was also observed using Agili-C scaffold (CartiHeal, Israel) in an equine model, where BMC steadily improved collagen orientation and collagen type II content, including the deposition of a hyaline-like tissue [27]. Therefore, allografts supplemented with BMC or PRP in the osseous portion of the graft might be a promising option to minimize treatment failures, to improve graft survivorship and integration, and thus patient outcomes.

20.4 Tendon Allograft

Several tendon allograft sources are available, including patellar, semitendinosus and Achilles tendons [28]. Compared with autograft ACL reconstruction, allograft incorporation proceeds with a similar but slower progression [28] characterized by distinct biological stages. Initially, during acute inflammation, transforming growth factor-β1 is released by platelets and attracts neutrophils and monocytes that generate chemokines and components of the proinflammatory cascade [29]. Until the fourth postoperative week, necrosis increases in the centre of the graft [30] and is accompanied by the release of growth factors able to stimulate cell migration (including MSC from the synovial fluid) [31]. Then, revascularization starts on the fourth postoperative week promoted by monocytes [30]. Between 4 and 12 weeks, a strong proliferation phase occurs and host fibroblasts with synovial cells repopulate the transplanted tendon after donor fibroblast necrosis [32]. IL-1 produced by macrophages, fibroblasts, and neutrophils induces matrix metallo-proteinases (MMP-1, -3 and -13) to initiate the degradation of collagen fibrils [32]. In a second step, metalloproteases continue collagen degradation preparing the tendon for remodelling [33]. Further, PDGF and TGF-β, released by degranulation of platelets, contribute to increased fibroblast proliferation and production of extracellular matrix components to generate a connective tissue scar [34]. From 12 weeks onwards, tendon allograft is actively remodelling and acquires its maximum properties in 1 year. In this time frame, cellularity returns to values of the intact tendon with vessels becoming evenly distributed throughout the entire graft [30], although the central portion of the graft remains essentially acellular [25].

Fresh tendons stimulate an immunologic reaction, because of the expression of major histocompatibility markers [28]. Therefore, fresh allografts have been abandoned with the use of freezing procedures that do not alter their mechanical and structural properties (architecture, fibre orientation, matrix, cell infiltration, fibroblast proliferation, edema and vascularization) [28]. Further, sterilization and irradiation to inactivate bacterial and viral pathogens are commonly used techniques although high doses of gamma irradiation (>2.5 Mrad) may have adverse effects on the biological and mechanical properties (30% average decrease in load to failure) [35], prompting the use of multiple stranded tendons to increase the mean peak load to failure [36]. To overcome this limitation, fractionation of irradiation doses has led to improved properties of patellar [37] and flexor digitorum superficialis tendons [38].

20.5 Conclusions

Allografts are effective in response to patients' clinical, biological and functional demands. Many biological issues such as incorporation, remodelling and immune responses are still to be further assessed. It clearly emerges that cell types, growth factors and cytokines are involved in a coordinated fashion during the early inflammatory and advanced remodelling phases. A better understanding of the complex biological events occurring at the host–implant interface will lead to improved biologically driven strategies for allogeneic implants.

References

1. Chiarello E, Cadossi M, Tedesco G, Capra P, Calamelli C, Shehu A, Giannini S. Autograft, allograft and bone substitutes in reconstructive orthopedic surgery. Aging Clin Exp Res. 2013;25(Suppl 1):S101–3.
2. McCormick F, Harris JD, Frank RM, Hussey KE, Wilson H, Gupta AK, Abrams GD, Bach BR, Cole BJ. Meniscal allograft transplantation reoperation rates, operative findings, and survival analysis: a review of 200 consecutive transplants at minimum two-year follow-up. Orthop J Sports Med. 2014;2(1 Suppl):2325967114S00003.
3. Chahal J, Gross AE, Gross C, Mall N, Dwyer T, Chahal A, Whelan DB, Cole BJ. Outcomes of osteochondral allograft transplantation in the knee. Arthroscopy. 2013;29(3):575–88.
4. Barber FA, Cowden CH 3rd, Sanders EJ. Revision rates after anterior cruciate ligament reconstruction using bone-patellar tendon-bone allograft or autograft in a population 25 years old and younger. Arthroscopy. 2014;30(4):483–91.

5. van der Wal RJ, Thomassen BJ, van Arkel ER. Long-term clinical outcome of open meniscal allograft transplantation. Am J Sports Med. 2009;37(11):2134–9.
6. von Lewinski G, Wirth CJ. Meniscal reconstruction: allograft. 10.1. Basic science. In: Beaufils P, Verdonk R, editors. The meniscus. Berlin: Springer; 2010. p. 303–15.
7. Schubert T, Cornu O, Delloye C. Organization: type of grafts, conservation, regulation. In: Beaufils P, Verdonk R, editors. The meniscus. Berlin: Springer; 2010. p. 315–20.
8. Jackson DW, Simon TM, Kurzweil PR, Rosen MA. Survival of cells after intra-articular transplantation of fresh allografts of the patellar and anterior cruciate ligaments. DNA-probe analysis in a goat model. J Bone Joint Surg Am. 1992;74(1):112–8.
9. Wada Y, Amiel M, Harwood F, Moriya H, Amiel D. Architectural remodeling in deep frozen meniscal allografts after total meniscectomy. Arthroscopy. 1998;14(3):250–7.
10. Arnoczky SP, DiCarlo EF, O'Brien SJ, Warren RF. Cellular repopulation of deep-frozen meniscal autografts: an experimental study in the dog. Arthroscopy. 1992;8(4):428–36.
11. Debeer P, Decorte R, Delvaux S, Bellemans J. DNA analysis of a transplanted cryopreserved meniscal allograft. Arthroscopy. 2000;16:71–5.
12. Farrar CA, Kupiec-Weglinski JW, Sacks SH. The innate immune system and transplantation. Cold Spring Harb Perspect Med. 2013;3(10):a015479.
13. Khoury MA, Goldberg VM, Stevenson S. Demonstration of HLA and ABH antigens in fresh and frozen human menisci by immunohistochemistry. J Orthop Res. 1994;12:751–7.
14. Wada Y. Meniscal transplantation using fresh and cryopreserved allografts. An experimental study in the genetically defined rat. J Jpn Orthop Assoc. 1993;67:677–83.
15. Binnet MS, Akan B, Kaya A. Lyophilised medial meniscus transplantations in ACL-deficient knees: a 19-year follow-up. Knee Surg Sports Traumatol Arthrosc. 2012;20:109–13.
16. De Bruycker M, Verdonk PCM, Verdonk RC. Meniscal allograft transplantation: a meta-analysis. SICOT J. 2017;3:33.
17. Shapiro F, Koide S, Glimcher MJ. Cell origin and differentiation in the repair of full-thickness defects of articular cartilage. J Bone Joint Surg Am. 1993;75(4):532–53.
18. DiBartola AC, Everhart JS, Magnussen RA, Carey JL, Brophy RH, Schmitt LC, Flanigan DC. Correlation between histological outcome and surgical cartilage repair technique in the knee: a meta-analysis. Knee. 2016;23(3):344–9.
19. LaPrade RF, Botker J, Herzog M, Agel J. Refrigerated osteoarticular allografts to treat articular cartilage defects of the femoral condyles. A prospective outcomes study. J Bone Joint Surg Am. 2009;91(4):805–11.
20. Bugbee WD, Pallante-Kichura AL, Görtz S, Amiel D, Sah R. Osteochondral allograft transplantation in cartilage repair: graft storage paradigm, translational models, and clinical applications. J Orthop Res. 2016;34(1):31–8.
21. Pallante AL, Görtz S, Chen AC, Healey RM, Chase DC, Ball ST, Amiel D, Sah RL, Bugbee WD. Treatment of articular cartilage defects in the goat with frozen versus fresh osteochondral allografts: effects on cartilage stiffness, zonal composition, and structure at six months. J Bone Joint Surg Am. 2012;94(21):1984–95.
22. Williams RJ 3rd, Dreese JC, Chen CT. Chondrocyte survival and material properties of hypothermically stored cartilage: an evaluation of tissue used for osteochondral allograft transplantation. Am J Sports Med. 2004;32(1):132–9.
23. Judas F, Rosa S, Teixeira L, Lopes C, Ferreira MA. Chondrocyte viability in fresh and frozen large human osteochondral allografts: effect of cryoprotective agents. Transplant Proc. 2007;39(8):2531–4.
24. Garrity JT, Stoker AM, Sims HJ, Cook JL. Improved osteochondral allograft preservation using serum-free media at body temperature. Am J Sports Med. 2012;40(11):2542–8.
25. Gitelis SL, Bodker A, Laurent MP, Kirk SS, Filardo G, Meyer MA, Hakimiyan AA, Rappoport L, Wimmer MA, Cole BJ, Chubinskaya S. The effect of surgical insertion and proinflammatory cytokines on osteochondral allograft survival and metabolism. Cartilage. 2018;9(3):284–92.
26. Stoker AM, Baumann CA, Stannard JP, Cook JL. Bone marrow aspirate concentrate versus platelet rich plasma to enhance osseous integration potential for osteochondral allografts. J Knee Surg. 2017;31(4):314–20.
27. Fortier LA, Potter HG, Rickey EJ, Schnabel LV, Foo LF, Chong LR, Stokol T, Cheetham J, Nixon AJ. Concentrated bone marrow aspirate improves full-thickness cartilage repair compared with microfracture in the equine model. J Bone Joint Surg Am. 2010;92(10):1927–37.
28. Eagan MJ, McAllister DR. Biology of allograft incorporation. Clin Sports Med. 2009;28(2):203–14.
29. Leask A, Holmes A, Abraham DJ. Connective tissue growth factor: a new and important player in the pathogenesis of fibrosis. Curr Rheumatol Rep. 2002;4:136–42.
30. Scheffler SU, Unterhauser FN, Weiler A. Graft remodeling and ligamentization after cruciate ligament reconstruction. Knee Surg Sports Traumatol Arthrosc. 2008;16:834–42.
31. Yoshikawa T, Tohyama H, Katsura T. Effects of local administration of vascular endothelial growth factor on mechanical characteristics of the semitendinosus tendon graft after anterior cruciate ligament reconstruction in sheep. Am J Sports Med. 2006;34:1918–25.
32. Knauper V, Will H, Lopez-Otin C, Smith B, Atkinson SJ, Stanton H, Hembry RM, Murphy G. Cellular

mechanisms for human procollagenase-3 (MMP-13) activation: evidence that MT1-MMP (MMP-14) and gelatinase a (MMP-2) are able to generate active enzyme. J Biol Chem. 1996;271:17124–31.
33. Sharma P, Maffulli N. Biology of tendon injury: healing, modeling and remodeling. J Musculoskelet Neuronal Interact. 2006;6(2):181–90.
34. Eppley BL, Woodell JE, Higgins J. Platelet quantification and growth factor analysis from platelet-rich plasma: implications for wound healing. Plast Reconstr Surg. 2004;114:1502–8.
35. Seto AU, Culp BM, Gatt CJ Jr, Dunn M. Radioprotection provides functional mechanics but delays healing of irradiated tendon allografts after ACL reconstruction in sheep. Cell Tissue Bank. 2013;14:655–65.
36. Vinagre G, Kennedy NI, Chahla J, Cinque ME, Hussain ZB, Olesen ML, LaPrade RF. Hamstring graft preparation techniques for anterior cruciate ligament reconstruction. Arthrosc Tech. 2017;6(6):e2079–84.
37. Hoburg A, Keshlaf S, Schmidt T, Smith M, Gohs U, Perka C, Pruss A, Scheffler S. Fractionation of high-dose electron beam irradiation of BPTB grafts provides significantly improved viscoelastic and structural properties compared to standard gamma irradiation. Knee Surg Sports Traumatol Arthrosc. 2011;19(11):1955–61.
38. Wei W, Liu Y, Yang X, Tian S, Liu C, Zhang Y, Xu Z, Hu B, Tian Z, Sun K. Fractionation of 50 kGy electron beam irradiation: effects on biomechanics of human flexor digitorum superficialis tendons treated with ascorbate. J Biomech. 2013;46:658–61.

21 Surgical Technique: What We Would Do in Different Situations—Graft Choice, One or Two Steps, Fixation, Associated Lesions

Kazumi Goto and Jacques Menetrey

21.1 Introduction

Anterior cruciate ligament (ACL) tears continue to be one of the most common sports injuries. ACL reconstruction (ACLR) are also common, and the number of ACL reconstruction (ACLR) has increased over the last years [1, 2]. Despite improved methods and techniques for primary ACLR, graft re-rupture rates have been reported between 0 and 5.6% [3]. Subsequently, the number of ACL revision surgeries has increased [4]. Outcomes after revision ACLR are generally inferior to those after primary ACLR. Only 43% of patients have been reported to return to their previous activity level, a significantly lower figure than that reported for primary ACLR [5]. In addition, the rates of re-revision ACLR after revision ACLR are higher than after primary ACLR (6.5% at 5 years and 9.0% at 8 years) [6]. The exact reasons why revision ACLR results in inferior outcomes are not completely known. However, it is a common perception for surgeons that revision ACLR is a challenging operation.

K. Goto
Centre for Sports Medicine and Exercise, Hirslanden Clinique La Colline, Geneva, Switzerland
e-mail: kazumi@kgorthop.com

J. Menetrey (✉)
Centre for Sports Medicine and Exercise, Hirslanden Clinique La Colline, Geneva, Switzerland

Orthopaedic Surgery Service, University Hospital of Geneva, Geneva, Switzerland
e-mail: Jacques.Menetrey@hirslanden.ch

21.2 Preoperative Planning

Preoperative planning, including comprehensive clinical and radiological evaluation, is the first and most important step. It is necessary to adequately understand the patient's symptoms such as instability, swelling, locking, stiffness, and pain. The history of previous injuries, how it occurred, pre-injured activity level (the competition and its level), the postoperative course, information on the mechanism and timing of reinjuries, is also crucial. Blood tests provide surgeons with information about possible infections as a routine preoperative examination. It is prerequisite to know the complete details of the primary surgery, the presence of the concomitant lesions and their treatment, and the type of graft and fixation methods.

Routine clinical examinations are conducted to assess anterior instability, rotational instability, and associated complications as before the primary surgery. Imaging evaluation should include X-ray, MRI, and CT scan. X-ray is a comprehensive imaging test that is very useful for understanding the overall condition. It is important to carefully observe the alignment evaluation, especially varus alignment and/or increased posterior slope of the tibia. Those conditions can provoke

M. T. Hirschmann et al. (eds.), *ESSKA Instructional Course Lecture Book*,
https://doi.org/10.1007/978-3-662-61264-4_21

ACL instability and the risk of graft failure [7]. In those cases, it should be considered to perform proximal tibial osteotomy concurrently in order to obtain suitable alignment. The position of the bone tunnel and previous device may also be observed, and if there is tunnel lysis or expansion, the decision of the revision surgical procedure will be affected. The CT scan can provide more detailed information related to tunnel position, size of tunnels, miserable tunnel expansion, and the presence of hardware. The MRI is useful to perceive the status of the graft, cartilage, meniscal lesion, and the surrounding soft tissues.

21.3 Graft Choice

The graft choice for revision surgery depends upon the graft used for primary ACLR and the placement of the tunnel and tunnel size. The surgeon's preferences and concepts are also influenced by the decision. Which of the graft is superior for primary or revision ACLR is still controversial [8, 9]. However, recent large cohort studies of revision ACLR reported that autograft is superior to allografts in terms of lower re-revision rate, lower postoperative laxity, patient reported outcome (IKDC and KOOS) at 2-year postoperatively, and the rate of return to sports (RTS) [10–15]. On the other hand, there is no clear consensus on what type of autograft should be selected in the revision ACLR, which depends mainly on experience and local conditions. Our most frequent graft choice in primary or revision is quadriceps tendon (QT). In certain cases, hamstring tendon (HT) or bone-patellar tendon-bone (BPTB) may also be considered, and surgeons need to master several techniques. Table 21.1 summarizes our algorithm for autograft management in revision ACLR.

Graft choice for revision ACLR was quite variable between large cohorts in France, Norway, and North America (Table 21.2) [9]. In the Multicenter ACL Revision study (MARS) cohort, allografts (49.4%) and autografts (47.9%) were used with similar frequency (hybrid were used for the remaining 2.6%), with BPTB autografts (26.2%) used slightly more than HT autografts (20.1%). In the Norwegian Knee Ligament Registry (NKLR), HT autograft (56.0%) was the most commonly used graft followed by BPTB autograft (32.4%). Other graft types were rare. In the Société Française d'Arthroscopie (SFA) survey, BPTB autograft (55.9%) was most common, followed by hamstring autograft (38.6%). QT autografts were used in 1–2% of cases in each cohort. However, interestingly, the analysis of MARS cohort [16] demonstrated that extrinsic factors (age, gender, previous graft choice) significantly influence graft choice, but finally the most important factor in revision ACL R graft choice is the surgeon.

Table 21.1 Algorithm for autograft choice in revision ACLR

Primary graft	Revision graft
Quadriceps tendon (QT)	Ipsilateral bone-patellar tendon-bone (BPTB)
BPTB, Hamstring tendon (HT)	Ipsilateral QT
Re-revisions for both BPTB and HT harvested	Ipsilateral QT
Re-revisions for both QT and BPTB harvested	Ipsilateral HT or allograft

Table 21.2 The data of graft choice between large cohorts in France, Norway, and North America [9]

	MARS ($n = 1216$)	NKLR ($n = 793$)	SFA ($n = 277$)
BPTB autograft	318 (26.2%)	257 (32.4%)	155 (55.9%)
HT autograft	245 (20.1%)	444 (56.0%)	107 (38.6%)
QT autograft	19 (1.6%)	13 (1.6%)	6 (2.2%)
Other	1 (0.1%)	5 (0.6%)	6 (2.2%)
Allograft	601 (49.4%)	30 (3.8%)	
Hybrid	32 (2.6%)		
Not reported		44 (5.5%)	3 (1.1%)

21.4 Quadriceps Tendon (QT)

Recently, the quadriceps tendon (QT) autograft (Fig. 21.1a.) has been discussed as a potential alternative graft for ACLR. Although the QT

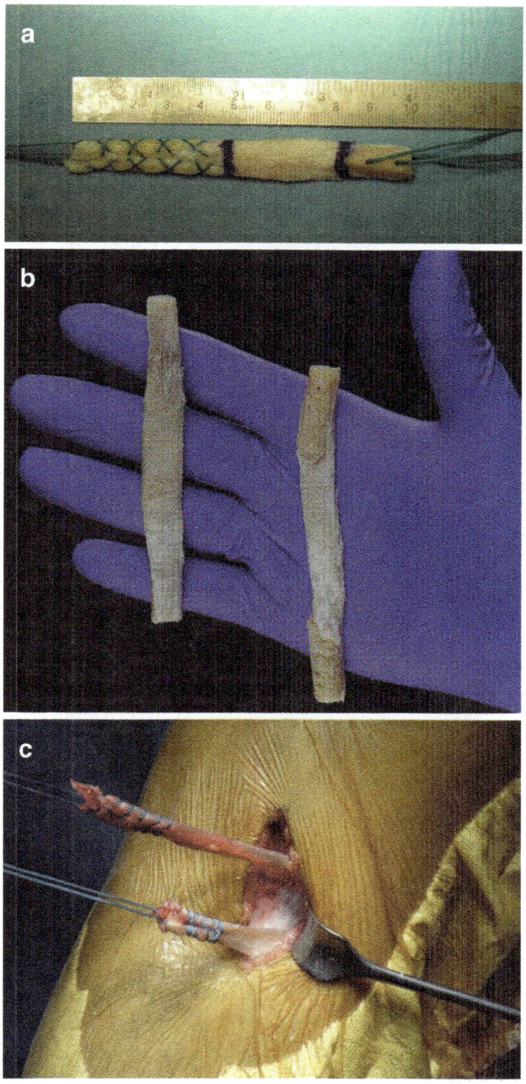

Fig. 21.1 The type of autografts. (a) Quadriceps tendon autograft. (b) Bone-patellar tendon-bone autograft. (c) Hamstring tendon autograft

autograft is the least studied and least used autograft, its use is expected to increase [17]. In 2010, 2.5% of all anatomic ACLR were performed with QT autografts [18], but increased to 11% in 2014 [19]. The biomechanical study showed that QT graft has a clear advantage because it provided a thicker graft with more advantageous tensile properties compared with BPTB and HT grafts [20–23]. Several studies found that the cross-sectional area of the QT was nearly twice that of the BPTB [20–23]. Shani et al. [21]. reported that ultimate load to failure (2186 vs. 1581 N) and stiffness (466 vs. 278 N/mm) were significantly higher for the QT graft compared with BPTB, respectively. Harris et al. [20] demonstrated that the load to failure of the QT was 1.36 times higher than that of a BPTB graft of comparable width. The most recent meta-analysis reported that QT autograft had comparable clinical and functional outcomes and graft survival rate compared with BPTB and HT autografts, with QT autograft showing significantly less harvest site pain compared with BPTB autograft and better functional outcome scores (Lysholm) compared with HT autograft [24].

In terms of cosmetic aspects, Bartlett et al. [25] noted that taking QT can cause unsightly wounds. In addition, Kim et al. [26] in his series, 7 patients out of 21 treated with ACLR using QT autografts required cosmetic surgery for scars that impair the appearance. However, Cavaignac et al. [27] reported that the appearance of the scar and the length of the incision were significantly better in QT versus BPTB and tended to be better without reaching the significant threshold of 2.5% in QT versus HT patients. Moreover, in this study, the harvesting of QT autograft for ACLR produces less area of hypoesthesia than both BPTB and HT autografts with statistical significance [27].

While many primary clinical outcomes have been reported, there are not many reports on the use of QT for revision ACLR. Wright et al. [28] reported that the systematic review of 766 patients showed autograft was used in 89.4% (685) and consisted of BPTB in 48%, HT in 40%, and QT in 12%. Barié et al. [29] reported that revision ACLR using QT autografts provides good objective knee stability in over 90% of the patients. This level of stability is comparable with that after primary ACLR, as indicated in previous studies. It is able to restore the function to a good or very good level in over 50% of the patients as previously reported in the literature. Nonetheless, there is still little data on the use of QT in revision ACLR and further research is required.

21.5 Bone-Patellar Tendon-Bone (BPTB)

BPTB (Fig. 21.1b) is one of the most commonly harvested autologous tissues used as grafts for primary or revision ACLR [9, 28]. In primary reconstruction, some authors suggest that BPTB autograft is the most favorable graft choice because of faster graft incorporation [30] a higher proportion of patients returning to preinjury activity levels [31], and potentially a lower risk of graft rupture [32]. A recent large Scandinavian registry study [33] reported a higher risk of graft rupture with HT than BPTB. The most recent meta-analysis found that patients undergoing primary ACLR with BPTB autograft were less likely to experience graft rupture and/or revision ACLR than patients treated with HT autograft [34].

In terms of revision surgery using BPTB, good results have also been reported in the literatures [35, 36]. Keizer et al. [37] reported that there was a significant difference in rate of return to sports (RTS) type in favor of using an ipsilateral BPTB autograft over a patellar tendon allograft (43.3% versus 75.0%, respectively) in patients undergoing revision ACLR after a minimum follow-up of 2 years.

However, disadvantages of using a BPTB autograft tendon might include anterior knee pain [38], donor site morbidity, quadriceps weakness [39, 40], and therefore a lower knee extensor moment [41].

21.6 Hamstring Tendon (HT)

HT (Fig. 21.1c) is also one of the common grafts used for both primary and revision surgery as well as BPTB [9]. Denti et al. [42] reported similar outcomes between HT and BPTB autografts in revision surgery. On the other hand, Grassi et al. [12] reported that HT autografts had better outcomes than BPTB autografts in revision ACLR, with IKDC score, Lysholm score, Tegner score and lower rates of complications and reoperations, while HT and BPTB autografts had similar outcomes in terms of laxity and pivot-shift. Legnani et al. [13] demonstrated that the use of contralateral HT autografts for ACL revision surgery produced similar subjective and objective outcomes at 5.2 years follow-up compared to revision with allograft patellar or Achilles tendon. With regard to RTS, patients undergoing revision surgery with autografts experienced a quicker RTS compared to patients who underwent allograft revision surgery.

Nevertheless, there are many reports that HT is higher risk of graft failure than BPTB in primary ACLR [32–34], therefore it is important to consider graft choice according to the individual characteristics.

21.7 Allograft

An allograft is still the preferred graft used in North America for revision ACLR [9, 43]. An allograft has the greatest advantage of being able to avoid donor site morbidity [43]. In addition, it can provide a large bone block that helps to fill the bone gap [44]. However, consideration should be given to infection, disease transmission risk, late re-cellularization, possibility of late failure, and the increased cost with this option [43–47].

However, a recent systematic review of graft type and the outcomes of revision ACLR reported autografts to have better results than allografts with lower postoperative laxity, and lower rates of reoperation and complications [12]. Some previous studies described allograft is inferior to autograft in terms of RTS [13, 36]. The Danish registry [14, 15] also showed that the re-revision rate was significantly higher for allograft compared with autograft (12.7% vs. 5.4%; $P < 0.001$), leading to a hazard ratio for re-revision of 2.2 (95% CI, 1.4–3.4) for allografts compared with autografts when corrected for age. Otherwise, Condello et al. [48] reported that the use of allografts for ACL revision can be regarded as a safe and effective approach: data from several studies have shown that the infection and overall complication rate, is similar with respect to primary procedures with autografts [49], and also clinical outcomes are satisfactory in terms of durable knee stability after revision and RTS [5, 7]. Additionally, Kay et al. [35] reported that there was no significant influence of graft choice on the rate of RTS after revision anterior cruciate ligament reconstruction identified between BPTB autografts (67%), HT autografts (55%), and allografts (64%).

21.8 One-Stage or Two-Stage Surgery?

Once all the necessary information has been obtained, the surgeon can choose a one- or a two-stage revision. One-stage revision can be considered when graft healing and fixation will not be influenced by previous surgery. Therefore, one-stage revision can be performed in a patient in whom previous tunnel did not interfere with the new tunnel, the tunnel did not significantly expand, no tunnel lysis or void bony defect, no associated injuries (malalignments, meniscal and chondral lesion, unless treated simultaneously), and no hardware removal problem. The two-stage procedure is performed in 6–9% of all ACL revision cases [48]. Even if the previous tunnel is correctly placed, if there is a significant tunnel enlargement or a void bony defect (Fig. 21.2), a two-stage revision is recommended [50]. The amount of tunnel enlargement required for two-stage surgery is still contentious. In general, it is accepted that two-stage surgery may be required when tunnel enlargement greater than 15–16 mm or 100% larger than the original tunnel [51, 52]. Even a 10–15 mm anatomically correct tunnel may require two-stage surgery depending on the shape of the tunnel or anticipated graft choice, while tunnels measuring less than 10 mm usually may be reused without grafting (permitting single-stage surgery) [52] (Fig. 21.3).

If a two-stage revision is deemed necessary, the first stage consists of removal of the old graft, and the metalwork from the primary repair. Some authors now advocate that metalwork should be left in situ if possible because screw and graft removal can leave large defect obtained between 3 and 6 months (3–4 months for autograft, 4–6 months for allograft) to assess the bone quality and the degree of graft incorporation. If these are deemed satisfactory, the second stage of the procedure consists of a standard graft repair.

Other indications for a two-stage revision are loss of range of motion, and concomitant surgery such as repair for locked bucket-handle meniscal tear or proximal tibial osteotomy that would slow down the postoperative recovery [48].

21.9 Fixation

The fixation method should be considered during planning, along with the suspected reason of previous graft failure. A variety of devices for bone and soft tissue fixation must be available aiming to not restrict the choice of the graft and use the best bone support [53]. The role of graft fixation in ACLR is to maintain sufficient graft stability in the early stages of healing to allow incorporation. The graft is completely reliant on the fixation device for its strength until it becomes incorporated into the tunnel wall. There are multiple types of fixation devices (interference screw, staples, buttons, post-screw, etc.) for the femur or tibia, and in some difficult revision cases these methods may be combined to increase primary resistance [52, 53].

One of the commonest methods is the interference screw technique [52], and we also prefer this technique. This may be metallic or biodegradable and works on the "press fit" principle, jamming the graft tightly against the tunnel wall so it may be eccentrically placed within the tunnels. The disadvantage of this technique was that interference screw tends to slip, especially with HT grafts. This slippage might provoke the graft laxity or graft migration. The EndoButton is also useful technique, which has advantage to adjust the length of the graft easily and keep bone stock. However, tunnel widening is commoner

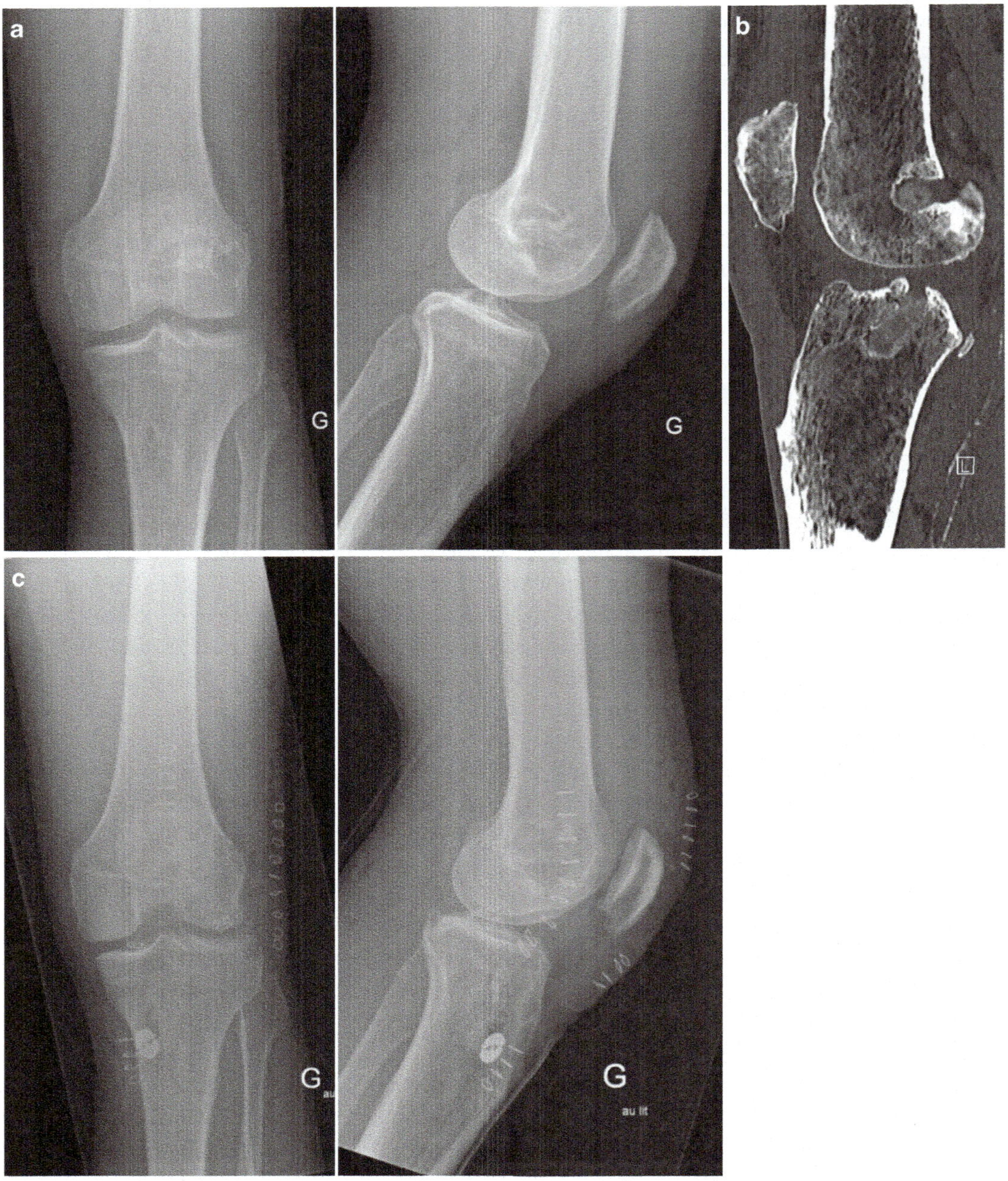

Fig. 21.2 The radiological evaluation of bone tunnel placement. (**a**) X-ray shows a posteriorly placed tibial tunnel placed. In this case, we decided to perform staged surgery in order be able to safely place the tibial tunnel and to assure a good fixation. (**b**) CT image after first step surgery for bone grafting. In this particular case, you should await 6 months before performing the second stage surgery. (**c**) Postoperative X-ray shows that previous bone tunnel was well filled up with grafted bone and allows for a proper placement of the tibial tunnel and a primary fixation with interference screw + post fixation as a safe backup

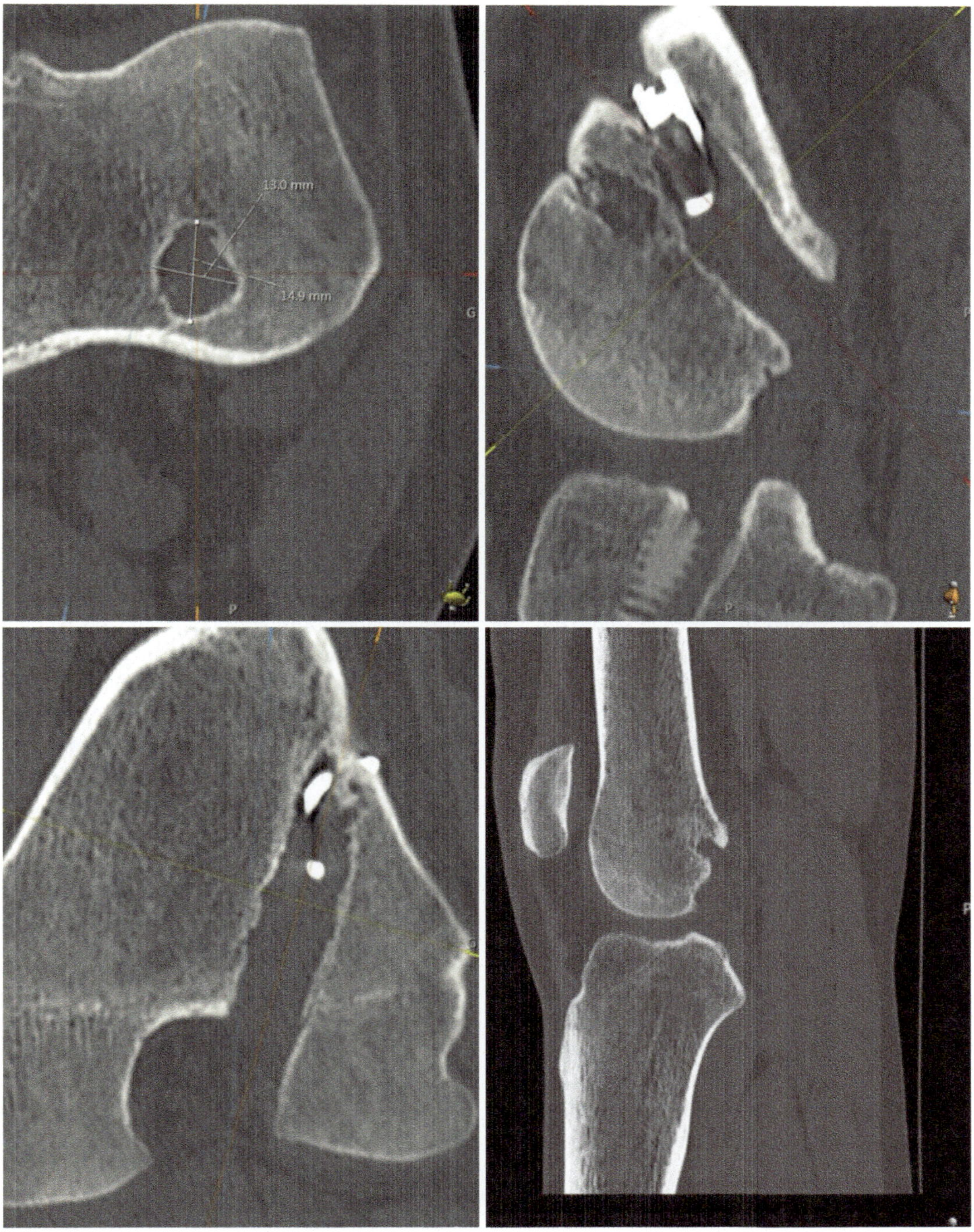

Fig. 21.3 CT image is able to provide more detailed information about bone tunnel enlargement

following the use of EndoButton fixation devices, and some authors have postulated that the delay in incorporation of these types of fixation method allows for micromotion to erode the adjacent tunnel wall during knee motion [54].

These techniques for graft fixation are mainly dependent on the remaining bone stock and the chosen graft [53, 55], thus, surgeons need to be familiar with each of these types of characteristics and must be trained in their use.

21.10 Associated Lesions

The most commonly reported associated injuries were meniscal tears and chondral lesions [36, 37, 56]. These associated lesions are very important. Revision procedures are able to restore knee stability, but symptoms and pain reduce knee function, resulting in poorer subjective outcome. As suggested by a French study, this can most likely be explained by concomitant meniscal and cartilage injuries in the revision reconstruction patients [57]. In the MARS ACL revision cohort, meniscal and cartilage injuries were seen in 90% of patients, and meniscal injury at the primary reconstruction resulted in an increased risk of cartilage deterioration at the time of revision surgery [58–60]. Wu et al. [61] obtained similar findings in 63 patients who had undergone ACLR and meniscectomy. These patients had significantly lower subjective function scores and ability to perform a single-leg hop test compared with patients with intact menisci at an average 10.4 years of follow-up. Therefore, it is extremely important to provide appropriate treatment for these combined injuries since the approach for meniscal injuries and/or chondral lesions should affect outcome of revision ACLR.

Recently, the presence of ramp lesion and posterolateral corner (PLC) injuries associated with ACL injury has been reported. Their incidence in primary ACLR is reported as high as 23.9% [62] to 19.7% [63].

Ramp lesion is a specific type of meniscal tear, which were defined as longitudinal tears of the peripheral attachment of the posterior horn of the medial meniscus (Fig. 21.4a). The posterior horn is recognized as a critical stabilizer in the ACL-deficient knee [64]. In a more recent cadaveric study, sectioning of the posteromedial meniscocapsular junction in an ACL- deficient knee resulted in a significant increase in anterior tibial translation and external rotation [65].

Also, many studies have established that missing the diagnosis of posterolateral corner (PLC) injury can increase the varus load on the ACL graft and the risk of graft failure [63, 66, 67]. The anatomy of the PLC is complicated, and injury is overlooked in many cases (50–76%) [63, 68, 69]. Thus, PLC-deficient condition after ACLR may be one of reason of graft failure or poor outcome. Furthermore, dysfunction of PLC should be overlooked again in revision surgery so that it is quite important to familiar with this pathology and strive to repair in both primary and revision surgery. We perform either mini-open or arthroscopic technique for these abnormal conditions which may lead to knee laxity (Fig. 21.4b, c).

Both ramp lesions and PLC injuries play a role in disrupting an important secondary stabilizer of the knee, and arthroscopic examination of the posterior structures and PLC of the knee and repair of these lesions must always be undertaken when revision ACL surgery is performed.

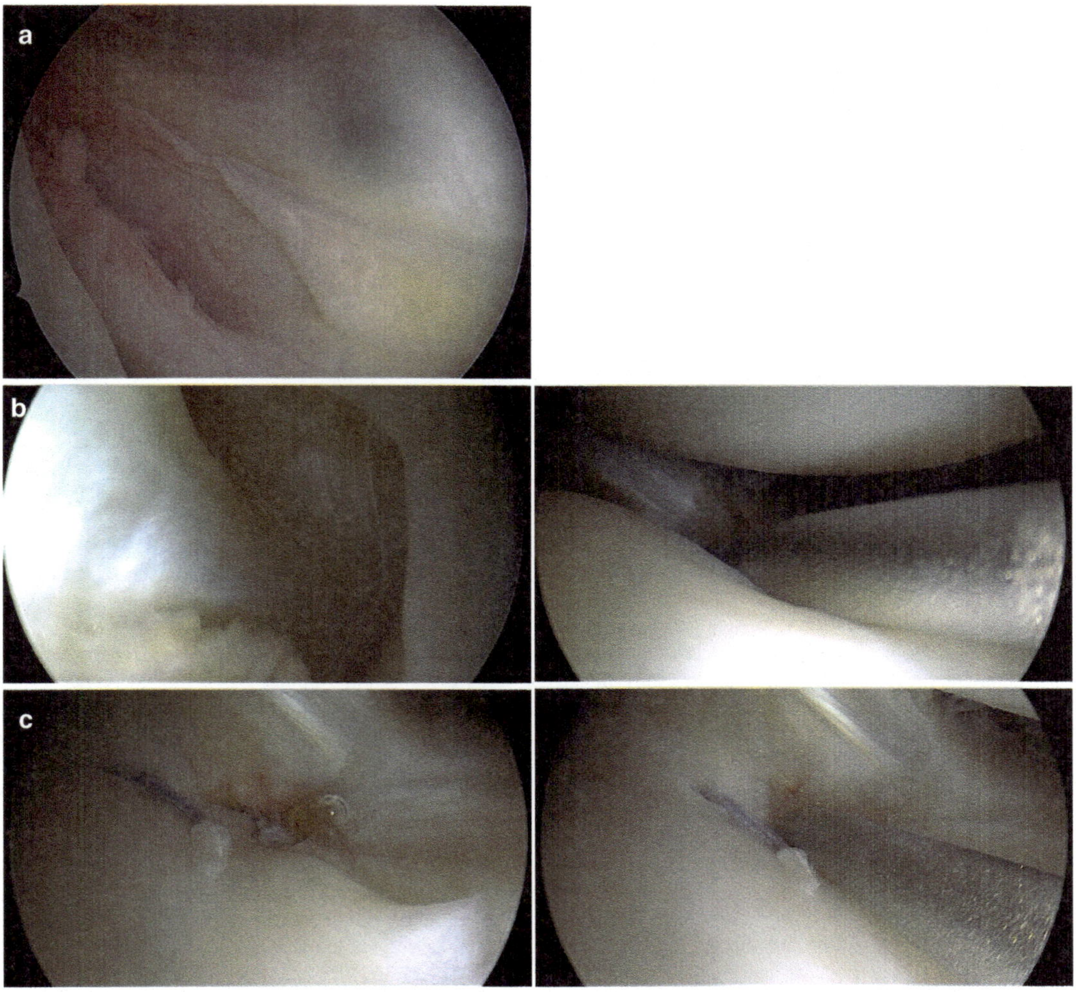

Fig. 21.4 Arthroscopic findings of associated lesions. (**a**) Ramp lesion. (**b**) PLC lesion provokes a positive lateral drive-through test and hypermobile lateral meniscus. (**c**) Lateral meniscus was fixed after arthroscopic repair of PLC

21.11 Summary

- The preoperative planning is the first and most important step.
- Autografts are superior to allograft for revision ACL surgery in many aspects.
- The evaluation of bone tunnel position and its enlargement is very important to determine whether to indicate one- or two-stage surgery.
- Don't overlook the associated lesions, especially ramp lesion and PLC injury.

References

1. Buller LT, Best MJ, Baraga MG, Kaplan LD. Trends in anterior cruciate ligament reconstruction in the United States. Orthop J Sports Med. 2015;3:2325967114563664.
2. Sanders TL, Maradit Kremers H, Bryan AJ, Larson DR, Dahm DL, Levy BA, et al. Incidence of anterior cruciate ligament tears and reconstruction: a 21-year population-based study. Am J Sports Med. 2016;44:1502–7.
3. Hurley ET, Calvo-Gurry M, Withers D, Farrington SK, Moran R, Moran CJ. Quadriceps tendon autograft in anterior cruciate ligament reconstruction: a systematic review. Arthroscopy. 2018;34(5):1690–8.

4. Hettrich CM, Dunn WR, Reinke EK, MOON Group, Spindler KP. The rate of subsequent surgery and predictors after anterior cruciate ligament reconstruction: two- and 6-year follow-up results from a multicenter cohort. Am J Sports Med. 2013;41:1534–40.
5. Andriolo L, Filardo G, Kon E, Ricci M, Della Villa F, Della Villa S, Zaffagnini S, Marcacci M. Revision anterior cruciate ligament reconstruction: clinical outcome and evidence for return to sport. Knee Surg Sports Traumatol Arthrosc. 2015;23:2825–45.
6. Vap AR, Persson A, Fenstad AM, Moatshe G, LaPrade RF, Engebretsen L. Re-revision anterior cruciate ligament reconstruction: an evaluation from the Norwegian knee ligament registry. Arthroscopy. 2019;35(6):1695–701.
7. Crawford MD, Diehl L, Amendola A. Surgical management and treatment of the anterior cruciate ligament–deficient knee with malalignment. Clin Sports Med. 2017;36(1):119–33.
8. Kim HS, Seon JK, Jo AR. Current trends in anterior cruciate ligament reconstruction. Knee Surg Relat Res. 2013;25(4):165–73.
9. Magnussen RA, Trojani C, Granan LP, Neyret P, Colombet P, Engebretsen L, Wright RW, Kaeding CC, MARS Group; SFA Revision ACL Group. Patient demographics and surgical characteristics in ACL revision: a comparison of French, Norwegian, and North American cohorts. Knee Surg Sports Traumatol Arthrosc. 2015;8:2339–48.
10. Wright RW, Huston LJ, Haas AK, Spindler KP, Nwosu SK, et al.; MARS Group. Effect of graft choice on the outcome of revision anterior cruciate ligament reconstruction in the multicenter ACL revision study (MARS) cohort. Am J Sports Med. 2014;42(10):2301–10.
11. Niki Y, Matsumoto H, Enomoto H, Toyama Y, Suda Y. Single-stage anterior cruciate ligament revision with bone-patellar tendon-bone: a case-control series of revision of failed synthetic anterior cruciate ligament reconstructions. Arthroscopy. 2010;26(8):1058–65.
12. Rosenberg TD, Franklin JL, Baldwin GN, Nelson KA. Extensor mechanism function after patellar tendon graft harvest for anterior cruciate ligament reconstruction. Am J Sports Med. 1992;20(5):519–26.
13. Denti M, Lo Vetere D, Bait C, et al. Revision anterior cruciate ligament reconstruction: causes of failure, surgical technique, and clinical results. Am J Sports Med. 2008;36:1896–902.
14. Pascual-Garrido C, Carbo L, Makino A. Revision of anterior cruciate ligament reconstruction with allografts in patients younger than 40 years old: a 2 to 4 year results. Knee Surg Sports Traumatol Arthrosc. 2014;22(5):1106–11.
15. Cerulli G, Placella G, Sebastiani E, Tei MM, Speziali A, Manfreda F. ACL reconstruction: choosing the graft. Joints. 2013;1(1):18–24.
16. MARS Group. Factors influencing graft choice in revision ACL reconstructions: a propensity analysis of the MARS cohort. J Knee Surg. 2016;29(6):458–63.
17. Lubowitz JH. Editorial commentary: quadriceps tendon autograft use for anterior cruciate ligament reconstruction predicted to increase. Arthroscopy. 2016;32(1):76–7.
18. Van Eck CF, Schreiber VM, Mejia HA, et al. "Anatomic" anterior cruciate ligament reconstruction: a systematic review of surgical techniques and reporting of surgical data. Arthroscopy. 2010;26(9 suppl):S2–S12.
19. Middleton KK, Hamilton T, Irrgang JJ, et al. Anatomic anterior cruciate ligament (ACL) reconstruction: a global perspective, part 1. Knee Surg Sports Traumatol Arthrosc. 2014;22(7):1467–82.
20. Harris NL, Smith DA, Lamoreaux L. Central quadriceps tendon for anterior cruciate ligament reconstruction, part I: morphometric and biomechanical evaluation. Am J Sports Med. 1997;25(1):23–8.
21. Shani RH, Umpierez E, Nasert M. Biomechanical comparison of quadriceps and patellar tendon grafts in anterior cruciate ligament reconstruction. Arthroscopy. 2016;32(1):71–5.
22. Stäubli HU, Schatzmann L, Brunner P. Mechanical tensile properties of the quadriceps tendon and patellar ligament in young adults. Am J Sports Med. 1999;27(1):27–34.
23. Hersekli MA, Akpinar S, Ozalay M, et al. Tunnel enlargement after arthroscopic anterior cruciate ligament reconstruction: comparison of bone-patellar tendon-bone and hamstring autografts. Adv Ther. 2004;21(2):123–31.
24. Mouarbes D, Menetrey J, Vincent Marot V, Courtot L, Berard E, Cavaignac E. Anterior cruciate ligament reconstruction. A systematic review and meta-analysis of outcomes for quadriceps tendon autograft versus bone–patellar tendon–bone and hamstring-tendon autografts. Am J Sports Med. 2019;21:363546518825340. [Epub ahead of print].
25. Bartlett RJ, Clatworthy MG, Nguyen TNV. Graft selection in reconstruction of the anterior cruciate ligament. J Bone Joint Surg Br. 2001;83-B(5):625–3.
26. Kim SJ, Kumar P, Oh KS. Anterior cruciate ligament reconstruction: autogenous quadriceps tendon- bone compared with bone-patellar tendon-bone grafts at 2-year follow-up. Arthroscopy. 2009;25(2):137–44.
27. Cavaignac E, Mouarbes D, Chiron P, Peque E, Dagneaux L, Matthieu O. Cutaneous and neurological complications of anterior cruciate ligament (ACL) reconstruction with quadriceps tendon (QT), bone patellar-tendon bone (BPTB) or Hamstring tendon (HT). 2019. In press.
28. Wright RW, Gill CS, Chen L, Brophy RH, Matava MJ, Smith MV, Mall NA. Outcome of revision anterior cruciate ligament reconstruction: a systematic review. J Bone Joint Surg Am. 2012;94(6):531–6.
29. Barié A, Ehmann Y, Jaber A, Huber J, Streich NA. Revision ACL reconstruction using quadriceps or hamstring autografts leads to similar results after 4 years: good objective stability but low rate of return to pre-injury sport level. Knee Surg Sports Traumatol

Arthrosc. 2019;27:3527–35. https://doi.org/10.1007/s00167-019-05444-z. [Epub ahead of print].
30. Papageorgiou CD, Ma CB, Abramowitch SD, Clineff TD, Woo SL. A multidisciplinary study of the healing of an intraarticular anterior cruciate ligament graft in a goat model. Am J Sports Med. 2001;29:620–6.
31. Xie X, Liu X, Chen Z, Yu Y, Peng S, Li Q. A meta-analysis of bone-patellar tendon-bone autograft versus four-strand hamstring tendon autograft for anterior cruciate ligament reconstruction. Knee. 2015;22:100–10.
32. Mohtadi NG, Chan DS, Dainty KN, Whelan DB. Patellar tendon versus hamstring tendon autograft for anterior cruciate ligament rupture in adults. Cochrane Database Syst Rev. 2011;9:CD005960.
33. Gifstad T, Foss OA, Engebretsen L, Lind M, Forssblad M, Albrektsen G, Drogset JO. Lower risk of revision with patellar tendon autografts compared with hamstring autografts: a registry study based on 45,998 primary ACL reconstructions in Scandinavia. Am J Sports Med. 2014;42:2319–28.
34. Samuelsen BT, Webster KE, Johnson NR, Hewett TE, Krych AJ. Hamstring autograft versus patellar tendon autograft for ACL reconstruction: is there a difference in graft failure rate? A meta-analysis of 47,613 patients. Clin Orthop Relat Res. 2017;475(10):2459–68.
35. Kay J, Naji L, Simunovic N, Peterson D, Samuelsson K, Musahl V, Ayeni OR. Graft choice has no significant influence on the rate of return to sport at the preinjury level after revision anterior cruciate ligament reconstruction: a systematic review and meta-analysis. J ISAKOS. 2016;2:21. https://doi.org/10.1136/jisakos-2016-000113.
36. Keizer MNJ, Hoogeslag RAG, van Raay JJAM, Otten E, Brouwer RW. Superior return to sports rate after patellar tendon autograft over patellar tendon allograft in revision anterior cruciate ligament reconstruction. Knee Surg Sports Traumatol Arthrosc. 2018;26(2):574–81.
37. Victor J, Bellemans J, Witvrouw E, Govaers K, Fabry G. Graft selection in anterior cruciate ligament reconstruction-pro- spective analysis of patellar tendon autografts compared with allografts. Int Orthop. 1997;21(2):93–7.
38. Hart JM, Turman KA, Diduch DR, Hart JA, Miller MD. Quadriceps muscle activation and radiographic osteoarthritis following ACL revision. Knee Surg Sports Traumatol Arthrosc. 2011;19(4):634–40.
39. Victor J, Bellemans J, Witvrouw E, Govaers K, Fabry G. Graft selection in anterior cruciate ligament reconstruction-prospective analysis of patellar tendon autografts compared with allografts. Int Orthop. 1997;21(2):93–7.
40. Grassi A, Kim C, Marcheggiani MGM, Zaffagnini S, Amendola A. What is the mid-term failure rate of revision ACL reconstruction? A systematic review. Orthop Relat Res. 2017;475(10):2484–99.
41. Legnani C, Zini S, Borgo E, Ventura A. Can graft choice affect return to sport following revision anterior cruciate ligament reconstruction surgery? Arch Orthop Trauma Surg. 2016;136(4):527–31.
42. Arianjam A, Inacio MCS, Funahashi TT, Maletis GB. Analysis of 2019 patients undergoing revision anterior cruciate ligament reconstruction from a community-based registry. Am J Sports Med. 2017;45(7):1574–80.
43. Thomas N, Carmichael J. Failure in ACL reconstruction: etiology, treatment, and results. In: Bonnin M, Amendola A, Bellemans J, MacDonald S, Ménétrey J, editors. The knee joint. Paris: Springer; 2012. p. 343–53.
44. Prodromos CC, Joyce BT. Allograft complications and risk factors. In: Prodromos C, Brown C, Fu FH, et al., editors. The anterior cruciate ligament reconstruction and basic science. Philadelphia: Saunders-Elsevier; 2008. p. 561–4.
45. Pereira H, Sevivas N, Pereira R, Espregueira-Mendes J, et al. Systematic approach from Porto School. In: Siebold R, Dejour D, Zaffagnini S, editors. Anterior cruciate ligament reconstruction: a practical surgical guide. Heidelberg: Springer; 2014. p. 367–86.
46. Lind M, Menhert F, Pedersen AB. Incidence and outcome after revision anterior cruciate ligament reconstruction: results from the Danish registry for knee ligament reconstructions. Am J Sports Med. 2012;40(7):1551–7.
47. Nissen KA, Eysturoy NH, Nielsen TG, Lind M. Allograft use results in higher re-revision rate for revision anterior cruciate ligament reconstruction. Orthop J Sports Med. 2018;6(6):2325967118775381.
48. Condello V, Zdanowicz U, Di Matteo B, et al. Allograft tendons are a safe and effective option for revision ACL reconstruction: a clinical review. Knee Surg Sports Traumatol Arthrosc. 2019;27(6):1771–81.
49. Maletis GB, Inacio MC, Reynolds S, Desmond JL, Maletis MM, Funahashi TT. Incidence of postoperative anterior cruciate ligament reconstruction infections: graft choice makes a difference. Am J Sports Med. 2013;41:1780–5.
50. Erickson BJ, Cvetanovich G, Waliullah K, Khair M, Smith P, Bach B Jr, Sherman S. Two-stage revision anterior cruciate ligament reconstruction. Orthopedics. 2016;39(3):e456–64.
51. Rizer M, Foremny GB, Rush A, Singer AD, Baraga M, Kaplan LD, Jose J. Anterior cruciate ligament reconstruction tunnel size: causes of tunnel enlargement and implications for single versus two-stage revision reconstruction. Skelet Radiol. 2017;46(2):161–9.
52. Groves C, Chandramohan M, Chew C, Subedi N. Use of CT in the management of anterior cruciate ligament revision surgery. Clin Radiol. 2013;68(10):e552–9.
53. Harvey A. Fixation of the graft in reconstruction of the anterior cruciate ligament. J Bone Joint Surg Br. 2005;87:593–603.
54. Cheung P, Chan WL, Yen CH, et al. Femoral tunnel widening after quadrupled hamstring anterior cruciate ligament reconstruction. J Orthop Surg (Hong Kong). 2010;18:198–202.

55. Thomas NP. Revision anterior cruciate ligament. In: Prodromos C, Brown C, Fu FH, Georgoulis AD, Gobbi A, Howell SM, Johson DL, Paulos LE, Shelbourne KD, editors. The anterior cruciate ligament: reconstruction and basic science. Philadelphia: Saunders Elsevier; 2008. p. 443–57.
56. Garofalo R, Djahangiri A, Siegrist O. Revision anterior cruciate ligament reconstruction with quadriceps tendon-patellar bone autograft. Arthroscopy. 2006;22(2):205–14.
57. Trojani C, Sbihi A, Djian P, et al. Causes for failure of ACL reconstruction and influence of meniscectomies after revision. Knee Surg Sports Traumatol Arthrosc. 2011;19(2):196–201.
58. Borchers JR, Kaeding CC, Pedroza AD, Huston LJ, Spindler KP, Wright RW. Intra-articular findings in primary and revision anterior cruciate ligament reconstruction surgery: a comparison of the MOON and MARS study groups. Am J Sports Med. 2011;39(9):1889–93.
59. Wright R, Spindler K, Huston L, et al. Revision ACL reconstruction outcomes: MOON cohort. J Knee Surg. 2011;24(4):289–94.
60. Wright RW, Huston LJ, Spindler KP, et al. Descriptive epidemiology of the multicenter ACL revision study (MARS) cohort. Am J Sports Med. 2010;38(10):1979–86.
61. Wu WH, Hackett T, Richmond JC. Effects of meniscal and articular surface status on knee stability, function, and symptoms after anterior cruciate ligament reconstruction a long-term prospective study. Am J Sports Med. 2002;30(6):845–50.
62. Sonnery-Cottet B, Praz C, Rosenstiel N, Blakeney WG, Ouanezar H, Kandhari V, Vieira TD, Saithna A. Epidemiological evaluation of meniscal ramp lesions in 3214 anterior cruciate ligament-injured knees from the SANTI study group database: a risk factor analysis and study of secondary meniscectomy rates following 769 ramp repairs. Am J Sports Med. 2018;46(13):3189–97.
63. Temponi EF, de Carvalho Júnior LH, Saithna A, Thaunat M, Sonnery-Cottet B. Incidence and MRI characterization of the spectrum of posterolateral corner injuries occurring in association with ACL rupture. Skelet Radiol. 2017;46(8):1063–70.
64. Musahl V, Citak M, O'Loughlin PF, Choi D, Bedi A, Pearle AD. The effect of medial versus lateral meniscectomy on the stability of the anterior cruciate ligament-deficient knee. Am J Sports Med. 2010;38(8):1591–7.
65. Stephen JM, Halewood C, Kittl C, Bollen SR, Williams A, Amis AA. Posteromedial meniscocapsular lesions increase tibiofemoral joint laxity with anterior cruciate ligament deficiency, and their repair reduces laxity. Am J Sports Med. 2016;44(2):400–8.
66. Shon OJ, Park JW, Kim BJ. Current concepts of posterolateral corner injuries of the knee. Knee Surg Relat Res. 2017;29(4):256–68.
67. LaPrade RF, Resig S, Wentorf F, et al. The effects of grade III posterolateral knee complex injuries on anterior cruciate ligament graft force. A biomechanical analysis. Am J Sports Med. 1999;27:469–75.
68. Pacheco RJ, Ayre CA, Bollen SR. Posterolateral corner injuries of the knee: a serious injury commonly missed. J Bone Joint Surg Br. 2011;93:194–7.
69. LaPrade RF, Wentorf FA, Fritts H, et al. A prospective magnetic resonance imaging study of the incidence of posterolateral and multiple ligament injuries in acute knee injuries presenting with a hemarthrosis. Arthroscopy. 2007;23:1341–7.

22 Cell-Free Biomaterials: Indications and Borders

Giuseppe Filardo

22.1 Introduction

Articular cartilage defects have poor self-healing potential and their treatment is a challenge in the orthopaedic practice. Moreover, if left untreated, they may increase in size and favour the development of degenerative processes, eventually leading to osteoarthritis (OA) in the long term [1], which prompts the development of effective strategies to restore the articular surface. In fact, traditional cartilage repair procedures, such as bone marrow stimulation techniques, showed the ability to improve symptoms and function in selected patients, but also presented several limitations related to the inferior quality of the repair tissue, questioning the benefit of these techniques especially for the treatment of large lesions [2]. More ambitious regenerative procedures have been therefore developed with the aim to overcome these limitations. Autologous chondrocytes implantation (ACI) was introduced in the early 1990s and showed promising outcomes, which were later confirmed up to long-term follow-up [3] also for the treatment of large defects. However, some drawbacks were reported, mainly related to a high rate of hypertrophy of the periosteal graft, and the need for two different surgeries for cartilage harvesting and subsequent implantation after culture expansion [4]. Further improvements of the technique involved the combination of cultured chondrocytes with biomaterials used as temporary three-dimensional scaffolds able to better support the tissue regeneration process. Some of these bioengineered tissues also offered the possibility to be implanted through an arthroscopic procedure, providing good and long-lasting clinical results [5–7]. Nevertheless, the practical and economic limitations related to the need of cell processing were still present.

Thus, thanks to the advances in biomaterials science, cell-free approaches have been introduced. These procedures involve the implantation of biomaterials capable of allowing the adhesion and differentiation of resident cells, in order to support tissue regeneration. This kind of matrices can be applied to cover the site of marrow stimulation, in order to stabilize the blood clot, and enhance the differentiation of cell precursors towards the chondrogenic lineage [8]. At the same time, the status of subchondral bone has been recognized as a key factor with regard to conditions affecting the overlying articular cartilage [9]. Therefore, a new treatment rationale was developed aimed at addressing both the chondral and osteochondral tissues: innovative bilayer constructs were tested and introduced into the clinical use, to be used as one-step procedures and provide a regenerative support for resident cells to proliferate and differentiate into both

G. Filardo (✉)
Rizzoli Orthopaedic Institute, Bologna, Italy
e-mail: ortho@gfilardo.com

M. T. Hirschmann et al. (eds.), *ESSKA Instructional Course Lecture Book*,
https://doi.org/10.1007/978-3-662-61264-4_22

subchondral bone and cartilage tissues [10]. The following chapter aims at summarizing the evidence about the clinical use of acellular scaffolds for the treatment of chondral and osteochondral lesions of the knee.

22.2 Chondral Scaffolds

The use of biocompatible and bioresorbable chondral scaffolds aims at ensuring coverage to the cartilage defect favouring the homogeneous distribution of the cell population coming from the bone marrow. This allows to stabilize the blood clot and exploit the body limited self-regenerative potential [8]. Autologous matrix-induced chondrogenesis (AMIC) [11, 12] was first introduced by Benthien and Behrens for the treatment of lesions up to 1.5 cm^2 [12]. Subsequently, the possibility to perform the procedure [13] also by dry arthroscopy using fibrin glue for the fixation was introduced. Different authors reported a significant clinical improvement at short-term follow-up, with a satisfaction rate up to 87% [14, 15]. Gille et al. confirmed the effectiveness of the procedure at long-term, with a further mild improvement of the clinical scores compared to the mid-term evaluation [7, 15, 16].

Despite the positive clinical results, some controversies emerged regarding the quality of the regeneration offered by this approach as seen by MRI. In fact, different authors reported an incomplete filling of the defects [17] or the presence of residual subchondral bone oedema at follow-up [14]. Augmentation procedures, such as the one-step combination with autologous bone marrow concentrate (BMC) or platelet rich-plasma (PRP), were therefore investigated in order to improve the potential of these procedures, with promising results up to mid-term follow-up [18, 19].

More recently, another approach to improve the outcomes of marrow stimulation techniques has been proposed. Chitosan is a biodegradable hydrogel which showed optimal biocompatibility in the animal model [20]. This material can be mixed with autologous peripheral whole blood, in order to provide stabilization to the blood cloth and in the end to improve the quality of tissue regeneration [21]. Similar clinical results were reported in a RCT compared to MF at short-term follow-up, but with a greater coverage of the lesions with hyaline-like tissue at T2 mapping [22], as well as better macroscopic and histologic scores [23] were observed with the hydrogel application. Recently, these findings were confirmed as stable at 5 years of follow-up [24].

A recent systematic review and meta-analysis has investigated the clinical results improvement over time of cell-free cartilage scaffold implantation [25]. Sixteen studies were identified and included in the meta-analysis, showing a significant improvement from basal score at 1, 2, and ≥3 years' follow-up. The improvement reached at 1 year remained stable up to the last follow-up for all scores. Therefore, the current literature suggests that cell-free scaffolds may provide good clinical short-/mid-term results. However, the low evidence of the published studies and their short/mean follow-up demand further evidence before more definitive conclusions can be drawn on their real potential over time and on their advantages and disadvantages compared to the cell-based strategies.

22.3 Osteochondral Scaffolds

Biphasic scaffolds were introduced with the aim to address the regeneration of both subchondral bone and cartilage at the same time [26]. These constructs are organized in different layers, in order to mimic the different anatomical and functional properties of these two different tissues. Several osteochondral devices were investigated at preclinical level, but only a few of them have been reported for clinical use.

The first one developed and introduced into clinical use was a resorbable biphasic polymer of PLGA-PGA (*Trufit CB*™, Smith & Nephew, USA), originally intended to fill donor sites of osteochondral grafting (OAT) [27], showing controversial preliminary findings at the imaging evaluation [28, 29] and no clinical improvement compared with donor sites left empty at mid-term after OAT [30]. Several reports studied the application of this device for the treatment of osteochondral defects, and reported promising early clinical findings [31–33], which were not confirmed by later reports. In fact, Dhollander et al. [34] observed only a slight clinical benefit paired with 20% failure rate within the first 12 months after surgery. Joshi et al. reported seven failures out of ten patients treated for patellar defects and evaluated at 24 months of follow-up [35]. Finally, Hindle et al. found a higher short-term improvement in patients treated with mosaicplasty compared with Trufit implantation [36].

A nanostructured biomimetic scaffold made of type I collagen and hydroxyapatite (HA) organized in three gradient layers was later introduced, with the rational to mimic extracellular cartilage and subchondral bone matrices [37] (*MaioRegen*™, Finceramica, Faenza, Italy) and provide a more effective osteochondral regeneration. The results of a pilot study showed a promising mid-term clinical improvement up to 60 months follow-up, which was faster in patients with higher pre-injury activity level [38–40]. This implant showed positive clinical results also for the treatment of osteochondritis dissecans (OCD), in a study with 5 years' follow-up [41], and for the treatment of patellar cartilage defects in a study with 24 months follow-up [42]. Long-term improvement was confirmed in a wider study on 79 patients, treated for defects of femoral condyles or trochlea. In this series, degenerative lesions had significantly lower results compared to traumatic ones [10]. However, positive findings were reported even in small series of patients treated for early [43] or unicompartmental OA, where the scaffold was implanted concurrently with combined procedures to address multiple comorbidities [44]. A further study confirmed the benefits of the osteochondral approach for this kind of degenerative disease by evaluating specifically the results of "complex" knee lesions, showing higher clinical scores when this osteochondral approach was used instead of a chondral one [45]. Other authors reported good clinical results also in case of large defects [46, 47], or explored different indications for this scaffold, such as spontaneous osteonecrosis of the knee [48]. The satisfactory clinical findings confirmed the versatility of this procedure for various conditions affecting the whole osteochondral unit. A possible exception is the treatment of patellar defects, where lower outcomes were reported, together with some abnormal findings at MRI [49].

Conversely with these positive clinical reports, imaging evaluation of the graft produced a less positive evidence. In fact, despite a good integration of the implant even at early postoperative evaluation [38], most of the authors observed abnormalities in the graft structure and a limited bone regeneration, which were improved but still present up to mid-term follow-up [10, 40, 41, 50, 51]. However, these issues seem not to affect the clinical outcomes [10, 40, 41, 50]. The limited tissue regeneration at MRI pushed further investigations to optimize the procedure, such as the improved fixation by using fibrin glue [52].

The last cell-free osteochondral scaffold applied in the clinical practice consists of aragonite, shaped in cylinders similar to mosaicplasty plugs (*Agili-C*™, CartiHeal (2009) Ltd., Israel). These rigid plugs have a bone phase made of calcium carbonate in the aragonite crystalline form, and a superficial layer of modified aragonite and hyaluronate. Positive findings in terms of safety and regeneration potential were reported at 6 months of follow-up in the animal model [10], with further improved tissue features and no degeneration occurred between 6 and 12 [53]. The first clinical report for this cell-free technique deals with a case of a 47-year-old who underwent to this scaffold implantation at the medial femoral condyle for a 2 cm^2 post-traumatic osteochondral defect. A complete recovery to the same level of pre-injury was reported at 18 months' follow-up, coupled with good integration of the bone layer and hyaline-like appearance of the cartilage layer at MRI [54]. Furthermore, a recent paper reported the preliminary results of a group of patients treated with this device, showing an overall clinical improvement after implantation of two different shapes for the plug, and highlighting the importance of this variable, being tapered implants safer than cylindrical ones in terms of early failure rate [55].

22.4 Conclusions

Various biopolymers are currently being tested in order to provide a temporary support for the proliferation and differentiation of resident cells. The most recent trend involves the use of one-step procedures, where the biomaterial can be implanted cell-free into the defect to maximize the regenerating potential of the tissue itself. Different devices, targeted either to chondral or osteochondral lesions, showed the ability to produce satisfactory clinical improvements but a limited quality of the regenerated tissues. Even though none of the authors found any correlation with the clinical results, these issues warrant further research in this kind of procedures. High-level studies are needed to assess the real benefits and the best indications of the available grafts, as well as ways to further improve and optimize the long-term outcomes of these cell-free scaffold-based procedures for the treatment of chondral and osteochondral lesions.

References

1. Madry H, Kon E, Condello V, et al. Early osteoarthritis of the knee. Knee Surg Sports Traumatol Arthrosc. 2016;24(6):1753–62.
2. Andrade R, Vasta S, Pereira R, et al. Knee donor-site morbidity after mosaicplasty—a systematic review. J Exp Orthop. 2016;3(1):31.
3. Brittberg M, Lindahl A, Nilsson A, et al. Treatment of deep cartilage defects in the knee with autologous chondrocyte transplantation. N Engl J Med. 1994;331(14):889–95.
4. Goyal D, Goyal A, Keyhani S, et al. Evidence-based status of second- and third-generation autologous chondrocyte implantation over first generation: a systematic review of level I and II studies. Arthroscopy. 2013;29(11):1872–8.
5. Peterson L, Vasiliadis HS, Brittberg M, et al. Autologous chondrocyte implantation: a long-term follow-up. Am J Sports Med. 2010;38(6):1117–24.
6. Aldrian S, Zak L, Wondrasch B, et al. Clinical and radiological long-term outcomes after matrix-induced autologous chondrocyte transplantation: a prospective follow-up at a minimum of 10 years. Am J Sports Med. 2014;42(11):2680–8.
7. Gille J, Behrens P, Schulz AP, et al. Matrix-associated autologous chondrocyte implantation: a clinical follow-up at 15 years. Cartilage. 2016;7(4):309–15.
8. Gille J, Kunow J, Boisch L, et al. Cell-laden and cell-free matrix-induced chondrogenesis versus microfracture for the treatment of articular cartilage defects: a histological and biomechanical study in sheep. Cartilage. 2010;1(1):29–42.
9. Pape D, Filardo G, Kon E, et al. Disease-specific clinical problems associated with the subchondral bone. Knee Surg Sports Traumatol Arthrosc. 2010;18(4):448–62.
10. Kon E, Filardo G, Perdisa F, et al. A one-step treatment for chondral and osteochondral knee defects: clinical results of a biomimetic scaffold implantation at 2 years of follow-up. J Mater Sci Mater Med. 2014;25(10):2437–44.
11. Benthien JP, Behrens P. Autologous matrix-induced chondrogenesis (AMIC). A one-step procedure for retropatellar articular resurfacing. Acta Orthop Belg. 2010;76(2):260–3.
12. Benthien JP, Behrens P. The treatment of chondral and osteochondral defects of the knee with autologous matrix-induced chondrogenesis (AMIC): method description and recent developments. Knee Surg Sports Traumatol Arthrosc. 2011;19(8):1316–9.
13. Piontek T, Ciemniewska-Gorzela K, Szulc A, et al. All-arthroscopic AMIC procedure for repair of cartilage defects of the knee. Knee Surg Sports Traumatol Arthrosc. 2012;20(5):922–5.
14. Schiavone Panni A, Cerciello S, Vasso M. The management of knee cartilage defects with modified AMIC technique: preliminary results. Int J Immunopathol Pharmacol. 2011;24(1 Suppl 2):149–52.
15. Gille J, Schuseil E, Wimmer J, et al. Mid-term results of autologous matrix-induced chondrogenesis for treatment of focal cartilage defects in the knee. Knee Surg Sports Traumatol Arthrosc. 2010;18(11):1456–64.
16. Gille J, Behrens P, Volpi P, et al. Outcome of autologous matrix induced chondrogenesis (AMIC) in cartilage knee surgery: data of the AMIC registry. Arch Orthop Trauma Surg. 2013;133(1):87–93.
17. Kusano T, Jakob RP, Gautier E, et al. Treatment of isolated chondral and osteochondral defects in the knee by autologous matrix-induced chondrogenesis (AMIC). Knee Surg Sports Traumatol Arthrosc. 2012;20(10):2109–15.
18. Gobbi A, Scotti C, Karnatzikos G, et al. One-step surgery with multipotent stem cells and hyaluronan-based scaffold for the treatment of full-thickness chondral defects of the knee in patients older than 45 years. Knee Surg Sports Traumatol Arthrosc. 2017;25(8):2494–501.
19. Gobbi A, Whyte GP. One-stage cartilage repair using a hyaluronic acid-based scaffold with activated bone marrow-derived mesenchymal stem cells compared with microfracture: five-year follow-up. Am J Sports Med. 2016;44(11):2846–54.
20. Rodriguez-Vazquez M, Vega-Ruiz B, Ramos-Zuniga R, et al. Chitosan and its potential use as a scaffold for tissue engineering in regenerative medicine. Biomed Res Int. 2015;2015:821279.

21. Steinwachs MR, Waibl B, Mumme M. Arthroscopic treatment of cartilage lesions with microfracture and BST-CarGel. Arthrosc Tech. 2014;3(3):e399–402.
22. Stanish WD, McCormack R, Forriol F, et al. Novel scaffold-based BST-CarGel treatment results in superior cartilage repair compared with microfracture in a randomized controlled trial. J Bone Joint Surg Am. 2013;95(18):1640–50.
23. Methot S, Changoor A, Tran-Khanh N, et al. Osteochondral biopsy analysis demonstrates that BST-CarGel treatment improves structural and cellular characteristics of cartilage repair tissue compared with microfracture. Cartilage. 2016;7(1):16–28.
24. Shive MS, Stanish WD, McCormack R, et al. BST-CarGel(R) treatment maintains cartilage repair superiority over microfracture at 5 years in a multicenter randomized controlled trial. Cartilage. 2015;6(2):62–72.
25. Andriolo L, Reale D, Di Martino A, Boffa A, Zaffagnini S, Filardo G. Cell-free scaffolds in cartilage knee surgery: a systematic review and meta-analysis of clinical evidence. Cartilage. 2019;5:1947603519852406.
26. Niederauer GG, Slivka MA, Leatherbury NC, et al. Evaluation of multiphase implants for repair of focal osteochondral defects in goats. Biomaterials. 2000;21(24):2561–74.
27. Slivka MA, Leatherbury NC, Kieswetter K, et al. Porous, resorbable, fiber-reinforced scaffolds tailored for articular cartilage repair. Tissue Eng. 2001;7(6):767–80.
28. Bedi A, Foo LF, Williams RJ 3rd, et al. The maturation of synthetic scaffolds for osteochondral donor sites of the knee: an MRI and T2-mapping analysis. Cartilage. 2010;1(1):20–8.
29. Barber FA, Dockery WD. A computed tomography scan assessment of synthetic multiphase polymer scaffolds used for osteochondral defect repair. Arthroscopy. 2011;27(1):60–4.
30. Quarch VM, Enderle E, Lotz J, et al. Fate of large donor site defects in osteochondral transfer procedures in the knee joint with and without TruFit plugs. Arch Orthop Trauma Surg. 2014;134(5):657–66.
31. Carmont MR, Carey-Smith R, Saithna A, et al. Delayed incorporation of a TruFit plug: perseverance is recommended. Arthroscopy. 2009;25(7):810–4.
32. Bekkers JE, Bartels LW, Vincken KL, et al. Articular cartilage evaluation after TruFit plug implantation analyzed by delayed gadolinium-enhanced MRI of cartilage (dGEMRIC). Am J Sports Med. 2013;41(6):1290–5.
33. Gelber PE, Batista J, Millan-Billi A, et al. Magnetic resonance evaluation of TruFit(R) plugs for the treatment of osteochondral lesions of the knee shows the poor characteristics of the repair tissue. Knee. 2014;21(4):827–32.
34. Dhollander AA, Liekens K, Almqvist KF, et al. A pilot study of the use of an osteochondral scaffold plug for cartilage repair in the knee and how to deal with early clinical failures. Arthroscopy. 2012;28(2):225–33.
35. Joshi N, Reverte-Vinaixa M, Diaz-Ferreiro EW, et al. Synthetic resorbable scaffolds for the treatment of isolated patellofemoral cartilage defects in young patients: magnetic resonance imaging and clinical evaluation. Am J Sports Med. 2012;40(6):1289–95.
36. Hindle P, Hendry JL, Keating JF, et al. Autologous osteochondral mosaicplasty or TruFit plugs for cartilage repair. Knee Surg Sports Traumatol Arthrosc. 2014;22(6):1235–40.
37. Tampieri A, Sandri M, Landi E, et al. Design of graded biomimetic osteochondral composite scaffolds. Biomaterials. 2008;29(26):3539–46.
38. Kon E, Delcogliano M, Filardo G, et al. A novel nano-composite multi-layered biomaterial for treatment of osteochondral lesions: technique note and an early stability pilot clinical trial. Injury. 2010;41(7):693–701.
39. Kon E, Delcogliano M, Filardo G, et al. Novel nano-composite multilayered biomaterial for osteochondral regeneration: a pilot clinical trial. Am J Sports Med. 2011;39(6):1180–90.
40. Kon E, Filardo G, Di Martino A, et al. Clinical results and MRI evolution of a nano-composite multilayered biomaterial for osteochondral regeneration at 5 years. Am J Sports Med. 2014;42(1):158–65.
41. Perdisa F, Kon E, Sessa A, Andriolo L, Busacca M, Marcacci M, Filardo G. Treatment of knee osteochondritis dissecans with a cell-free biomimetic osteochondral scaffold: clinical and imaging findings at midterm follow-up. Am J Sports Med. 2018;46(2):314–21.
42. Perdisa F, Filardo G, Sessa A, Busacca M, Zaffagnini S, Marcacci M, Kon E. One-step treatment for patellar cartilage defects with a cell-free osteochondral scaffold: a prospective clinical and MRI evaluation. Am J Sports Med. 2017;45(7):1581–8.
43. Di Martino A, Kon E, Perdisa F, et al. Surgical treatment of early knee osteoarthritis with a cell-free osteochondral scaffold: results at 24 months of follow-up. Injury. 2015;46(Suppl 8):S33–8.
44. Marcacci M, Zaffagnini S, Kon E, et al. Unicompartmental osteoarthritis: an integrated biomechanical and biological approach as alternative to metal resurfacing. Knee Surg Sports Traumatol Arthrosc. 2013;21(11):2509–17.
45. Filardo G, Kon E, Perdisa F, et al. Osteochondral scaffold reconstruction for complex knee lesions: a comparative evaluation. Knee. 2013;20(6):570–6.
46. Delcogliano M, de Caro F, Scaravella E, et al. Use of innovative biomimetic scaffold in the treatment for large osteochondral lesions of the knee. Knee Surg Sports Traumatol Arthrosc. 2014;22(6):1260–9.
47. Berruto M, Delcogliano M, de Caro F, et al. Treatment of large knee osteochondral lesions with a biomimetic scaffold: results of a multicenter study of 49 patients at 2-year follow-up. Am J Sports Med. 2014;42(7):1607–17.
48. Berruto M, Ferrua P, Uboldi F, et al. Can a biomimetic osteochondral scaffold be a reliable alternative to prosthetic surgery in treating late-stage SPONK? Knee. 2016;23(6):936–41.

49. Perdisa F, Filardo G, Sessa A, et al. One-step treatment for patellar cartilage defects with a cell-free osteochondral scaffold: a prospective clinical and MRI evaluation. Am J Sports Med. 2017;45(7):1581–8.
50. Christensen BB, Foldager CB, Jensen J, et al. Poor osteochondral repair by a biomimetic collagen scaffold: 1- to 3-year clinical and radiological follow-up. Knee Surg Sports Traumatol Arthrosc. 2016;24(7):2380–7.
51. Dhollander A, Verdonk P, Almqvist KF, et al. Clinical and MRI outcome of an osteochondral scaffold plug for the treatment of cartilage lesions in the knee. Acta Orthop Belg. 2015;81(4):629–38.
52. Kon E, Filardo G, Perdisa F, et al. Clinical results of multilayered biomaterials for osteochondral regeneration. J Exp Orthop. 2014;1(1):10.
53. Kon E, Filardo G, Shani J, et al. Osteochondral regeneration with a novel aragonite-hyaluronate biphasic scaffold: up to 12-month follow-up study in a goat model. J Orthop Surg Res. 2015;10:81.
54. Kon E, Drobnic M, Davidson PA, et al. Chronic posttraumatic cartilage lesion of the knee treated with an acellular osteochondral-regenerating implant: case history with rehabilitation guidelines. J Sport Rehabil. 2014;23(3):270–5.
55. Kon E, Robinson D, Verdonk P, et al. A novel aragonite-based scaffold for osteochondral regeneration: early experience on human implants and technical developments. Injury. 2016;47(Suppl 6):S27–32.

23 The Rationale for Using Navigation for Revision Total Knee Arthroplasty

Jean-Yves Jenny

23.1 Introduction

The number of revision total knee arthroplasty (RTKA) has dramatically increased in recent years and may account for 10% of all TKR [1]. Causes for RTKA include septic failure, knee instability, implant malpositioning, implant breakage, patellar maltracking and aseptic loosening or wear [2]. RTKA is a challenging procedure, especially because most of the standard bony and ligamentous landmarks are lost due to the primary implantation [3]. However, as for primary total knee arthroplasty (PTKA), restoration of the joint line, adequate limb axis correction and ligamentous stability are considered critical for the short- and long- term outcome of RTKA.

There is no available data about the range of tolerable leg alignment. However, it is logical to assume that the same range than after PTKA might be accepted, that is ±3° off the neutral alignment [4]. Conventional instruments with intra- or extra-medullary rods have been developed for primary replacement and adapted to revision cases. It has been demonstrated that their accuracy was less than optimal for primary cases [5]. One might assume that these conventional instruments, which rely on visual or anatomical alignments of intra- or extra-medullary rods, are associated with significant higher variation of the leg axis correction for revision cases. The efficiency of navigation systems has been extensively demonstrated for PTKA [6–9]. It was logical to adapt this technology for RTKA as well.

We are using for more than 10 years a non-image-based navigation system for PTKA [4]. We wanted to use the same operative technique for revision cases and to compare the accuracy of implantation of navigated RTKA to conventional RTKA and PTKA. We hypothesized that the rate of satisfactory implantation will be higher for navigated RTKA than for conventional RTKA.

23.2 Materials and Methods

1. Operative technique:
   (a) The navigated technique (OrthoPilot®, Aesculap Tuttlingen, FRG) has been described elsewhere (Jenny). Briefly, arrays were fixed by a screw on the distal femur and on the proximal tibia and strapped on the dorsal part of the foot. A kinematic registration of the hip, knee and ankle joints was performed. The data were implemented by the palpation of some relevant anatomical points with a navigated stylus. Then the system displayed the orientation of the mechanical

J.-Y. Jenny (✉)
Hôpitaux Universitaires de Strasbourg, Strasbourg, France
e-mail: jean-yves.jenny@chru-strasbourg.fr

M. T. Hirschmann et al. (eds.), *ESSKA Instructional Course Lecture Book*,
https://doi.org/10.1007/978-3-662-61264-4_23

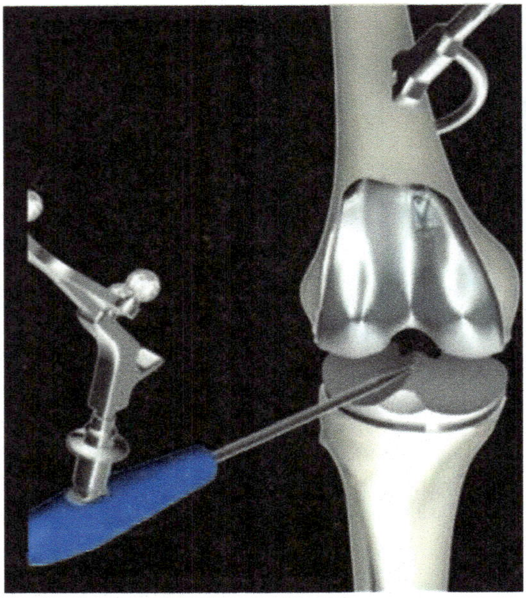

Fig. 23.1 Data registration with the index prosthesis in place

axes of the femur and the tibia. Navigated resection guides were oriented and fixed to the bones along these axes to the desired position. The bone resections were performed with a conventional saw blade.

The same software and the same instruments were used for RTKA. Kinematic and anatomic registration was performed with the index implants left in place (Fig. 23.1), without any difference in comparison to PTKA. Navigated resection guides were oriented and fixed to the bones along these axes to the desired position (Fig. 23.2). The bone resections were performed with a conventional saw blade. The prosthesis was implanted with either normal or extension stems as appropriate.

(b) The conventional technique involved intramedullary rods which were introduced into the femoral and tibial canal to provide the reference bone axis. Resection guides were oriented and fixed to the bones along these axes to the

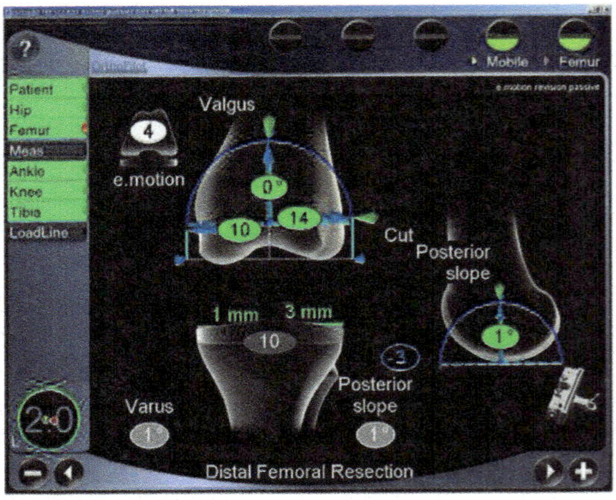

Fig. 23.2 Intra-operative navigated information

desired position. The bone resections were performed with a conventional saw blade. The prosthesis was implanted with either normal or extension stems as appropriate.

2. Two groups of cases were defined: navigated RTKA (group A) and conventional RTKA (group B). All RTKAs implanted during the period of the current study were included: 50 into group A and 36 into group B.
3. Data collection: We collected following preoperative items: age, gender, height, body weight, BMI, reason for revision, knee score and function score according to the Knee Society Scoring System [10], coronal femoro-tibial angle. The accuracy of implantation was retrospectively analyzed on postoperative long leg X-rays in unipodal support. Coronal mechanical femoro-tibial angle and coronal and sagittal orientations of both femoral and tibial components [11] were assessed. The RTKA was expected to be implanted with the following requirements: a coronal femoro-tibial mechanical angle of 0° ± 3°, a coronal angle between the horizontal axis of the femoral or tibial implant and the mechanical femoral or tibial axis of 90° ± 3°, and a sagittal angle between the horizontal axis of the tibial implant and the proximal posterior tibial cortex of 90° ± 3°. A prosthesis was considered optimally implanted when all criteria were fulfilled.

4. Data analysis: The primary criterion was the rate of optimally implanted prosthesis. Secondary criteria were the rate of outliers for each individual item. The comparison between the three groups was performed with a chi-squared test at a 0.05 level of significance for qualitative items and with a Student's *t*-test at a 0.05 level of significance for quantitative items.

23.3 Results

We selected 86 cases for the study: 50 navigated RTKA and 36 conventional RTKA. There were 57 female and 29 male patients, with a mean age of 70.6 ± 7.7 years (range, 44–88 years). The mean BMI was 31.1 ± 4.8 (range, 23.5–42.3). The main reasons for revision were aseptic loosening (52 cases) and infection (32 cases). The mean preoperative knee score was 49.9 ± 14.1 points (range, 4–90 points), the mean preoperative function score was 39.6 ± 13.4 points (range, 0–90 points). The mean preoperative coronal femoro-tibial angle was 175° ± 14° (range, 162°–203°). There was no significant difference for all these items between all subgroups.

There were 31 cases (62%) with an optimal global implantation in group A and 14 (39%) in group B ($p < 0.05$).

The mean postoperative coronal femoro-tibial angle was 181° ± 3° (range, 175°–188°) in group A and 179° ± 3° (range, 176°–187°) in group B (NS). There were nine outliers (18%) in group A and nine outliers (26%) in group B (NS).

The mean postoperative coronal femoral angle was 91° ± 2° (range, 88°–96°) in group A and 89° ± 3° (range, 82°–94°) in group B (NS). There were eight outliers (15%) in group A and nine outliers (25%) in group B (NS).

The mean postoperative coronal tibial angle was 90° ± 1° (range, 88°–92°) in group A and 90° ± 2° (range, 86°–93°) in group B (NS). There were three outliers (5%) in group A and four outliers (11%) in group B (NS).

The mean postoperative sagittal tibial angle was 91° ± 2° (range, 83°–95°) in group A and 91° ± 3° (range, 88°–99°) in group B (NS). There were 11 outliers (23%) in group A and 12 outliers (34%) in group B (NS).

23.4 Discussion

Navigation systems have been validated for PTKA. However, there are few papers about the use of such systems for RTKA [12–14].

Perlick et al. [14] hypothesized that a significantly better leg alignment and component orientation were achieved when using a navigation system in comparison to conventional technique. They compared two groups of 25 RTKAs operated on either with a CT-free navigation system or with the conventional manual technique. The postoperative alignment was measured on long leg coronal and sagittal X-rays. The mechanical limb axis was significantly better corrected in the navigated group (92% versus 76%). All navigated femoral components were well aligned in the coronal plane, against only 84% of the conventional group ($p < 0.05$). All navigated tibial components were well aligned in the coronal plane, against only 94% of the conventional group ($p > 0.05$). The sagittal alignment of both femoral and tibial implants was also improved in navigation group ($p > 0.05$). The level of the joint line was also more accurately restored with help of the navigation system.

Massin et al. [13] reported their experience about 19 RTKAs operated with a navigation system combining intra-operative surface bone registration and preoperative CT scan imaging, with a retrospective comparison to 10 non-navigated revision cases performed concomitantly by the same surgeon. Although they observed no significant difference in the number of outliers for the two series, navigation appeared to be a valuable aid in reconstructing both bone extremities, while controlling the level of the joint line.

Ochs et al. [15] reported the results of 18 RTKA operated with the same navigation system used in our study. Correction of the deformation was routinely obtained, and navigation helped controlling implant positioning and restoring the joint line.

Hoffart et al. [12] reported the development of a navigation software dedicated to RTKA, but did not document any clinical or radiological result. Meijer et al. [16] planned a prospective comparative study but did not report results.

We used the OrthoPilot® non-image-based navigation system for RTKA, and our results were similar to that already published. The global accuracy of implantation was improved when using this technology in comparison to conventional, manual technique. Differences, although not significant, were also observed for all individual items in favor of the navigated technique. We confirm the results of the two previous studies: navigation has the potential to enhance RTKA accuracy. However, the accuracy obtained for a primary implantation [17] was not achieved, although the same navigation software and technique has been used. We identified a major explanation for this discrepancy.

The standard navigation software did not allow navigating the stem extensions and bone defects. In several cases, we observed that the bone resection at the joint level was well oriented. But the axis of the bone medullary canal was not perpendicular to this resection. Consequently, the prosthesis implanted with a stem extension has been forced to the direction of the diaphyseal axis, with a mismatch with the articular resection.

Furthermore, the standard navigation software offers no possibility to deal with bone loss and reconstruction of the joint line height. Therefore, a dedicated application for RTKA, including all these improvements, was developed (Figs. 23.3 and 23.4), and the first experience as reported by the developing team is encouraging [18]. This new application is currently used on a routine basis, but it needs to be validated on a larger scale.

There might be some drawbacks to use a navigation system for RTKA, as it has been extensively discussed for PTKA [19]. These possible drawbacks include increased cost, increased operative time, and risk of fracture involving the holes for the trackers. We observed no complication related to the navigation use in the present study. We think that the improvement of the quality of implantation overweighs these possible disadvantages.

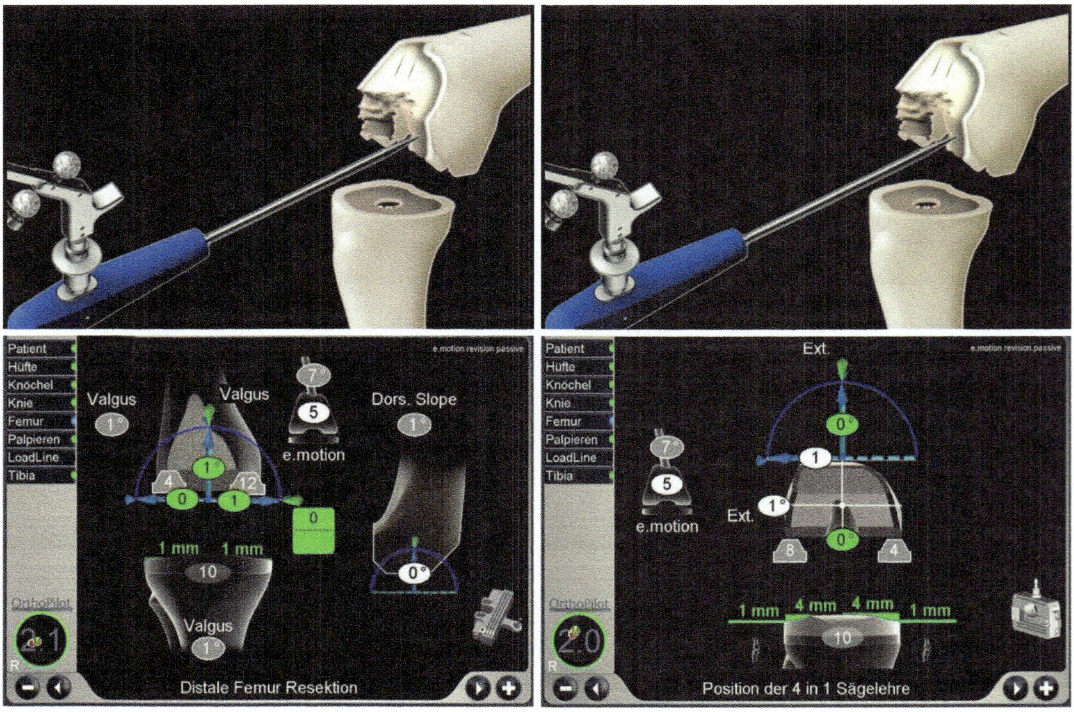

Fig. 23.3 Specific development—navigation of the bone defects

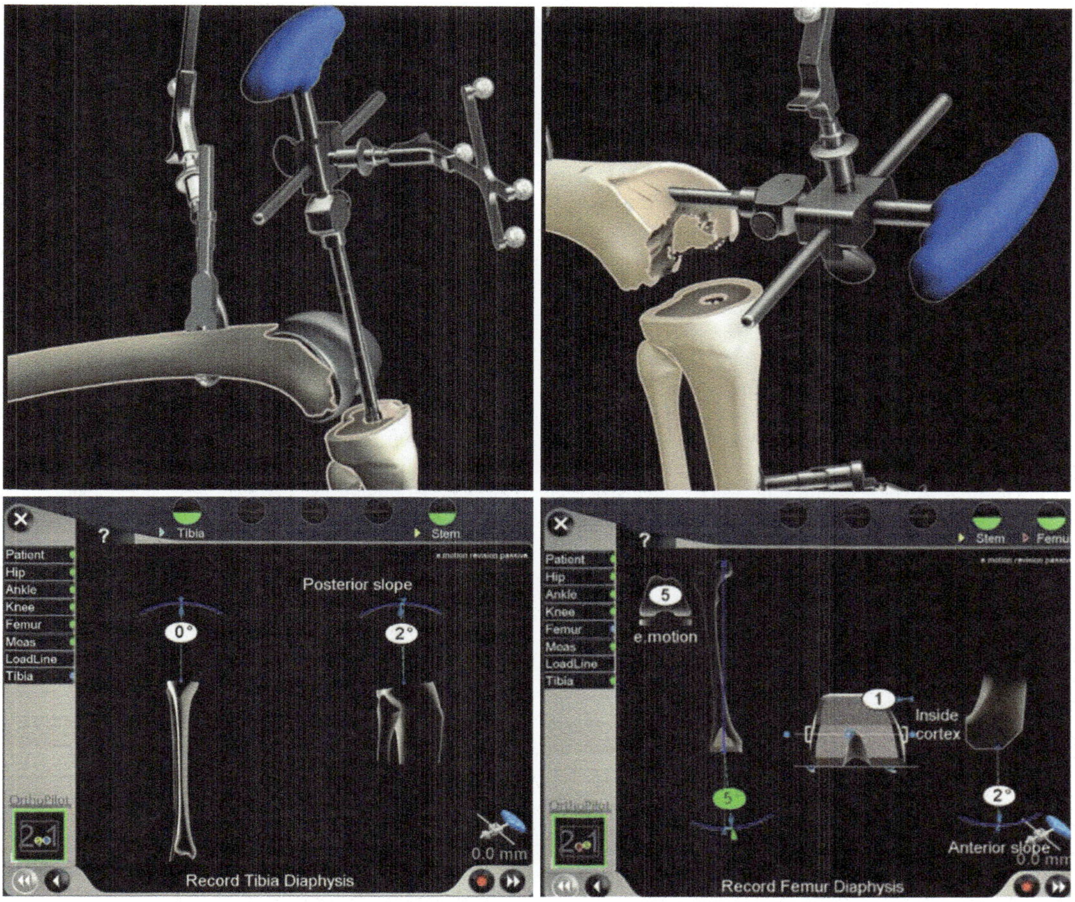

Fig. 23.4 Specific development—navigation of the stem extension

23.5 Conclusion

The use of a standard navigation software for RTKA allows a significant improvement of the accuracy of implantation. However, the use of a dedicated software allows addressing more precisely the specific features of a RTKA, such as stem extension positioning, defects filling, and joint line reconstruction.

References

1. Gofton WT, Tsigaras H, Butler RA, Patterson JJ, Barrack RL, Rorabeck CH. Revision total knee arthroplasty: fixation with modular stems. Clin Orthop. 2002;404:158–68.
2. Bozic KJ, Kurtz SM, Lau E, Ong K, Chiu V, Vail TP, Rubash HE, Berry DJ. The epidemiology of revision total knee arthroplasty in the United States. Clin Orthop. 2010;468:45–51.
3. Partington PF, Sawhney J, Rorabeck CH, Barrack RL, Moore J. Joint line restoration after revision total knee arthroplasty. Clin Orthop. 1999;367:165–71.
4. Jenny JY, Clemens U, Kohler S, Kiefer H, Konermann W, Miehlke RK. Consistency of implantation of a total knee arthroplasty with a non-image-based navigation system: a case-control study of 235 cases compared with 235 conventionally implanted prostheses. J Arthroplasty. 2005;20:832–29.
5. Teter KE, Bregman D, Colwell CW Jr. Accuracy of intramedullary versus extramedullary tibial alignment cutting systems in total knee arthroplasty. Clin Orthop. 1995;321:106–10.
6. Jones CW, Jerabek SA. Current role of computer navigation in total knee arthroplasty. J Arthroplasty. 2018;33:1989–93.
7. Saragaglia D, Picard F, Chaussard C, Montbarbon E, Leitner F, Cinquin P. Mise en place des prothèses totales du genou assistée par ordinateur: comparaison avec la technique conventionnelle. Rev Chir Orthop. 2001;87:18–28.

8. Sparmann M, Wolke B, Czupalla H, Banzer D, Zink A. Positioning of total knee arthroplasty with and without navigation support. A prospective, randomised study. J Bone Joint Surg. 2003;85B:830–5.
9. Victor J, Hoste D. Image-based computer-assisted total knee arthroplasty leads to lower variability in coronal alignment. Clin Orthop. 2004;428:131–9.
10. Insall JN, Dorr LD, Scott RD, Scott WN. Rationale of the knee society clinical rating system. Clin Orthop. 1989;248:13–4.
11. Siu D, Cooke TD, Broekhiven LD, Lam M, Fisher B, Saunders G, Challis TW. A standardized technique for lower limb radiography. Practice, applications, and error analysis. Invest Radiol. 1991;26:71–7.
12. Hoffart HE, Dinges H, Kolbeck S, Ritschl P, Hommel H. Novel computer-assisted method for revision arthroplasty of the knee. World J Orthop. 2015;6:821–8.
13. Massin P, Boyer P, Pernin J, Jeanrot C. Navigated revision knee arthroplasty using a system designed for primary surgery. Comput Aided Surg. 2008;13:179–87.
14. Perlick L, Bäthis H, Perlick C, Lüring C, Tingart M, Grifka J. Revision total knee arthroplasty: a comparison of postoperative leg alignment after computer-assisted implantation versus the conventional technique. Knee Surg Sports Traumatol Arthrosc. 2005;13:167–73.
15. Ochs BG, Schreiner AJ, de Zwart PM, Stöckle U, Gonser CE. Computer-assisted navigation is beneficial both in primary and revision surgery with modular rotating-hinge knee arthroplasty. Knee Surg Sports Traumatol Arthrosc. 2016;24:64–73.
16. Meijer MF, Stevens M, Boerboom AL, Bulstra SK, Reininga IH. The influence of computer-assisted surgery on rotational, coronal and sagittal alignment in revision total knee arthroplasty. BMC Musculoskelet Disord. 2014;15:94. https://doi.org/10.1186/1471-2474-15-94.
17. Jenny JY, Boeri C. Computer-assisted implantation of total knee prostheses: a case-control comparative study with classical instrumentation. Comput Aided Surg. 2001;6:217–20.
18. Thielemann FW, Clemens U, Hadjicostas PT. Computer-assisted surgery in revision total knee arthroplasty: early experience with 46 patients. Orthopedics. 2007;30(10 Suppl):S132–5.
19. Bonutti PM, Dethmers D, Ulrich SD, Seyler TM, Mont MA. Computer navigation-assisted versus minimally invasive TKA: benefits and drawbacks. Clin Orthop. 2008;466:2756–62.

24 Pearls, Pitfalls, and Complications (MPFL Reconstruction)

Phillip Schöttle

The MPFL is the most important passive stabilizer of the patellofemoral joint. Inadequate function plays a crucial role in the development of patellofemoral instability. According to current knowledge, an MPFL rupture or insufficiency is considered a prerequisite for patellofemoral instability. Several studies have shown that in more than 90% of patients who have had patellar dislocation, there is a ruptured or insufficient MPFL. Here, a distinction must be made between an acute, fresh rupture after traumatic dislocation event and a chronic insufficiency or MPFL underdevelopment in patients with already existing habitual patellar luxations. The latter group of patients may be based on a variety of predisposing factors. It is essential to know and consider these when choosing the treatment method. These factors include mainly trochlear dysplasia, patella alta, valgus deformity, internal femoral rotation, and more rarely external tibial rotation. In addition, the correct rupture localization of the MPFL patellar or femoral for the risk of redislocation in the treatment planning plays an important role.

Therefore, for the correct indication for the reconstruction of the MPFL, patients history, clinical examination, as well as the diagnostic imaging are decisive and demanding in order to determine the presence or the expression of the above-mentioned pathologies to filter out triggering factors. As a further orientation, the Patella Injury Severity Score (PISS) can be used, in which each predisposing factor is assigned to a score, and the sum can assess the risk of relocation.

Since MPFL reconstruction became the most common treatment option in patellofemoral instability (PFI), it is obvious that we will see an increase in number of failures and therefore revisions. Shah et al. [1], in a systematic review (meta-analysis level of evidence II) of complications and failures associated with the MPFL reconstruction in patients with a chronic PFI, found that the complication rate associated with this procedure (26%) is not at all insignificant even though MPFL has a high success rate. Therefore, it is important to inform the patient of the potential risks of this surgery beforehands. These authors also showed that instability represents 32% of all the complications (52/164) found in MPFL reconstruction [1].

It is the idea to help understanding and avoiding the main causes of failure after MPFL reconstruction which are:

1. Incorrect surgical indication or surgical technique/patient selection.
2. A surgical technical error.
3. An incorrect assessment of the additional risk factors.

P. Schöttle (✉)
Knee and Health Institute, Munchen, Germany

M. T. Hirschmann et al. (eds.), *ESSKA Instructional Course Lecture Book*,
https://doi.org/10.1007/978-3-662-61264-4_24

Surprisingly enough, almost half of those complications resulted from technical problems or surgical errors. Ultimately, most failed MPFL reconstructions result from surgeon-dependent factors.

24.1 Indication and Contraindication for MPFL Reconstruction

As in all surgical interventions, the perfect indication is crucial for an ideal outcome. Therefore, the indications and contraindications are pearl and pitfall at the same time.

An ideal candidate for an isolated MPFL reconstruction, without bony procedures, should have a history consistent with recurrent dislocation and a physical examination demonstrating excessive lateral patella translation, with minimal or absent pain between episodes of instability and a normal or low-grade dysplastic trochlea (e.g., type A Dejour classification). There should be no radiological evidence of an increased lateral PF load, tubercle sulcus angle between 0 and 5°, no excessive valgus, and no excessive patella height (reasonable overlap of patella and trochlea surfaces on sagittal MRI measured by patella-trochlea index). The Caton-Deschamps index up to 1.4 can be acceptable, except where there is a very short trochlea or significant knee hyperextension.

An MPFL reconstruction can be performed isolated as well as in combination with other procedures. An isolated MPFL reconstruction is used in patients with traumatic isolated rupture of MPFL without any of the above-mentioned concomitant pathologies with persistent instability and recurrence dislocations. In the case of purely traumatic patellar dislocation, a direct impact trauma can result in a patellar dislocation and rupture of the MPFL without the presence of a predisposing factor. However, this accident mechanism is rather inferior in number and is about less than 3% of all patella dislocations.

After a fresh dislocation event, the recognition of osteochondral detachments at the medial patellar facet or at the lateral femoral condyle in the sense of a "contre-coup" injury is of particular importance. These occur in about a quarter of all patella dislocations. In this case, there is a clear recommendation for prompt surgical treatment with refixation of the osteochondral flake and MPFL reconstruction. Without additional osteochondral injuries, the procedure may be conservative or, if indicated, at a later point. However, it is not recommended to have immediate surgical treatment in an acute posttraumatic condition, if there is no osteochondral flake, making this necessary.

Ultimately, surgical decisions involve a blend of imaging and physical examination features, combined with patient expectation and surgeon's experience and judgment.

The demanding tool in radiological diagnostics is an MRI assessment to determine different anatomical issues such as the degree of trochlear dysplasia and an eventually increased patellar tilt and shift as well as measure the TTTG. In addition, the condition of the femoropatellar articular cartilage as well as the integrity and rupture area of the MPFL can be estimated. In case of clinical suspicion of a high-grade valgus malalignment and persistent patellofemoral instability over 60° knee flexion, long leg axis images and, if necessary, a rotation CT must be completed.

Overall, more or less pronounced forms of dysplasia are found in up to 96% of all cases with patellofemoral instability. In patients with a minor degree of trochlear dysplasia, there is an instability in the approximate range from 0° to about 20° knee flexion. With increasing degrees of flexion, the patella is stabilized by the immersion in the trochlear groove. The correct anatomical reconstruction of the MPFL therefore allows the instability to be remedied close to extension.

The challenge in the indication for an operative approach is to achieve a sufficient stabilization of the patella, without provoking an increase in pressure on the femoropatellar articular surface. To select the optimal surgical procedure in patients with patella instability, the underlying pathologies must be correctly identified and classified. The following risk factors must be considered:

- Triggering event (minor trauma vs. chronic habitual patellar luxation without adequate trauma).
- Age at first luxation <14 years.

- Instability or dislocation on the opposite side.
- Multiple dislocation events.
- Positive family history.
- Type of trochlear dysplasia.

If there is no adequate traumatic event and several of the e.g. points are identified, a higher-grade, static instability with osseous pathomorphology has to be assumed. The risk of redislocation after an isolated MPFL reconstruction would be very high in these cases. So, according to an adequate complete examination of all involved risk factors is demanding and avoids failure after isolated MPFL reconstruction [4]. Here, the operative stabilization in combination with a correction of the existing accompanying bony pathology is indicated.

During the process selection for the respective patient, additional information by the clinical investigation as well as the radiological diagnostics are needed.

Evidence of the presence of osseous risk factors in the clinical examination is a valgus position prominent at the standing inspection, a positive apprehension sign in more then 30° knee flexion, and a positive J sign at over 30° knee flexion. In particular, the reversed J-sign indicates the presence of a pronounced osseous pathology. This phenomenon describes the insertion of the previously lateralized patella into the trochlea during the transition from extension to flexion, which is achieved by an accustomed trick movement. Likewise, an increased patella shift and tilt is a hint sign. If there is a pronounced patella alta in a patient, this is also clinically recognizable from the outside with a knee flexion of 80°.

If these signs occur during clinical examination, an isolated MPFL reconstruction should not be used.

Another diagnostic criterion is the differentiation between complaints caused by patellofemoral instability and patellofemoral pain. The anterior knee pain often occurs in patients with already existing problems, which may already be preexistent and may be an indication of an early patellofemoral arthritis. Therefore, an MPFL reconstruction is not indicated in patients with AKP without patellar instability.

In these situations, an isolated MPFL reconstruction can lead to an aggravation, since the patellar ridge would possibly be pressed into the already arthritically altered area of the trochlea.

Overall, an MPFL reconstruction is NOT indicated in patellofemoral pain patients—at least not in an isolated manner.

An MPFL reconstruction should not be performed if the patella cannot be laterally dislocated.

Last, but not least, the MPFL is not meant to pull, but rather to keep the patella in position and stabilize it, once the patellofemoral tracking has been corrected and the patella is in the correct position.

An MPFL reconstruction is not indicated in an isolated procedure to eliminate patella J-tracking.

Also it is very important to understand if the MPFL insufficiency was the trigger or the result of a lateralized patella—therefore, in a fixed lateral patella dislocation, the main problem is the retraction of the extensor mechanism of the knee and very often a flat lateral condyle, leading to secondary MPFL insufficiency.

Furthermore, an isolated MPFL reconstruction is not indicated in patients with patellofemoral arthrosis because it further increases patellofemoral pressure and increases arthrosis. In these cases, a pressure release and correction of the malalignment has to be addressed before the tracking is improved by performing an MPFL reconstruction.

24.2 Failure in the Surgical Technique

According to Parikh et al., 47% of the complications that occur after MPFL reconstructive surgery are related to technical errors.

The most frequent and significant technical mistake that can lead to MPFL reconstruction failure is a malposition, moreover at the femoral tunnel then the patellar insertion [4–7]. The femoral fixation point is crucial as it determines the length change behavior of the graft and therefore the graft tension at different angles of the full range of motion. Since it is an anatomical structure, there should be no length change pattern. Due to the knee anatomy and the shape of the femur, a normal MPFL is tighter in extension than in flexion. If the femoral fixation point is placed excessively anterior and/or superior, the graft tightens when the knee is flexed, and patellar overload will occur, creating pain, limited range of motion, stiffness, and scaring. In the mid-term, it may lead to an early onset of patellofemoral osteoarthritis. Therefore, the intraoperative accurate monitoring of the femoral tunnel placement is mandatory.

Unlike the femoral fixation point, accuracy in placing the patellar fixation has been shown to be less important.

24.2.1 Failure Due to Excessive Graft Tension

Therefore, one has to understand the concept of MPFL, which in its native state is NOT under constant tension. It only comes under tension when the patella starts displacing laterally due to an lateral acting vector. My preferred simile is a dog leash, which is loose most of the time, except when the dog (the patella) wants to run away (dislocate), and only then it becomes tight. But if I would have the leash (the MPFL) tight all the time, it would choke the dog and transferred into the patellofemoral joint, and it would create a high patellofemoral pressure leading to an early osteoarthritis. In vivo, MPFL kinematic studies have shown that MPFL length was longest from 0 to 60° of knee flexion and decreased significantly during flexion from 60 to 120°, thereby checking excessive patellofemoral compression force during high degrees of knee flexion [2].

To avoid hyperpression on the joint and hypertension on the graft, fix the graft when the patella is engaged fully into the trochlea at around 30° of flexion.

24.3 Failure Due to Insufficient Assessment of Concomitant Factors

Around 85% of PFI occur between 0 and 30° of flexion. In these ROM, patella stability relies mainly on the MPFL. Apprehension that is relieved at 30° of knee flexion suggests a good clinical result with an isolated MPFL reconstruction. Beyond 30°, bony factors such as the shape of the trochlea and/or rotational alignment become important. An apprehension beyond 60° of knee flexion suggests a severe trochlear dysplasia, a significant patella alta, and/or other bony malalignments or all.

While an isolated MPFL reconstruction may be sufficient in most cases in the first group of patients, failure may/will occur in the second group. This has been proven already in early studies, such as from Nelitz or Schoettle. Furthermore, Wagner et al. [6, 8] suggested that the MPFL graft might be overloaded in high degrees of trochlear dysplasia—correlated with poor clinical outcome given that there is more instability in dysplastic situations, additionally resulting in a PF overload. In these cases, an additional trochleoplasty has to be considered.

We also should remember that a trochleoplasty procedure not only corrects the trochlear dysplasia but according to Fucentese et al. also normalizes the TT–TG distance.

Dejour et al. [9, 10] have shown that the sulcus-deepening trochleoplasty is an acceptable revision option for the surgical treatment of patients with persisting patellar dislocation and high-grade trochlear dysplasia. According to Schoettle as well as Fucentese et al. [3, 8], trochleoplasty is a useful and reliable surgical technique to improve patellofemoral instability in patients with a dysplastic trochlea. However, while improved stability is predictable, pain is less predictable and may even increase following surgery. Interestingly, Schöttle et al. [3] have shown that the risk for cartilage damage after trochleoplasty is low. In conclusion, severe trochlear dysplasia can be successfully treated with a trochleoplasty.

Even more, then in dysplastic trochlea, there are significant controversies about other osteotomy indications such as femoral derotation or variation or the way and direction of the transfer of the tuberosity. According to Robert Teitge and Gerd Seitlinger, we may consider an osteotomy in cases with torsion greater than 20° above normal (femoral anteversion >35° and tibial external torsion >45°) that have failed after an isolated MPFL reconstruction.

24.4 Conclusion

The number and percentage of complications after MPFL reconstruction is higher not only due to the indication but also due to the still existing learning curve in the surgical technique. However, most of the patients do well anyhow, since they are relieved from their PFI. Nevertheless, failures in MPFL reconstruction lead to a limited range of motion and/or pain due to a patellofemoral overload and therefore early onset of arthritis. In these cases, an early revision has to be considered once the reason for failure is identified since conservative treatments are not successful and may additionally increase pain and degeneration.

To avoid these cases in the future, a national MPFL register, compared to those of the ACL should and most probably will be installed 1 day.

References

1. Shah JN, Howard JS, Flanigan DC, Brophy RH, Carey JL, Lattermann C. A systematic review of complications and failures associated with medial patellofemoral ligament reconstruction for recurrent patellar dislocation. Am J Sports Med. 2012;40:1916–23. [PMC free article] [PubMed] [Google Scholar].
2. Sanchis-Alfonso V, Ramirez-Fuentes C, Montesinos-Berry E, Domenech J, Martí-Bonmatí L. Femoral insertion site of the graft used to replace the medial patellofemoral ligament influences the ligament dynamic changes during knee flexion and the clinical outcome. Knee Surg Sports Traumatol Arthrosc. 2017;25(8):2433–41.
3. Schöttle PB, Schell H, Duda G, Weiler A. Cartilage viability after trochleoplasty. Knee Surg Sports Traumatol Arthrosc. 2007;15:161–7.
4. Sanchis-Alfonso V. Guidelines for medial patellofemoral ligament reconstruction in chronic lateral patellar instability. J Am Acad Orthop Surg. 2014;22:175–82.
5. Nelitz M, Theile M, Dornacher D, Wölfle J, Reichel H, Lippacher S. Analysis of failed surgery for patellar instability in children with open growth plates. Knee Surg Sports Traumatol Arthrosc. 2012;20:822–8.
6. Wagner D, Pfalzer F, Hingelbaum S, Huth J, Mauch F, Bauer G. The influence of risk factors on clinical outcomes following anatomical medial patellofemoral ligament (MPFL) reconstruction using the gracilis tendon. Knee Surg Sports Traumatol Arthrosc. 2013;21:318–24.
7. Schöttle PB, Schmeling A, Rosenstiel N, Weiler A. Radiographic landmarks for femoral tunnel placement in medial patellofemoral ligament reconstruction. Am J Sports Med. 2007;35:801–4.
8. Fucentese SF, Zingg PO, Schmitt J, Pfirrmann CW, Meyer DC, Koch PP. Classification of trochlear dysplasia as predictor of clinical outcome after trochleoplasty. Knee Surg Sports Traumatol Arthrosc. 2011;19:1655–61.
9. Dejour D, Byn P, Ntagiopoulos PG. The Lyon's sulcus-deepening trochleoplasty in previous unsuccessful patellofemoral surgery. Int Orthop. 2013;37:433–9.
10. Dejour D, Ferrua P, Ntagiopoulos PG, Radier C, Hulet C, Rémy F, Chouteau J, Chotel F, Boisrenoult P, Sebilo A, et al. The introduction of a new MRI index to evaluate sagittal patellofemoral engagement. Orthop Traumatol Surg Res. 2013;99:S391–8.

What to Do If It Goes Wrong? Solutions After Failure

25

F. Martetschläger and F. Zampeli

25.1 Introduction

Acromioclavicular (AC) joint injuries usually occur during sports participation or road traffic accidents and fall from height (high-energy trauma). They represent about 12% of all traumatic shoulder girdle injuries with reported incidence of 9.2 injuries per 1000 person-years in young athletes [1, 2]. Surgical management is recommended for patients with high-grade injury according to Rockwood classification (type IV–VI) [3, 4]. Although the management of type III injuries is still controversial, many authors advocate early surgical reconstruction in select high-functioning patients such as manual laborers and overhead-throwing athletes [5–8].

The surgical management of high-grade AC joint disruption has evolved from the classic Weaver–Dunn procedure [9] to its several modifications [5, 10–13] and during the last decade to the more anatomic coracoclavicular (CC) ligament reconstruction techniques. With the evolution of arthroscopic surgery and advances in implant designs, arthroscopically assisted ACJ stabilization anatomic procedures have gained popularity and carry advantages in terms of a minimally invasive approach, facilitating management of associated intra-articular lesions and good visualization of the coracoid [14–23]. Although there is no consensus about the "gold standard" technique, the overall principle of arthroscopic-assisted stabilization in acute ACJ injury is to use an internal bracing that provides reduction of the AC joint during the healing process of the CC and AC ligaments. The efficiency of such anatomic CC ligament reconstruction methods has been evaluated in both biomechanical [7, 24–29] and clinical studies, and the results have been good to excellent [14, 16, 23, 30].

However, the increasing popularity of such new methods has resulted in some distinct new complications that came to be added to the already known complications of loss of reduction and re-dislocation [31–34]. Due to the internal bracing concept, these techniques typically involve cortical fixation devices, heavy sutures, free tendon grafts, or combination, each of which requires drilling holes to the distal clavicle and/or the coracoid process. As a result, tunnel widening, as well as clavicle and coracoid fractures occurring through drill holes have been reported by several authors. Finally, persistent or recurrent horizontal instability has recently gained more attention. Complications may vary and be dependent on the implant and fixation method used during the index procedure. In fact, the diversity

F. Martetschläger (✉)
German Center for Shoulder Surgery, ATOS Clinic Munich, Munich, Germany
e-mail: frank.martetschlaeger@atos.de

F. Zampeli
Hand, Upper Limb and Microsurgery Department, General Hospital "KAT", Athens, Greece

M. T. Hirschmann et al. (eds.), *ESSKA Instructional Course Lecture Book*,
https://doi.org/10.1007/978-3-662-61264-4_25

of techniques, the decades of variations and modifications among surgeons, as well as the question "was the procedure performed correctly, or does this represent poor surgical technique?" may have largely affected the incidence and type of complications that have been reported [32, 35]. Except for the type of surgical technique, also patients aged >40 years have presented higher rates of complications while the increasing severity of AC joint injury did not correlate with an increased risk of surgical complications [32]. For the treatment of any complication (if required) and even more essential to the planning process in revision scenarios is understanding the contributing factors to failure and the type of surgery performed at the index procedure. The objective should be to identify a source or mode of failure from the prior procedure, such as pain from residual horizontal instability or loss of fixation due to coracoid or clavicle fracture. The ability to identify a clear source of failure increases the likelihood of success for revision surgery.

The purpose of this chapter is to focus on the reported complications related to these arthroscopically assisted anatomical reconstruction techniques and their treatment options.

25.2 Complications

25.2.1 Loss of Reduction

The loss of reduction problem after ACJ reconstruction procedures is a problem for which there is still no consensus about its definition and its clinical relevance. Clavert et al. and Shin et al. defined the loss of reduction (also named it as radiological failure) as a 50% loss of reduction at the final follow-up on AP radiographs of the clavicle corresponding to a 50% increase in the CC distance compared to the contralateral side [16, 31, 34]. However, this definition does not consider any "inadequate reduction" during the operation or in the immediate postoperative radiograph. For Choi et al. loss of reduction was defined as more than 25% increase of CC interspace, comparing the CC percentage of the injured shoulder between immediately postoperative visit and the final follow-up visit [36]. According to the authors, a value of 25% was chosen because a side-to-side CC interspace difference of more than 25% indicates complete disruption of the CC ligaments. Martetschläger et al. defined it as a side-to-side difference of CC distance of >10 mm while Milewski et al. defined it as more than 5-mm increased CC interval displacement on subsequent postoperative radiographs [37, 38]. Taking these variations into consideration in definitions, it is not safe to state about the exact incidence of this complication. In a systematic review, the range varied from 6.5 to 80%, and the pooled rate was 27% [39]. On the other hand, the rate of recurrent instability has been reported to be as high as 11% [32]. Whatever the definition, the resulting problem is a re-dislocation (partial or complete) during the healing phase.

Although failure modes leading to loss of reduction and/or recurrent instability and their prognostic factors have been widely described, they have not been assessed systematically so far for different surgical techniques. Possible problems and causes are implant failure (tear, loosening, cutout), malpositioning of tunnels and implants and subsequent implant migration, new trauma events, or compliance issues of the patient. The main reason for loss of reduction is thought to be migration or bony ingrowth of implants, loosening of knots, or breakage of sutures [40]. In their study, Scheibel et al. reported no correlation between implant migration and CC distance or difference of CC distance between affected and normal side [23]. This method of failure due to implant migration is considered secondary to inappropriate tunnel placement or small-diameter implants. Correct clavicular tunnel placement for appropriate implant positioning as well as positioning of implant centrally under the coracoid base are considered key steps in avoiding re-dislocation (Fig. 25.1) [40, 41]. Schliemann et al. investigated possible risk factors for failure and showed the negative impact of malpositioning of the coracoid bone tunnel on the outcome after their anatomic procedure [41]. If the coracoid button is not placed centrally under the coracoid base, failure of the reconstruction is likely to occur. For

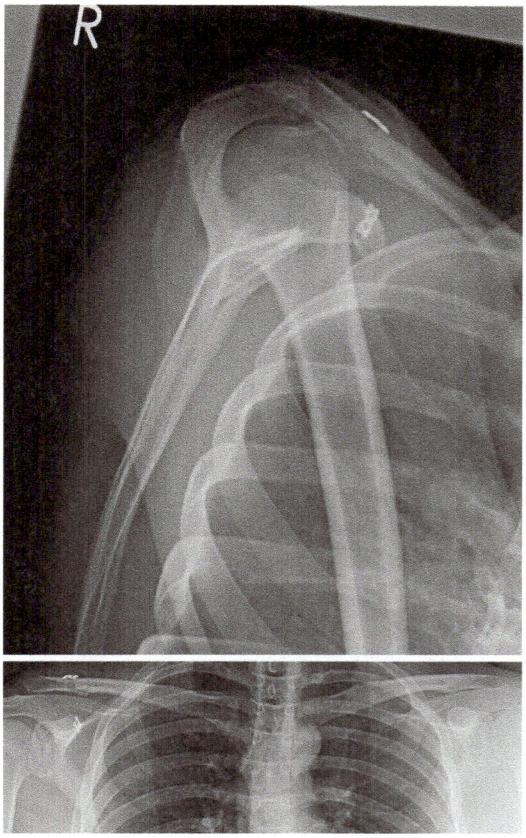

Fig. 25.1 Case of recurrent instability following arthroscopically ACJ stabilization. Several problems can be seen: (1) the clavicle shows an obvious tunnel widening; (2) The subcoracoid button is placed reverse close to the tip of the coracoid; (3) Horizontal and vertical instability results

patients with coracoid button placed laterally to the center of the coracoid base, an early failure of the reconstruction because of button dislocation may lead to surgical revision [27, 41]. For clavicular tunnel placement, it has been shown that very medial tunnel misplacement and very distal tunnels are both significant factors in risk for loss of reduction and early failures when performing anatomic CC ligament reconstructions [31, 42]. A further reason for re-dislocation or suture breakage might be a persistent horizontal instability of the AC joint after surgery [22, 40].

Not all patients are symptomatic, and the decision for revision should be based on patient's symptoms and not on radiographic findings [30, 33, 37, 43]. Patients who have minimal or no symptoms who are showing a loss of reduction

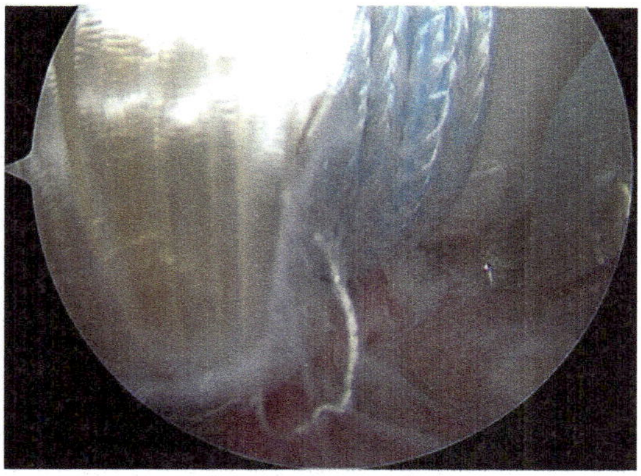

Fig. 25.2 Intraoperative picture of a revision case using a "loop technique" with two suture tapes and an autologous gracilis tendon graft since a large drill hole was already present inside the coracoid base

can be successfully managed conservatively. If the symptoms and pain remain and worsen, revision operation is recommended with tendon graft reconstruction/augmentation (open or arthroscopically assisted). Due to prior surgery, the drill holes and the status of the coracoid and clavicle should be evaluated preoperatively with CT scan to facilitate surgical planning. An intact coracoid allows the surgeon to have multiple options to secure alternate CC graft fixation. In the same way, an intact clavicle provides a stable structure by which fixation and a graft can be secured. If the coracoid base or the clavicle is compromised, then revision options will be limited and more challenging (see below). Due to recurrent instability in cases that this presents, biological reconstruction of the AC and CC ligaments protected by a suture tape construct as in chronic AC joint instability is proposed [44]. The graft and button-suture tape construct enhance horizontal and vertical stability of the AC joint. The graft and suture tapes can be looped around coracoid and clavicle without need for new drill holes if the bony situation is already critical (Fig. 25.2).

25.2.2 Fracture

25.2.2.1 Coracoid Fracture

Many of the anatomic CC ligament reconstruction techniques involve drill holes through the coracoid (for either graft placement or fixation), and this may increase the possibility of coracoid fracture and cutout. The reported incidence is 20% [38] and may occur in both single- and double-tunnel techniques [33, 38, 39, 45], while there is also one report for coracoid fracture following a coracoid loop fixation technique, that occurred 7 months postoperatively in an active baseball player while pitching [8]. The risk factors for this complication are pathological bone density, diameter of the drill tunnels, the number and positioning of tunnels, and the type of fixation [31]. Besides the loss of reduction, the revision surgical technique must be decided taking into consideration that anchoring in the coracoid is difficult or impossible.

In a cadaveric study by Martetschläger et al., the failure mechanism analysis showed that one 2.4-mm drill hole led to less destabilization of the coracoid than one or two 4-mm drill holes [46]. Therefore, minimization of the tunnel diameter may decrease the risk for coracoid fracture. This risk can also be minimized by the passage of the graft and/or suture around and under the coracoid without drilling [37, 38]. Furthermore, adequate visualization of the entire base of the coracoid is essential. Accurate coracoid tunnel placement particularly in the center-center or medial-center position in the coracoid minimizes bony failure risk [27].

Concerning the optimal treatment of coracoid fracture following AC joint reconstructions, most of the available evidence comes from expert opinion and case reports. Non-displaced or minimally displaced fractures can be treated conservatively, and after healing, ACJ stabilization can be performed if necessary, like in other chronic ACJ instability cases. In displaced fractures, open reduction and internal fixation of the coracoid fragment depending on the displacement and size of the distal fragment can be performed with screw fixation [47]. Furthermore, a hook plate with or without tendon graft can be a reasonable solution if any fixation to the fractured coracoid is impossible. In some cases of coracoid tip fractures, looping of a graft along with suture tapes around the coracoid base can be a feasible option.

25.2.2.2 Clavicle Fracture

Similar to coracoid fractures, the new arthroscopically assisted anatomic CC ligament reconstruction techniques raise the risk of clavicle fractures intraoperatively or during the postoperative period. In their biomechanical study, Spiegl et al. found that the graft reconstruction technique with 6.0-mm tunnels, grafts, and tenodesis screws caused significantly more reduction of clavicle strength compared with the cortical fixation button (CFB) technique with 2.4-mm tunnels and CFB device [48]. Besides, they found that relative tunnel width correlated highly with the strength reduction. Except from large drill holes, many clinical studies have also underlined that technical errors in tunnel placement are usually the reason for clavicle fractures [35, 37–39]. Specific recommendations have been made regarding minimization of the clavicular tunnel diameter along with adequate tunnel spacing of 20–25 mm between clavicular tunnels to reduce the incidence of clavicle fracture [25, 49].

The management of clavicle fractures after anatomic CC reconstruction may be conservative for minimally displaced fractures [49]. For displaced clavicle fractures with loss of AC joint reduction, open reduction and internal fixation are warranted with clavicle plates or hook plates depending on the location of the clavicle fracture [37].

25.2.3 Tunnel Widening

It has been shown that arthroscopic ACJ stabilization with the use of bone tunnels leads to significant increase of the clavicular tunnel size even during the early postoperative period. In a recent study, 90% of patients showed 67% (2 mm) increase in clavicular tunnel width during the first 4.5 months. This phenomenon carries a higher fracture risk, especially in high-impact athletes, which needs to be considered preoperatively [50, 51]. The use of sharp drills, continuous irrigation to dampen the heat produced along with perpendicular drill position, is paramount in reducing the possibility on initial tunnel widening. The occurrence of tunnel widening, and a possible fracture risk should be highlighted during informed consent procedure, and different surgical techniques avoiding bone tunnels should be discussed for high-risk individuals such as contact athletes.

25.2.4 Persistent Horizontal Instability

In a systematic review, Woodmass et al. (2015) evaluated 12 studies [39]. Only one by Scheibel et al. assessed horizontal instability clinically (cross-body test; resisted ACJ compression test) and radiographically (Alexander view: a modified scapular lateral view showing posterior displacement of the clavicle in AC joint injuries) [23]. An unstable pattern was identified radiographically in 42.9% of cases, and these patients had significantly lower TAFT scores and ACJI scores that show significantly inferior results in both AC joint–specific scoring systems. The cross-body test and resisted ACJ compression were negative in all patients [23].

Except from the inferior functional results, persistent horizontal (anteroposterior) instability of the AC joint may be the actual underlying cause for many complications as it increases the strain on the upper CFB and thus increases the risk of suture/hardware failure, clavicular fracture, passing the button through the clavicle, or clavicular bone erosion [31].

The underlying cause is the defect of the AC joint capsule and ligament even if the fascia is intact. Cadaveric studies have shown that only combined AC and CC reconstruction can adequately re-establish physiological horizontal ACJ stability [52, 53].

If there is no pain or functional disability for the patient, no specific treatment is needed. On the contrary, in cases that excessive horizontal instability is detected and related to patient's symptoms, revision of the AC joint and use of graft augmentation may be warranted. The best way to prevent this complication is to correctly examine the patient for horizontal instability and if indicated to use a surgical technique that addresses both the horizontal and vertical direction.

25.2.5 Other Complications

Cases of cutaneous hardware-related pain (knots, superior CFB devices) have been mentioned [31, 37]. Patients usually reported pain when wearing a backpack or carrying a handbag. Methods to prevent this is to use knotless implants or to create on purpose large knot that can be consequently "buried" and positioned horizontally under the fascia instead of being prominent vertically under fascia and skin. In cases of persistent pain, the removal of the implant may be warranted.

Development of ossifications of the coracoclavicular ligaments has been mentioned by several studies. Usually it may not have any clinical consequences.

References

1. Lemos MJ. The evaluation and treatment of the injured acromioclavicular joint in athletes. Am J Sports Med. 1998;26(1):137–44.
2. Pallis M, Cameron KL, Svoboda SJ, Owens BD. Epidemiology of acromioclavicular joint injury in young athletes. Am J Sports Med. 2012;40:2072–7.
3. Rockwood CA. Injuries to the acromioclavicular joint. In: Rockwood CA, Green DP, editors. Fractures in adults, vol. 1. 2nd ed. Philadelphia: JB Lippincott Co; 1984. p. 860.
4. Li X, Ma R, Bedi A, et al. Management of acromioclavicular joint injuries. J Bone Joint Surg Am. 2014;96(1):73–84.
5. Spencer EE Jr. Treatment of grade III acromioclavicular joint injuries: a systematic review. Clin Orthop Relat Res. 2007;455:38–44.
6. Tamaoki MJ, Belloti JC, Lenza M, et al. Surgical versus conservative interventions for treating acromioclavicular dislocation of the shoulder in adults. Cochrane Database Syst Rev. 2010;(8):CD007429.
7. Thomas K, Litsky A, Jones G, Bishop JY. Biomechanical comparison of coracoclavicular reconstructive techniques. Am J Sports Med. 2011;39(4):804–10.
8. Tomlinson DP, Altchek DW, Daavila J, Cordasco FA. A modified technique for arthroscopically assisted AC joint reconstruction and preliminary results. Clin Orthop Relat Res. 2008;466(3):639–45.
9. Weaver JK, Dunn HK. Treatment of acromioclavicular injuries, especially complete acromioclavicular separation. J Bone Joint Surg Am. 1972;54(6):1187–94.
10. Boileau P, Old J, Gastaud O, Brassart N, Roussanne Y. All-arthroscopic Weaver-Dunn-Chuinard pro-

cedure with double-button fixation for chronic acromioclavicular joint dislocation. Arthroscopy. 2010;26(2):149–60.
11. Millett PJ, Braun S, Gobeze R, Pacheco IH. Acromioclavicular joint reconstruction with coracoacromial ligament transfer using the docking technique. BMC Musculoskelet Disord. 2009;10:6.
12. Weinstein DM, McCann PD, McIlveen SJ, Flatow EL, Bigliani LU. Surgical treatment of complete acromioclavicular dislocations. Am J Sports Med. 1995;23(3):324–31.
13. Michlitsch MG, Adamson GJ, Pink M, Estess A, Shankwiler JA, Lee TQ. Biomechanical comparison of a modified Weaver-Dunn and a free-tissue graft reconstruction of the acromioclavicular joint complex. Am J Sports Med. 2010;38(6):1196–203.
14. Cook JB, Krul KP. Challenges in treating acromioclavicular separations: current concepts. J Am Acad Orthop Surg. 2018;26(19):669–77.
15. Hann C, Kraus N, Minkus M, Maziak N, Scheibel M. Combined arthroscopically assisted coraco- and acromioclavicular stabilization of acute high-grade acromioclavicular joint separations. Knee Surg Sports Traumatol Arthrosc. 2018;26(1):212–20.
16. Shin SJ, Jeon YS, Kim RG. Arthroscopic-assisted coracoclavicular ligament reconstruction for acute acromioclavicular dislocation using 2 clavicular and 1 coracoid cortical fixation buttons with suture tapes. Arthroscopy. 2017;33(8):1458–66.
17. Sirin E, Aydin N, Mert Topkar O. Acromioclavicular joint injuries: diagnosis, classification and ligamentoplasty procedures. EFORT Open Rev. 2018;3(7):426–33.
18. Tauber M, Valler D, Lichtenberg S, Magosch P, Moroder P, Habermeyer P. Arthroscopic stabilization of chronic acromioclavicular joint dislocations: triple- versus single-bundle reconstruction. Am J Sports Med. 2016;44(2):482–9.
19. Martetschläger F, Tauber M, Habermeyer P, Selim HA. Arthroscopic coracoclavicular and acromioclavicular stabilization of acute acromioclavicular joint dislocation by suspensory fixation system. Arthrosc Tech. 2019;8(6):e611–5. https://doi.org/10.1016/j.eats.2019.02.002. PMID: 31334018.
20. Braun S, Beitzel K, Buchmann S, Imhoff AB. Arthroscopically assisted treatment of acute dislocations of the acromioclavicular joint. Arthrosc Tech. 2015;4(6):e681–5.
21. Baumgarten KM, Altchek DW, Cordasco FA. Arthroscopically assisted acromioclavicular joint reconstruction. Arthroscopy. 2006;22(2):228.e1–6.
22. Salzmann GM, Walz L, Buchmann S, Glabgly P, Venjakob A, Imhoff AB. Arthroscopically assisted 2-bundle anatomical reduction of acute acromioclavicular joint separations. Am J Sports Med. 2010;38(6):1179–87.
23. Scheibel M, Dröschel S, Gerhardt C, Kraus N. Arthroscopically assisted stabilization of acute high-grade acromioclavicular joint separations. Am J Sports Med. 2011;39(7):1507–16.
24. Beitzel K, Obopilwe E, Chowaniec DM, et al. Biomechanical comparison of arthroscopic repairs for acromioclavicular joint instability: suture button systems without biological augmentation. Am J Sports Med. 2011;39(1):2218–25.
25. Carofino BC, Mazzocca AD. The anatomic coracoclavicular ligament reconstruction: surgical technique and indications. J Shoulder Elbow Surg. 2010;19(2 Suppl):37–46.
26. Clevenger T, Vance RE, Bachus KN, Burks RT, Tashjian RZ. Biomechanical comparison of acromioclavicular joint reconstructions using coracoclavicular tendon grafts with and without coracoacromial ligament transfer. Arthroscopy. 2011;27(1):24–30.
27. Ferreira JV, Chowaniec D, Obopilwe E, Nowak MD, Arciero RA, Mazzocca AD. Biomechanical evaluation of effect of coracoid tunnel placement on load to failure of fixation during repair of acromioclavicular joint dislocations. Arthroscopy. 2012;28(9):1230–6.
28. Nuchtern JV, Sellenschloh K, Bishop N, Jauch S, et al. Biomechanical evaluation of 3 stabilization methods of acromioclavicular joint dislocations. Am J Sports Med. 2013;41(6):1387–94.
29. Walz L, Salzmann GM, Fabbro T, Eichhorn S, Imhoff AB. The anatomic reconstruction of acromioclavicular joint dislocations using 2 TightRope devices: a biomechanical study. Am J Sports Med. 2008;36(12):2398–406.
30. Venjakob AJ, Salzmann GM, Gabel F, Buchmann S, Walz L, Spang JT, et al. Arthroscopically assisted 2-bundle anatomic reduction of acute acromioclavicular joint separations: 58-month findings. Am J Sports Med. 2013;41(3):615–21.
31. Clavert P, Meyer A, Boyer P, Gastaud O, Barth J, Duparc F, SFA. Complication rates and types of failure after arthroscopic acute acromioclavicular dislocation fixation. Prospective multicenter study of 116 cases. Orthop Traumatol Surg Res. 2015;101(8 Suppl):S313–6.
32. Hippensteel KJ, Brophy R, Smith M, Wright R. Surgical volume and postoperative complications of acromioclavicular joint separations: analysis of the ABOS part II examination. Am J Sports Med. 2018;46(13):3174–81.
33. Ma R, Smith PA, Smith MJ, Sherman SL, Flood D, Li X. Managing and recognizing complications after treatment of acromioclavicular joint repair or reconstruction. Curr Rev Musculoskelet Med. 2015;8(1):75–82.
34. Shin SJ, Kim NK. Complications after arthroscopic coracoclavicular reconstruction using a single adjustable-loop-length suspensory fixation device in acute acromioclavicular joint dislocation. Arthroscopy. 2015;31(5):816–24.
35. Brand JC, Lubowitz JH, Provencher MT, Rossi MJ. Acromioclavicular joint reconstruction: complications and innovations. Arthroscopy. 2015;31(5):795–7. https://doi.org/10.1016/j.arthro.2015.03.001.
36. Choi NH, Lim SM, Lee SY, Lim TK. Loss of reduction and complications of coracoclavicular ligament

reconstruction with autogenous tendon graft in acute acromioclavicular dislocations. J Shoulder Elbow Surg. 2017;26(4):692–8. https://doi.org/10.1016/j.jse.2016.09.014.
37. Martetschläger F, Horan MP, Warth RJ, Millett PJ. Complications after anatomic fixation and reconstruction of the coracoclavicular ligaments. Am J Sports Med. 2013;41(12):2896–903.
38. Milewski MD, Tompkins M, Giugale JM, et al. Complications related to anatomic reconstruction of the coracoclavicular ligaments. Am J Sports Med. 2012;40:1628–34.
39. Woodmass JM, Esposito JG, Ono Y, Nelson AA, Boorman RS, Thornton GM, Lo IK. Complications following arthroscopic fixation of acromioclavicular separations: a systematic review of the literature. Open Access J Sports Med. 2015;6:97–107. https://doi.org/10.2147/OAJSM.S73211.
40. Rush LN, Lake N, Stiefel EC, Hobgood ER, Ramsey JR, O'Brien MJ, Field LD, Savoie FH. Comparison of short-term complications between 2 methods of coracoclavicular ligament reconstruction: a multicenter study. Orthop J Sports Med. 2016;4(7):2325967116658419. https://doi.org/10.1177/2325967116658419. PMCID: PMC4962340.
41. Schliemann B, Roßlenbroich SB, Schneider KN, et al. Why does minimally invasive coracoclavicular ligament reconstruction using a flip button repair technique fail? An analysis of risk factors and complications. Knee Surg Sports Traumatol Arthrosc. 2015;23:1419–25.
42. Cook JB, Shaha JS, Rowles DJ, et al. Clavicular bone tunnel malposition leads to early failures in coracoclavicular ligament reconstructions. Am J Sports Med. 2013;41:142–8.
43. Sandmann GH, Martetschläger F, Mey L, Kraus TM, Buchholz A, Ahrens P, Stöckle U, Freude T, Siebenlist S. Reconstruction of displaced acromioclavicular joint dislocations using a triple suture-cerclage: description of a safe and efficient surgical technique. Patient Saf Surg. 2012;6(1):25. https://doi.org/10.1186/1754-9493-6-25. PMID: 23098339.
44. Martetschläger F, Tauber M, Habermeyer P, Hawi N. Arthroscopically assisted acromioclavicular and coracoclavicular ligament reconstruction for chronic acromioclavicular joint instability. Arthrosc Tech. 2016;5(6):e1239–46. https://doi.org/10.1016/j.eats.2016.07.014. PMID: 28149720.
45. Gerhardt DC, VanDerWerf JD, Rylander LS, et al. Postoperative coracoid fracture after transcoracoid acromioclavicular joint reconstruction. J Shoulder Elbow Surg. 2011;20:e6–10.
46. Martetschläger F, Buchholz A, Sandmann G, Siebenlist S, Döbele S, Hapfelmeier A, Stöckle U, Millett PJ, Elser F, Lenich A. Acromioclavicular and coracoclavicular PDS augmentation for complete AC joint dislocation showed insufficient properties in a cadaver model. Knee Surg Sports Traumatol Arthrosc. 2013;21(2):438–44. https://doi.org/10.1007/s00167-012-2067-6.
47. Kawasaki Y, Hirano T, Miyatake K, et al. Safety screw fixation technique in a case of coracoid base fracture with acromioclavicular dislocation and coracoid base cross-sectional size data from a computed axial tomography study. Arch Orthop Trauma Surg. 2014;134:913–8.
48. Spiegl UJ, Smith SD, Euler SA, et al. Biomechanical consequences of coracoclavicular reconstruction techniques on clavicle strength. Am J Sports Med. 2014;42:1724–30.
49. Turman KA, Miller CD, Miller MD. Clavicular fractures following coracoclavicular ligament reconstruction with tendon graft: a report of three cases. J Bone Joint Surg Am. 2010;92:1526–32.
50. Thangaraju S, Tauber M, Habermeyer P, Martetschläger F. Clavicle and coracoid process periprosthetic fractures as late post-operative complications in arthroscopically assisted acromioclavicular joint stabilization. Knee Surg Sports Traumatol Arthrosc. 2019;27(12):3797–802. https://doi.org/10.1007/s00167-019-05482-7. [Epub ahead of print]. PMID: 30900030.
51. Thangaraju S, Cepni S, Magosch P, Tauber M, Habermeyer P, Martetschläger F. Arthroscopically assisted acromioclavicular joint stabilization leads to significant clavicular tunnel widening in the early post-operative period. Knee Surg Sports Traumatol Arthrosc. 2019;27(12):3821–6. https://doi.org/10.1007/s00167-019-05662-5. [Epub ahead of print]. PMID: 31410526.
52. Saier T, Venjakob AJ, Minzlaff P, Föhr P, Lindell F, Imhoff AB, Vogt S, Braun S. Value of additional acromioclavicular cerclage for horizontal stability in complete acromioclavicular separation: a biomechanical study. Knee Surg Sports Traumatol Arthrosc. 2015;23(5):1498–505. https://doi.org/10.1007/s00167-014-2895-7.
53. Beitzel K, Obopilwe E, Apostolakos J, Cote MP, Russell RP, Charette R, Singh H, Arciero RA, Imhoff AB, Mazzocca AD. Rotational and translational stability of different methods for direct acromioclavicular ligament repair in anatomic acromioclavicular joint reconstruction. Am J Sports Med. 2014;42(9):2141–8. https://doi.org/10.1177/0363546514538947.

Advanced Hip Arthroscopy: What's New?

26

Oliver Marin-Peña, Ali Bajwa, Athanasios V. Papavasiliou, Christoph Gebhart, Bent Lund, Vikas Khanduja, Olufemi R. Ayeni, Luis Perez-Carro, Nolan S. Horner, Adrian Z. Kurz, Karadi H. Sunil Kumar, and Ankit Rai

Hip arthroscopy technique is evolving rapidly in the last years. Concepts and technical aspects become old in only 3–4 years. Therefore, along present chapter our goal is to update the current concepts about main hot topics in hip arthroscopy. We divide the chapter into six topics:

- Arthroscopic management of cam deformity
- Modern approach to pincer deformity
- Management of labral injuries
- Update on chondral repair techniques
- Soft tissue management in hip instability
- Arthroscopic management of deep gluteal syndrome

O. Marin-Peña (✉)
Orthopedic Department, Hip Surgery Unit, University Hospital Infanta Leonor, Madrid, Spain

A. Bajwa
The Villar Bajwa Practice, The Princess Grace Hospital, London, UK

A. V. Papavasiliou
Hip Arthroscopy Centre, Interbalkan European Medical Centre, Thessaloniki, Greece

C. Gebhart
Privatklinik Döbling, Vienna, Austria

B. Lund
Department of Orthopaedic Surgery, Aarhus University Hospital, Aarhus, Denmark

V. Khanduja
Addenbrookes Hospital, Cambridge, UK

University of Cambridge, Cambridge, UK

O. R. Ayeni · N. S. Horner
Division of Orthopaedic Surgery, McMaster University, Hamilton, ON, Canada

L. Perez-Carro
Orthopedic Surgery Department, Clinica Mompia, Santander, Cantabria, Spain

A. Z. Kurz
Kelowna Orthopaedics, Kelowna Bone and Joint Health, Kelowna, BC, Canada

K. H. Sunil Kumar
Addenbrookes Hospital, Cambridge, UK

A. Rai
University of Cambridge, Cambridge, UK

M. T. Hirschmann et al. (eds.), *ESSKA Instructional Course Lecture Book*,
https://doi.org/10.1007/978-3-662-61264-4_26

26.1 Arthroscopic Management of "Cam" Deformity

Cam deformity treatment options include open surgical dislocation, direct anterior mini open approach, and arthroscopy [1–3]. The rates of good to excellent outcomes are comparable between open and arthroscopic techniques, although reported complications may be slightly less with arthroscopy [4–7]. The management of the femoral head–neck junction is one of the commonest arthroscopic hip procedures, and the 2018 UK Non Arthroplasty Hip Registry (http://www.nahr.co.uk/) accounts for 89.4% of all femoral procedures performed. There are many published surgical variations of how to approach the cam in planning, portals, and use of fluoroscopy, and we believe as many anecdotal variations as the number of surgeons performing hip arthroscopy since every physician has their own tricks and routine [8–10]. We provide some basic principles where the surgeons can evolve their own routine (Table 26.1).

26.1.1 Imaging to Evaluate "Cam" Deformity

Although three-dimensional (3D) imaging using CT and magnetic resonance imaging (MRI) are effective for visualizing cam morphology, there are increased costs and, in the case of CT, exposure to ionizing radiation. Thus, radiographs should serve as the primary means of imaging cam morphology [11].

Plain radiographs are used as the sole means to evaluate hip morphology in nearly one third of patients with cam-type FAI [12]. The ability to understand a 3D spherical dynamic pathology from 2D imaging is difficult, so routine imaging involves multiple radiographic views. It is suggested by a number of studies that a complete radiographic series in evaluating cam-type FAI should include an anteroposterior pelvis, 45° lateral Dunn, cross-table lateral, and frog-leg lateral [13–16].

CT scanning with three-dimensional (3D) reconstruction (Fig. 26.1) and analysis of the femoral version can be invaluable in providing a

Table 26.1 Principles for planning and performing head–neck osteoplasty

	Principles for planning and performing osteoplasty
Imaging	Preoperative radiographs should include anteroposterior pelvis, 45° lateral Dunn views
	A 3D CT can further help to evaluate the extent of cam lesion and its relation to the lateral retinacular vessels
Fluoroscopy	Pre-arthroscopy fluoroscopy should be used in a number of limp positions as dynamic imaging to confirm FAI and assist as a baseline to monitor bone resection
Surgical tips and tricks	If preoperative imaging studies show cam-type pathology but intraoperative findings do not confirm the pathology, bony resection should be debated
	Sclerotic and discolored bone is commonly encountered on the femoral neck in areas of impingement
	The presence of a femoral neck cyst/herniation pit confirms the area of impingement and can be used as a guide on the depth of resection
	The 5.5-mm round burr which is used for the osteoplasty can be used as a visual aid to quantify the amount of bone removed
	Sphericity of the head is not easy to judge arthroscopically; the supplement use of fluoroscopy in leg positions used at the beginning of the procedure can verify the visual findings
	If the perineal post or the tractions boot interferes with the neck osteoplasty, it can be removed when traction is no longer required
	A T-capsulotomy should be used for increased visualization, as needed, but capsular resection should be avoided
	If a capsulotomy is performed, it should not extend through the zona orbicularis
	The superolateral synovial fold is the site of the superolateral retinacular vessels and should be carefully protected throughout the case
	It is important to periodically and dynamically assess for impingement during the cam resection to avoid over-resection and resultant loss of the labral seal

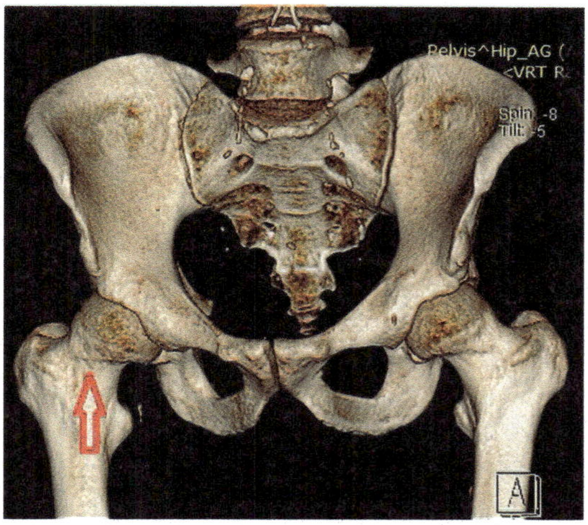

Fig. 26.1 3D CT reconstruction of right hip (arrow shows cam lesion)

detailed assessment of the proximal femoral and acetabular geometry in order to define intra- and extra-articular sources of impingement [17, 18]. Precise localization of the maximal deficiency of offset is a principal benefit of 3D CT analysis. Without knowing the site of the maximum prominence, surgical decompression may be incomplete [19]. 3D dynamic CT has tremendous future potential for identifying additional causes and locations of extra-articular impingement [20].

Magnetic resonance imaging (MRI) is the imaging modality of choice in the preoperative and postoperative assessment of patients undergoing hip arthroscopy. MRI especially after the introduction of 3 T MRI is considered the most sensitive and specific modality to diagnose labral pathology and associated bony and soft tissue abnormalities associated with FAI as well as those independent of FAI (i.e., osteonecrosis, bone tumors, synovial chondromatosis) [20, 21]. Recent approaches to quantify the glycosaminoglycan (GAG) content of hip joint cartilage with a contrast-based MR, delayed gadolinium enhanced MRI of cartilage (dGEMRIC), are very promising into detecting early cartilage lesions [22].

26.1.2 Surgical Technique

The authors perform hip arthroscopy in the supine position with the use of two to three portals depending on the location of the lesion, with the workhorse being the antero-lateral (ALP) and mid-anterior (MAP) portals. Once the central compartment pathology has been addressed, attention is turned to the peripheral compartment and the cam lesion. This is performed without traction by either releasing the traction or taking the foot out of the traction boots. Usually we prefer to the keep the foot in the boot rather than freeing it. It is advisable though to relax the strapping of the boot which could be tight since, complications have been described secondary to this [23, 24]. The traction is removed in order to gain access to the peripheral compartment because this relaxes the anterior capsule-ligamentous structures, thus making the compartment more spacious allowing easier access and maneuverability. This is further achieved when the hip is flexed 20–45° and the central post removed.

26.1.2.1 Identification of Cam Lesion

During arthroscopy, the femoral head and acetabular rim are visualized regionally through multiple portals. This regional assessment can make global evaluation of the bony pathology and subsequent resection difficult. Thus, the cam lesion needs to be defined both arthroscopically and radiographically. Arthroscopically, the cam is identifiable as a sclerotic, discolored (purplish/gray), or peel-off lesion (fibrillation/flap/fissure) that distinctly demarcates it from the rest normal-appearing articular cartilage of the head–neck junction (Fig. 26.2). During a dynamic examination, the scope can visualize FAI as excessive displacement of the labrum and simultaneous levering of the femoral head out of the socket, indicating loss of the suction seal. The amount of flexion for this to happen can be as early as 40°, particularly in patients with large anterior deformities [25].

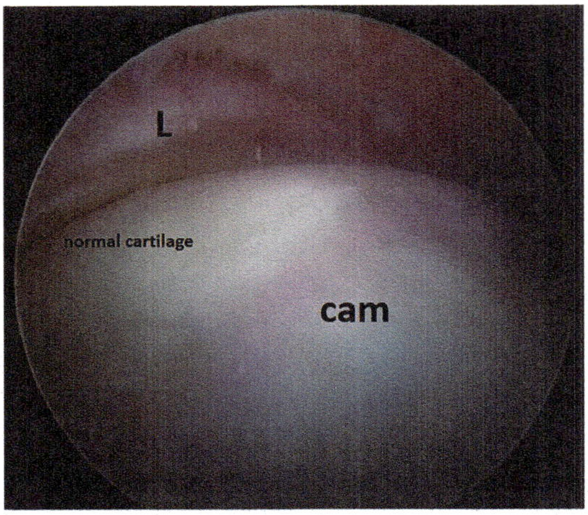

Fig. 26.2 Note the discoloration of cam in comparison to normal cartilage (*L* labrum)

26.1.2.2 Dynamic Examination

It starts by moving the hip from full extension into flexion in neutral position while directly visualizing the motion with the arthroscope (the 70° arthroscope is placed in the MAP). Through the ALP, the capsule can be elevated to improve visualization. Next, the hip is abducted, and a 45° abduction test is performed in both extension and in 90° of flexion to evaluate possible superolateral impingement [26]. The hip is then maneuvered into flexion, adduction, and maximal internal rotation in order to verify anterior impingement. The majority of cam lesions are almost exclusively anterior, anterolateral, or lateral, so this basic dynamic assessment will allow the surgeon to visualize the majority of the bony morphology of interest and the areas requiring resection. In general, the anteroinferior head–neck junction is best accessed with the hip in flexion external rotation, and the supero-posterior head–neck junction is best accessed with the hip in extension, internal rotation.

26.1.2.3 Intraoperative Fluoroscopy

It can help to identify the lesion and verify the arthroscopic findings as well as to monitor how much bone is removed during the procedure since under- or over-resection is one of the most frequent problems seen with the technique [19, 27, 28]. A number of intraoperative fluoroscopic techniques have been published to guide the femoral osteoplasty during arthroscopy. The "around-the-world" evaluation suggests six fluoroscopic images pre- and post-procedure in every case in order to better define the head–neck junction and adequacy of the resection. Three views are taken in 20–40 degrees of flexion with the hip in neutral, 30° external rotation, and 60° external rotation to better evaluate the anterior and posterior head–neck junction. Furthermore, another three views are taken in full-hip extension with the hip in 30° internal rotation, neutral rotation, and 30° external rotation in order to better define the lateral and medial femoral head–neck junction [10, 27, 29]. The concern that radiation exposure during fluoroscopy-assisted hip arthroscopy is high enough in its own right to repeatedly use image for conformation of the osteoplasty for both surgeon and patient is largely unfounded. Our opinion is that the use of fluoroscopy is mandatory to achieve the best result, but the exposure largely depends on physician comfort and experience [30, 31].

26.1.2.4 Cam Resection

Initially, the proximal extent of the osteoplasty can be demarcated with radiofrequency as a line that begins at the inferior head–neck junction and runs roughly perpendicular to the femoral neck to the superior head–neck junction (Fig. 26.3). This

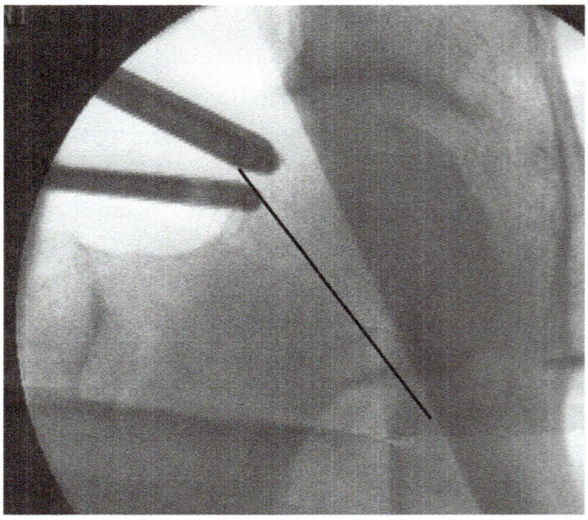

Fig. 26.3 Area where the cam is usually located from to the superior head–neck junction

can help as a visual aid to the area that needs to be resected. The magnitude of femoral osteoplasty is variable and should be estimated by preoperative radiographs and confirmed with intraoperative findings but as a rule of a thump the 5.5-mm round burr which is used for the osteoplasty can quantify the amount of bony resection. If visualization is limited, an additional "T" incision can be made down the anterior femoral neck with care not to extend it through the zona orbicularis although this is rarely required. Typically, the resection is performed from the medial synovial fold (the most inferior extent of cam) to the lateral retinacular vessels. The blood supply to the femoral head, the posterior circumflex vessels, travels within the lateral synovial fold, and femoral neck posterolaterally, so the resection should stay at a safe distance. If working beyond the lateral synovial fold because more superior areas of femoral head need to be reached, this can be achieved with the hip in extension, the foot maximally internally rotated, and the use of traction. With the arthroscope in the MAP and a 5.5-mm round burr in the ALP, the osseous lesion is gradually removed and the head–neck junction recontoured, working medially toward the lateral retinacular vessels and proximal to distal in order to recreate the normal shape and offset of the hip. Frequent switching between portals can aid in visualization and orientation. One needs to be careful not to remove too much bone proximally because it will create a defect ("apple bite") (Fig. 26.4) at the head–neck junction which, when it articulates with the acetabulum during flexion, will break the suction seal of the labrum. Care should be taken not to make too sharp a ledge approaching the articular surface because this could compromise the labral suction seal. Anecdotally, and in order to give a 'smoother' contour to the proximal edge of the osteoplasty, the author finds it helpful to use a small curved rasp. When the procedure is complete, a dynamic examination should show elimination of the bony impingement. At the completion of the procedure, the joint is irrigated to remove bony debris, and radiofrequency is used to provide hemostasis at the site of bone resection in order to minimize the risk of heterotopic ossification and adhesions, respectively. Capsular closure is performed in selected cases [8, 24, 32, 33] (Fig. 26.5).

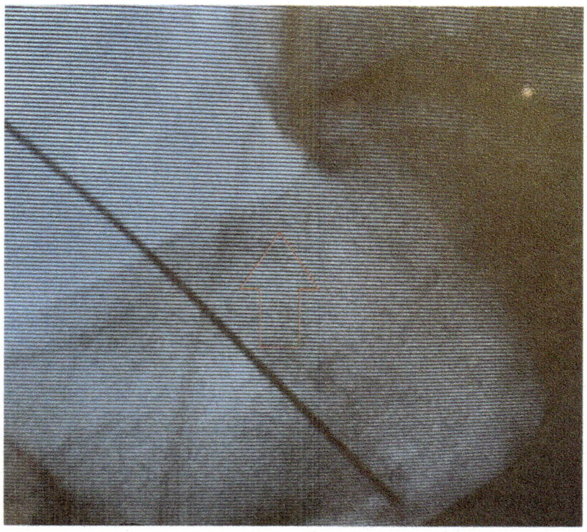

Fig. 26.4 Revision case. Note the osteoplasty, was not fully performed from proximal to distal creating an "apple bite"-type resection

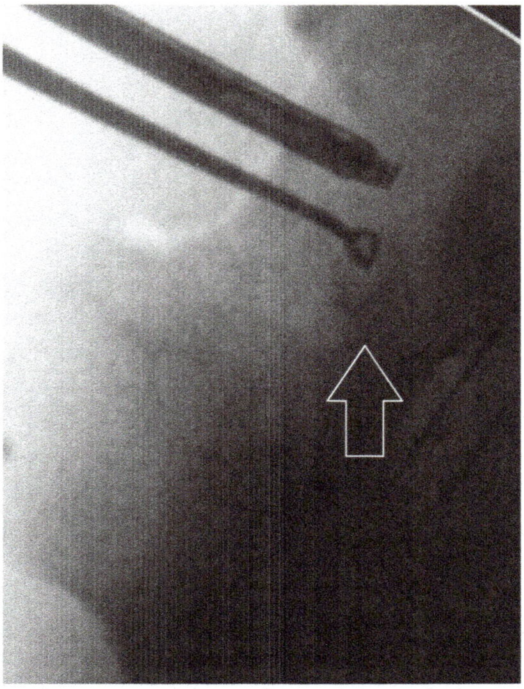

Fig. 26.5 Herniation pit is often seen in the area of impingement—it confirms the lesion. It is advisable to curettage the cyst—usually the depth of the cyst can aid in the estimation of the bone that needs to be resected

26.1.3 Future Directions

The contemporary definition of FAI syndrome is "a motion-related clinical disorder of the hip with a triad of symptoms, clinical signs and imaging findings" [11]. The fact that the prevalence of cam morphology is common in the general population, with or without the presence of symptoms casts doubts on the ability of contemporary imaging to diagnose a dynamic condition further reinforcing the dictum "treat the patient, not the MRI" [34, 35]. The debate thus needs to move forward to establish who, when, and what to treat rather on how to surgically approach the hip joint. So, the future seems to rely on dynamic imaging and possibly in computer-assisted hip arthroscopy two parts that are by definition interlinked [36, 37].

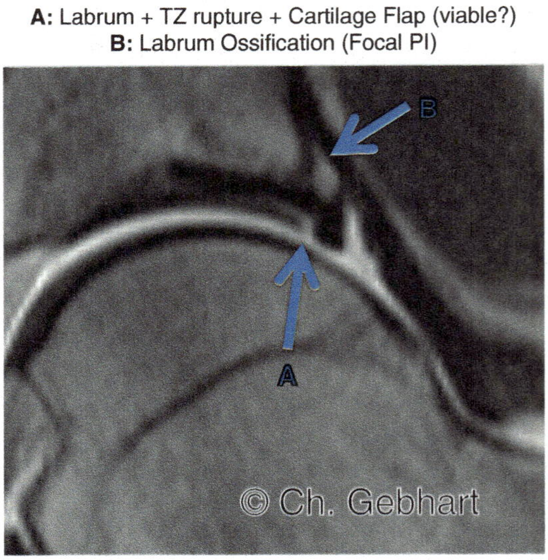

Fig. 26.6 Chondrolabral complex lesion. (**a**) Chondrolabral disruption. (**b**) Bone apposition at the extra-articular labral side

26.2 Modern Approach to Handling Pincer Impingement with Hip Arthroscopy

Due to current anatomical studies as well as three- and four-dimensional computer analyses of hip joint kinematics, an improved understanding of involved bones and contact points has evolved. Recently knowledge about rotational disorders of acetabulum and femur and bone appositions at the acetabular site ("pincer") or at the femur ("cam") demonstrated a reduction of range of hip joint motion. This can lead to painful tissue overuse and destruction of involved structures at the acetabular side (labrum, cartilage, bone) and thereby cause early osteoarthritis (Fig. 26.6).

If we revise the current literature, we could find several attempts to establish an approach and algorithms for individual pincer classification and treatment [38, 39]. All algorithms take into account the chondrolabral complex. Several parameters have been proposed to describe shape, orientation, and position of the hip acetabulum and its relation with proximal femur. Assessment of pincer deformities should be initiated with standard radiological projections (at least two views). To evaluate the relationship between anterior and posterior rim, a well-done AP pelvis view should be carefully analyzed [40]. However, despite a correct evaluation of the acetabular position (inclination, version, LCE, ACE, AI), the determination of the exact location and amount of required acetabular bone resection for reestablishment of impingement-free range of motion remains sometimes unclear. A worldwide concern seems to be the differentiation between global and segmental overcoverage situations [41]. The threshold when a segmental pincer turns into a global overcoverage deformity is still lacking. It is definitely clear that focal overcoverage can occur either at the anterior or at the posterior part of the acetabulum.

26.2.1 Anterior Overcoverage

A normal acetabulum is anteverted and therefore projects the anterior acetabular rim medial to the posterior wall margin. In contrast, overcoverage of a prominent anterior acetabular rim results in a projected overlap of the posterior wall, resulting in the so-called cross-over sign [42]. Anterior overcoverage could clinically result in anterior painful limited flexion and internal rotation.

Whether the anterior acetabular wall is prominent or the posterior wall is deficient can be distinguished by detailed analysis of the posterior wall that normally descends directly through the center of rotation of the femur head.

26.2.2 Posterior Acetabular Overcoverage

This can be seen when the posterior wall line is projected lateral to the femoral center of rotation in an AP pelvis X-ray, resulting in the so-called posterior wall sign. Posterior focal pincer impingement clinically results in a posterior painful hip in external rotation and extension. Overall, anterior or posterior overcoverage develops a pressure increase at chondrolabral complex and could progress to labral and acetabular cartilage damage.

26.2.3 Acetabular Malrotation

True malrotation of the acetabulum is a clear contraindication for an arthroscopic approach. Pelvic rotational disorders require detailed three-dimensional pelvic analysis with a meticulous preoperative evaluation of the bone deformities to plan a pelvic osteotomy correction. Compared to these open osteotomies, arthroscopically procedures are usually less invasive and have developed sophisticated techniques for soft tissue repair over recent years.

26.2.4 Arthroscopic Treatment

Once these true malrotations have been excluded, an arthroscopic approach could be selected. It seems to be generally accepted that the aim of arthroscopic treatment should be to restore normal function and the original interaction of the anatomical structures. The main goal of arthroscopic treatment should be to focus on restoring labrum functions of sealing mechanism, stability, and proprioception. Cartilage repair should also be done as it plays an important role to prevent the development of early osteoarthritis.

The chondrolabral complex or transition zone (TZ), where the labrum shall be connected to the facies lunata hyaline cartilage, is a key player in the osteoarthritis development. Therefore, arthroscopically repair of the chondrolabral complex damage is the basis of an algorithm for arthroscopic treatment of "pincer" deformity (Fig. 26.7).

Labrum width is an important feature for the decision-making process in the surgical treatment. According to literature, there is a minimum labral width of about 5 mm for normal labrum function. Furthermore, "pincer" impingement with ossified labrum are not always able to be repaired and are tended to develop progressive joint degeneration. The aim is to resume normal chondrolabral complex function with free range of motion. Restoring acetabular normal anatomy should prevent cartilage delamination and joint degeneration.

Technical tips should include rim trimming with a 4.5–5 mm burr with or without previous labrum taking down to expose acetabular bone overcoverage (Fig. 26.7). Frequently, the labrum has not to be completely taken down to remove pincer deformity in order to keep chondrolabral complex intact. Following pincer deformity removal, impingement-free range of motion should be tested and labral anatomical position should be restored using anchors and sutures. When massive labral damage appears, only labral resection or labral reconstruction should be performed.

Contraindication of arthroscopic treatment of chondrolabral complex lesions should be established in case of global pincer deformity (more than 50% of acetabular clockwise) that requires deep inferior-anterior or posterior bone resections and labral repair. In this special situation, open surgical approach might still have to be considered.

26.3 Labral Lesions: When to Repair or Graft?

26.3.1 Labral Anatomy

The acetabular labrum is a fibrocartilaginous structure at the bony margin of the acetabulum. The capsular side of the labrum is thicker and is composed

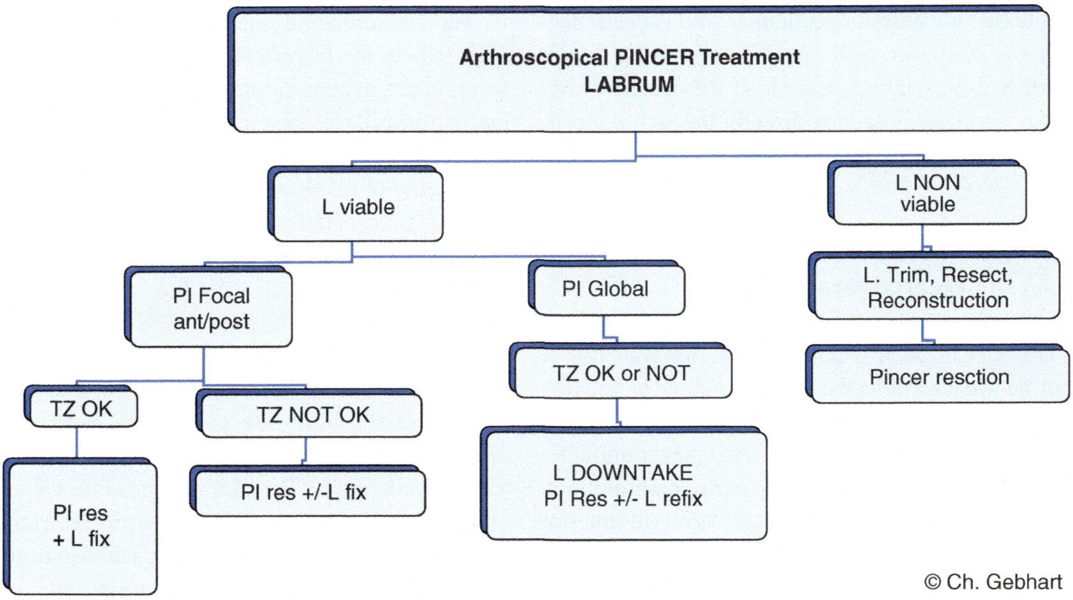

Fig. 26.7 Algorithm of arthroscopic treatment of pincer deformity. *L* Labrum, *PI* pincer impingement, *TZ* transition zone or chondrolabral complex, *PI res* pincer resection, *L fix* labral fixation, *Resect* partial labral resection, *L refix* labral refixation

of dense connective tissue, whereas the articular side of the labrum is composed of type II collagen fibrocartilage [43]. The cross section of the acetabular labrum is triangular in shape, and the osseous rim of the acetabulum penetrates into this triangle for attachment to the labrum (Fig. 26.8). The acetabular labrum has no intrinsic blood supply [44], and an anastomotic ring surrounding the capsular attachment of the labrum provides the blood supply to the labrum. The vascularity of the labrum is greater at the capsular portion attached to the osseous acetabulum, and therefore, the healing potential is greatest at the peripheral capsule–labral junction. An important factor to consider is whether a labral tear is repairable or should be resected or even grafted. The normal size of labrum is between 4 and 6 mm in width.

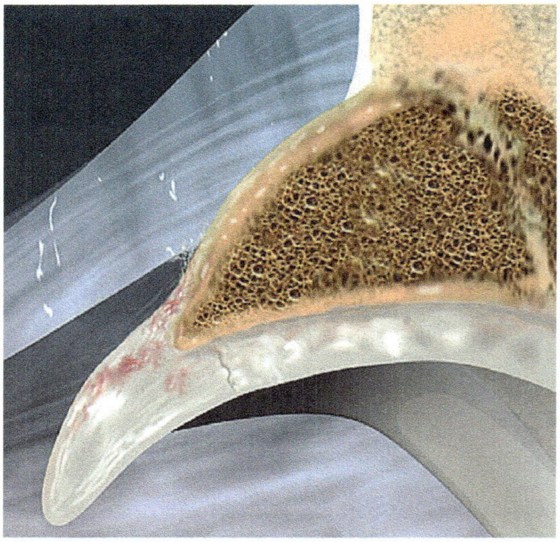

Fig. 26.8 Acetabular labrum anatomy (with kind permission from Marc Safran)

26.3.2 Labral Tear Classification

In 1996 Lage et al. came up with a labral tear classification and divided the tears into four distinct etiological and four distinct morphological groups [45] (Fig. 26.9).

A modification of this classification has been used by the Danish Hip Arthroscopy Registry since 2012, and it divides the labral tears and damage into five subgroups [46] (Table 26.2).

In younger patients, the most common type of labral tear is a longitudinal peripheral tear along

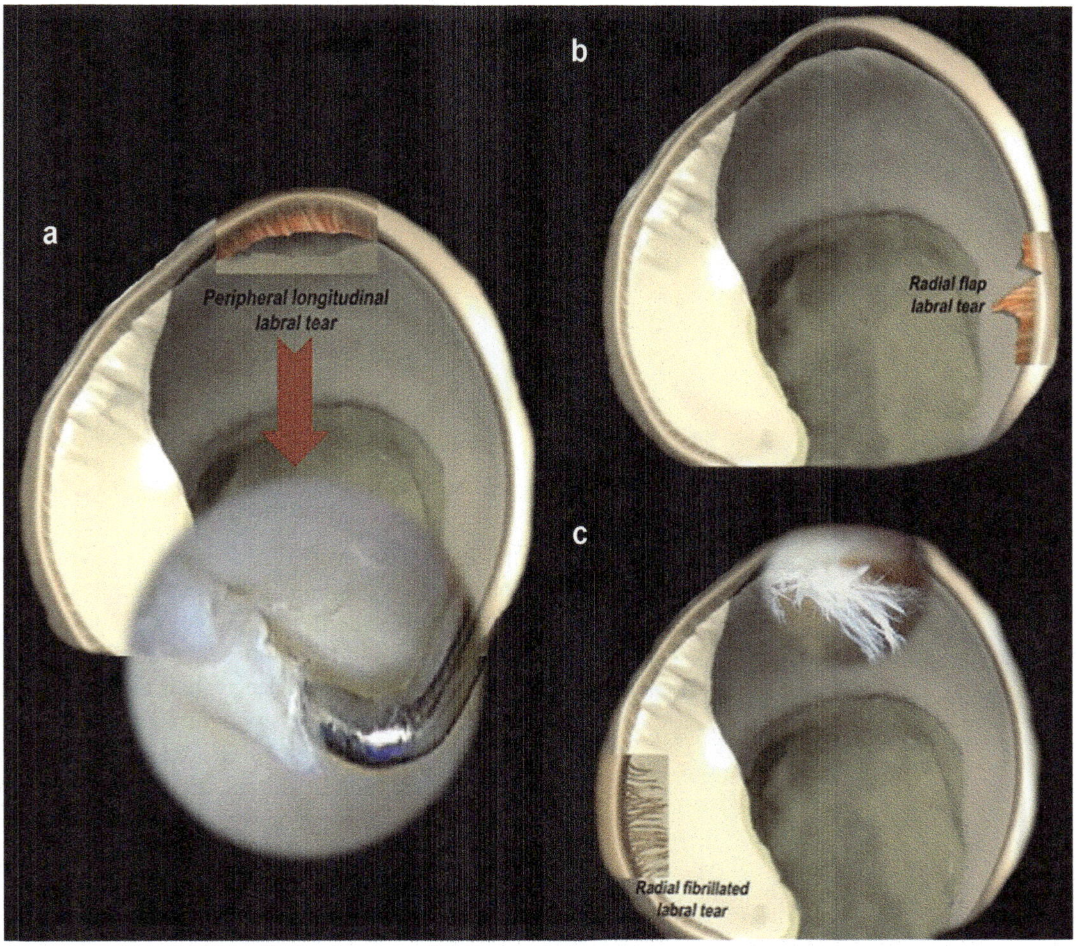

Fig. 26.9 Labral tear types from Lage classification: (**a**) Peripheral longitudinal labral tear, (**b**) Radial flap labral tear and (**c**) Radial fibrillated labral tear

Table 26.2 Labral tear and damage types (Danish Hip Arthroscopy Registry)

1	Radial fibrillated tear at the free margin of the labrum
2	Longitudinal peripheral tear, along the acetabular insertion of the labrum
3	Bucket-handle-type tear
4	Degenerative-type tear
5	Ossification of labrum

the acetabular insertion of the labrum (Fig. 26.10), whereas in older patients, the labral tears tend to become more degenerative with fatty infiltration (Fig. 26.11) or calcified labrum (Fig. 26.12).

Patients with developmental dysplasia of the hip (DDH) very often have a very large and hypertrophic labrum as it functions as a second-

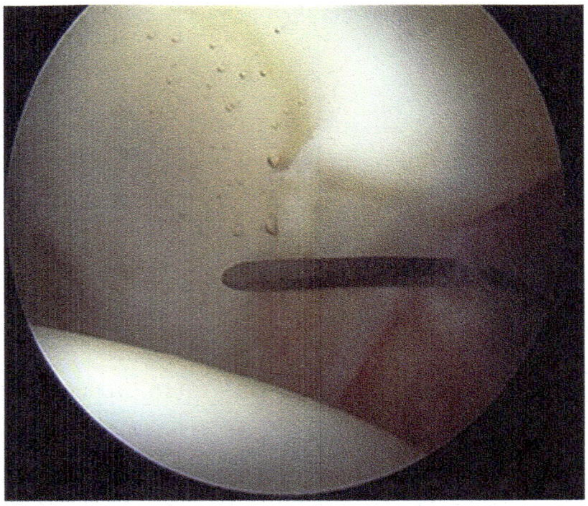

Fig. 26.10 Longitudinal peripheral tear (younger patients)

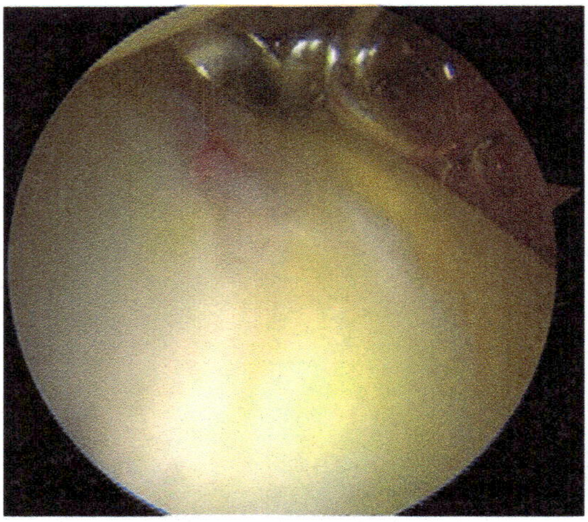

Fig. 26.11 Fatty degeneration in the labral substance and even ossification of the labral tissue is seen (older patients)

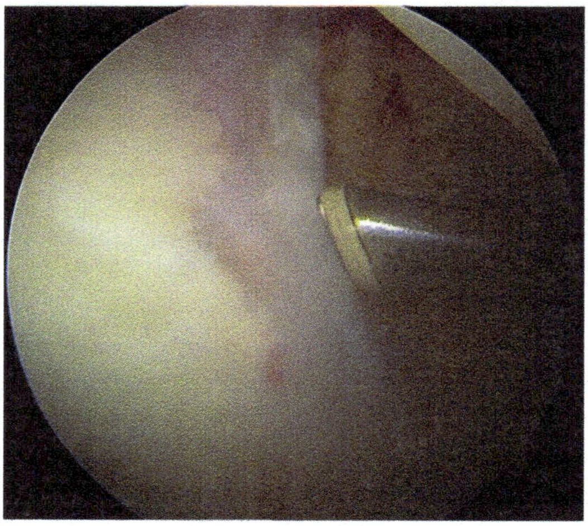

Fig. 26.12 Ossified labrum (older patients)

ary stabilizer of the hip joint, because of the undercoverage of the femoral head (Fig. 26.13).

26.3.3 Diagnosis and Preoperative Evaluations

Patients with labral tears very often present with groin pain, and most patients have a positive FADIR (Flexion-Adduction-Internal-Rotation) test. Sometimes they present with clicking and catching of the hip joint and pain on especially internal rotation. In any standard screening

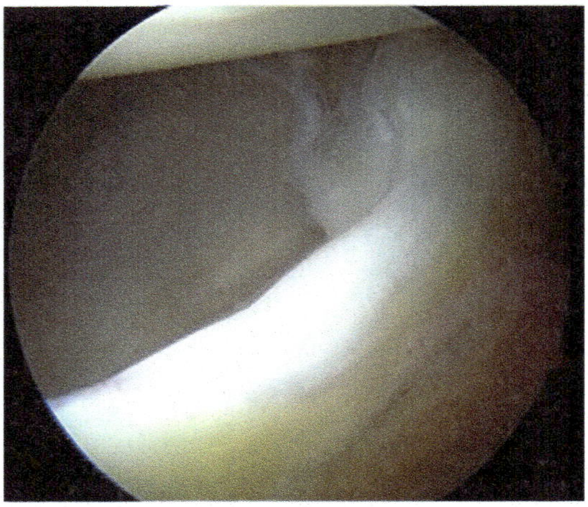

Fig. 26.13 Hypertrophic labrum with large tear

program, a standing AP-pelvis X-ray is recommended to diagnose possible osteoarthritis, femoroacetabular impingement (FAI) or hip dysplasia (DDH). Sometimes a partially or fully ossified rim can be seen, which means that the labrum might be ossified and non-repairable. MRI (3 T) or an MRI-arthrogram is commonly used for diagnosing labral tears and here the classification by Czerny is very useful [47].

26.3.4 Surgical Tips and Tricks

In most cases of femoroacetabular impingement, the symptomatic patients will have a labral tear at the time of surgery, and most of these patients will have concomitant injuries to the cartilage and some also to the ligamentum teres. Cartilage lesions can range from minor fibrillations (grade I) to full-thickness (grade IV) lesions with cartilage defect. The labral tears in association with pincer-type FAI are more likely to be Czerny type IIA (Fig. 26.14), whereas the cam or mixed-type lesions are more likely to be Czerny type IIIA (Fig. 26.15).

But there is a mix of types and extension of lesions depending on the severity of the FAI. In the more degenerate-type lesions, paralabral cysts are seen quite commonly. Nowadays most FAI patients are treated arthroscopically, and in order to be able to treat the labral tears and repair them, it is essential to debride the perilabral

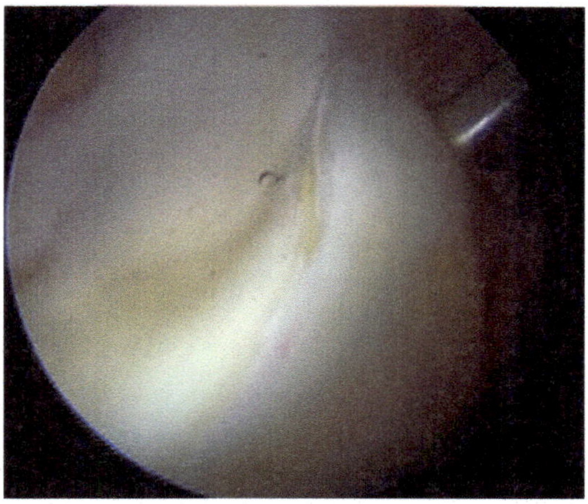

Fig. 26.14 Labral damage Czerny type IIA (frequently seen in "pincer" type)

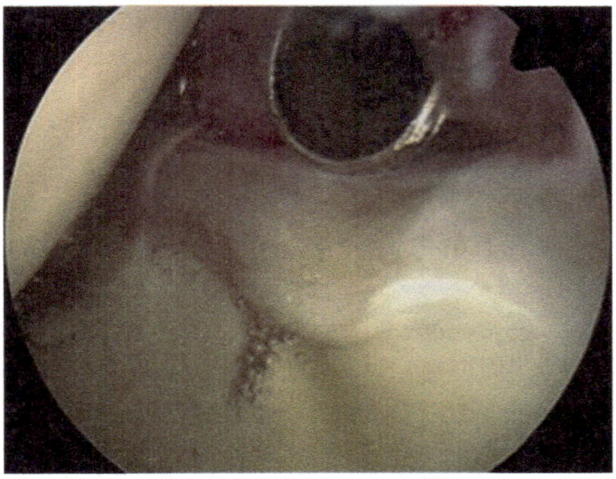

Fig. 26.15 Labral tear Czerny type IIIA (frequently seen in "mixed" type)

sulcus. This area is the sulcus between the capsule and the labrum on the capsular side. Some authors prefer to use a synovial resector/shaver blade, while others use a radiofrequency ablator to remove synovial tissue in order to expose the pincer deformity. The bony deformity can then be removed with a motorized burr and the labrum can be refixated using bone anchors or debrided if it is too degenerated.

Labral reconstruction with either autografts or allografts is used to reconstruct or augment poor labral tissue. A systematic review highlights the patients who are candidates for labral reconstruction, and they are young, active individuals with an irreparable or degenerative labrum, prior labral resection, and a minimum of 2 mm of joint space [46]. The reconstruction is done when the labral damage is too severe or the tissue itself is too large or degenerative (>10 mm) or too small or diminutive (<3 mm) [48]. The labral reconstruction is a technically demanding procedure, and various techniques have been described [46, 49, 50]. Labral reconstruction should only be performed in high-volume centers and by experienced hip surgeons.

26.3.5 Outcomes

There is a scarcity in the literature of high-level publications regarding labral debridement versus labral repair and clinical outcome. Most relevant literature is based on level III case reports, and a systematic review from 2016 by Forster-Horvath et al. illustrates that [51]. The conclusion in the systematic review was that clinical outcomes after labral debridement/segmental resection versus labral reconstruction were found to be comparable. Regarding labral reconstructions, both with autografts or allografts, only short-term outcomes are available, and there remains a paucity of literature supporting clinical justification for labral reconstruction. A systematic review supports the use of labral reconstruction as a viable treatment option for advanced labral pathology and with equivalent clinical efficacy to debridement [51].

26.4 Update on Chondral Repair Techniques in Hip Arthroscopy

Cartilage injuries in the hip commonly occur as a result of femoroacetabular impingement (FAI), trauma, developmental dysplasia, slipped capital femoral epiphysis, and osteonecrosis to name a few. FAI is a condition described in the 1990s by Ganz et al., which was postulated to cause arthritis in the hip [52]. Increasingly femoroacetabular impingement (FAI) is found to be associated with cartilage damage with up to 67% having acetabular cartilage lesions and 90% having labral tears, as described by Nepple [53]. The common theme in FAI mechanism is the abnormal contact between bony surfaces and the acetabular labrum. This impaction predisposes to labral and cartilage fissuring and delamination [54]. In the last couple of decades, there has been a great progress in hip arthroscopy alongside developments in imaging techniques, especially high-resolution MRI scanning. This has aided early identification and in turn progression of treatment strategies [53].

26.4.1 Articular Cartilage Structure and Healing

Articular cartilage has poor healing potential due to its avascularity and the scarcity of chondrocytes [55]. However, when there is an injury to the subchondral bone, multipotent stem cells are released from the bone marrow to fill the defect that promotes the formation of fibrocartilage [55]. This newly introduced fibrocartilage, however, has an inferior mechanical profile when compared to hyaline cartilage [55, 56]; hence, various repair techniques have been developed to try to create hyaline or hyaline-like cartilage at the site of the injury.

26.4.2 Cartilage Repair Techniques

The majority of cartilage repair techniques have been described in the knee joint, in part because it is the most widely arthroscoped joint, and their outcomes have been extrapolated and used in other joints. However, in the hip, the use of cartilage repair techniques is limited and can be broadly divided into four types (Table 26.3).

Table 26.3 Different cartilage repair techniques

Type of procedure	Repair technique
Cartilage palliation	Debridement chondroplasty
Cartilage repair	Direct cartilage suture repair Fibrin adhesive
Cartilage regeneration	Microfracture Autologous chondrocyte implantation Matrix-associated chondrocyte implantation Autologous matrix-induced chondrogenesis Osteochondral autograft transplantation (mosaicplasty) Osteochondral allograft transplantation
Biological approaches	Intra-articular BM-MSC injection

26.4.3 Cartilage Palliation: Symptomatic Treatment

Debridement is the main technique used for cartilage palliation. Chondral defects lead to an abnormal biomechanical environment encompassing the opposing cartilage surfaces precipitating symptoms of increased matrix metalloproteinase production. The aim of the debridement is to remove all unstable cartilage up to the calcified layer to form a new layer. Hubbard et al. [57] produced results showing that excising the damaged cartilage in the knee led to the improvement of symptoms for 5 years. Notably, however, although debridement is useful in superficial cartilage defects, the results gradually deteriorated over a 5-year period. A pilot study in 2012 demonstrated that debridement carried out after hip arthroscopy was not better than autologous chondrocyte transplantation (ACT). In a cohort of patients presenting with posttraumatic hip chondral injury of grade 3 or 4 according to the Outerbridge classification, with the cartilage defect measuring at least 2 cm^2 [58], Harris hip scores (HHS) were significantly better postoperatively in those who underwent ACT than those who received debridement alone (Fig. 26.16).

26.4.4 Cartilage Repair

26.4.4.1 Direct Cartilage Suture Repair

In the case of a full-thickness isolated chondral flap, direct repair of the chondral flap has been described with excellent outcomes [59]. Full-thickness flaps are at risk of complete detachment but, if picked up early, may be amenable to

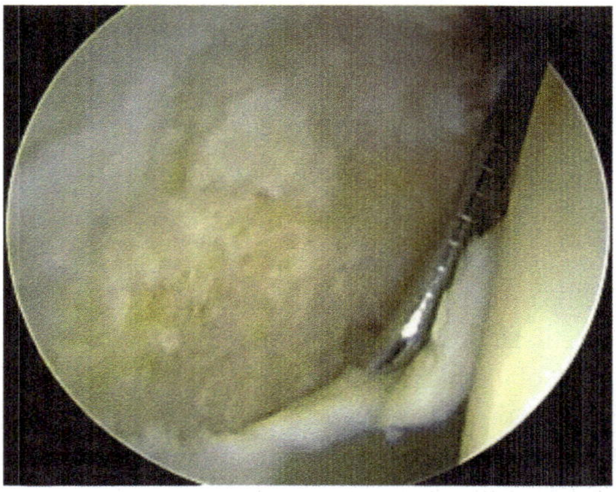

Fig. 26.16 Unstable flap in a grade IV cartilage lesion

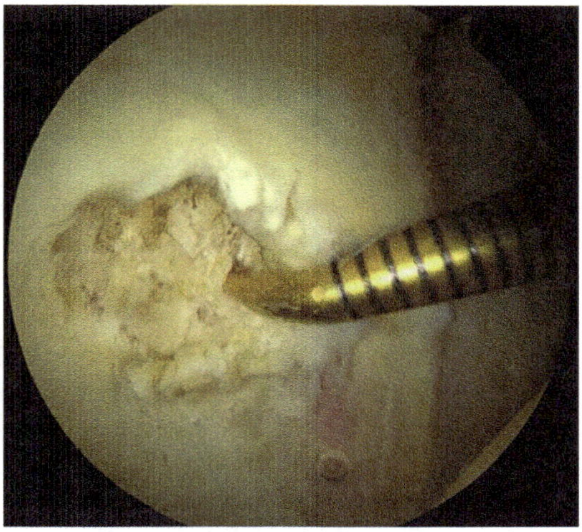

Fig. 26.17 Cartilage microfracture technique in a 3 cm^2 cartilage lesion

repair with sutures [60]. Sekiya et al. reported the case of a 17-year-old male with a full-thickness chondral flap that was repaired following a microfracture procedure underneath the cartilage flap in order to generate some mesenchymal stem cells (MSCs) into the defect [59].

26.4.4.2 Fibrin Adhesive

Chondral flaps develop after delamination of the cartilage from the subchondral bone [61]. Fibrin glue has been used to stick down the delaminated cartilage to avoid debriding the flap and thus preserves the source of chondrocytes. Tzaveas reported a significant improvement in modified HHS in 19 patients treated with fibrin glue [62] as well as excellent results in 40 out of 43 patients treated with fibrin glue repair. The remaining three patients had to undergo further arthroscopic procedures for persisting symptoms [63].

26.4.5 Cartilage Regeneration

26.4.5.1 Microfracture

A technique introduced by Richard Steadman in 1990s combines total debridement of all unstable cartilage in the defect with making multiple holes in the defect up to the subchondral bone, allowing for filling in the defect by multipotent bone marrow stem cells which subsequently differentiate to form cartilage. Microfracture has been shown to provide medium- to long-term symptomatic improvement [64–66] and, in a systematic review, demonstrated good to excellent clinical outcomes in active patients with small (<2–4 cm^2) defects at short-term follow-up [67]. Microfracture is a commonly performed procedure without any donor side morbidity with a low cost, but the regeneration of hyaline cartilage post-procedure is not a certainty and is dependent on several variables [68], for instance, age, the chondrogenic potential of the mesenchymal cells decreases with age [69]. Philippon and Karthikeyan have reported satisfactory outcomes of hip microfracture [70, 71], and a study by Zaltz and Leunig has supported the use of microfracture for hip chondral defects with patients returning to the preoperative functional level [72]. In their study, at the latest follow-up, there was no evidence of narrowing of the joint space or asymmetry on radiographic examination (Fig. 26.17).

26.4.5.2 Autologous Chondrocyte Implantation

In 1994, Britberg et al. described the use of autologous cultured chondrocytes in the treatment of full-thickness cartilage defects in the knee with good mid-term results. Since then, there have been numerous studies showing the efficacy of autologous chondrocyte transplantation (ACT) in the treatment of cartilage defects in the knee but very few studies on its efficacy for hip cartilage defects [73]. Pestka et al. reported good outcomes with the use of ACT after failure of microfracture for well-contained chondral defects between 2 and 10 cm^2 [74]. Furthermore, Oleander and Minas revealed a favorable outcome following ACT in a 19-year-old female for a hip chondral defect of 10 cm^2. Postoperative MRI in this patient demonstrated that the defect had repaired, and joint space was maintained. Also, as detailed above, Fontana et al. have purported that ACT may be more effective in posttraumatic chondral injuries [58].

26.4.5.3 Matrix-Associated Chondrocyte Implantation (MACI)

MACI is an advancement of ACT wherein the cultured chondrocytes are inserted into and supported by absorbable scaffolds to regenerate the cartilage. Associated donor site morbidity is a possible consequence, but unlike ACT, MACI requires an open surgical dislocation of the hip in the second stage of the procedure, which is not a procedure without complications. Mancini and Fontana compared the results of autologous matrix-induced chondrogenesis (AMIC) and MACI for all cartilage defects between 2 and 4 cm^2 and found that both the groups of patients continued to improve after 2 years [75]. They did not find any statistical difference between these two groups.

26.4.5.4 Autologous Matrix-Induced Chondrogenesis (AMIC)

This is a technique for well-contained chondral defects, which utilizes the aforementioned microfracture technique following debridement of the cartilage defect to stable edges. The defect is then covered with a Chondro-Gide matrix patch, made up of protein collagen that helps to stabilize the fibrin clot in the defect with a view to forming new cartilage. The advantage is that it can be performed as a one-stage procedure with no donor site morbidity. Several authors have shown good results with AMIC in the short to medium term for chondral defects of Outerbridge grade 3 and 4 [72, 76–78]. In addition, Fontana, in a comparative study between microfracture and AMIC techniques, showed that the AMIC group remained stable after 4 years when compared to microfracture [76].

26.4.5.5 Osteochondral Autograft Transplantation (Mosaicplasty)

This technique aims to transplant healthy hyaline cartilage from non-weight-bearing areas to the site of cartilage defect. Due to the autologous nature of this procedure, the donor sites are limited to the inferior aspect of femoral head, femoral head–neck junction, and periphery of femoral trochlea [69]. This has the advantages of transferring hyaline cartilage to the defect, better integration of autograft and no risk of disease transmission. However, there is a limit to the donor sites, and it carries a risk of donor site morbidity [69]. Among several case reports showing good results with this procedure, Girard et al. have reported significantly improved clinical outcomes following mosaicplasty in ten patients at 29 months follow-up [79].

26.4.5.6 Osteochondral Allograft Transplantation

Mosaicplasty is useful in providing a functional hyaline cartilage for immediate transfer to the defect. However, there are limitations in autograft mosaicplasty. To overcome these, allograft tissues have been used with the ability to obtain a larger area of tissue to cover larger cartilage defects and also avoid unnecessary donor site morbidity [69]. Krych et al. reported two cases that underwent allograft mosaicplasty for acetabular chondral defects with successful incorporation of the allograft as demonstrated on the MRI scan at 18 months. These cases also exhibited hip outcome scores of 100 points each at 2 years [80].

26.4.6 Biological Approaches

Intra-articular BM-MSC injection is gaining importance due to its potential to differentiate into different tissues, including cartilage, depending on specific signals released by the injury site. As well as several animal studies reporting good outcomes, a case series of 29 patients, who underwent hip arthroscopy for focal chondral defects and three intra-articular injections of bone marrow MSCs at 4–6 week intervals, showed good clinical outcomes and VAS scores [81].

26.4.7 Conclusion

Although there are many different cartilage restoration techniques available, current best evidence does not support any one surgical technique as a superior method for treating cartilage injuries in the hip. While microfracture, AMIC and mosaicplasty are well-reported techniques with reasonable short-term outcomes, the future perhaps holds a move toward biological approaches to treat these defects.

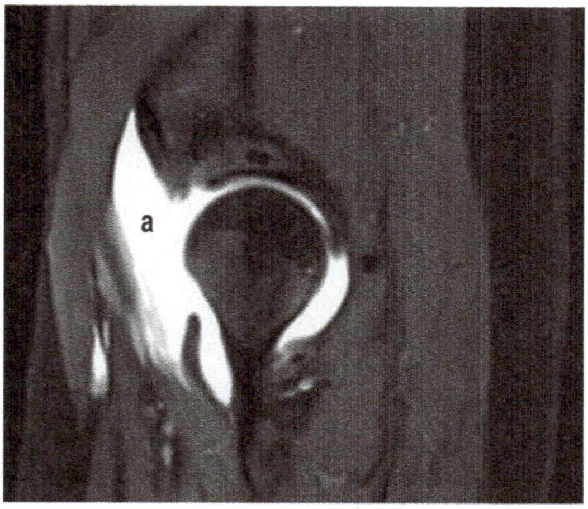

Fig. 26.18 MRI of a healthy 30-year-old female who experienced an anterior hip dislocation after hip arthroscopy with an unrepaired interportal capsulotomy. The MRI shows significant contrast extravasation through a gross capsular defect (a) (Image reproduced with permission from Yeung et al. [83])

26.5 Hip Instability: Soft Tissue Management with Hip Arthroscopy

Native hip instability after hip arthroscopy is a rare but devastating complication. The severity of instability can vary from micro-instability with vague symptoms to hip dislocations. One study found that 3.0% of patients developed symptoms of instability after hip arthroscopy requiring revision surgery. A systematic review of over 6000 hip arthroscopy patients found a 0.07% rate of gross hip instability (i.e., hip dislocations) [82]. Female gender, hip dysplasia, generalized ligamentous laxity, and connective tissue disorders are patient risk factors for hip instability after hip arthroscopy [83]. Surgical factors that potentially cause instability include over-resection of the acetabular rim, unrepaired capsulotomy, and excessive labral resection [84].

26.5.1 Imaging Evaluation

Although AP radiographs will typically be normal appearing, evidence of acetabular dysplasia, such as a decreased center-edge angle (CEA), may be present. False profile views may show widening of the posterior joint space, eccentric positioning of the femoral head, or anterior under coverage [85]. Evaluation with CT may be useful, particularly in the setting of suspected acetabular dysplasia. Magnetic resonance imaging (MRI) may show subtle capsular deficiencies or a clear defect in the iliofemoral ligament (Fig. 26.18).

26.5.2 Role of Capsular Management

One systematic review found that 78% of patients who experienced gross instability after hip arthroscopy had an unrepaired capsulotomy [83].

26.5.2.1 Capsulotomy in Hip Arthroscopy

It can be useful to improve access to the joint, allow working space for instrumentation, and improve visualization. The most commonly performed capsulotomy techniques are the interportal capsulotomy and T-capsulotomy. An interportal capsulotomy involves a transverse incision in the capsule running parallel to the labrum which connects the anterior (or modified anterior) and anterolateral portals. A

T-capsulotomy involves a second incision joining perpendicular to the interportal capsulotomy in line with the femoral neck (Fig. 26.19). In many cases, the interportal capsulotomy provides sufficient access to the joint for central compartment diagnosis and treatment. The T-capsulotomy allows improved access to the peripheral compartment and better visualization of the head–neck junction during CAM resection [87]. Minimally invasive capsulotomies and puncture capsulotomies that cause minimal disruption of the capsule have also been described [88, 89].

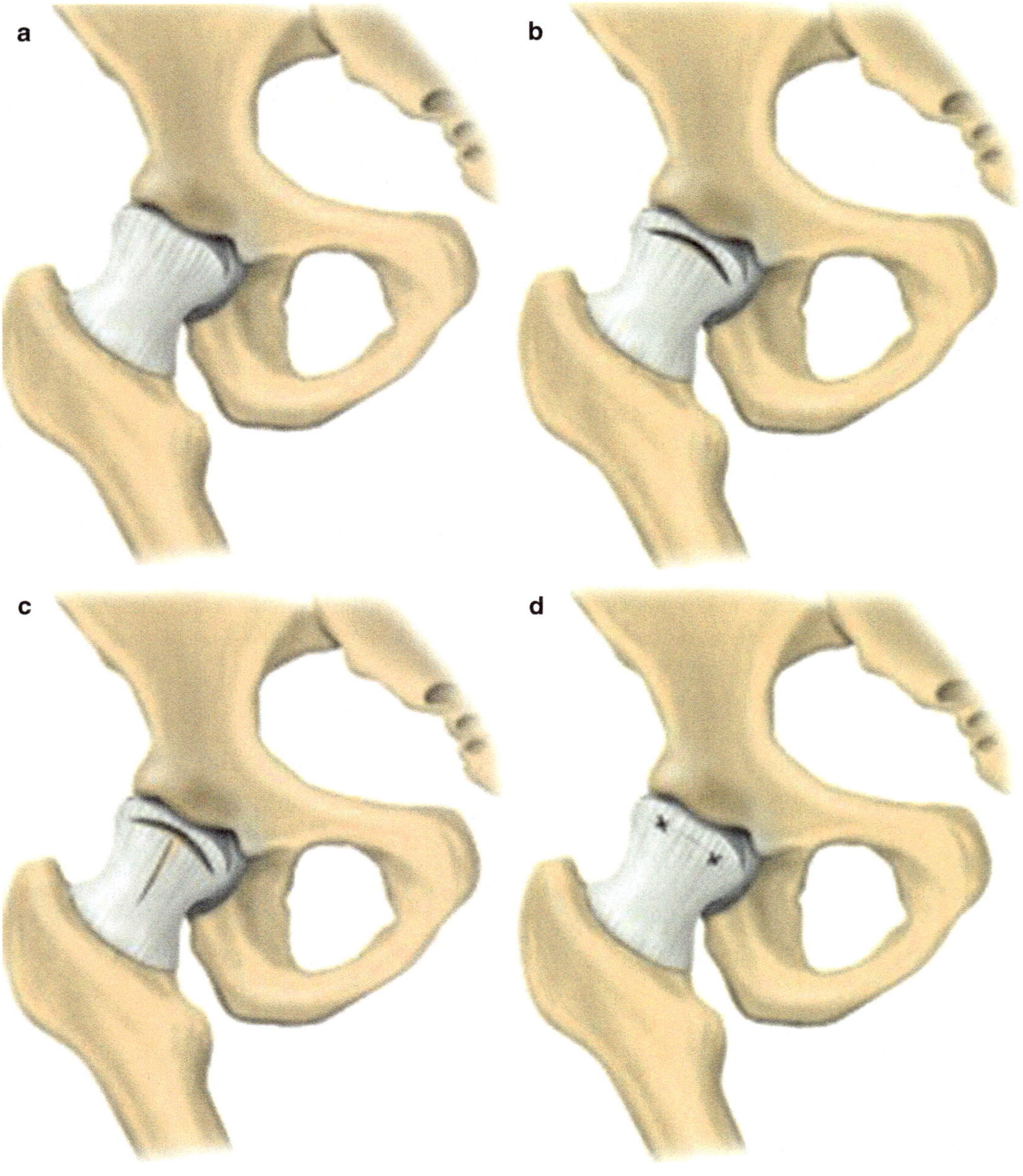

Fig. 26.19 Illustration of the commonly used capsulotomy and capsular repair techniques. (**a**) Normal hip joint; (**b**) Interportal capsulotomy; (**c**) T-capsulotomy; (**d**) Repaired interportal capsulotomy; (**e**) Partially repaired T-capsulotomy; (**f**) Completely repaired T-capsulotomy (Image reproduced with permission from Ekhtiari et al. [86]. Original image by Pontus Andersson)

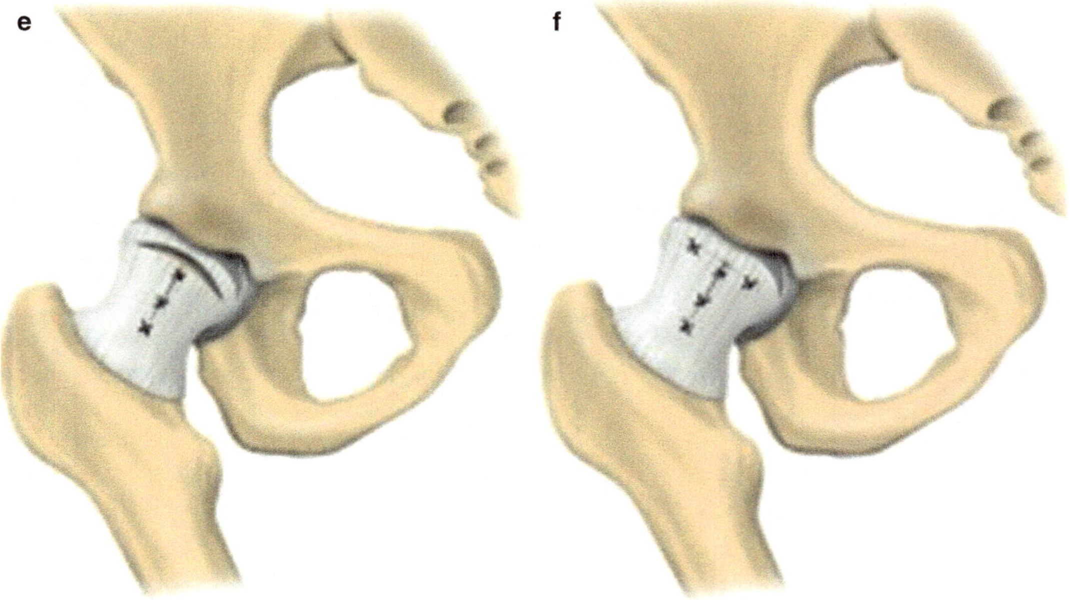

Fig. 26.19 (continued)

The hip capsule represents an important soft tissue stabilizer. The capsule is made up of three ligaments (iliofemoral, pubofemoral, and ischiofemoral) and the zona orbicularis [90]. The iliofemoral ligament, the thickest portion of the capsule, is partially transected during an interportal or T-capsulotomy [90]. Cadaveric studies have found that capsulotomies result in increased joint mobility. Larger capsulotomies and T-capsulotomies result in larger increases in rotation [91]. Cadaveric studies have also shown that hip rotation can be restored to normal ranges through appropriate capsular repair [91].

26.5.2.2 Capsule Closure

Options for post-capsulotomy capsular management include leaving the capsulotomy unrepaired, partial closure (closing only one of the perpendicular limbs in a T-capsulotomy), complete closure, or capsular plication. One survey of high-volume hip arthroscopists found that all respondents routinely performed capsulotomies but that 78% only selectively performed capsular repairs [92]. Surgeons stated that they base their decision on whether to perform a capsular repair on factors including the presence of preoperative stiffness or instability and intraoperative findings. Capsular plication may be preferred over capsular repair in patients with connective tissue disorders such as Ehlers–Danlos syndrome [93]. The thickness of the capsule can be measured using MRI and may be helpful in guiding capsular management. Patients with thicker capsules are known to have less laxity in their hip compared to patients with thinner capsules [94]. Table 26.4 summarizes the common indications and contraindications for capsular closure.

Belemmi et al. compared two groups of patients undergoing hip arthroscopy that had a T-capsulotomy [86]. One group had their capsulotomy repaired, whereas the other group did not. No significant difference in functional outcome scores was found between the groups. In contrast, another study found a significantly greater improvement in the Sport Specific Hip Outcome Score in patients with a T-capsulotomy treated with complete capsular repair versus those treated with partial repair [95]. Multiple studies report that capsular repair in revision hip arthroscopy was a positive predictor of improved outcomes [96, 97]. This finding is likely explained by the fact that a high percentage of patients undergoing

Table 26.4 Indications and contraindications for capsular closure

Indications	Contraindications
Female	Preoperative stiffness
Generalized hyperlaxity	Adhesive capsulitis
Connective tissue disorders	Inflammatory arthritis
Gross instability	Capsular hypertrophy and thickening
Micro-instability	
Acetabular dysplasia	
Revision surgery	
Impaired neuromuscular function	
Concern for excessive rim resection	
Concern for excessive labral resection	
Ligamentum teres tear	

revision surgery for reasons other than residual impingement are known to have capsular defects [98]. Patients who experience instability after hip arthroscopy can generally be treated with revision hip arthroscopy for capsular repair with positive outcomes. In cases of hip dislocation after hip arthroscopy, patients can be treated with urgent closed reduction prior to capsular repair. However, in patients with persistent hip instability after arthroscopic repair, generalized ligamentous laxity, connective tissue disorders, or large capsule-ligamentous defects, an open capsular reconstruction may be necessary [99, 100].

26.5.3 Conclusions

Most patients with hip instability after hip arthroscopy have had an unrepaired capsulotomy. However, currently the literature has not shown that capsular repair results in significantly improved functional outcomes compared to no capsular repair. Therefore, it remains unclear if routine capsular repair is indicated in primary surgery. Capsular repair should be strongly considered in those with risk factors for instability including females, acetabular dysplasia, generalized ligamentous laxity, and connective tissue disorders. In patients undergoing revision surgery, capsular repair is a positive predictor of an improved outcome and should be performed if there is any concern for micro-instability contributing to the patient's symptoms.

26.6 Deep Gluteal Pain Syndrome (DGS) and Role of Hip Arthroscopy

26.6.1 Concept and Definition

Deep gluteal syndrome describes the presence of pain in the subgluteal space caused from non-discogenic and extrapelvic entrapment of the sciatic nerve. The subgluteal space is the cellular and fatty tissue located between the middle and deep gluteal aponeurosis layers [101, 102].

26.6.2 Etiology

Multiple orthopedic and non-orthopedic conditions may manifest as a DGS [103–105]. Although deep gluteal syndrome and piriformis syndrome were considered synonymous in the past, it has since become clear that piriformis syndrome is just one of many different causes that may be responsible for sciatic nerve entrapment causing pain in the buttock. In fact, in only one-fourth of the patients in a systematic review was the piriformis found to be causing entrapment of the sciatic nerve intraoperatively [106].

26.6.2.1 Fibrous and Fibro-Vascular Bands

Diminished or absent sciatic mobility during hip and knee movements due to these bands is the precipitating cause of sciatic neuropathy (ischemic neuropathy) [107]. From the point of view of its macroscopic structure, there are three primary types of bands: fibro-vascular bands, pure fibrous bands, and pure vascular bands [108]. Depending on the pathogenic mechanism, bands can be classified as follows:

1. Compressive or bridge-type bands (type 1), which limit the movement compressing the

nerve from anterior to posterior (type 1A) or from posterior to anterior (type 1B).

2. Adhesive bands or horse-strap bands (type 2), which bind strongly to the sciatic nerve structure, anchoring it in a single direction and not allowing it to perform its normal excursion during hip movements. These bands can be attached to the sciatic nerve laterally from the major trochanter (type 2A) or medially from the sacro-tuberous ligament (type 2B).
3. Bands anchored to the sciatic nerve with undefined distribution (type 3). These kinds of bands with an erratic distribution are characterized by anchoring the nerve in multiple directions.

26.6.2.2 Piriformis Syndrome

Hypertrophy of the Piriformis Muscle

Asymmetry associated with sciatic nerve hyperintensity at the sciatic notch revealed a specificity of 93% and sensitivity of 64% in patients with piriformis syndrome distinct from that which had no similar symptoms [109].

Dynamic Sciatic Nerve Entrapment by the Piriformis Muscle

Often the only finding at imaging that can be shown is nerve signal hyperintensity in edema-sensitive sequences.

Anomalous Course of the Sciatic Nerve (Anatomical Variations)

Six categories of anatomic variations of the relationship between the piriformis muscle and sciatic nerve were originally reported in 1938 by Beaton and Anson. The anomaly itself may not always be the etiology of DGS symptoms as some asymptomatic patients present these variations, and some symptomatic patients do not. A subsequent event such as any etiology reported in this chapter or prolonged sitting, direct trauma to the gluteal region, prolonged stretching, overuse, pelvic/spinal instability or orthopedic conditions may then precipitate sciatic nerve neuropathy [110].

26.6.2.3 Gemelli-Obturator Internus Syndrome

Dynamic compression of the sciatic nerve caused by a stretched or altered dynamic of the obturator internus muscle should be included as a possible diagnosis for DGS. As the sciatic nerve passes under the belly of the piriformis and over the superior gemelli/obturator internus, a scissor-like effect between the two muscles can be the source of entrapment.

26.6.2.4 Quadratus Femoris and Ischiofemoral Pathology

Ischiofemoral impingement syndrome (IFI) is an under-recognized form of atypical, extra-articular hip impingement defined by hip pain related to narrowing of the space between the ischial tuberosity and the femur. Characteristic findings are a decreased ischiofemoral space compared to healthy controls (the ischiofemoral space measures 23 ± 8 mm and femoral space 12 ± 4 mm) and altered signals from the quadratus femoris muscle, which results in edema, muscular rupture, or atrophy [111]. The ischiofemoral space should be understood as a gait-related dynamic area with several contributing and predisposing factors [112] (Table 26.5).

Table 26.5 Potential etiologies and predisposing factors of IFI according to the pathophysiological mechanisms [112]

Primary or congenital (orthopedic disorders)	Secondary or acquired
Congenital posteromedial femoral position	Functional disorders (hip instability, pelvic/spinal instability, abductor/adductor imbalance)
Prominence of the lesser trochanter	Traumatic, overuse, extreme motion
Abnormal femoral antitorsion	Iatrogenic causes
Coxa breva	Tumors
Variations of the pelvic bony anatomy	Other etiologies (genu valgum, leg discrepancy, pronated foot)
Coxa Valga	Ischial tuberosity enthesopathies
Larger cross section of the femur	

26.6.2.5 Hamstring Conditions

The sciatic nerve can be affected by a wide spectrum of hamstring origin enthesopathies appearing either isolated or in combination: partial/complete hamstring strain (acute, recurrent, or chronic), tendon detachment avulsion fractures (acute or chronic/non-united), apophysitis, non-united apophysis, proximal tendinopathy, calcifying tendinosis, and contusions result in entrapment during hip motion (ischial tunnel syndrome) [110].

26.6.3 Clinical Examination and Symptoms

26.6.3.1 Deep Gluteal Syndrome/Sciatic Nerve Entrapment: Pain by Palpation at the Sciatic Notch

The active piriformis and seated piriformis stretch tests reveal higher sensitivity and specificity for the diagnosis of sciatic nerve entrapments than the other tests, especially when both are used in combination [107].

26.6.3.2 Ischiofemoral Impingement: Pain by Palpation Lateral to the Ischium

The specific physical examination test included the long-stride walking test and ischiofemoral impingement test [101, 110, 113].

26.6.3.3 Hamstring Conditions: Pain by Palpation Lateral and/or Posterior to the Ischium

Hamstring active test at 30° knee flexion in seated position (hip 90°) [114].

26.6.4 Imaging Evaluation

Plain radiography, ultrasound (US), computed tomography (CT), and magnetic resonance imaging (MRI) have all been used to assess posterior hip anatomy and pathologies [102]. Nerve stiffness associated with limb movements in the diagnosis of sciatic nerve entrapment in deep gluteal syndrome can give us crucial information about the degree of nerve entrapment.

26.6.5 Surgical Treatment: Endoscopic

The technique of endoscopic decompression of the sciatic nerve requires significant hip arthroscopy experience with familiarity with the gross and endoscopic anatomy of the subgluteal space [102, 115].

26.6.5.1 Position

Supine position in a traction table, standard preparation for hip arthroscopy, no traction, and 20° of contralateral tilt. Leg is abducted to about 15–20° in order to open the interval between the trochanter and the iliotibial band, and the leg is internally rotated 20–40° for the same reason. This procedure can also be done in the lateral decubitus position [116, 117].

26.6.5.2 Portals

(1) Standard portals redirected to the peritrochanteric space (anterolateral, anterior, and posterolateral portals) and (2) portals described to access the peritrochanteric space [118] (proximal anterolateral accessory portal, distal anterolateral accessory portal, peritrochanteric space portal, and auxiliary posterolateral portal). Auxiliary distal portals at the level of the lesser trochanter are crucial for the treatment of ischiofemoral impingement (IFI portals) [113] (Figs. 26.20 and 26.21).

26.6.5.3 Distal Dissection

Inspection of the sciatic nerve begins distal to the quadratus femoris, just above the gluteal sling. Inspect the ischial tunnel hamstring origin and sacrotuberous ligament, releasing any fibers from the sciatic nerve. Assess the lateral, medial, and posterior borders of the sciatic nerve to ensure the distal release is complete and identify the posterior cutaneous nerve.

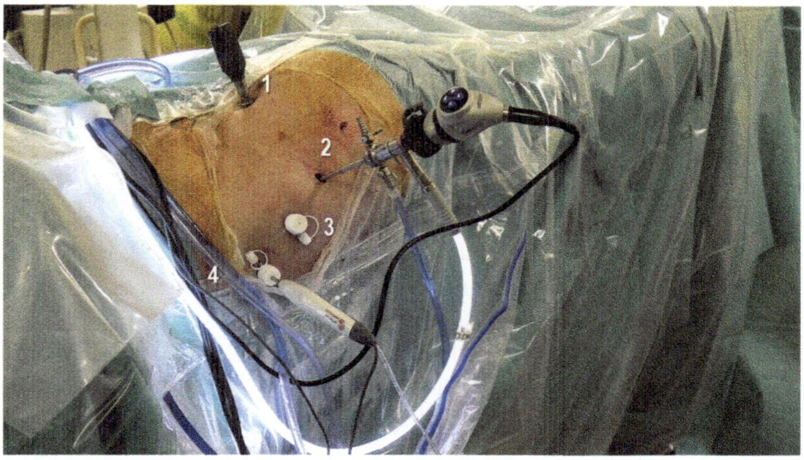

Fig. 26.20 Right gluteal region showing portal placement for subgluteal endoscopy. (1) Mid-anterior portal, (2) anterolateral distal portal, (3) posterolateral portal, and (4) auxiliary posterolateral portal

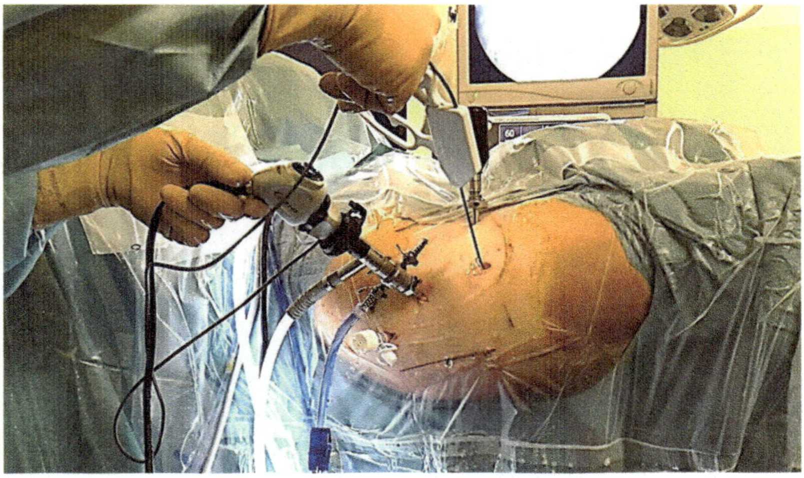

Fig. 26.21 Right gluteal region showing portal placement for ischiofemoral impingement decompression. Scope in the midanterior portal. Radiofrequency in the anterolateral distal portal. Cannula in the posterolateral portal. Rod in the posterior ischiofemoral proximal portal

26.6.5.4 Proximal Dissection

After the distal dissection, move proximal. When the piriformis tendon is identified, it should be possible to identify the tendons of the gemellus and obturator internus muscles. Constant attention must be paid to the branches of the inferior gluteal artery lying in proximity to the piriformis muscle. A rotatory shaver can be used to shave the distal border of the piriformis muscle to gain adequate access to the piriformis tendon. Finally probe the sciatic nerve up to the sciatic notch. The kinematic excursion of the sciatic nerve is then assessed with the leg in flexion with internal/external rotation and full extension with internal/external rotation.

26.6.5.5 Lesser Trochanter Approach for IFI Syndrome

Arthroscopic access to decompress the IFS, as an alternative to an open approach, has been recently described with high success rates because it managed to significantly improve clinical scores [113, 119–121]. Due to the location of the lesser trochanter (LT), the arthroscopic procedure can be approached either anteriorly or posteriorly and with partial or complete resection of the LT. The goal of surgery is to restore a normal distance, which may not require a complete resection of the lesser trochanter. We agree with other authors that the posterolateral transquadratus approach seems to be the most appropriate route [110, 113]. The anatomy of vascular structures suggests increased safety of posterior access to the lesser trochanter [122]. Another advantage of this approach is that allows simultaneous assessment of the sciatic nerve and hamstring repair if needed. Resection of the ischium could be done through this approach if necessary. The aim of the osteoplasty of the posterior one third of the lesser trochanter is to obtain a minimum IFS distance of 17 mm, leaving non-impingement bone and the iliopsoas insertion intact. Access to the lesser trochanter is achieved via a small window in the quadratus femoris muscle (Fig. 26.22).

26.6.6 Results

26.6.6.1 Deep Gluteal Syndrome Outcomes

Overall, 33 studies evaluating the surgical management (open and endoscopic) of deep gluteal syndrome were identified in the literature [106, 110, 123]. Outcomes were positive, with an improvement in pain at final follow-up.

26.6.6.2 Ischiofemoral Syndrome Outcomes

A systematic review by Nakano et al. found 17 relevant papers, with five studies reported on the

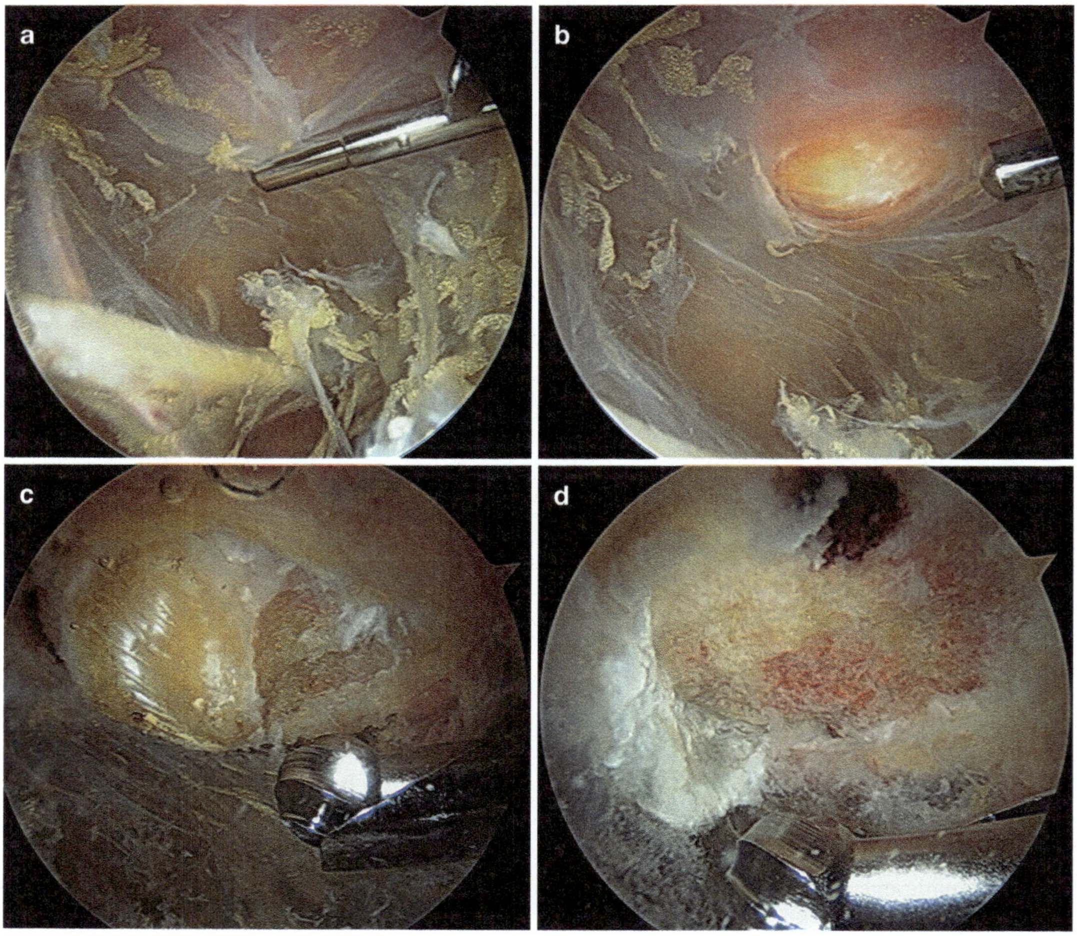

Fig. 26.22 Right hip. Endoscopic view showing ischiofemoral impingement decompression. Access to resection of the lesser trochanter through the posterolateral trans-quadratus approach. Identification of lesser trochanter (**a**, **b**) and posterior partial resection with a 4.5 mm burr (**c**, **d**)

use of endoscopic surgical management. All of them reported on partial or entire resection of the LT and good short- to medium-term outcomes without any neurological or vascular complication [124]. We have reviewed and evaluated our results for this publication, 14 patients (15 hips) (14 female) (9 right and 6 left) treated in our clinic for ischiofemoral impingement and endoscopic posterolateral trans-quadratus approach decompression of the lesser trochanter between November 2011 and April 2018. Mean age was 38 years (20–52 years). The mean modified Harris Hip Score increased from 58 points preoperatively to 92 points at the final follow-up. No complications or adverse effects were found.

References

1. Cohen SB, Huang R, Ciccotti MG, Dodson CC, Parvizi J. Treatment of femoroacetabular impingement in athletes using a mini-direct anterior approach. Am J Sports Med. 2012;40(7):1620–7. PubMed PMID: 22562788. Epub 2012/05/09.
2. Steppacher SD, Anwander H, Zurmuhle CA, Tannast M, Siebenrock KA. Eighty percent of patients with surgical hip dislocation for femoroacetabular impingement have a good clinical result without osteoarthritis progression at 10 years. Clin Orthop Relat Res. 2015;473(4):1333–41. PubMed PMID: 25367110. Pubmed Central PMCID: 4353536.
3. Bedi A, Kelly BT, Khanduja V. Arthroscopic hip preservation surgery: current concepts and perspective. Bone Joint J. 2013;95-B(1):10–9. PubMed PMID: 23307667. Epub 2013/01/12.
4. Bedi A, Chen N, Robertson W, Kelly BT. The management of labral tears and femoroacetabular impingement of the hip in the young, active patient. Arthroscopy. 2008;24(10):1135–45. PubMed PMID: 19028166. Epub 2008/11/26.
5. Ng VY, Arora N, Best TM, Pan X, Ellis TJ. Efficacy of surgery for femoroacetabular impingement: a systematic review. Am J Sports Med. 2010;38(11):2337–45. PubMed PMID: 20489213. Epub 2010/05/22.
6. Matsuda DK, Carlisle JC, Arthurs SC, Wierks CH, Philippon MJ. Comparative systematic review of the open dislocation, mini-open, and arthroscopic surgeries for femoroacetabular impingement. Arthroscopy. 2011;27(2):252–69. PubMed PMID: 21266276. Epub 2011/01/27.
7. Botser IB, Smith TW Jr, Nasser R, Domb BG. Open surgical dislocation versus arthroscopy for femoroacetabular impingement: a comparison of clinical outcomes. Arthroscopy. 2011;27(2):270–8. PubMed PMID: 21266277. Epub 2011/01/27.
8. Aoki SK, Beckmann JT, Wylie JD. Arthroscopic femoral osteochondroplasty for cam-type femoroacetabular impingement: the trough technique. Arthrosc Tech. 2016;5(4):e743–e9. PubMed PMID: 27709031.
9. Nogier A, Boyer T, Khan MT. Hip arthroscopy: less invasive technique. Arthrosc Tech. 2014;3(1):e101–6. PubMed PMID: 24749026. Pubmed Central PMCID: 3986488. Epub 2014/04/22.
10. Lee CB, Clark J. Fluoroscopic demonstration of femoroacetabular impingement during hip arthroscopy. Arthroscopy. 2011;27(7):994–1004. PubMed PMID: 21693351. Epub 2011/06/23.
11. Griffin DR, Dickenson EJ, O'Donnell J, Agricola R, Awan T, Beck M, et al. The Warwick agreement on femoroacetabular impingement syndrome (FAI syndrome): an international consensus statement. Br J Sports Med. 2016;50(19):1169–76. PubMed PMID: 27629403.
12. Haldane CE, Ekhtiari S, de Sa D, Simunovic N, Ayeni OR. Preoperative physical examination and imaging of femoroacetabular impingement prior to hip arthroscopy-a systematic review. J Hip Preserv Surg. 2017;4(3):201–13. PubMed PMID: 28948032. Pubmed Central PMCID: 5604278.
13. Nepple JJ, Martel JM, Kim YJ, Zaltz I, Clohisy JC. Do plain radiographs correlate with CT for imaging of cam-type femoroacetabular impingement? Clin Orthop Relat Res. 2012;470(12):3313–20. PubMed PMID: 22930210. Epub 2012/08/30.
14. Nho SJ, Beck EC. Editorial commentary: if you can't see it, you can't treat it: proper hip radiographic views are critical. Arthroscopy. 2019;35(6):1807–8. PubMed PMID: 31159965.
15. Hipfl C, Titz M, Chiari C, Schopf V, Kainberger F, Windhager R, et al. Detecting cam-type deformities on plain radiographs: what is the optimal lateral view? Arch Orthop Trauma Surg. 2017;137(12):1699–705. PubMed PMID: 28918517.
16. Saito M, Tsukada S, Yoshida K, Okada Y, Tasaki A. Correlation of alpha angle between various radiographic projections and radial magnetic resonance imaging for cam deformity in femoral head-neck junction. Knee Surg Sports Traumatol Arthrosc. 2017;25(1):77–83. PubMed PMID: 26878850.
17. Heyworth BE, Dolan MM, Nguyen JT, Chen NC, Kelly BT. Preoperative three-dimensional CT predicts intraoperative findings in hip arthroscopy. Clin Orthop Relat Res. 2012;470(7):1950–7. PubMed PMID: 22528376. Pubmed Central PMCID: 3369089. Epub 2012/04/25
18. Milone MT, Bedi A, Poultsides L, Magennis E, Byrd JW, Larson CM, et al. Novel CT-based three-dimensional software improves the characterization of cam morphology. Clin Orthop Relat Res. 2013;471(8):2484–91. PubMed PMID: 23361933. Epub 2013/01/31.
19. Ross JR, Larson CM, Adeoye O, Kelly BT, Bedi A. Residual deformity is the most common reason for revision hip arthroscopy: a three-dimensional CT

study. Clin Orthop Relat Res. 2015;473(4):1388–95. PubMed PMID: 25475714. Pubmed Central PMCID: 4353554.
20. Gupta AK, Abrams GD, Nho SJ. What's new in femoroacetabular impingement surgery: will we be better in 2023? Sports Health. 2014;6(2):162–70. PubMed PMID: 24587868. Pubmed Central PMCID: 3931340. Epub 2014/03/04.
21. Linda DD, Naraghi A, Murnaghan L, Whelan D, White LM. Accuracy of non-arthrographic 3T MR imaging in evaluation of intra-articular pathology of the hip in femoroacetabular impingement. Skelet Radiol. 2017;46(3):299–308. PubMed PMID: 27975135.
22. Mamisch TC, Kain MS, Bittersohl B, Apprich S, Werlen S, Beck M, et al. Delayed gadolinium-enhanced magnetic resonance imaging of cartilage (dGEMRIC) in Femoacetabular impingement. J Orthop Res. 2011;29(9):1305–11. PubMed PMID: 21437964. Epub 2011/03/26.
23. Said HG, Steimer O, Kohn D, Dienst M. Vascular obstruction at the level of the ankle joint as a complication of hip arthroscopy. Arthroscopy. 2011;27(11):1594–6. PubMed PMID: 21958670. Epub 2011/10/01.
24. Papavasiliou AV, Bardakos NV. Complications of arthroscopic surgery of the hip. Bone Joint Res. 2012;1(7):131–44. PubMed PMID: 23610683. Pubmed Central PMCID: 3629445.
25. Fernquest S, Arnold C, Palmer A, Broomfield J, Denton J, Taylor A, et al. Osseous impingement occurs early in flexion in cam-type femoroacetabular impingement: a 4D CT model. Bone Joint J. 2017;99-B(4 Suppl B):41–8. PubMed PMID: 28363893.
26. Locks R, Chahla J, Mitchell JJ, Soares E, Philippon MJ. Dynamic hip examination for assessment of impingement during hip arthroscopy. Arthrosc Tech. 2016;5(6):e1367–72. PubMed PMID: 28149735. Pubmed Central PMCID: 5263892.
27. Larson CM, Wulf CA. Intraoperative fluoroscopy for evaluation of bony resection during arthroscopic management of femoroacetabular impingement in the supine position. Arthroscopy. 2009;25(10):1183–92. PubMed PMID: 19801295. Epub 2009/10/06.
28. Philippon MJ, Schenker ML, Briggs KK, Kuppersmith DA, Maxwell RB, Stubbs AJ. Revision hip arthroscopy. Am J Sports Med. 2007;35(11):1918–21. PubMed PMID: 17703000. Epub 2007/08/19.
29. Matsuda DK. Fluoroscopic templating technique for precision arthroscopic rim trimming. Arthroscopy. 2009;25(10):1175–82. PubMed PMID: 19801294. Epub 2009/10/06.
30. Budd H, Patchava A, Khanduja V. Establishing the radiation risk from fluoroscopic-assisted arthroscopic surgery of the hip. Int Orthop. 2012;36(9):1803–6. PubMed PMID: 22588691. Pubmed Central PMCID: 3427451.
31. Gaymer CE, Achten J, Auckett R, Cooper L, Griffin D. Fluoroscopic radiation exposure during hip arthroscopy. Arthroscopy. 2013;29(5):870–3. PubMed PMID: 23538042. Epub 2013/03/30.
32. Jackson TJ, Stake CE, Trenga AP, Morgan J, Domb BG. Arthroscopic technique for treatment of femoroacetabular impingement. Arthrosc Tech. 2013;2(1):e55–9. PubMed PMID: 23767009. Pubmed Central PMCID: 3678601. Epub 2013/06/15.
33. Byrd JW, Jones KS. Arthroscopic femoroplasty in the management of cam-type femoroacetabular impingement. Clin Orthop Relat Res. 2009;467(3):739–46. PubMed PMID: 19096902. Pubmed Central PMCID: 2635454. Epub 2008/12/20.
34. Martin HD, Kelly BT, Leunig M, Philippon MJ, Clohisy JC, Martin RL, et al. The pattern and technique in the clinical evaluation of the adult hip: the common physical examination tests of hip specialists. Arthroscopy. 2010;26(2):161–72. PubMed PMID: 20141979. Epub 2010/02/10.
35. Frank JM, Harris JD, Erickson BJ, Slikker W 3rd, Bush-Joseph CA, Salata MJ, et al. Prevalence of femoroacetabular impingement imaging findings in asymptomatic volunteers: a systematic review. Arthroscopy. 2015;31:1199–204. PubMed PMID: 25636988.
36. Burke CJ, Walter WR, Gyftopoulos S, Pham H, Baron S, Gonzalez-Lomas G, et al. Real-time assessment of femoroacetabular motion using radial gradient echo magnetic resonance arthrography at 3 tesla in routine clinical practice: a pilot study. Arthroscopy. 2019;35(8):2366–74. PubMed PMID: 31395172.
37. Kobayashi N, Inaba Y, Kubota S, Higashihira S, Choe H, Ike H, et al. Computer-assisted hip arthroscopic surgery for femoroacetabular impingement. Arthrosc Tech. 2018;7(4):e397–403. PubMed PMID: 29868411. Pubmed Central PMCID: 5983053.
38. Hadeed MM, Cancienne JM, Gwathmey FW. Pincer impingement. Clin Sports Med. 2016;35(3):405–18. PubMed PMID: 27343393.
39. Malahias MA, Alexiades MM. The clinical outcome of chondrolabral-preserving arthroscopic acetabuloplasty for pincer- or mixed-type femoroacetabular impingement: a systematic review. Musculoskelet Surg. 2019;103:207–14. PubMed PMID: 30850935.
40. Mascarenhas VV, Rego P, Dantas P, Caetano AP, Jans L, Sutter R, et al. Can we discriminate symptomatic hip patients from asymptomatic volunteers based on anatomic predictors? A 3-dimensional magnetic resonance study on cam, pincer, and spinopelvic parameters. Am J Sports Med. 2018;46(13):3097–110. PubMed PMID: 30379583.
41. Sanders TL, Reardon P, Levy BA, Krych AJ. Arthroscopic treatment of global pincer-type femoroacetabular impingement. Knee Surg Sports Traumatol Arthrosc. 2017;25(1):31–5. PubMed PMID: 27506809.

42. Rego P, Beaule PE, Ayeni OR, Tey M, Marin-Pena O, Dantas P, et al. Femoroacetabular impingement: what the surgeon wants to know. Semin Musculoskelet Radiol. 2019;23(3):257–75. PubMed PMID: 31163501.
43. Petersen W, Petersen F, Tillmann B. Structure and vascularization of the acetabular labrum with regard to the pathogenesis and healing of labral lesions. Arch Orthop Trauma Surg. 2003;123(6):283–8. PubMed PMID: 12802599.
44. McCarthy J, Noble P, Aluisio FV, Schuck M, Wright J, Lee JA. Anatomy, pathologic features, and treatment of acetabular labral tears. Clin Orthop Relat Res. 2003;406:38–47. PubMed PMID: 12578998.
45. Lage LA, Patel JV, Villar RN. The acetabular labral tear: an arthroscopic classification. Arthroscopy. 1996;12(3):269–72. PubMed PMID: 8783819. Epub 1996/06/01.
46. Ayeni OR, Alradwan H, de Sa D, Philippon MJ. The hip labrum reconstruction: indications and outcomes—a systematic review. Knee Surg Sports Traumatol Arthrosc. 2014;22(4):737–43. PubMed PMID: 24318405. Epub 2013/12/10.
47. Czerny C, Hofmann S, Neuhold A, Tschauner C, Engel A, Recht MP, et al. Lesions of the acetabular labrum: accuracy of MR imaging and MR arthrography in detection and staging. Radiology. 1996;200(1):225–30. PubMed PMID: 8657916.
48. White BJ, Herzog MM. Labral reconstruction: when to perform and how. Front Surg. 2015;2:27. PubMed PMID: 26217668. Pubmed Central PMCID: 4489330.
49. White BJ, Stapleford AB, Hawkes TK, Finger MJ, Herzog MM. Allograft use in arthroscopic labral reconstruction of the hip with front-to-Back fixation technique: minimum 2-year follow-up. Arthroscopy. 2016;32(1):26–32. PubMed PMID: 26422708.
50. Bhatia S, Chahla J, Dean CS, Ellman MB. Hip labral reconstruction: the "kite technique" for improved efficiency and graft control. Arthrosc Tech. 2016;5(2):e337–42. PubMed PMID: 27354954. Pubmed Central PMCID: 4912620.
51. Forster-Horvath C, von Rotz N, Giordano BD, Domb BG. Acetabular labral debridement/segmental resection versus reconstruction in the comprehensive treatment of symptomatic femoroacetabular impingement: a systematic review. Arthroscopy. 2016;32(11):2401–15. PubMed PMID: 27475898.
52. Ganz R, Parvizi J, Beck M, Leunig M, Notzli H, Siebenrock KA. Femoroacetabular impingement: a cause for osteoarthritis of the hip. Clin Orthop Relat Res. 2003;417:112–20. PubMed PMID: 14646708. Epub 2003/12/04.
53. Nepple JJ, Carlisle JC, Nunley RM, Clohisy JC. Clinical and radiographic predictors of intra-articular hip disease in arthroscopy. Am J Sports Med. 2011;39(2):296–303. PubMed PMID: 21098820. Epub 2010/11/26.
54. Yen YM, Kocher MS. Chondral lesions of the hip: microfracture and chondroplasty. Sports Med Arthrosc Rev. 2010;18(2):83–9. PubMed PMID: 20473126.
55. Gikas PD, Bayliss L, Bentley G, Briggs TW. An overview of autologous chondrocyte implantation. J Bone Joint Surg. 2009;91(8):997–1006. PubMed PMID: 19651824.
56. Mankin HJ. The response of articular cartilage to mechanical injury. J Bone Joint Surg Am. 1982;64(3):460–6. PubMed PMID: 6174527.
57. Hubbard MJ. Articular debridement versus washout for degeneration of the medial femoral condyle. A five-year study. J Bone Joint Surg Br. 1996;78(2):217–9. PubMed PMID: 8666628.
58. Fontana A, Bistolfi A, Crova M, Rosso F, Massazza G. Arthroscopic treatment of hip chondral defects: autologous chondrocyte transplantation versus simple debridement—a pilot study. Arthroscopy. 2012;28(3):322–9. PubMed PMID: 22142720. Epub 2011/12/07.
59. Sekiya JK, Martin RL, Lesniak BP. Arthroscopic repair of delaminated acetabular articular cartilage in femoroacetabular impingement. Orthopedics. 2009;32(9). PubMed PMID: 19750994. Epub 2009/09/16.
60. Beaule PE, Zaragoza EJ. Surgical images: musculoskeletal acetabular cartilage delamination demonstrated by magnetic resonance arthrography: inverted "Oreo" cookie sign. Can J S. 2003;46(6):463–4. PubMed PMID: 14680355. Pubmed Central PMCID: 3211760.
61. Beck M, Leunig M, Parvizi J, Boutier V, Wyss D, Ganz R. Anterior femoroacetabular impingement: part II. Midterm results of surgical treatment. Clin Orthop Relat Res. 2004;418:67–73. PubMed PMID: 15043095. Epub 2004/03/27.
62. Tzaveas AP, Villar RN. Arthroscopic repair of acetabular chondral delamination with fibrin adhesive. Hip Int. 2010;20(1):115–9. PubMed PMID: 20235074. Epub 2010/03/18.
63. Stafford GH, Bunn JR, Villar RN. Arthroscopic repair of delaminated acetabular articular cartilage using fibrin adhesive. Results at one to three years. Hip Int. 2011;21(6):744–50. PubMed PMID: 22117261. Epub 2011/11/26.
64. Steadman JR, Rodkey WG, Rodrigo JJ. Microfracture: surgical technique and rehabilitation to treat chondral defects. Clin Orthop Relat Res. 2001;(391 Suppl):S362–9. PubMed PMID: 11603719.
65. Steadman JR, Briggs KK, Rodrigo JJ, Kocher MS, Gill TJ, Rodkey WG. Outcomes of microfracture for traumatic chondral defects of the knee: average 11-year follow-up. Arthroscopy. 2003;19(5):477–84. PubMed PMID: 12724676.
66. Steadman JR, Miller BS, Karas SG, Schlegel TF, Briggs KK, Hawkins RJ. The microfracture technique in the treatment of full-thickness chondral lesions of the knee in National Football League players. J Knee Surg. 2003;16(2):83–6. PubMed PMID: 12741420.

67. Goyal D, Keyhani S, Lee EH, Hui JH. Evidence-based status of microfracture technique: a systematic review of level I and II studies. Arthroscopy. 2013;29(9):1579–88. PubMed PMID: 23992991.
68. Payne KA, Didiano DM, Chu CR. Donor sex and age influence the chondrogenic potential of human femoral bone marrow stem cells. Osteoarthritis Cartilage. 2010;18(5):705–13. PubMed PMID: 20171308. Pubmed Central PMCID: 2862807.
69. Nakano N, Gohal C, Duong A, Ayeni OR, Khanduja V. Outcomes of cartilage repair techniques for chondral injury in the hip—a systematic review. Int Orthop. 2018;42(10):2309–22. PubMed PMID: 29536127.
70. Philippon MJ, Schenker ML, Briggs KK, Maxwell RB. Can microfracture produce repair tissue in acetabular chondral defects? Arthroscopy. 2008;24(1):46–50. PubMed PMID: 18182201. Epub 2008/01/10.
71. Karthikeyan S, Roberts S, Griffin D. Microfracture for acetabular chondral defects in patients with femoroacetabular impingement: results at second-look arthroscopic surgery. Am J Sports Med. 2012;40(12):2725–30. PubMed PMID: 23136178. Epub 2012/11/09.
72. Zaltz I, Leunig M. Parafoveal chondral defects associated with femoroacetabular impingement. Clin Orthop Relat Res. 2012;470(12):3383–9. PubMed PMID: 22777588. Epub 2012/07/11.
73. Brittberg M, Lindahl A, Nilsson A, Ohlsson C, Isaksson O, Peterson L. Treatment of deep cartilage defects in the knee with autologous chondrocyte transplantation. N Engl J Med. 1994;331(14):889–95. PubMed PMID: 8078550.
74. Pestka JM, Bode G, Salzmann G, Sudkamp NP, Niemeyer P. Clinical outcome of autologous chondrocyte implantation for failed microfracture treatment of full-thickness cartilage defects of the knee joint. Am J Sports Med. 2012;40(2):325–31. PubMed PMID: 22056348.
75. Mancini D, Fontana A. Five-year results of arthroscopic techniques for the treatment of acetabular chondral lesions in femoroacetabular impingement. Int Orthop. 2014;38(10):2057–64. PubMed PMID: 24951948. Epub 2014/06/22.
76. Fontana A, de Girolamo L. Sustained five-year benefit of autologous matrix-induced chondrogenesis for femoral acetabular impingement-induced chondral lesions compared with microfracture treatment. Bone Joint J. 2015;97-B(5):628–35. PubMed PMID: 25922456.
77. Leunig M, Tibor LM, Naal FD, Ganz R, Steinwachs MR. Surgical technique: second-generation bone marrow stimulation via surgical dislocation to treat hip cartilage lesions. Clin Orthop Relat Res. 2012;470(12):3421–31. PubMed PMID: 22773396. Epub 2012/07/10.
78. Fontana A. Autologous membrane induced chondrogenesis (AMIC) for the treatment of acetabular chondral defect. Muscles Ligaments Tendons J. 2016;6(3):367–71. PubMed PMID: 28066742. Pubmed Central PMCID: 5193527.
79. Girard J, Roumazeille T, Sakr M, Migaud H. Osteochondral mosaicplasty of the femoral head. Hip Int. 2011;21(5):542–8. PubMed PMID: 21948031.
80. Krych AJ, Lorich DG, Kelly BT. Treatment of focal osteochondral defects of the acetabulum with osteochondral allograft transplantation. Orthopedics. 2011;34(7):e307–11. PubMed PMID: 21717995.
81. Mardones R, Via AG, Jofre C, Minguell J, Rodriguez C, Tomic A, et al. Cell therapy for cartilage defects of the hip. Muscles Ligaments Tendons J. 2016;6(3):361–6. PubMed PMID: 28066741. Pubmed Central PMCID: 5193526.
82. Harris JD, McCormick FM, Abrams GD, Gupta AK, Ellis TJ, Bach BR Jr, et al. Complications and reoperations during and after hip arthroscopy: a systematic review of 92 studies and more than 6,000 patients. Arthroscopy. 2013;29(3):589–95. PubMed PMID: 23544691. Epub 2013/04/03.
83. Yeung M, Memon M, Simunovic N, Belzile E, Philippon MJ, Ayeni OR. Gross instability after hip arthroscopy: an analysis of case reports evaluating surgical and patient factors. Arthroscopy. 2016;32(6):1196–204.e1. PubMed PMID: 27013107.
84. Matsuda DK. Acute iatrogenic dislocation following hip impingement arthroscopic surgery. Arthroscopy. 2009;25(4):400–4. PubMed PMID: 19341927. Epub 2009/04/04.
85. Crim J. Imaging evaluation of the hip after arthroscopic surgery for femoroacetabular impingement. Skelet Radiol. 2017;46(10):1315–26. PubMed PMID: 28466104. Pubmed Central PMCID: 5559574.
86. Ekhtiari S, de Sa D, Haldane CE, Simunovic N, Larson CM, Safran MR, et al. Hip arthroscopic capsulotomy techniques and capsular management strategies: a systematic review. Knee Surg Sports Traumatol Arthrosc. 2017;25(1):9–23. PubMed PMID: 28120020.
87. Bedi A, Galano G, Walsh C, Kelly BT. Capsular management during hip arthroscopy: from femoroacetabular impingement to instability. Arthroscopy. 2011;27(12):1720–31. PubMed PMID: 22047925. Epub 2011/11/04.
88. Conaway WK, Martin SD. Puncture capsulotomy during hip arthroscopy for femoroacetabular impingement: preserving anatomy and biomechanics. Arthrosc Tech. 2017;6(6):e2265–9. PubMed PMID: 29349029. Pubmed Central PMCID: 5765917.
89. Forster-Horvath C, Domb BG, Ashberg L, Herzog RF. A method for capsular management and avoidance of iatrogenic instability: minimally invasive capsulotomy in hip arthroscopy. Arthrosc Tech. 2017;6(2):e397–400. PubMed PMID: 28580258. Pubmed Central PMCID: 5443139.

90. Telleria JJ, Lindsey DP, Giori NJ, Safran MR. An anatomic arthroscopic description of the hip capsular ligaments for the hip arthroscopist. Arthroscopy. 2011;27(5):628–36. PubMed PMID: 21663720. Epub 2011/06/15.
91. Abrams GD, Hart MA, Takami K, Bayne CO, Kelly BT, Espinoza Orias AA, et al. Biomechanical evaluation of capsulotomy, capsulectomy, and capsular repair on hip rotation. Arthroscopy. 2015;31(8):1511–7. PubMed PMID: 25882176.
92. Gupta A, Suarez-Ahedo C, Redmond JM, Gerhardt MB, Hanypsiak B, Stake CE, et al. Best practices during hip arthroscopy: aggregate recommendations of high-volume surgeons. Arthroscopy. 2015;31(9):1722–7. PubMed PMID: 25980403.
93. Larson CM, Stone RM, Grossi EF, Giveans MR, Cornelsen GD. Ehlers-Danlos syndrome: arthroscopic management for extreme soft-tissue hip instability. Arthroscopy. 2015;31:2287–94. PubMed PMID: 26198768.
94. Kay J, Memon M, Rubin S, Simunovic N, Nho SJ, Belzile EL, et al. The dimensions of the hip capsule can be measured using magnetic resonance imaging and may have a role in arthroscopic planning. Knee Surg Sports Traumatol Arthrosc. 2018. PubMed PMID: 30259148.
95. Frank RM, Lee S, Bush-Joseph CA, Kelly BT, Salata MJ, Nho SJ. Improved outcomes after hip arthroscopic surgery in patients undergoing T-capsulotomy with complete repair versus partial repair for femoroacetabular impingement: a comparative matched-pair analysis. Am J Sports Med. 2014;42(11):2634–42. PubMed PMID: 25214529.
96. Larson CM, Giveans MR, Samuelson KM, Stone RM, Bedi A. Arthroscopic hip revision surgery for residual femoroacetabular impingement (FAI): surgical outcomes compared with a matched cohort after primary arthroscopic FAI correction. Am J Sports Med. 2014;42:1785–90. PubMed PMID: 24875469. Epub 2014/05/31.
97. Newman JT, Briggs KK, McNamara SC, Philippon MJ. Revision hip arthroscopy: a matched-cohort study comparing revision to primary arthroscopy patients. Am J Sports Med. 2016;44(10):2499–504. PubMed PMID: 27307496.
98. McCormick F, Slikker W 3rd, Harris JD, Gupta AK, Abrams GD, Frank J, et al. Evidence of capsular defect following hip arthroscopy. Knee Surg Sports Traumatol Arthrosc. 2014;22(4):902–5. PubMed PMID: 23851921. Epub 2013/07/16.
99. Yeung M, Khan M, Williams D, Ayeni OR. Anterior hip capsuloligamentous reconstruction with Achilles allograft following gross hip instability post-arthroscopy. Knee Surg Sports Traumatol Arthrosc. 2017;25(1):3–8. PubMed PMID: 27492383.
100. Gehrman M, Cornell M, Seeley M. Iatrogenic hip instability after hip arthroscopy: is there a role for open capsular reconstruction?: a case report. JBJS Case Connect. 2019;9(2):e0091. PubMed PMID: 31233426.
101. Martin HD, Shears SA, Johnson JC, Smathers AM, Palmer IJ. The endoscopic treatment of sciatic nerve entrapment/deep gluteal syndrome. Arthroscopy. 2011;27(2):172–81. PubMed PMID: 21071168. Epub 2010/11/13.
102. Martin HD, Gómez Hoyos JC. Posterior hip disorders. In: Clinical evaluation and management. xv, 365p.
103. Nho SJ, Leunig M, Larson CM, Bedi A, Kelly B. Hip arthroscopy and hip joint preservation surgery. 2 volumes (xxx, 1205p).
104. Kulcu DG, Naderi S. Differential diagnosis of intraspinal and extraspinal non-discogenic sciatica. J Clin Neurosci. 2008;15(11):1246–52. PubMed PMID: 18789864.
105. Ergun T, Lakadamyali H. CT and MRI in the evaluation of extraspinal sciatica. Br J Radiol. 2010;83(993):791–803. PubMed PMID: 20647515. Pubmed Central PMCID: 3473399.
106. Kay J, de Sa D, Morrison L, Fejtek E, Simunovic N, Martin HD, et al. Surgical management of deep gluteal syndrome causing sciatic nerve entrapment: a systematic review. Arthroscopy. 2017;33(12):2263–78.e1. PubMed PMID: 28866346.
107. Martin HD, Kivlan BR, Palmer IJ, Martin RL. Diagnostic accuracy of clinical tests for sciatic nerve entrapment in the gluteal region. Knee Surg Sports Traumatol Arthrosc. 2014;22(4):882–8. PubMed PMID: 24217716.
108. Hernando MF, Cerezal L, Perez-Carro L, Abascal F, Canga A. Deep gluteal syndrome: anatomy, imaging, and management of sciatic nerve entrapments in the subgluteal space. Skelet Radiol. 2015;44(7):919–34. PubMed PMID: 25739706.
109. Lewis AM, Layzer R, Engstrom JW, Barbaro NM, Chin CT. Magnetic resonance neurography in extraspinal sciatica. Arch Neurol. 2006;63(10):1469–72. PubMed PMID: 17030664.
110. Carro LP, Hernando MF, Cerezal L, Navarro IS, Fernandez AA, Castillo AO. Deep gluteal space problems: piriformis syndrome, ischiofemoral impingement and sciatic nerve release. Muscles Ligaments Tendons J. 2016;6(3):384–96. PubMed PMID: 28066745. Pubmed Central PMCID: 5193530.
111. Torriani M, Souto SC, Thomas BJ, Ouellette H, Bredella MA. Ischiofemoral impingement syndrome: an entity with hip pain and abnormalities of the quadratus femoris muscle. AJR Am J Roentgenol. 2009;193(1):186–90. PubMed PMID: 19542413.
112. Hernando MF, Cerezal L, Perez-Carro L, Canga A, Gonzalez RP. Evaluation and management of ischiofemoral impingement: a pathophysiologic, radiologic, and therapeutic approach to a complex diagnosis. Skelet Radiol. 2016;45(6):771–87. PubMed PMID: 26940209.
113. Hatem MA, Palmer IJ, Martin HD. Diagnosis and 2-year outcomes of endoscopic treatment

for ischiofemoral impingement. Arthroscopy. 2015;31(2):239–46. PubMed PMID: 25278353.
114. Gomez-Hoyos J, Martin RL, Martin HD. Current concepts review: evaluation and management of posterior hip pain. J Am Acad Orthop Surg. 2018;26(17):597–609. PubMed PMID: 30080760.
115. Kim Y-J, Mamisch TC. Hip magnetic resonance imaging. xiii, 230p.
116. Knudsen JS, McConkey MO, Brick MJ. Endoscopic sciatic neurolysis. Arthrosc Tech. 2015;4(4):e353–8. PubMed PMID: 26759776. Pubmed Central PMCID: 4680922.
117. Ilizaliturri VM Jr, Arriaga R, Villalobos FE, Suarez-Ahedo C. Endoscopic release of the piriformis tendon and sciatic nerve exploration. J Hip Preserv Surg. 2018;5(3):301–6. PubMed PMID: 30393558. Pubmed Central PMCID: 6206698.
118. Robertson WJ, Kelly BT. The safe zone for hip arthroscopy: a cadaveric assessment of central, peripheral, and lateral compartment portal placement. Arthroscopy. 2008;24(9):1019–26. PubMed PMID: 18760209. Epub 2008/09/02.
119. Jo S, O'Donnell JM. Endoscopic lesser trochanter resection for treatment of ischiofemoral impingement. J Hip Preserv Surg. 2015;2(2):184–9. PubMed PMID: 27011837. Pubmed Central PMCID: 4718495.
120. Safran M, Ryu J. Ischiofemoral impingement of the hip: a novel approach to treatment. Knee Surg Sports Traumatol Arthrosc. 2014;22(4):781–5. PubMed PMID: 24346740.
121. Wilson MD, Keene JS. Treatment of ischiofemoral impingement: results of diagnostic injections and arthroscopic resection of the lesser trochanter. J Hip Preserv Surg. 2016;3(2):146–53. PubMed PMID: 27583151. Pubmed Central PMCID: 5005049.
122. Crock HV. Anatomy of the medial femoral circumflex artery and its surgical implications. J Bone Joint Surg Br. 2001;83(1):149–50. PubMed PMID: 11245526.
123. Aguilera-Bohorquez B, Cardozo O, Brugiatti M, Cantor E, Valdivia N. Endoscopic treatment of sciatic nerve entrapment in deep gluteal syndrome: clinical results. Rev Esp Cir Ortop Traumatol. 2018;62(5):322–7. PubMed PMID: 29807785. Manejo endoscopico del atrapamiento del nervio ciatico en el sindrome de gluteo profundo: resultados clinicos.
124. Nakano N, Shoman H, Khanduja V. Treatment strategies for ischiofemoral impingement: a systematic review. Knee Surg Sports Traumatol Arthrosc. 2018. PubMed PMID: 30426139.

Platt's Syndrome: A Nerve Complication Associated with Ligament Injuries

27

M. Llusa, P. Alvarez, J. Casañas, X. Cusco, M. R. Morro, R. Seijas, E. Alentorn, D. Barastegui, and R. Cugat

27.1 Introduction

Common peroneal nerve (CPN) palsy is associated with acute trauma injuries in the lower extremity, especially around the knee. The occurrence rate of CPN palsy in the general population with knee dislocation or bicruciate ligament injury ranges from 10 to 40% [1]; the peroneal nerve injury associated with sports-related knee injury has been reported to account for 18%. Cho [2] retrospectively reviewed 84 cases, evaluated for injury mechanism and other items and found 84 of 448 cases of peroneal nerve injury, all of which were found to be sports related (skiing 42 cases, football 23 cases, soccer 8 cases, basketball 6 cases, ice hockey 2 cases, track 2 cases, and volleyball 1 case). Sports that are more related to knee injury and peroneal nerve lesion are skiing, American football and soccer. The high prevalence is due to the risks associated not only with particular sport but also with the biomechanics of the trauma. These biomechanics could be direct or indirect such as a common occurrence in football in which injury happens when the foot is fixed on the ground with a typical varus and hyperextension of the knee. In Spain of course,

M. Llusa (✉)
Department of Orthopaedic and Traumatology, Hospital Clínic, Barcelona, Spain

Department of Human Anatomy, University of Barcelona, Barcelona, Spain

Trauma Unit, Teknon University Hospital, Barcelona, Spain
e-mail: mllusa@ub.edu

P. Alvarez
Mutualidad Catalana de Futbolistas, Barcelona, Spain

Artroscopia GC, Quirón University Hospital, Barcelona, Spain

Fundación García Cugat, Barcelona, Spain

Universitat Internacional de Catalunya, Barcelona, Spain

J. Casañas
Trauma Unit, Teknon University Hospital, Barcelona, Spain

X. Cusco
Artroscopia GC, Quirón University Hospital, Barcelona, Spain

Fundación García Cugat, Barcelona, Spain

M. R. Morro
Department of Orthopaedic and Traumatology, Hospital Clínic, Barcelona, Spain

Department of Human Anatomy, University of Barcelona, Barcelona, Spain

R. Seijas
Artroscopia GC, Quirón University Hospital, Barcelona, Spain

Fundación García Cugat, Barcelona, Spain

Universitat Internacional de Catalunya, Barcelona, Spain

E. Alentorn · D. Barastegui · R. Cugat
Mutualidad Catalana de Futbolistas, Barcelona, Spain

Artroscopia GC, Quirón University Hospital, Barcelona, Spain

Fundación García Cugat, Barcelona, Spain

M. T. Hirschmann et al. (eds.), *ESSKA Instructional Course Lecture Book*,
https://doi.org/10.1007/978-3-662-61264-4_27

Table 27.1 Nerve injury classification and pathology correlation

Classification	Seddon	Sunderland	Pathology
	Neuroapraxia	Grade 1	Myelin injury or ischemia
	Axonotmesis	Grade 2	Axon loss, internal derangement Endo, peri, and epineurium intact
		Grade 3	Endoneurium disrupted
		Grade 4	Perineurium disrupted
	Neurotmesis	Grade 5	Epineurium disrupted

Adapted from Birch [5]

soccer is the main cause of nerve lesion and sport-related knee injury. Our group, Mutualitat Catalana de Futbolistes (soccer players' mutual insurance in Catalonia) includes 150,000 athletes and performs medical assistance to 26,000 soccer players per year.

From the neurological point of view, when evaluating patients, the orthopedic surgeon must take into account the *extension* of the lesion, the *level* of the lesion, and the *severity* of the lesion. *Extension* determines the extent of the injury. Does it affect only the peroneal nerve, or does the damage reach the tibialis nerve and/or other related nerves as well; *level* refers to the affected area. This may be distal or proximal (or very proximal) to the fibular head, the latter being the most frequent and difficult. The *severity* of the injury is related to the degree of structural disruption of the peripheral nerve.

Seddon [3] classified nerve injuries, and structural disruption, into three major groups: neuroapraxia, which involves myelin damage with delayed conduction and intact structural components; axonotmesis, characterized by axon discontinuity, with the development of Wallerian degeneration; and neurotmesis, being the most severe injury characterized by a complete disruption of the nerve, including separation of the axons and/or the epineurium. Sunderland [4] describes a more extensive nerve injury classification in which grade 1 corresponds to Seddon's neuroapraxia, grade 2 corresponds to axonotmesis; grade 3, however, represents an endoneurial disruption, grade 4 a perineurium disruption, and grade 5 equivalent to a Seddon neurotmesis. Grades 3 and 4 reflect a functional nerve disruption but with the epineurium intact, leaving only the epineurium sheath in continuity (Table 27.1) [5].

Traumatic knee-level sport-related peroneal nerve injury is usually due to stretching or contusion, with or without fracture/dislocation [1]. Not all the nerve injuries are of this type. When the onset is not acute but progressive, the most common is compressive neuropathy around the fibular neck [6]. Likewise, not all the acute paralysis with foot drop are due to direct nerve injury. Keep in mind to always rule out the devastating compartment syndrome, with its symptoms of intense disproportionate pain and a severe swelling or an associated vascular injury, usually without pulse in the main distal vessels [7].

27.2 Anatomy

CPN is a part of the sciatic nerve. In the thigh, the peroneal division is located in the lateral and posterior areas of the common sciatic nerve. At mid-level of the thigh, the peroneal nerve supplies the innervation to the short head of the biceps femoris muscle before separating from the tibial nerve in the upper part of the popliteal fossa. At that level, the nerve crosses posterior to the lateral head of the gastrocnemius muscle through the posterior intermuscular septum and gives off the lateral sural cutaneous branch that is going to join the main sural nerve in the calf. After that, the peroneal nerve becomes subcutaneous for a short segment, to proceed deep to the peroneus longus muscle while it curves around the fibular head (Fig. 27.1). Just at this level the nerve divides into the superficial peroneal neve (SPN), deep peroneal nerve (DPN), and articular branch for the proximal tibiofibular joint. The SPN travels distally in the lateral compartment of the leg, innervating the peroneus longus and peroneus brevis muscles. Approximately 8–12 cm above the lateral malleolus, the superficial branch pierces the sural fascia over the lateral compartment, becomes subcutaneous, and divides into its terminal branches as the intermediate and medial

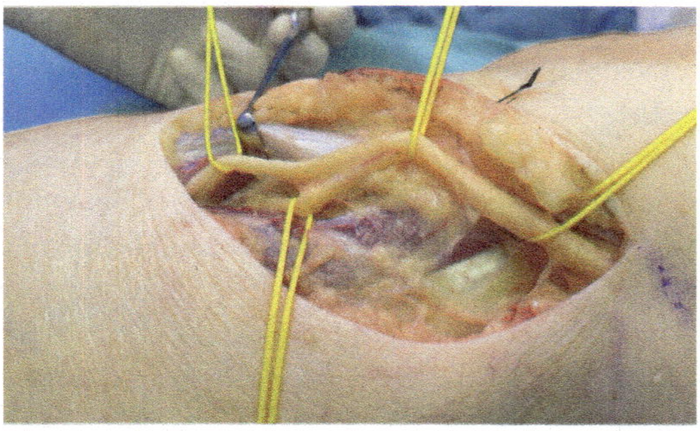

Fig. 27.1 Posterolateral view of a left knee. Course of the common peroneal nerve and its main branches SPN and DPN, just behind the biceps femoris muscle and tendon unit and around the fibular neck

dorsal cutaneous nerves on the dorsum of the foot and toes for sensory innervation (except sensory innervation of the dorsal first web space) [5, 6, 8].

The DPN courses from 2 to 4 cm along the anterior cortex of the fibula and then travels distally to pierce the intermuscular septum between the anterior and lateral compartment to join the anterior tibial artery at the upper part of the calf. Distally the DPN supplies innervation to the most powerful foot dorsiflexor, the tibialis anterior muscle (through the first branch of the DPN very close to the fibular neck) and the toe dorsiflexors including the hallux (extensor digitorum longus, peroneus tertius, extensor hallucis longus). Finally, at the ankle level, the nerve passes under the extensor retinaculum and terminates as a sensory branch in the dorsal first web space.

27.3 Pathomechanics of the Platt Syndrome

The peroneal nerve is relatively fixed at the level of the lateral intermuscular septum, especially under the long peroneus fibrous arch origin around the fibular head and, finalizes when the deep branch pierces the intermuscular septum between the anterior and lateral compartments [5, 8]. That is because in all these areas the nerve is vulnerable to stretch forces, such as varus and hyperextension that result in posterolateral knee complex lesions. In this kind of varus knee injury, Harry Platt recognized the relation between fibular head avulsion through the biceps tendon insertion and lateral collateral insertion on the

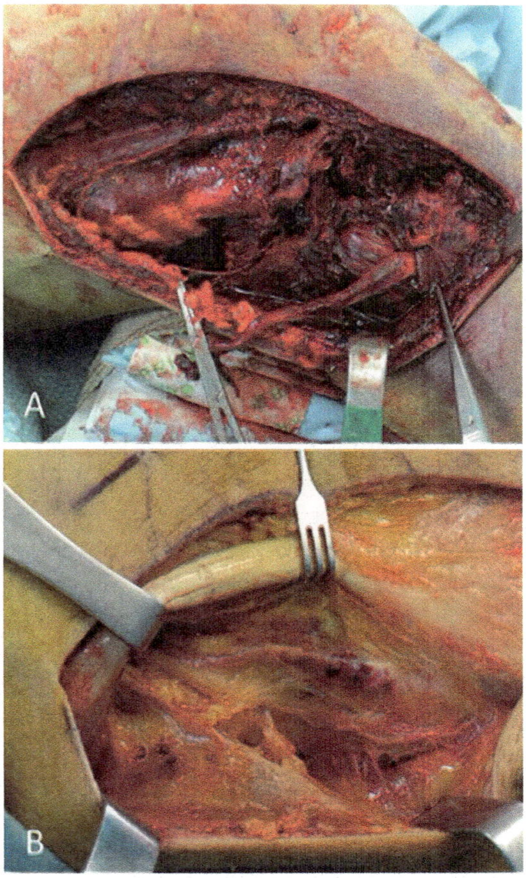

Fig. 27.2 Macroscopic anatomopathological findings in the Platt syndrome: fibular head avulsion, through the biceps tendon insertion and lateral collateral insertion on the styloid apophysis, and proximal stretch lesion (frank nerve rupture) of the peroneal nerve very distant from the fibular head (**a**). Severe stretch injuries can lead to an initial intraneural hematoma due to the rupture of the vasa nervorum and subsequent fibrosis and scar formation inside the nerve over time (**b**)

styloid apophysis and stretch lesion of the peroneal nerve [5, 9] (especially at proximal part of the nerve, extended far proximal to the fibular head, with frank nerve rupture or long neuroma in continuity (Fig. 27.2a).

CPN palsy depends on the direction and degree of the initial displacement causing the different ligament ruptures, which depend on knee position, trauma velocity, and strength of the structures involved. Besides, peroneal nerve connective tissue damage may occur with severe stretch injuries, which can lead to intraneural and extraneural tissue destruction, intraneural hematoma, subsequent fibrosis, and scar formation (Fig. 27.2b).

The basic biomechanical role played by the posterolateral structures in this mechanism are varus laxity, mainly contained by lateral collateral ligament, regardless of the degree of knee flexion, and secondarily by the popliteal complex and posterolateral capsule; injury of the posterolateral structures increases lateral tibial rotation, maximum at 30° of flexion. The cruciate ligaments also play a considerable role in controlling varus and lateral rotation; when posterioanterior forces (hyperextension) are applied, the tibia tends to turn in lateral rotation [2, 10, 11].

Isolated injuries of the posterolateral structures account for 5.7% of the knee sprains [10]. The frequency of posterolateral lesions associated with anterior cruciate ligament tear is as high as 10% and those with posterior cruciate ligament tear 27%. The fibular nerve is involved in 15% of cases [10].

There is a consensus as to the parallel nature of the neurologic and ligament lesions: The more extensive and severe the latter, the more frequent and severe the CPN palsy [1]. However, the knee position and direction of the applied force are essential; the degree of varus deformity seems to be the more important in developing a true Platt syndrome [11].

27.4 Diagnosis

The general clinical evaluation and radiographic studies for posterolateral instabilities were covered previously in this ICL and is out of the scope of this presentation. Just remember Platt syndrome is associated with fibular head avulsion because of the severe varus force applied through the biceps tendon insertion and lateral collateral insertion on the styloid apophysis. This should be an alarm sign to suspect this devastating injury. In fact, the final prognosis of the injury and surgical repair or reconstruction depends on the functional recovery of the nerve lesion if it coexist in the injury [12–15].

27.4.1 Clinical Diagnosis

Clinical diagnosis of a CPN palsy is obvious; the characteristic foot drop with paralyzed ankle dorsiflexors and anesthetic cutaneous area over the dorsum of the foot and toes and hallux is evident. That, with acute onset related to a knee trauma seem to be enough for a clinical diagnosis. A more detailed exploration and physical examination focusing on the elements of each component of the nerve, superficial and deep main branches, should be done to define the extent of the injury and to localize the level of nerve injury. Numbness or dysesthesias in the upper lateral leg and paralysis or paresis of the anterior compartment muscles (extensor digitorum longus and peroneus tertius, extensor hallucis longus, the main ankle dorsiflexor, and tibialis anterior muscle) and lateral compartment muscles (peroneus lateralis longus and peroneus lateralis brevis) indicates a proximal injury to the fibular head. Paralysis of the short head of the biceps femoris muscle (muscle contraction over the short head of the biceps may be difficult to appreciate clinically but can be assessed by electro-neurological studies) indicates an even more proximal injury. Decreased or abnormal sensation in the first web space (with preservation of the sensation in the lower lateral leg and dorsum of the foot and toes) and anterior compartment muscles paralysis or paresis with preservation of lateral compartment muscles function indicate a DPN injury [2, 5, 6, 9]. The less frequent but tricky situation is decreased or abnormal sensation in the lower lateral leg and dorsum of the foot and toes (with preservation of the first web space sensation) and lateral compartment muscles paralysis or paresis (with preservation of anterior compartment muscles), indicating an SPN injury. This last situation could be missed if enough attention is not paid because ankle dorsiflexion is functioning (but is dorsiflexion with varus).

It should be emphasized that in these cases of acute trauma around the knee, it is mandatory to explore the vascular status of the lower extremity, looking for and ruling out a vascular injury of the popliteal artery, tibialis anterior artery, or tibialis posterior. The results should be written down in the medical report very clearly as such injuries may raise legal problems [14, 16, 17]. Assessment of vascular lesions in knee injuries is initially based on clinical examination, pulse-taking and Doppler exploration of the main vessels, popliteal artery and pedis artery (as a continuation of the tibialis anterior artery) and tibialis posterior at the retromalleolar sulcus. In case of doubt, a mandatory angioTC and consult a vascular surgeon [16, 18, 19]. The problem is not only the acute rupture or the artery but the intimal lesions of the vessel that can be initially present even with some peripheral pulse but could induce a secondary ischemic problem in hours by clotting around the intimal flap. It seems the popliteal artery rupture is more frequently associated with trauma while the knee is 90° flexed and the fearsome intimal lesion occurs in knee hyperextension injuries, as in posterolateral ligament injuries. According to available literature, the incidence of associated vascular injuries in biligamentous cruciate injuries of the knee ranges from 16 to 64% with a mean rate of 30% [19, 20]. In a report from the French Society of Orthopedic Surgery and Traumatology (SOFCOT) published by Boisrenoulte in 2009, a multicenter prospective study was conducted where among 67 patients with dislocation or bicruciate injury of the knee [16], nine were vascular injuries (12%) and that the absence of vascular lesion could be confirmed in 58 of the 59 patients with peripheral pulse at initial examination.

On the contrary, it is possible to detect peripheral pulses initially, even though the patient would have suffered an intimal lesion with a secondary ischemia. This is especially true for the tibialis artery in the area close to the intermembranous space. At that level the artery presents a marked angulation while it is fixed at the popliteal muscle point where the popliteal artery divides into the tibioperoneal trunk and the ramification of the tibialis anterior artery is almost 90° (Fig. 27.3).

It seems commonsensical to distinguish a common peroneal palsy from a compartment syndrome, but some cases prove to be more complicated. Paralysis of the foot dorsiflexors is a common fact for both conditions but disproportionated pain, hard swelling with tightness of compartment, is pathognomonic of the last condition. The trick is that some vascular lesion with intima flap in the artery, characteristically in the tibialis anterior artery, could lead to secondary ischemia by clotting and a subsequent compartment syndrome [16].

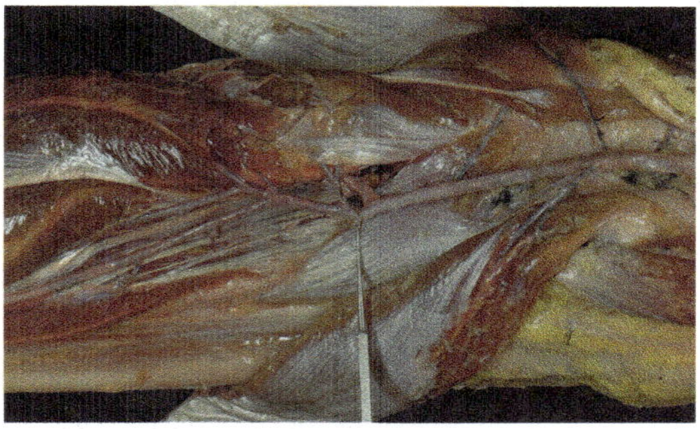

Fig. 27.3 Left knee. Posterior view of anatomic preparation showing the popliteal artery and its division in common tibioperoneal trunk and the ramification of the tibialis anterior artery coming off at almost 90° angle at this level. High risk of intimal lesion of the artery

27.4.2 CT

A CT scan may be used to evaluate further bony abnormalities.

In any case of abnormal pulse, emergency imaging is essential (angioscan or angio-TC). In cases of uncertain clinical situations, some surgeons advocate selective indications for angio-TC [16, 21–23] or echo-Doppler, with a high diagnostic sensitivity, specificity, and 98% diagnostic accuracy [24, 25]. This last technique, however, is operator-dependent. The reason for this attitude is that there are many reports of initially normal pulse associated with popliteal artery lesions [26, 27].

27.4.3 MRI

Assessment of knee injuries generally includes an MRI scan in the outpatient evaluation (in some centers, this may be included in the emergency departments) to evaluate the ligaments, meniscus, other soft tissues, and associated fractures [28, 29]. The radiologist must be instructed to evaluate especially the CPN, not only in close relation with the fibular head and neck but also in the proximal part around the intermuscular septum were most Platt injuries are seen. Some authors even order an angio-MRI to assess vascular around the knee before surgery [28, 30].

27.4.4 Ultrasonography

Ultrasonography is considered to evaluate not only the soft tissues as the ligaments, capsule, meniscus, and in some degree cartilage involvement but also, as mentioned before, the peripheral nerve relationships, especially nerve continuity, swelling and intraneural hematomas [25, 31], and if the specialist is familiar with the technique, the echo-Doppler could assess the vascular status of the main vessels.

27.4.5 Electrodiagnostic Studies

Electrodiagnostic studies are not useful and should not be performed during the initial 2–3 weeks. Nerve conduction velocity (NCV) studies and electromyography (EMG) are valuable tools for diagnosing nerve palsy, helping the surgeon evaluate the motor end sensory axons of the peroneal nerve and its branches, localizing the site of injury, and determining the severity of an injury [32, 33]. Specific study of the posterolateral cutaneous nerve of the calf may help to localize the level of the injury, and it is important to rule out Platt syndrome [6]. Of course, the studies should include the common sciatic nerve, the tibial nerve, and the sural nerve to diagnose or exclude other nerve injuries. Needle EMG helps to identify location and severity of CPN lesion. Besides the muscle innervated by the DPN (anterior compartment) and SPN (lateral compartment), studies of the short head of the biceps femoris muscle and muscles innervate by the tibial nerve distal to the knee help to identify injuries of the sciatic nerve proximally or the tibia nerve at the popliteal level. The tibial nerve is most often injured in association with knee dislocation or very severe cases of posterolateral injuries [2].

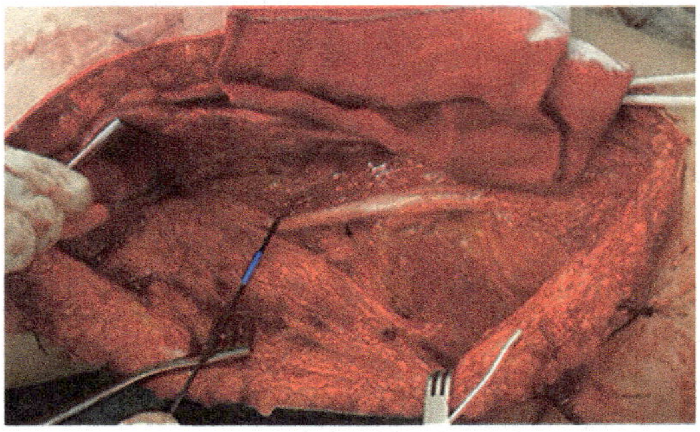

Fig. 27.4 Intraoperative nerve action potentials (NAPs) have a specific place in the surgical treatment of nerve lesions; intraoperative NAP studies in a CPN with a neuroma in continuity

Electrodiagnostic studies are also used for monitoring recovery after a nerve injury or after its surgical treatment. The results of the NCV and EMG studies could help to determine the course treatment and prognosis, and when surgical intervention is necessary. An electrophysiology study should be performed in all patients with a nerve lesion to obtain a baseline in all cases [5, 6, 33]. The study may be repeated every 6 weeks or 3 months to monitor improvement or spontaneous recovery, or to monitor the surgical treatment of the nerve lesion (repair or neurolysis). On the other hand, intraoperative electrophysiological studies have a specific place in the surgical treatment of nerve lesions in continuity; nerve action potential (NAP) studies are done along the course of the nerve when there is a lesion in continuity, even if there is a visible neuroma (Fig. 27.4). If NAP studies are flat, the segment of the nerve is resected and the nerve ends prepared for graft repair [32–35]. When the nerve is initially without continuity, then it is clear that we should proceed with grafting the gap, usually with the contralateral sural nerve.

27.5 Treatment

Initial treatment of peroneal nerve lesions and palsy in the common population involved a nonsurgical approach as it resulted in partial or full spontaneous recovery returns over time. In this group of patients, the etiologies for nerve palsy are numerous, compression being the most common cause. Even traumatic cases and direct blunt trauma injuries are managed non-surgically as they tend to result in positive prognosis and spontaneous recovery in most of them. A period of observation and nonoperative treatment is initially performed, utilizing a rehabilitation program and orthotic devices to avoid drop foot [36] and avoiding the imbalance between the functional plantar flexors of the ankle (triceps sural, tibialis posterior, flexor digitorum longus of the toes and flexor hallucis longus muscles) and the paralyzed dorsiflexors or extensors that could result in fixed or hard to reduce equinovarus position. The only exception is lacerations or fractures around the knee when the surgical approach for the osteosynthesis is in close vicinity with the nerve.

On the other hand, in the population group with CPN and sports-related knee injury, the attitude of the orthopedic surgeon is very different in the initial treatment of this type of lesion, especially when there is a posterolateral anatomic structure damage or a knee dislocation. This is not only because we are dealing with special group of very active individuals, most of them being professional athletes, but also because the severity of the injuries used to be much more intense, equivalent to a high energy car accident or fall from height. The energy released during the sporting accident is so high that it produces a real soft tissue explosion with severe damage, including peripheral nerves. To remark that there are reports of a higher incidence of nerve lesion in obese and sedentary patients with ultra-low-velocity dislocations of the knees, surgical ligament reconstruction of posterolateral corner and nerve appears to improve outcomes [37, 38]. Biomechanics of a combination of varus, external rotation and hyperextension forces across the knee predispose it to the stretch or avulsion injury of all the soft tissues including peroneal nerve stretch injury or rupture. The other reason for initial surgical treatment of the nerve injury is because most surgeons agree to treat primarily these complex posterolateral instabilities in the acute period when it is relatively easy to localize and anatomically repair or reconstruct the damaged structures and the nerve is in close relation.

27.5.1 Nonoperative Treatment

In cases where non-surgical treatment is selected, the patient needs to follow a rehabilitation program adapted to each injury and personal situation. In general, rehabilitation includes a physical therapy program, the use of orthotic devices at knee level, and anti-drop foot orthosis (Rancho Los Amigos orthosis or new adapted orthosis). It is important that the patient be educated of the importance of preserving ankle joint flexibility and avoid any contracture of the Achilles tendon, tibialis posterior tendon, or flexor digitorum tendons that could compromise any recovery of the innervation of the ankle dorsiflexor and evertors [2, 37]. Physical therapy should insist on stretching all these muscles. Electrical stimulation could be considered to maintain some muscle trophism and biomechanical properties. It may have a limited role in the initial period but could be very useful if the nerve recovers its functions using the electrical stimulation to fire muscle contraction. During all the recovery period, the surgeon must control the reinnervation of the muscles by EMG studies every 6 weeks to 3 months [5, 6, 33]. In cases when there is no appropriated progression in the reinnervation, the surgeon should consider surgical options for the nerve injury (neurolysis, nerve grafts, tendon transfers or even the new option of nerve transfer, or nerve allograft, depending on each particular situation and case).

27.5.2 Operative Treatment

Early surgical ligament repair or reconstruction is uncommon in isolated ligament injury. Even so, posterolateral complex structural injuries, especially in association with posterior cruciate ligament injury, are better managed by surgical treatment. Immediate or early surgical repair or reconstruction is reportedly superior to late reconstruction [10, 36]. Most of the ICL is dedicated to this specific topic and is beyond our scope. In clinical practice, our team has a clear idea that these cases must be tackled using a multidisciplinary approach among specialized orthopedic surgeons, sport and knee surgeons, and neuro orthopedic surgeons. In our institution, because we are a close-related working team sharing offices and operating rooms, the collaboration is always between the sport and knee specialist and neuro orthopedic surgeon. In fact, most of the time we preoperative joint visits and evaluations, we collaborate during the procedure, and again, postoperative together; and when secondary surgery is needed for neurolysis, nerve grafting, tendon or nerve transfer if nerve recovery was not adequate. Collaboration between surgical teams could be a little tricky; you must know well each other's way of work and organize and coordinate the operation. Our experience includes 14 patients with knee ligamentous injury, and CPN palsy has been treated in two different centers.

The time from trauma to repair has been found to be important on good functional outcome of the injured CPN [2, 33]. Although most neurosurgeons recommend follow-up for the first 3 months before operating [6, 39], we disagree with this idea and prefer to review the nerve at the same time that the posterolateral structures repair and reconstruction in the acute period.

27.5.2.1 Operative Treatment in Acute Cases

In case of an acute ligament repair or reconstruction in patients with CPN palsy, the first thing we do is discuss how to position on the operating table and agree on a surgical approach that permits to do our technique for repair of the posterolateral structures and reconstruction (sport and knee team) and to explore and treat the CPN lesion (neuro orthopedic team) in the same operation. Usually we agree in placing the patient in a supine position with the knee and leg straight on a support unit, but with the possibility to flex the knee and holding this position. Generally, a lateral incision along the posterior biceps tendon that curve towards the Gerdy tubercle is selected (Fig. 27.5). With that approach we can elevate a vascularized cutaneous flap to expose the peroneal nerve along all its course from the intermuscular septum in the upper part to the fibular neck in the inferior part. This allows for a Gerdy tubercle osteotomy for ligament reconstruction and posterolateral complex structure repair. Once the approach is done, the next step is to evaluate all the soft tissue lesions and associated fractures and plan how to proceed to repair and reconstruct. After that, it is the time for nerve exploration and evaluation and to trace a plan for treatment or reconstruction. At this moment, we stop for a while and expose our specialized requirements and make a conjoint strategy to follow.

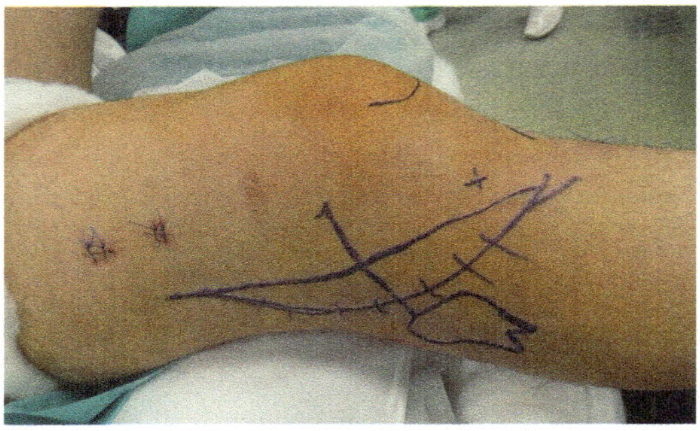

Fig. 27.5 Patient position in the table and surgical approach after agreement between sport and knee team and neuro orthopedic team that permits repair/reconstruction of the posterolateral structures and exploration and treatment of the CPN lesion in the same intervention

In our practice we found *different clinical situations in the acute period.*

The CPN is located and inspected, and *nerve is in continuity* with any sign of partial rupture. Usually there is an important diffuse or fusiform hematoma inside the epineurium of the nerve due to the rupture of the vasa nervorum. We palpate the nerve looking for internal disruption [40]. At this moment, it is only possible to electroestimulate the nerve or, if you have the adequate team of electroneurophysiologist, an intraoperative electroneurography may be performed looking for the nerve action potentials (NAP) along all the course of the nerve, from very high close to the intermuscular septum or even from the common sciatic nerve before it divides into peroneal and tibial, until the fibular neck level [32–35, 39, 41]. If NAP studies are correct and are transmitted across the lesion, then we only perform an external neurolysis, but also, very important, a longitudinal epineurotomy and internal neurolysis just to clean the hematoma inside the nerve (Fig. 27.6a–d). This hematoma acts as a compressive force inside the nerve and is similar to an intraneural compartment syndrome

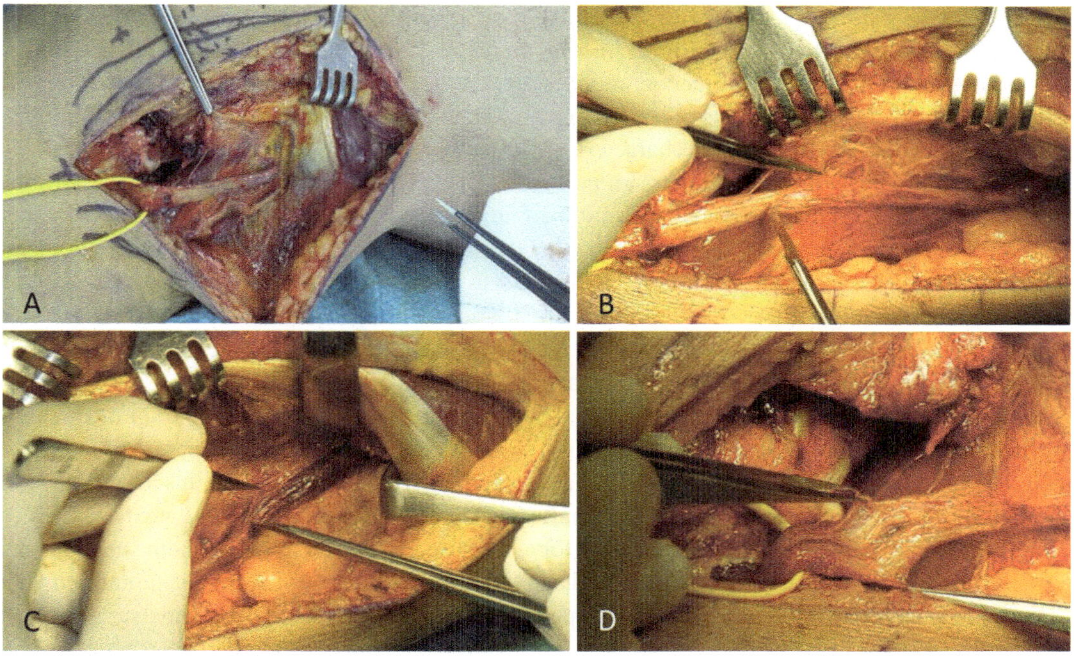

Fig. 27.6 Left knee. Peroneal nerve with important epineural thickening and fibrosis. After external neurolysis (**a**), a longitudinal epineurotomy is done (**b**) and limited internal neurolysis just to clean the hematoma inside the nerve and release the fascicles is performed (**c**). Final appearance (**d**). Hematoma, after some weeks leads to a fibrous tissue and scar formation, precluding nerve regeneration

and, after some weeks, leads to a fibrous tissue and scar formation, precluding nerve regeneration. This is the main reason we prefer to review the nerve early on. Nothing more is done, other than clinical follow-up, checks and electroneurophysiologic studies every 3 months. Kim and Kline [39] report their results of neurolysis performed at 6 months after injury in patients with different mechanism of lesion including stretch injury where 71–80 patients (89%) with transmittable NAP across lesions in continuity recovered useful function. If the NAP traces are negative or flat, the segment of nerve is resected, and a repair is done with a graft (depending on the length, we use the lateral cutaneous branch for short defects or the contralateral sural nerve for longer defects). At present nerve allograft is an option to consider, but promising experience with this technique is only at the initial stages. Allografts have a limitation in width (4–5 mm) and length (70 mm).

A second situation is when the *nerve is in continuity, but after exploration and release a partial rupture is suspected.* Again, electrostimulation and NAP studies are done to try to localize the non-functioning fascicles. Whenever possible we proceed to a partial graft using the lateral sural cutaneous branch as donor (with a vascularized pedicle or not) or an allograft. This situation is very infrequent.

Finally, the worst situation is when the *nerve is in discontinuity*. It could be *a frank discontinuity* or a tricky appearance where all the *intraneural structures are in discontinuity but the epineurium is in continuity* (a Sunderland grade 4 lesion); the latter, in delayed cases, looks as a *neuroma in continuity*. You must inspect very carefully all the length of the nerve, from the proximal part, close to the sciatic division, to the nerve division into superficial and deep peroneal branches, distal to the fibular neck. In the literature there are reports of neurolysis around the fibular head vicinity, but, if there is no recovery of the nerve, a second operation verified a very proximal nerve rupture [40].

Experience recommends not to trust the first impression and macroscopic aspect and to discard rupture of the nerve all along its course by direct visualization, palpation, and opening the epineurium to rule out a Sunderland grade 4 lesion (all the axons and perineurium are disrupted but the epineurium is still in continuity as shown in Fig. 27.7a–d)). This type of lesion is not suitable for nerve suture due to the characteristic pathological changes of traction or stretch nerve injuries [5, 32, 35], and the nerve ends should be trimmed until normal nerve tissue appears in order to receive an autograft from the contralateral sural nerve (Fig. 27.8a–d). At present, in some countries, there is a possibility to use an allograft (limitation in width (4–5 mm) and length (70 mm)).

In cases where the nerve is in discontinuity, initially the surgical attitude is to graft the gap; but at this point the defect length and graft length are very important in the prognosis for recovery of function of the nerve and muscles. There are many reports dealing with this specific topic [42, 43].

According to Bleton [44], 20 cm is the limit, beyond which functional regeneration is no longer obtained; other surgeons set this limit at 15 cm [45] and some others [33] at 6 cm. For our team, it is not only the length of the graft but also when you graft, because time is a very important factor in nerve regeneration and recovery. Kim [32] analyzes 318 CPN lesions with different injury mechanisms, and graft repair was performed in 138 patients at 6 months after diagnosis. Useful function was achieved in 75% of patients with grafts less than 6 cm, in 38% with grafts between 6 and 12 cm, and in 16% in grafts longer that 13 cm.

In our practice we proceed to graft the nerve gaps up to 12 cm in the acute cases but only up to 6 cm in the chronic cases. In this acute period we refuse to graft nerve defects longer than 12 cm because you need to recollect both sural nerves if you use autograft (allograft maximum length is 7 cm); besides, the risks (more surgical time, sural graft from both legs, etc.) and benefits (poor functional outcomes, not useful motor recovery, etc.) is not clear. Graft length is one of the main

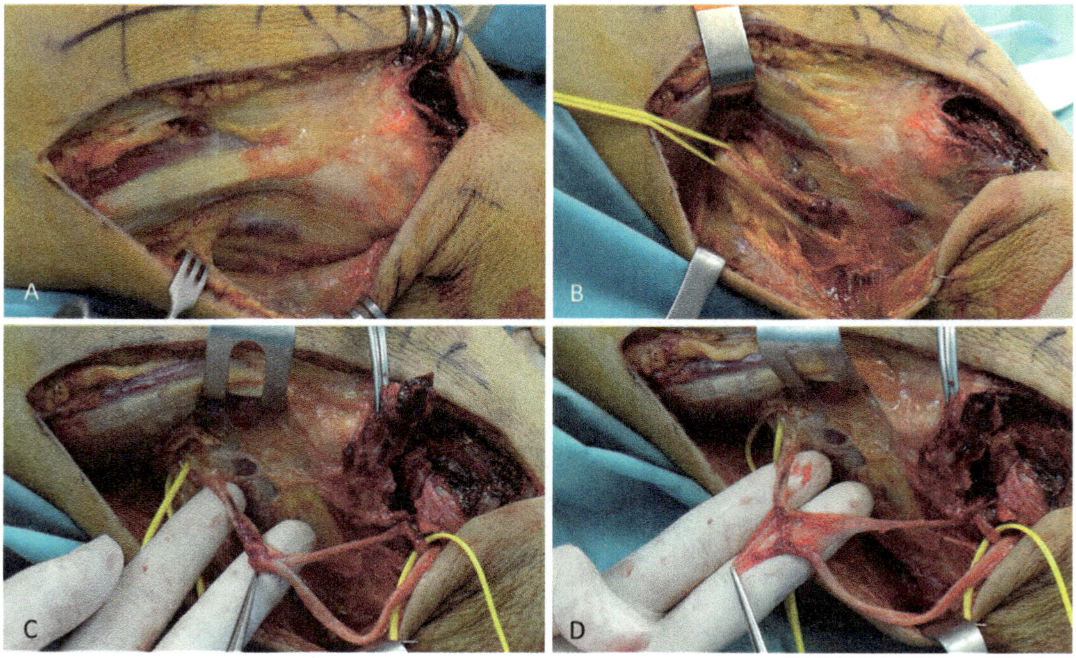

Fig. 27.7 Right knee. Harry Platt syndrome typical intraoperative anatomopathological findings: fibular head avulsion, through the biceps tendon insertion (upper and right corner), and a hematoma in relation to CPN (**a**) just behind the biceps femoris tendon; diffuse or fusiform hematoma inside the epineurium and stretch lesion of the peroneal nerve (**b**). Connective tissue damage occurs with intraneural tissue destruction (**c**). Even though it seems the CPN was initially in continuity in fact it was a Sunderland grade 4 injury, epineurium in continuity but perineurium and endoneurium totally disrupted (**d**)

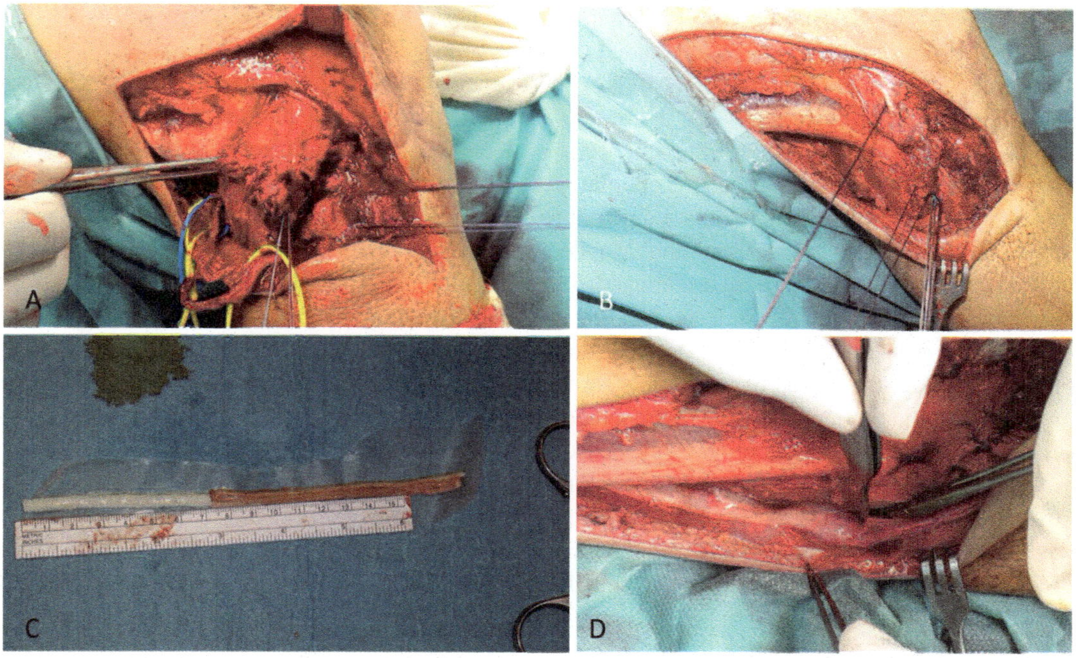

Fig. 27.8 Clinical case. Mechanism of injury: severe varus and hyperextension of the right knee. Typical avulsion of fibular head, biceps (marked with a suture) and lateral collateral ligament, and stretching of the peroneal nerve at the proximal part (marked with yellow vessel loops) (**a**). Aspect after ligament repair and reconstruction, and remaining a long nerve defect (**b**). Sural nerve autograft (right) for insertion and comparison with a nerve allograft (left) (**c**); In this patient we used conventional sural nerve graft with 9-0 nylon suture and fibrin adhesive (**d**)

factors to be considered in the recovery prognosis of nerve repair but time and patient age need to be considered too [33, 39]. Our group of patients use to be young, healthy and active sportsman but we must be realistic; We should clearly informed the patient and his family (before the operation) about the possibility of this severe and extensive nerve destruction and the possible future palliative treatments (poor results of long nerve graft and acceptable results of tendon transfers); in that cases, we put sutures as a reference at the nerve ends, just in case the patient decided to try a long grafting in the near future, associated or not to a tendon transfer.

The immediate postoperative treatment in case of neurolysis do not interfere with the general recommendations for the ligament repair and reconstruction. In case of nerve grafting, we only recommend limitation of the flexo-extension for 2 weeks and that do not interfere neither, except to take some care at dressing the wounds.

Depending on what surgical technique we used to manage the nerve lesion, we control the recovery with clinical examination every 6 weeks, and we order the first electrodiagnostic studies at 3 months, and from that on every 3-month intervals. Nerve recovery used to be very slow and depends on the initial severity of the injury, time to repair, quality of the repair, length of the lesion, the graft if used, associated vascular injury, and patient age [5, 34, 35], but usually it takes months or 1–2 years to recover. And some partial recovery is not useful enough or sometimes there is no recovery at all. That is a very negative situation for young active sportsmen, and you should be cautions when answering questions about the prognosis for nerve recovery.

Between 6 and 9 months, we need to reevaluate the whole situation. Sometimes a second-stage surgery for posterior cruciate or anterior cruciate ligament was planned, but very frequently this reconstruction is no longer needed because the nerve lesion sequela precluded their indication. This is one important factor to consider: evolution and recovery.

In cases with nerve revision in the acute period but with nerve defect longer than 12 cm that we refuse to graft initially, now is a good moment to explain to the patient the real situation. Maybe a good option could be to discard a nonmandatory surgery on the cruciate ligaments and try to improve the nerve palsy dysfunction. In our practice, we explain the option of long grafts for the nerve defect but without expecting a great recovery, perhaps some proprioception, some sensory improvement, and maybe some muscular function but probably not useful for dorsiflexing the ankle, and at the same time perform tendon transfers for ankle dorsiflexion and toe and hallux extension in a single stage.

27.5.2.2 Operative Treatment in Chronic Cases

In cases that the patient arrived to us at the chronic stage, the initial planification for posterolateral instability and nerve injury is similar to that in the acute stage. The nerve used to be difficult to individualize, and there is no hematoma to decompress, instead we found an important fibrosis around the nerve. We use intraoperative NAP across the lesion in the nerve in continuity and proceed in the same way as in the acute cases [33–35, 39]. The main difference is that we do not use grafts alone if the defect is longer than 6 cm; in that case we propose a one-stage nerve repair and tendon transfers [46–49] once the patient has recovered from the ligament repair or reconstruction [50], once rehabilitation of the knee is finished and trophic changes, and swelling and edema of the foot and leg have subside resolve. Acquired flatfoot does not appear to be a significant long-term complication despite the loss of a functioning tibialis posterior tendon [51] maybe in relation with the tendency to rigid deformity in equinovarus position or technical modifications [52]. The new tendency of nerve transfers advocates for using a branch of the tibial nerve to the motor branch of the tibialis anterior muscle [53–55] or a lateral gastrocnemius branch to tibialis anterior too [56–58]; we have a limited experience of one case with the latter technique, and we think it is better because of the synergism between gastrocnemius and tibials anterior (knee flexion and ankle dorsiflexion). Some authors proposed a free functional muscle transfer (latissimus dorsi, gracilis or rectus femoris muscle), but this is a very complex microsurgical procedure [59, 60], with a new donor area, and not useful strength for active sport practice. Even though we use this microsurgical technique in brachial plexus cases, in this paralysis we prefer tibialis posterior tendon transfer to the second cuneiform for reanimation of ankle dorsiflexion, and hemiabductor hallucis to extensor hallucis longus for hallux extension (Fig. 27.9a–d).

27.6 Take Home Message

As a general consideration, we would like to remark that nerve repair is one of the most important priorities to consider, and a timely operation and thorough evaluation and treatment by a multidisciplinary team are essential for good results. We recommend early exploration at the same time that of ligament reconstruction or repair. The anatomic appearance of a nerve in continuity in case of a possible stretch injury should be evaluated very carefully, and NAP studies be done. The length of the contusion or elongation in a non-ruptured nerve is predictive of recovery; If NAP traces are negative, the segment of nerve should be resected (if less than 6 cm) and grafted in the acute phase. Graft length is a prognostic factor for regrowth after interfascicular graft.

Functional prognosis for sport-related ligament knee injury associated with CPN palsy depends not only on ligament repair and healing but also on neurologic recovery; early intraneural hematoma decompression is a factor that could improve better recovery avoiding intraneural scar formation and permanent paralysis.

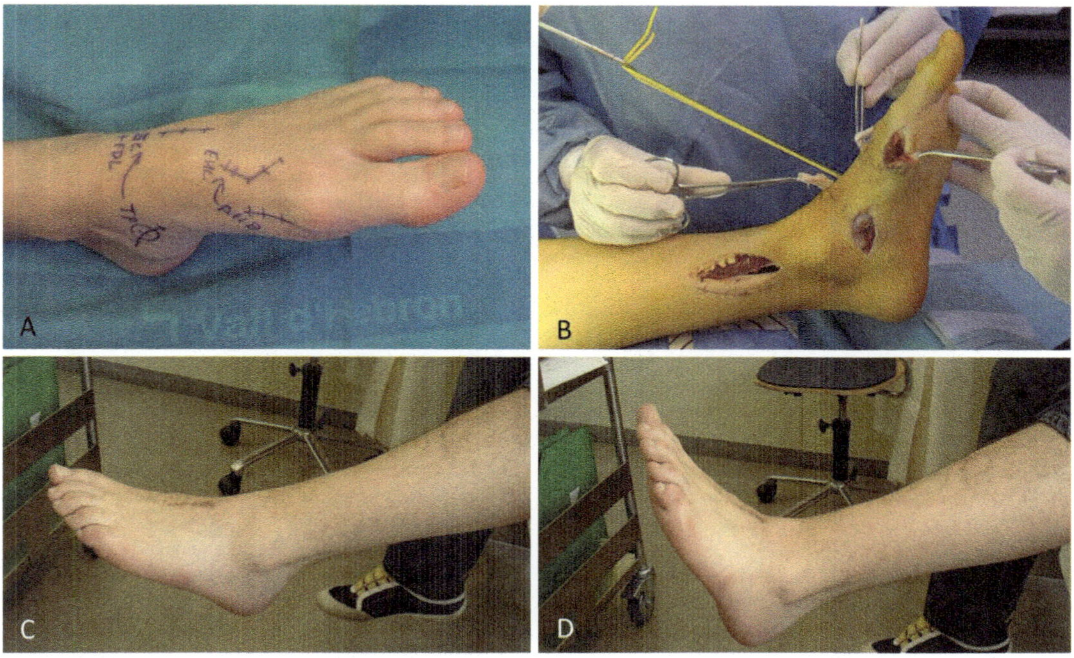

Fig. 27.9 Our tendon transfer technique of choice for CPN palsy: tibialis posterior tendon transfer to the second cuneiform for reanimation of ankle dorsiflexion and hemi-abductor hallucis to extensor hallucis longus for hallux extension. Left foot and ankle. Skin incisions (**a**). Tendon donors and receptors, before fixation (**b**). Clinical result in extension (**c**) and ankle dorsiflexion (**d**); notice de hallux position in both movements

References

1. Bonnevialle P, Dubrana F, Galau B, Lustig S, Barbier O, Neyret P, Rosset P, Saragaglia D, French Society of Orthopedic Surgery and Traumatology (SOFCOT). Common peroneal nerve palsy complicating knee dislocation and bicruciate ligaments tears. Orthop Traumatol Surg Res. 2010;96:64–9.
2. Cho D, Saetia K, Lee S, Kline DG, Kim DH. Peroneal nerve injury associated with sports-related knee injury. Neurosurg Focus. 2011;31:1–8.
3. Seddon HJ. A classification of nerve injuries. Br Med J. 1942;2:237–9.
4. Sunderland S. A classification of peripheral nerve injuries producing loss of function. Brain. 1951;74:491–516.
5. Birch R. Surgical disorders of the peripheral nerves. 2nd ed. London: Springer; 2011. isbn:978-1-84882-107-1.
6. Poage C, Roth C, Scott B. Peroneal nerve palsy: evaluation and management. J Am Acad Orthop Surg. 2016;24:1–10.
7. Bonnevialle P, Chaufour X, Loustau O, Mansat P, Pidhorz L, Mansat M. Traumatic knee dislocation with popliteal vascular disruption: retrospective study of 14 cases. Rev Chir Orthop Reparatrice Appar Mot. 2006;92:768–77.
8. Llusa M, Meri A, Ruano D. Manual y atlas fotográfico de anatomía del aparato locomotor. 1st ed. Madrid: Editorial Panamericana; 2004. isbn-10: 8479037849.
9. Platt H. On the peripheral nerve complications of certain fractures. J Bone Joint Surg. 1928;10:403–14.
10. Djian P. Posterolateral knee reconstruction. Orthop Traumatol Surg Res. 2015;101:s159–70.
11. Oshima T, Nakase J, Numata H, Takata Y, Tsuchiya H. Common peroneal nerve palsy with multiple-ligament knee injury and distal avulsion of the biceps femoris tendon. Case Rep Orthop. 2015;2015:306260, 6 pages.
12. Yeh WL, Tu YK, Su JY, Hsu RW. Knee dislocation: treatment of high-velocity knee dislocation. J Trauma. 1999;46:693–701.
13. Bonnevialle N, Delannis Y, Beaulieu JY, Martinel V, Mansat P, Bonnevialle P. Paralysie du nerf fibulaire commun dans les lux-ations traumatiques du genou. Rev Chir Orthop. 2006;92(Suppl. VI):3S131.
14. Johnson ME, Foster L, de Lee JC. Neurologic and vascular injuries associated with knee ligament injuries. Am J Sports Med. 2008;36:2448–62.
15. Niall DM, Nutton RW, Keating JF. Palsy of the common peroneal nerve after traumatic dislocation of the knee. J Bone Joint Surg Br. 2005;87:664–7.
16. Boisrenoult P, Lustig S, Bonneviale P, Leray E, Versier G, Neyret P, Rosset P, Saragaglia D, the French Society of Orthopedic Surgery and Traumatology

(SOFCOT). Vascular lesions associated with bicruciate and knee dislocation ligamentous injury. Orthop Traumatol Surg Res. 2009;95:621–6.
17. Wascher DC, Dvirnak PC, De Coster TA. Knee dislocation: initial assessment and implications for treatment. J Orthop Trauma. 1997;11:525–9.
18. Koffler KM, Kelly JD IV. Neurovascular trauma in athletes. Orthop Clin North Am. 2002;33:523–34.
19. Green NE, Allen BL. Vascular injuries associated with dislocation of the knee. J Bone Joint Surg Am. 1977;59:236–9.
20. Hegyes MS, Richardson MW, Miller MD. Knee dislocation. Complication of non-operative and operative management. Clin Sports Med. 2000;19:519–43.
21. Gakhal MS, Sartip KA. CT angiography signs of lower extremity vascular trauma. AJR Am J Roentgenol. 2009;193:49–57.
22. Redmond JM, Levy BA, Dajani KA, Cass JR, Cole PA. Detecting vascular injury in lower-extremity orthopedic trauma: the role of CT angiography. Orthopedics. 2008;31:761–7.
23. Peng PD, Spain DA, Tataria M, Hellinger JC, Rubin GD, Brundage SI. CT angiography effectively evaluates extremity vascular trauma. Am Surg. 2008;74:103–7.
24. Gable DR, Allen JW, Richardson JD. Blunt popliteal artery injury: is physical examination alone enough for evaluation. J Trauma. 1997;43:541–4.
25. Bynoe RP, Miles WS, Bell RM, Greenwold DR, Sessions G, Haynes JL, et al. Noninvasive diagnosis of vascular trauma by duplex ultrasonography. J Vasc Surg. 1991;14:346–52.
26. Miranda FE, Dennis JW, Veldenz HC, Dovgan PS, Frykberg ER. Confirmation of the safety and accuracy of physical examination in the evaluation of knee dislocation for injury of the popliteal artery: a prospective study. J Trauma. 2002;52:247–52.
27. McCutchan JD, Gilham NR. Injury to the popliteal artery associated with dislocation of the knee: palpable distal pulses do not negate the requirement for arteriography. Injury. 1989;20:307–10.
28. Twaddle BC, Hunter JC, Chapman JR, Simonian PT, Escobedo EM. MRI in acute knee dislocation. A prospective study of clinical, MRI, and surgical findings. J Bone Joint Surg Br. 1996;78:573–9.
29. Yu JS, Goodwin D, Salonen D, Pathria MN, Resnick D, Dardani M, et al. Complete dislocation of the knee; spectrum of associated soft-tissue injuries depicted by MR imaging. AJR Am J Roentgenol. 1995;164:135–9.
30. Potter HG, Weinstein M, Allen AA, Wickiewicz TL, Helfet DL. Magnetic resonance imaging of the multiple-ligament injured knee. J Orthop Trauma. 2002;16:330–9.
31. Gruber H, Peer S, Meirer R, Bodner G. Peroneal nerve palsy associated with knee luxation: evaluation by sonography initial experience. AJR Am J Roentgenol. 2005;185:1118–25.
32. Kim DH, Murovic JA, Tiel RL, Kline DG. Management and out-comes in 318 operative common peroneal nerve lesions at the Louisiana State University Health Sciences Center. Neurosurgery. 2004;54:1421–8.
33. Kline DG. Surgical repair of peripheral nerve injury. Muscle Nerve. 1990;13:843–52.
34. Kim D, Midha R, Murovic JA, Spinner RJ. Kline and Hudson's nerve injuries. 2nd ed. Philadelphia: Saunders; 2007. isbn: 9780721695372.
35. Kline DG, Hudson AR, Kim DH. Atlas of peripheral nerve lesions. 1st ed. Philadelphia: Saunders; 2000. isbn-10: 721679889.
36. Krych AJ, Giuseffi SA, Kuzma SA, Stuart MJ, Levy BA. Is peroneal nerve injury associated with worse function after knee dislocation? Clin Orthop Relat Res. 2014;472:2630–6.
37. Azar FM, Brandt JC, Miller RH III, Phillips BB. Ultra-low-velocity knee dislocations. Am J Sports Med. 2011;39:2170–4.
38. Georgiadis AG, Guthrie ST, Shepard AD. Beware of ultra-low-velocity knee dislocation. Orthopedics. 2014;37:656–8.
39. Kim DH, Kline DG. Management and results of peroneal nerve lesions. Neurosurgery. 1996;39:319–20.
40. Tomaino M, Day C, Pagageorgiou C, Harner C, Fu FH. Peroneal nerve palsy following knee dislocation: patho-anatomy and implications for treatment. Knee Surg Sports Traumatol Arthrosc. 2000;8:163–5.
41. Prasad AR, Steck JK, Dellon AL. Zone of traction injury of the common peroneal nerve. Ann Plast Surg. 2007;59:302–6.
42. Peskun C, Chahal J, Steinfeld Z, Whelan D. Risk factors for peroneal nerve injury and recovery in knee dislocation. Clin Orthop Relat Res. 2012;470:74–7.
43. Verdú E, Ceballos D, Vilches JJ, Navarro X. Influence of aging on peripheral nerve function and regeneration. J Peripher Nerv Syst. 2000;5:191–208.
44. Bleton R, Alnot JY, Oberlin C. Les lésions traumatiques du tronc du nerf sciatique et ses branches terminales. Rev Chir Orthop Reparatrice Appar Mot. 1993;79:205–17.
45. Piton C, Fabre T, Lasseur E, Andre D, Geneste M, Durandeau A. Les lésions du nerf fibulaire commun: approche diagnostiqueet thérapeutique. Rev Chir Orthop Reparatrice Appar Mot. 1997;83:515–21.
46. Garozzo D, Ferraresi S, Buffatti P. Common peroneal nerve injuries in knee dislocations: results with one-stage nerve repair and tibialis posterior tendon transfer. J Orthop Traumatol. 2002;2:135–7.
47. Ferraresi S, Garozzo D, Buffati P. Common peroneal nerve injuries; results with one-stage nerve repair and tendon transfer. Neurosurg Rev. 2003;26:175–9.
48. Garozzo D, Ferraresi S, Buffatti P. Surgical treatment of common peroneal nerve injuries: indications and results. A series of 62 cases. J Neurosurg Sci. 2004;48:105–12.
49. Hove LM, Nilsen PT. Posterior tibial tendon transfer for drop foot. Acta Orthop Scand. 1998;69:608–10.
50. Ohkoshi Y, Nagasaki S, Shibata N, Yamamoto K, Hashimoto T, Yamane S. Two stage reconstruction

with auto grafts for knee dislocations. Clin Orthop. 2002;398:169–75.
51. Yeap JS, Birch R, Singh D. Long-term results of tibialis posterior tendon transfer for drop-foot. Int Orthop. 2001;25:114–8.
52. Vigasio A, Marcoccio I, Patelli A, Mattiuzzo V, Prestini G. New tendon transfer for correction of drop-foot in common peroneal nerve palsy. Clin Orthop Relat Res. 2008;466:1454–66.
53. Nath RK, Lyons AB, Paizi M. Successful management of foot drop by nerve transfers to the deep peroneal nerve. J Reconstr Microsurg. 2008;24:419–27.
54. Giuseffi SA, Bishop AT, Shin AY, Dahm DL, Stuart MJ, Levy BA. Surgical treatment of peroneal nerve palsy after knee dislocation. Knee Surg Sports Traumatol Arthrosc. 2010;18:1583–6.
55. Ninković M, Ninković M. Neuromusculotendinous transfer: an original surgical concept for the treatment of drop foot with long-term follow-up. Plast Reconstr Surg. 2013;132:438e–45e.
56. Bodily KD, Spinner RJ, Bishop AT. Restoration of motor function of the deep fibular (peroneal) nerve by direct nerve transfer of branches from the tibial nerve: an anatomical study. Clin Anat. 2004;17:201–5.
57. Flores LP. Proximal motor branches from the tibial nerve as direct donors to restore function of the deep fibular nerve for treatment of high sciatic nerve injuries: a cadaveric feasibility study. Neurosurgery. 2009;65:218–24.
58. Strazar R, White CP, Bain J. Foot reanimation via nerve transfer to the peroneal nerve using the nerve branch to the lateral gastrocnemius: case report. J Plast Reconstr Aesthet Surg. 2011;64:1380–2.
59. Wechselberger G, Ninkovic M, Pülzl P, Schoeller T. Free functional rectus femoris muscle transfer for restoration of knee extension and defect coverage after trauma. J Plast Reconstr Aesthet Surg. 2006;59:994–8.
60. Lin CH, Lin YT, Yeh JT, Chen CT. Free functioning muscle transfer for lower extremity posttraumatic composite structure and functional defect. Plast Reconstr Surg. 2007;119:2118–26.

28 Biological Therapies in Orthopedics and Sports Medicine

Gonzalo Samitier, Eduard Alentorn-Geli, Giuseppe Filardo, Rocco Aicale, Filippo Rosati Tarulli, Nicola Maffulli, Ewa Trams, Katarzyna-Kozar Kaminska, Stanislaw Pomianowski, Rafal Kaminski, Mikel Sánchez, Diego Delgado, Ane Garate, Pello Sánchez, Ane Miren Bilbao, Nicolás Fiz, Ignacio Dallo, Vetri Kumar, Alberto Gobbi, and Ramón Cugat

G. Samitier (✉) · E. Alentorn-Geli · R. Cugat
Instituto Cugat, Hospital Quirónsalud Barcelona, Barcelona, Spain
e-mail: gsamitier@sportstrauma.com; ealentorn@sportrauma.com; info@fundaciongarciacugat.org

G. Filardo
Rizzoli Orthopaedic Institute, Bologna, Italy
e-mail: ortho@gfilardo.com

R. Aicale · F. R. Tarulli
Department of Musculoskeletal Disorders, Faculty of Medicine and Surgery, University of Salerno, Baronissi, Italy

Clinica Ortopedica, Ospedale San Giovanni di Dio e Ruggi D'Aragona, Salerno, Italy

N. Maffulli
Department of Musculoskeletal Disorders, Faculty of Medicine and Surgery, University of Salerno, Baronissi, Italy

Clinica Ortopedica, Ospedale San Giovanni di Dio e Ruggi D'Aragona, Salerno, Italy

Queen Mary University of London, Barts and the London School of Medicine and Dentistry, Centre for Sports and Exercise Medicine, Mile End Hospital, London, UK

Keele University, School of Medicine, Institute of Science and Technology in Medicine, Guy Hilton Research Centre, Stoke-on-Trent, UK
e-mail: n.maffulli@qmul.ac.uk

E. Trams · K.-K. Kaminska · S. Pomianowski
R. Kaminski
Department of Musculoskeletal Trauma Surgery and Orthopaedics, Postgraduate Center for Medical Education, Professor A. Gruca Teaching Hospital, Otwock, Poland

Department of Medical Biology, The Cardinal Stefan Wyszynski Institute of Cardiology, Warsaw, Poland

M. Sánchez
Arthroscopic Surgery Unit, Hospital Vithas San José, Vitoria-Gasteiz, Spain

Advanced Biological Surgery Unit, Hospital Vithas San José, Vitoria-Gasteiz, Spain
e-mail: mikel.sanchez@ucatrauma.com

D. Delgado · A. Garate · P. Sánchez
Advanced Biological Surgery Unit, Hospital Vithas San José, Vitoria-Gasteiz, Spain

A. M. Bilbao · N. Fiz
Arthroscopic Surgery Unit, Hospital Vithas San José, Vitoria-Gasteiz, Spain

I. Dallo
Unit of Regenerative Therapy and Arthroscopic Surgery, Sanatorio Garay, Santa Fe, Argentina

V. Kumar · A. Gobbi
Orthopaedic Arthroscopic Surgery International (OASI), Bioresearch Foundation, Milan, Italy
e-mail: gobbi@cartilagedoctor.it

M. T. Hirschmann et al. (eds.), *ESSKA Instructional Course Lecture Book*,
https://doi.org/10.1007/978-3-662-61264-4_28

28.1 Understanding What PRPs Are and How They Work

Platelet-rich plasma (PRP) is a blood derivative, produced by centrifugation or filtration of the whole blood to concentrate or isolate platelets to a level higher (generally considered 3–5 times more) than normal plasma levels [1]. The reason for this variability in platelet concentration is explained by the many different methods available to produce PRP (e.g., different centrifugation protocols and the development of several commercial kits) [2]. This contributed to generate confusion in literature, as there are several products which may differ in terms of effects and indications, which hampers the possibility to compare studies and understand the real effectiveness of PRP in the several applications and study conditions.

Regardless of the production methods and the platelet concentration, PRP is characterized by a high concentration of a large composition of growth factors and cytokines involved in both healing process and immunoregulation. These biological mediators are released by exocytosis of the platelet α-granules (as well as by the membrane disruption which might occur during manipulation of this blood derivative) after their activation with an initial burst followed by further sustained release. To this regard, there are actually different methods to activate PRP, which might influence the release curve, but calcium chloride is currently the most common. In particular, 5% calcium chloride seems to be effective to obtain a high concentration of biological mediators in PRP, although some products are also promoted without the use of an activator, relying on the spontaneous activation induced in by the contact with the collagen in situ once PRP is injected [3].

The high amount of GFs released is responsible for the multiple effects of PRP, such as the anabolic effect and the enhancement of cell proliferation and differentiation, vessels remodeling, modulation of inflammation and immunoregulation, promotion of cell migration and synthesis of extracellular matrix proteins [4–7]. In particular, among the most studied GFs secreted by platelets are included vascular endothelial growth factor (VEGF), fibroblast growth factor (FGF), platelet-derived growth factor (PDGF), insulin-like growth factor-1 (IGF-1), interleukin-10 (IL-10), transforming growth factor-β1 (TGF-β1), epidermal growth factor (EGF), hepatocyte growth factor (HGF), etc. [2, 8].

The effects of these GFs have been extensively analyzed through in vitro and in vivo studies [2, 4–10]: TGF-β1 has been shown to enhance matrix deposition and induce chondrogenic differentiation and cell proliferation, and it downregulates type-I collagen gene expression and upregulates type-II collagen (like in hyaline cartilage) and proteoglycans expression in contrast to the effect of IL-1; moreover, it induces migration toward the site of injury, proliferation, and chondrogenic differentiation of bone marrow stromal cells (BMSCs). VEGF is a signal protein involved in angiogenesis, together with other angiogenic factors.

FGF stimulates the proliferation of fibroblasts and contributes to angiogenesis.

PDGF stimulates cell proliferation and angiogenesis, and it has a mitogenic role for fibroblast. IGF-1 enhances matrix deposition and stimulates cell proliferation and fibroblast differentiation; moreover, it is a mediator in growth and repair of skeletal muscle; recent evidences has identified in the IGF-1 a possible inhibitor of apoptosis, regulating the expression of the PDCD 5 protein [11]. EGF stimulates proliferation and migration of mesenchymal and epithelial cells. HGF stimulates angiogenesis and proliferation of endothelial cells, and it has an anti-fibrotic role and increases the level of anti-inflammatory cytokines. IL-10 is an anti-inflammatory cytokine.

Besides the biological rationale, current evidence further supports the role of PRP in modulating the intra-articular environment by affecting inflammation in degenerative joint diseases: after an initial pro-inflammatory action, with the stimulation of synoviocytes to release metalloproteinases and cytokines, a following phase of modulation and reduction of the inflammatory response has been demonstrated, with a decrease in pro-inflammatory cytokines, contrasting the chemotaxis of monocyte-like cells [12]. Moreover, pre-clinical literature also showed an analgesic effect of PRP, possibly by increasing cannabinoid receptors [13]. Based on this evidence, it is important to underline that PRP may not directly promote tissue regeneration, but it may rather act through its different bioactive molecules affecting tissue homeostasis, slowing down the catabolic and degenerative processes, and offering a benefit in terms of symptom relief and functional improvement.

Thanks to these biological effects, PRPs have found different clinical applications over the years, from dentistry, maxillo-facial surgery, plastic surgery, dermatology, to even orthopedic surgery with different evidences of effectiveness. The confusion regarding the effectiveness of PRPs mostly derives from the aforesaid different procedures for its production, with different features in terms of platelets, leucocytes, and fibrin content, which may cause different biological and mechanical characteristics. For this reasons, in 2009 Dohan Ehrenfest et al. divided PRP into four categories according to the fibrin architecture and the leucocyte content: pure platelet-rich plasma (P-PRP), leukocyte- and platelet-rich plasma (L-PRP), pure platelet-rich fibrin (P-PRF), leukocyte- and platelet-rich fibrin (L-PRF) [14]. Each category presents some major specificities, but also inside the same category, each different product has its own individual identity. For example, several studies evaluated the different behavior of PRF and PRP, revealing that PRF remains solid and intact and continues to release a large quantity of growth factors produced by the cell population longer. PRP, instead, releases most of its growth factors in the first hours, although a sustained release has been demonstrated by some more concentrated blood derivatives [14, 15].

Another parameter of this classification is the presence/absence of leukocytes. Some authors argue that the presence of leukocytes can provide a stimulation of the inflammatory process, while other authors argue that the presence of leukocyte [16] in PRP may increase growth factors and anti-pain mediators production [17, 18], also providing an antimicrobical activity [19]; in general, leukocytes have a key role in the regulation of inflammatory and healing processes, but this remains nowadays one of the most important discussed point about PRPs. Regardless of these differences, PRPs have been applied in clinical practice, showing promising results as minimally invasive treatments for knee osteoarthritis, where it seems to provide a short-term symptomatic benefit [20]. However, although the general biological rationale for the use of PRPs is known, and despite some promising clinical findings, further studies are still needed to better understand the different biological and clinical effects of the different formulations, as well as the best way to exploit PRP properties to provide better clinical results and to identify the best indications for the use of PRPs.

28.2 Growth Factors for the Treatment of Myotendinous Injuries

With the increasing prevalence of acute muscle injuries associated with competitive sport, there has been an increased interest in optimizing treatment strategies for athletes who suffered these lesions. Clinical examination and imaging are the bases for the diagnosis of muscle injury, in particular magnetic resonance imaging (MRI) and ultrasound (US) are mainstay of imaging, and both modalities have demonstrated good specificity and sensitivity for tendinopathy or tears [21–23]. During the last few years, platelet-rich plasma (PRP) used to speed up and improve the healing of muscles and tendons, modulate inflammation mediators, decrease time to return to sports, and improve activities of daily living [24] and has become popular.

As we explained previously, PRP is obtained centrifuging autologous blood to separate it into layers based on the density of the contents. Platelets and leukocytes are separated from erythrocytes, and further centrifuging increases the concentration of each component. In addition, thrombin and calcium, which are activating agents, can be added to serum to begin the release of growth factors, or PRP can be injected and activation occurs when it comes into contact with collagen [24, 25].

The main component of PRP are the platelets, which can mediate the release of several growth factors essential in the healing process. Various formulations of PRP are on the market, and there is speculation regarding the benefit of leukocyte-rich (LR) versus leukocyte-poor (LP) PRP [25]. A recent study comparing LR and LP PRP formulations for tendinopathy demonstrated a better histologic healing response with LP PRP, possibly from a higher concentration of catabolic cytokine such as IL-6, in LR preparations [26].

During the healing response, the inflammatory phase is important, but an excessive reaction and duration of this phase can increase pain, fibrosis, and ring scar [27]. For this reason, the optimal platelet and leukocyte concentrations actually remain unclear.

In orthopedic practice, benefits have been shown with the use of PRP for the management of conditions such as lateral epicondylitis, knee osteoarthritis, rotator cuff tendinopathy, patellar tendinopathy, Achilles tendinopathy, and plantar fasciitis [28–33]. Conversely, surgical repair such as anterior cruciate ligament reconstruction, rotator cuff repair, Achilles tendon repair, and fracture healing have not been shown to benefit from the application of PRP [34–36].

Basic science research demonstrated that muscle regeneration and myogenesis depend on paracrine growth factors such as insulin-like growth factor-1 (IGF-1), hepatocyte growth factor (HGF), fibroblast growth factor 2 (FGF-2), transforming growth factor-ß1 (TGF-ß1), tumor necrosis factor-a (TNF-a), platelet-derived growth factor (PDGF), and prostaglandins (PG). Moreover, a single study demonstrated that the addition to PRP of an antifibrotic agent, such as Losartan, enhances muscle healing by stimulating regeneration and angiogenesis and preventing fibrosis [37].

A recent work [27] has investigated the time of return to sport and the risk for reinjury after acute grade 2 muscle lesions in recreational group of patients and competitive athletes treated with or without PRP. Statistically significant difference ($p = 0.001$) was found between these two groups with a mean time to return to sport of 21.1 days for the PRP group and 25 days for the control group [27]. Delos et al. reported no complications from PRP injections and a return to sport in half the time compared to athletes not treated with PRP, but no control group was available for comparison [38]. In 2014, a randomized controlled trial [39] examined outcomes for the use of PRP in acute grade 2 hamstring injuries, with a return to play of 26.7 days compared to 42.5 days for the control groups ($p < 0.001$), but no statistical significance was found in the overall VAS pain scores [39]. A recent systematic review [40] evaluated return to sport in 268 athletes (mean age 25 years) treated with or without PRP for acute muscle injuries in different sports, with 12 months follow-up. Soccer was the most common sport for acute muscle injury at 69.2%, the difference in time to return to sport between the groups was 6 days in favor of PRP [40]. Furthermore, while for acute 1 or 2 muscle strains, there was a significant reduction in time to return to sport with no increased risk for re-rupture at 6 months, acute grade 1 or 2 hamstring strains showed no difference in time of return to sport compared with the control group [40].

Conversely, some additional studies challenge the clinical utility of this treatment, for example, Hamilton et al. [41] comparing the use of PRP injection, platelet-poor plasma (PPP) injection, and no injection, reported that the mean time of return to sport was 21 days in the first group, 27 days in the PPP group, and 25 days in the no injection group. Comparing PRP and PPP, there was a significant difference in favor of PRP ($p = 0.01$), with no significant difference between PRP and no injection groups ($p = 0.210$). Reinjury rate at 6 months posttreatment showed no difference between the groups. A meta-analysis evaluated six studies, among which only two were randomized controlled trials, analyzing the effect of PRP for the management of acute muscle injuries comparing the use of placebo injection or physical therapy [42]. The time to return to sport was significantly shorter in patients treated with PRP with a mean difference of 7.17 days ($p < 0.05$). However, considering that in this meta-analysis only studies ($n = 3$) dealt with hamstring injuries, no significant differences were found between the groups [42].

In summary little evidence and a low number of studies exist demonstrating a clear benefit of PRP, and the comparisons between outcomes studies are limited by variability in design, PRP preparation, or application techniques; moreover, reinjury rates are reported only in some studies. More studies are needed to better understand the role of PRP in the management of acute muscle and tendon strains.

28.3 Growth Factors for the Treatment of Ligamentous Injuries

28.3.1 Ligament Structure and Composition

Ligaments are key joint elements since they connect the bones to each other and provide stability to the joint. However, these bands of fibrous tissue have a structure and composition that condition their regenerative properties and therefore their ability to repair. Said composition is characterized by a high water content compared to the solid material, most of which is extracellular matrix dotted with a small number of fibroblasts that are also responsible for the maintenance and repair of this tissue.

The most predominant protein in the ligament is collagen, which is mostly organized in collagen fibers type I, with a much lower presence of fibers type 3. Due to the torsion and traction forces to which the ligaments are subjected, these collagen fibers adopt a wide variety of directions and orientations. Other extracellular matrix proteins present in ligaments are proteoglycans, elastin, actin, laminins, and integrins [43].

Microvascularity and nerve ending reach the ligaments through the epiligament providing proprioception and nociception. All these structural characteristics allow the ligaments an optimal mechanical and visco-elastic behavior for their stabilization function in addition to detect and control the position and the movement of the knee.

However, this excellent organization for the performance of joint functions is limited in terms of regenerative properties, which are also hampered by the poor vascularization of the ligaments. Consequently, they are structures with little capacity for repair after injury and that also are susceptible to relapse. Thus, the use of biological therapies that stimulate the regenerative processes is a promising tool in this kind of lesions [44].

28.3.2 Ligament Repair Process

In the manner of other musculoskeletal injuries and PRP applications, it is necessary to understand the repair processes that occur in the ligament after an injury in order to maximize the therapeutic properties of PRP. Actions such as strong impacts or abrupt direction changes cause the rupture of ligaments due to the large excess of mechanical energy they generate. As a consequence of this rupture, both the extracellular matrix and vascularization are affected, generating extravasation of plasma in the injured tissue as well as in the adjacent areas [45]. The signals generated at this stage attract cellular elements, namely endothelial cells, macrophages, platelet, and mesenchymal stem cells (MSCs), which are activated and migrate from their niches to the injured site. Because of biomolecules, growth factors, and cytokines released by these cells, symptoms such as heat, edema, pain, and dysfunction appear to protect the knee from further damage. Along with this cell migration, an angiogenesis occurs through which new vessels as well as new extracellular matrix are synthesized. Next, a fibrin clot is formed where platelet and MSCs are anchored, releasing more biomolecules that favor repair process [46]. All these steps lead to the formation of a scar of granular tissue in which the proteins, mainly the collagen type I and III, are synthesized by fibroblasts. The last and longest stage is the remodeling of the tissue where cellularity and vascularity decrease.

Therefore, the biological element is essential in ligament repair, and it is necessary to take it into consideration for an optimal healing. Biological therapies such as PRP or MSCs contain or synthetize biomolecules that can modulate and optimize these repair processes. Associating the biological therapies in the anterior cruciate ligament reconstruction surgery could be a great advance due to the great variability of results in this surgery [47]. They would help to enhance the key aspects that influence the failure or not of reconstruction such as the integration of anchor points or the remodeling of the graft, promoting safer rehabilitation and a faster return to activity.

28.3.3 Biological Action of Platelet-Rich Plasma in Ligament Injuries

The therapeutic action of PRP is based on increased concentrations of platelets with respect to blood levels and the absence of harmful elements for the articulation such as red blood cells. In addition, being an autologous product makes this therapy completely personalized with high patient safety. The activation of the platelets present in the PRP causes the active biomolecules that reside in their granules to be released and together with the circulating plasma molecules form a biological cocktail capable of mimicking and modulating the physiological process of tissue repair [44]. This biological regulation carried out by the growth factors takes place throughout all the phases of the healing process explained above.

Thus, an exaggerated initial inflammatory response in a ligament injury that could lead to fibrosis and limit recovery could be attenuated by growth factors such as hepatocyte growth factor (HGF) and insulin-like growth factor (IGF-1). These molecules act on the NF-kB cellular signaling pathway, inhibiting their inflammatory tissue stimulation and thereby generating an anti-inflammatory effect [48]. Other growth factors within the PRP enhance the processes related to the activity of the cells and their arrival at the area of the lesion. Platelet-derived growth factor (PDGF) and transforming growth factor-β (TGF-β), for instance, stimulate the activation, migration, and proliferation of different cell populations, including MSCs, and VEGF is a key protein in neovascularization [49]. Finally, in the new tissue formation phase, several studies have demonstrated the importance of fibroblast growth factor (FGF) in the stimulation of the processes that lead to the synthesis of collagen and in the proliferation of fibroblasts, both are key elements in the structure and composition of the ligaments [50, 51].

In vivo studies confirmed that the application of biological stimuli based on PRP improves the recovery and quality of repaired tissue. Hildebrand et al. observed that the application of growth factors in a rabbit model of acute collateral ligament injury favored the biomechanical properties of the ligament in the repair of early stages [52]. In another study carried out in a porcine model of anterior ligament reconstruction, the authors demonstrated that the application of a collagen-platelet composite improved the structural properties of the graft and reduced early knee laxity [53]. Zhang et al. also studied the application of PRP-based therapies for anterior cruciate ligament reconstruction in rabbits. They combined PRP with a gelatin sponge and achieved bone marrow MSC proliferation, osteogenic gene expression, and early healing process at the tendon–bone junction [54].

The translation of these findings achieved in basic research to clinical practice has generated variable although promising results [55]. This variability of the outcomes could be due to the early stage of the use of PRP in this type of surgery, whose protocols are neither optimized nor standardized, and their application is very heterogeneous. In some cases, the choice of PRP can be key since the use of leukocyte-rich plasma could hinder the anti-inflammatory action [56, 57] so the results when used in this surgery could not be as expected [58, 59]. In addition, the application of PRP is also an important factor to obtain the adequate result. When applying the PRP, it is necessary to cover all the elements of the surgery, injecting both the tunnels and the graft. This favors the ligamentization of the tendons used as graft, an antiapoptotic effect on it and a better bone integration [44]. The lack of application on any of these components could lead to a decrease in the effectiveness of the technique [36, 59, 60]. Authors of several works observed improvements in aspects such as bone tunnel [61], joint stability [59], and return to previous level of activity without surgery in patients without partial ACL tears [62]. More clinical studies are necessary to optimize both the type of PRP and the application protocol used in ligament injuries.

However, the outpatient or surgical application of this technique in a tissue with a low regenerative capacity is a promising tool in these pathologies. Its biological action together with the mechanical stimuli generated during physiotherapeutic work would achieve an optimal recovery. To that end, it is necessary both to understand the mechanism of action of PRP and to administrate it properly.

28.3.4 Application of Platelet-Rich Plasma in Ligament Injuries

28.3.4.1 Anterior Cruciate Ligament Reconstruction by Arthroscopy Associated with PRP

Next, the application of PRP at different times during the reconstruction of anterior cruciate ligament by arthroscopic surgery is described in order to leverage the biological stimuli in key aspects of the surgery (Fig. 28.1) [44, 63]. These points can also be transferred to other ligaments that require surgery.

Before inducing anesthesia, the volume of peripheral venous blood needed is withdrawn to obtain the required amount of PRP that will be applied during surgery. Part of the PRP will be activated with calcium chloride to allow a fibrin clot/membrane to form and place it at the end of surgery in the donor region of the tendon or bone-tendon-bone if it has been used as autograft.

The steps followed during surgery include the usual arthroscopic assessment of the joint, cleaned of remaining LCA, chondroplasty, and the obtention of autografts if their use has been selected. In addition, a bed of bleeding bone is created, which will provide cells and proteins that enhance the integration of the graft. Regardless of whether allografts or autografts are used, they are infiltrated with activated PRP as well as soaked in a recipient with PRP until implantation. The activation of PRP with calcium chloride prior to infiltrations performed during surgery not only causes the release of platelet content but also prevents local hypocalcemia.

When generating the tunnels, and in case the chosen surgical technique involves the use and extraction of bone plugs, these will also be

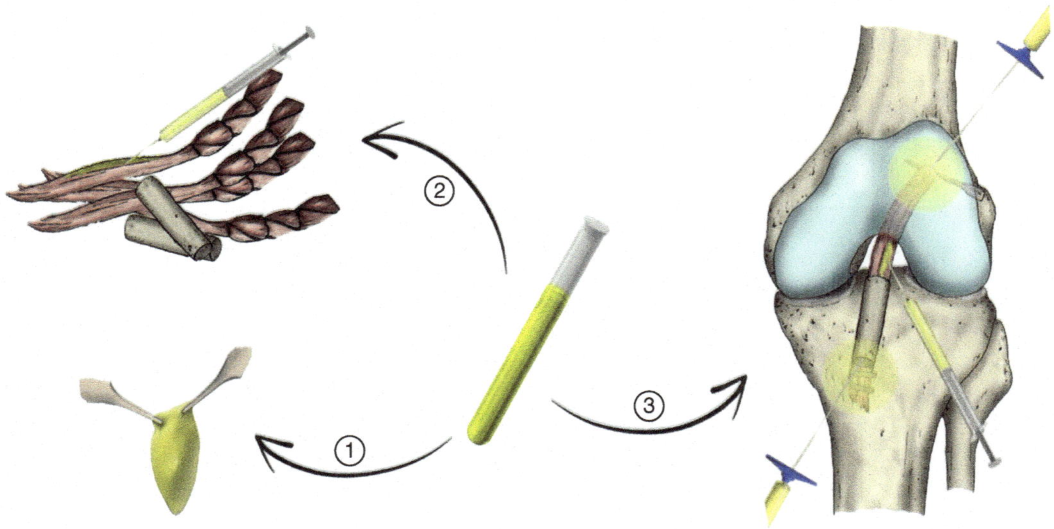

Fig. 28.1 Application of PRP in the reconstruction of the anterior cruciate ligament. The activation of PRP with calcium chloride at the beginning of surgery allows the formation of a fibrin clot to place it in the donor region of the autografts if these are used (1). The liquid formulation of activated PRP is used to infiltrate and soak grafts and bone plugs (if this technique is used) (2). At the end of the surgery, activated PRP is also injected into the grafts as well as into the tunnels intraosseously (3)

immersed in activated PRP and re-implanted when the graft is introduced, sealing the tibial tunnel. Moreover, the bone surrounding the tunnels is injected with PRP after graft fixation using trocar for bone biopsy, and graft is again infiltrated after placing. All this PRP application will provide a source of proteins and cells that enhance graft integration. Finally, a PRP intraarticular infiltration is conducted generating a biological anti-inflammatory environment.

For the optimal recovery of the patient, it is necessary that we follow a physiotherapy plan so that the mechanical stimulation generates the mechanotransduction phenomena [64]. The synergy between these and the biological action of the PRP will achieve a better and faster healing.

28.3.4.2 Ultrasound-Guided Platelet-Rich Plasma Injections for Ligament Injuries

In both the cases of acute injuries and chronic conditions that do not require surgery, the outpatient application of PRP may help the patient improve symptomatically and accelerate their recovery. This technique is in demand in the injuries of knee lateral ligaments, and lesions may be located into the ligament body or insertions (Fig. 28.2) [58].

Prior to infiltration, all the interventions will be conducted under aseptic conditions, cleaning and sterilizing the intervention area and using a sterile protector on the ultrasound probe. Local anesthesia is normally not necessary and the volume of injected PRP could vary from 3 to 8 mL depending on the size of the ligament.

When ligament lesion is located by ultrasound examination, activated PRP is also performed under ultrasound guidance with the probe in the long axis. It is applied both in the area of the damaged tissue and in the adjacent healthy areas, whose biological stimulation will help repair the damaged area. The needle should be inserted as parallel as possible to the ligament to ensure a proper distribution and diffusion of the PRP along the ligament. After infiltration, it is advisable to apply ice for a few minutes to relieve both pain and inflammation.

This infiltration could be repeated weekly depending on the clinical evolution of the injury which is assessed by ultrasound or magnetic resonance. As mentioned in the anterior cruciate ligament reconstruction, in these outpatient cases a good physiotherapy work is also key to achieving an optimal recovery.

28.4 Growth Factors for the Treatment of Meniscal Injuries

28.4.1 Anatomy and Biomechanical Aspects of the Meniscus

The term meniscus is derived from the Greek "meniskos" (crescent), adopted because of the structures' semilunar shape when seen from the

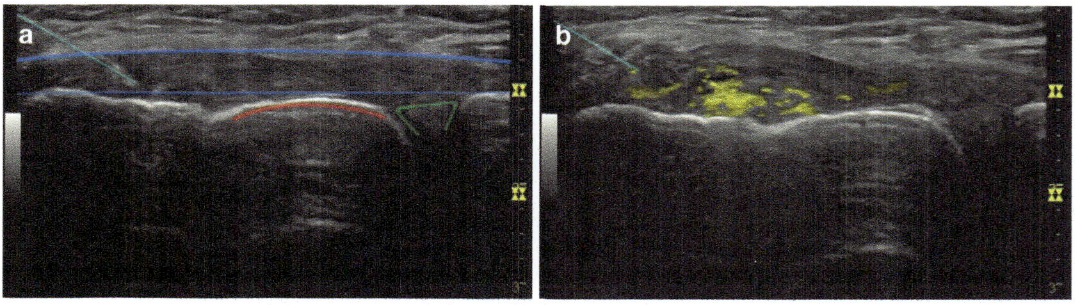

Fig. 28.2 Ultrasound-guided percutaneous PRP injections into medial collateral injection. The infiltration of the ligament is performed with the ultrasound probe in the long axis, allowing to observe the ligament (blue) as well as reference structures such as the distal femur (red) and the meniscus (green) (**a**). Placing the needle parallel to the ligament allows diffusion along this structure, which thickens when the PRP infiltrates (yellow) (**b**)

top [65]. The knee joint has two menisci, the largest in the human body—a C-shaped medial meniscus covering approximately 50–60% of the medial tibial plateau, and the lateral meniscus with a more circular shape, covering approximately 70–80% of the lateral tibial plateau [65, 66].

The menisci constitute a part of the "meniscus-meniscal ligament complex" consisting of the menisci, their bone attachments (anterior and posterior roots) and the ligaments attached to the respective meniscus bodies (menisco-tibial, menisco-femoral, menisco-patellar, transverse meniscal, oblique meniscomeniscal) [65, 67]. Their histological structures change in accordance with age, injuries, pathological conditions, and other factors. About 70% of a meniscus is water, with the remaining 30% dry weight composed of collagens, glycosaminoglycans, DNA, and glycoproteins [65, 66]. About 75–80% of the organic matter is collagen, predominantly collagen type I, with low content of collagen II, III, V, VI, and XVIII [65, 66, 68].

The important factors fostering meniscal development and healing are the structure and proximity to the perimeniscal capillary plexus. Based on the observation described, menisci were divided into zones [69]: red-red (vascularized part, fibroblast-like cells, Cooper zone 0 or 1) characterized by a good healing potential, white-red (transition part, Cooper zone 2) with intermediate healing potential, and white-white (avascular part, chondrocite-like cells, Copper zone 3) with very low healing potential. [65, 68]

A classification of meniscal tears was developed by ISAKOS, containing the following components: (1) tear depth, (2) rim width (zone 1, 2, 3), (3) radial location, (4) location according to popliteal hiatus, (5) tear pattern, (6) tissue quality, (7) length of tear, (8) the amount of meniscal tissue excised, (9) the percentage of meniscus excised (surface area) [70–74].

Risk factors from a meta-analysis by Snoeker et al. showed a strong evidence that age (older than 60 years), gender (male), work-related kneeling and squatting, and climbing stairs (greater than 30 flights) constituted risk factors for degenerative meniscal tears [75]. Playing soccer or rugby was also connected to higher incidence of acute meniscal tears. Knee instability for a period longer than 12 months constituted a strong risk factor for a medial meniscal tear but not for lateral meniscus injuries [75]. Medial meniscal tears were also associated with advanced age, female gender, higher BMI, increased Kellgren-Lawrence grade, varus mechanical axis angle, and low sports activity level [76].

The meniscus plays pivotal role for biomechanics of the knee. Its major roles include load transfer, shock absorption, lubrication, and nutrition of joint cartilage [68, 70]. As menisci are involved in so many different processes, their injuries are very common, with annual incidence estimates at 0.33–10.08 per 1000 person-years [75, 77–81]. Arthroscopy is the procedure of choice for most of these patients, with arthroscopic partial meniscectomy performed most typically. The data available regarding the early osteoarthritis onset after meniscectomy has not changed the routine for many years [67]. Currently, meniscal repair is considered "a gold standard" for young and active patients, but an increasing volume of data shows that even in patients aged 40 years and older, meniscal repair yields very good healing rates and patient-reported outcome measures (PROMs) [82].

Approximately 52–93% of meniscal repairs have been reported to heal, with many factors influencing the process already identified. The most important seems to include tear type, time from injury, chronic vs. acute injury, knee load bearing, medial vs. lateral meniscus injury. A subgroup of patients with failed meniscal repairs still remains, though. So far, many techniques have been used to improve the healing rates after meniscus repair. A limited number of clinical trials have provided evidence for the use of biological augmentation: vascular access channel formation, fibrin clot/fibrin glue technique, platelet-rich plasma, or bone marrow venting procedures. Still, extending our knowledge of current methods fostering meniscus healing and developing new ones continue to be of high importance [65, 66, 83].

28.4.2 Patient Assessment

28.4.2.1 Clinical Examination

Physical examination and medical history are essential for correct diagnosis, constituting the initial step in clinical evaluation for meniscal tears [65, 67]. Within a short time after the injury and before seeing a doctor, the patient may complain of pain when bending the knee, climbing stairs or squatting, decreased range of motion, locking, swelling, popping, catching, etc. Patients with degenerative meniscal tears report mild catching, snapping or clicking, occasional pain, or mild swelling [66, 67, 83, 84].

Uncovering the injury mechanism is important. Most meniscal injuries occur when the knee is partially flexed and a rotational force is applied to the joint. Then the menisci may become impaled between two condyles [65, 66, 71, 84], and patients usually report having heard or felt a "pop" followed by acute pain [65, 67].

A physician examines general knee structures and then proceeds to specific tests to exclude associated injuries, e.g., of cruciate ligaments or collateral ligaments [65, 66, 71]. The final diagnosis is then confirmed with specific meniscal tests. There are several provocative tests used for meniscal tear detection: palpation tests (joint line tenderness, McMurray's) and rotation tests (Apley's, Thessaly's, Childress, etc.). There is no single perfect test for meniscal injury (summarized in Table 28.1), with most satisfactory results possibly achieved by performing 2–3 different tests and comparing the results, taking medical history and personal experience into account [65, 71, 84].

28.4.3 Radiological Assessment

Imaging techniques also play an important role in confirming meniscal tear diagnoses. Standard X-ray images (anteroposterior and lateral) should be made after acute injury to exclude bone fractures and other bone pathologies [71, 84]. Ultrasonography may be useful in diagnosing meniscal tears because of low cost and high availability. The sensitivity of meniscus ultrasonography is 85%, while specificity ranges around 69% [89, 90].

Currently, magnetic resonance imaging constitutes a gold standard for meniscal tear imaging with its high sensitivity of 79% for lateral meniscus and 93% for medial meniscus and specificity of 96% for lateral meniscus and 88% for medial meniscus [65, 72].

MRI for meniscal pathologies should consist of three planes: sagittal, coronal, and axial, high spatial resolution, a typical field of view of 14 cm × 16 cm, and slice thickness of no more than 3 mm. It should be performed in two sequences: T1-weighted proton density sequences, sagittal, to evaluate anatomy and morphology of ligaments, menisci and osteochondral structures,

Table 28.1 Meniscal test specificity and sensitivity [85–88]

Test	Examination	Sensitivity (%)	Specificity (%)
Joint line tenderness	Pain while pressing on the medial/lateral joint line, bent knee	83	83
McMurray's test	Pain with flexed knee and twisting the foot in external and internal rotation, patient supine	61	84
Apley's test	Pain with foot pressed forced and rotated internally and externally, patient prone, knee is flexed at 90°	60	70
Thessaly's test	Discomfort and locking sensation when patient stands on one foot with the other knee flexed at 5° and then 20°. Perform knee and body rotation three times internally and externally	75	87
Childress sign (squat test)	Pain while doing squats and "duck walk"	68	66
Steinmann I test	Pain during external and internal rotation of foot while patient sits on the table with legs dangling	48	89

with the view providing high sensitivity to meniscal tears, followed by T2-weighted fast spin-echo with specific fat suppression or STIR, to evaluate pathology of intra-articular structures, exhibiting lower sensitivity but higher specificity. A 3-grade scale of abnormal meniscal signal is also available, with third grade identified in arthroscopy in 90% of cases. The scanner used for meniscal tear imaging should operate at no less than 1.5 T, and 3.0 T yields somewhat more detailed images, but several studies already compared 1.5 T and 3.0 T and demonstrated no significant difference [65, 71, 91–94].

MRI Meniscal Tears Classification includes orientation within the meniscus (longitudinal, radial, parrot-beak tears) and the spatial plane (horizontal, vertical). Additionally, special types of meniscal tears like bucket handle, flipped meniscus, complex tear, or meniscal root tear are included [71].

When patients are not able to get an MRI, usually because of medical contraindications (heart pacemakers—especially older types, insulin pumps, implanted hearing aids, neurostimulators, ferromagnetic metal clips, metallic bodies in the eye), computer tomography arthrography could be performed. The CT arthrography has sensitivity of 86% and specificity of 100% for the evaluation of meniscal lesions, surpassing an ultrasound scan [65, 91].

28.4.4 Orthobiological Techniques

Injury of the meniscus occurring in close proximity to the perimeniscal capillary plexus (red-red zone) is amenable to repair. Unfortunately, tears in the avascular part (white-white zone) are very unlikely to heal. These patients often undergo partial meniscectomy to preserve the undamaged meniscus part, relieve pain and regain range of motion in the locked knee. Disadvantages of the treatment include bigger load on knee cartilage and erosion of articular surface leading to osteoarthritis development and usually total knee replacement in the near future [65, 95, 96]. The progression encouraged orthopedic surgeons to develop new options for the treatment of tears located in red-white or white-white zone, starting with simple options such as rasping of the injury site and the synovium [97]. Throughout the years, many orthobiological techniques have been demonstrated to enhance meniscal tear healing in clinical trials, including vascular access channels and synovial abrasion, fibrin clot, platelet-rich plasma (PRP), and bone marrow venting procedures (BMVP) [66, 96].

28.4.4.1 Vascular Access Channels and Synovial Abrasion

These simple methods were developed in the 1980s. First evidence was provided by Arnotzky et al. [98] and Gao [99] on a canine meniscal tear model. Later on Fox et al. [100] analyzed the efficacy of incomplete meniscal lesion trephination with good to excellent results in 90% of patients. Additional evidence was provided by Zhang et al., who demonstrated significantly smaller retear rate of repaired menisci when performed concomitantly with meniscal trephination [101]. In addition to creating vascular access channels, the increasing rate of synovial attachment to the meniscus also increases blood supply. In animal studies, this technique was found successful and valuable in the treatment of meniscal lesions [102]. A modified technique was developed to create a synovial flap [103, 104]. Interestingly, synovial abrasion was effective in clinical setting [105] and capable of inducing meniscal healing without surgical fixation [106].

28.4.4.2 Fibrin Clot (FC)

Studies have demonstrated that extra-articular tissues heal following a predefined sequence of events. At the beginning, a blood extravasation and formation of a primary fibrin–platelet clot occurs, which then fills the gap between the torn tissue ends. This process creates scaffold for the cells to migrate to and remodel the primary clot. In the next steps, a scar forms, filling the defect. In contrast, an injury to the joint tissues activates synoviocytes and upregulates urokinase plasminogen activator (PA) expression, which is excreted to the intra-articular environment. As a result, the plasminogen present in the synovial fluid is converted into its plasmin [72], which degrades fibrin. Therefore, fibrin in the intra-articular space is unable to form a stable clot [73–75]. This early loss of this provisional scaffold is considered as a reason why tissues within joints fail to heal [73, 74, 107].

The use of exogenous fibrin clot represents an initial augmentation technique in meniscal repair. It was demonstrated successful in preclinical and clinical studies [108, 109].

Injuries occurring within the meniscus red-red zone lead to the activation of coagulation processes in damaged vessels. Initiation of extruding and intrinsic coagulation pathways results in thrombin formation and conversion of fibrinogen into an FC, releasing inflammatory cells and growth factors as well as distributing undifferentiated mesenchymal cells. The white-white zone of the meniscus does not possess vascular supply to provide healing factors [109–111]. An FC made from peripheral blood and supplied close to the meniscus tear could imitate the process which occurs in response to injury in the vascular zone and supports the healing cascade [109, 112].

The mechanism of autologous FC action is still unsure. It is presumed that injury exposes collagen fibers and attaches FC to them enabling a gradual release of growth factors (GF)—the transforming growth factor (TGF-β1), platelet-derived growth factor (PDGF), and vascular endothelial growth factor (VEGF)—into the local environment. GFs exhibit chemotactic activity as well as stimulate angiogenesis, fibroblast proliferation, and collagen synthesis [95, 110, 113]. FCs form fibrin matrices, highly organized structures to better stimulate the healing process and stem cell migration [110, 114]. Studies have demonstrated that FC releases growth factors gradually and in small concentrations over a longer period of time as compared to platelet-rich plasma (PRP) [110]. The former may be also prepared faster and cheaper, as there is no need for special equipment [112].

In 1988 Arnoczky et al. made FC more popular when he examined 12 dogs with full-thickness meniscus injury and revealed that supplying FC to the meniscal lesion supports healing by stimulating proliferation of fibrous connective tissue that eventually develops into fibrocartilaginous tissue [115]. Sethi et al. modified the technique and successfully applied it in clinical practice [113]. Later on, studies by Henning et al. showed that application of the fibrin clot technique in meniscal repair may decrease the failure rate from 41 to 8% [116]. Jang et al. repaired 41 meniscal tears by supplying FC through a cannula inserted under the meniscus and sutures. Eight months after the initial surgery, they performed second-look arthroscopy or MRI. Interestingly, 39 out of 41 menisci were healed (95%) [112]. Similar results were obtained when FC was applied to the repair site of radial meniscal tears [117]. Chrystanthal et al. treated 24 patients with meniscus tear arthroscopically along with FC injected into the joint through a cannula and then placed into the meniscal gap reduced by tightening the sutures [108]. Another study by Ra et al. involving 12 patients provided evidence for augmentation of radial meniscal tears with fibrin clot. Postoperative MRI after 11 ± 3 months showed 11 completely and 1 incompletely healed menisci. Postoperative Lysholm and IKDC subjective knee scores were improved significantly at a mean of 30 ± 4 months after surgery [118].

28.4.5 The Use of Platelet-Rich Plasma (PRP) in Meniscal Injuries

PRP is a concentration of blood platelets and growth factors in a small volume of plasma. Platelets, called thrombocytes, are cytoplasmic fragments of mature megakaryocytes in bone marrow. If the defect site is small, platelet clotting is sufficient, but larger wounds may require mature blood clots. A blood clot is activated via intrinsic and extrinsic pathways. Coagulation occurs by polymerization of fibrinogen monomers. The fibrin clot provides a matrix environment for migration of fibroblasts and other tissue-forming cells, including endothelial cells, leukocytes, etc. [119]. They stimulate tissue regeneration and wound healing and release GF locally. TGF-β, PDGF, VEGF, EGF, and IGF-1 are associated with the healing cascade leading to cellular chemotaxis, promotion of angiogenesis, collagen matrix production, cell proliferation, and stimulation of bone tissue regeneration.

Platelet-rich plasma clots also stimulate DNA synthesis, extracellular matrix (ECM) synthesis, and mRNA expression of biglycan and decorin [95, 107, 119–122]. PRP is made from patient's own blood. Centrifugation separates whole blood into three fractions: platelet-poor plasma (PPP), platelet-rich plasma, and red blood cells [119–123].

Ishida et al. carried out in vitro and in vivo studies to verify a hypothesis of PRP enhancing meniscal tissue regeneration. The in vitro study showed that concentration of growth factors was higher in the PRP sample than in the PPP sample. PRP was found to promote meniscal cell proliferation by stimulating higher expression of biglycan and decorin mRNA and synthesis of TGF-β1, VEGF, and SGAG. The in vivo study in rabbits with injury in the avascular meniscus zone showed that PRP stimulated higher expression of biglycan and decorin mRNA as well as higher synthesis of DNA and ECM [124].

Several clinical trials have been carried out with PRP as an adjuvant to the operative meniscal repair. In a study by Pujol et al., 51 young patients underwent open meniscal repair. Seventeen of them received an additional PRP injection during the procedure. After 1 year, MRI was performed and five cases were observed without hypersignal within the repaired meniscus (chronic tear) in the group with PRP injection contrasted with no cases as described above in the group without PRP. After minimum 2 years of follow-up, improved scores were reported for PRP group in KOOS and IKDC scales [125]. A study by Kaminski et al. showed a significant improvement in the rate of meniscal healing of complete vertical meniscal tears after arthroscopy [126]. The recorded improvement was from 47% (no PRP) to 85% of repaired menisci treated with PRP supported arthroscopy. Similarly to previous studies, a significant improvement in PROM scores was noticed. Griffin et al. performed a retrospective analysis, with a second-look surgery and the Lysholm score as the main outcomes analyzed, with minimum 2 years of follow-up. The authors failed to show any benefit of PRP augmentation in the treatment of meniscal tears [127]. Furthermore, in a non-randomized study, platelet-rich fibrin and PRP were incorporated into 17 arthroscopic meniscal repairs, with five patients in the control group [110]. The PROMs recorded were comparable in both groups, and no benefits of biological augmentation use were observed. Similarly, a recent study of lateral discoid meniscus lesion arthroscopic repair demonstrated no significant differences in pain relief, functional improvement, or failure rate between the groups at mid-term follow-up [128]. However, all these studies were small in terms of participant numbers, with the risk of having been underpowered for all the outcomes. Additionally, tear type and location differed for each of the studies.

PRP was also used to augment meniscal transplants. Recently Zhang et al. [129] reported the outcomes of 31 patients who underwent a meniscal allograft transplant procedure, with 90.7% improving in terms of pain and PROMs. Unfortunately, the efficacy of the PRP could not be identified as no control group was included. Everhart et al. performed a study on 550 patients undergoing meniscal repair with or without PRP administration as well as with or without ACL reconstruction. Results after 3 years showed that meniscal repair with PRP (14% failures) has better outcomes than the same procedure performed without PRP (17% and 20% for isolated meniscal repairs), but no differences were recorded when the surgery was performed with a concomitant ACL reconstruction [130]. Another study by Kemmochi et al. involved 22 patients with meniscal tears. Seventeen underwent meniscus repair with platelet-rich plasma and platelet-rich fibrin. Five patients were assigned to a control group with the menisci merely sutured. After 6 months follow-up, a comparison of pre- and postoperative MRIs and functional assessments (Tegner Activity Level Score, Lysholm Knee Scoring Scale, International Knee Documentation Committee Score) was carried out. There were no significant difference between both groups in terms of PROMs, but both showed gradual improvement in functional assessment. MRIs did not indicate any significant improvements, either [110].

Some studies were also carried out on chronic meniscal lesions. *Blanke* et al. revealed that percutaneous injections of PRP were able to provide pain relief and stop the progression of intrasubstance meniscal lesions on MRI over the period of 6 months [131]. A recent report by Betancourt et al. described a favorable outcome of PRP treatment in a patient with grade 3 medial meniscus tear over a 30 months follow-up [132]. Another study by Strümper et al. demonstrated that intra-articular PRP injection was an effective option in knee pain associated with meniscal lesions [133]. The study showed significantly improved function in 83% patients. Additionally, concomitant PRP injection lowered the need for a future arthroscopy during the 6-month observation period. No progression of meniscal lesions in MRI, measured by Boston Leeds Osteoarthritis Knee Score, was noticed. Kaminski et al. carried out a prospective, randomized, double-blind, parallel-group, placebo-controlled study with 72 patients who underwent meniscal trephination with or without PRP injection. Failures controlled by MRI/second-look arthroscopy were rarer in the group with concomitant PRP injection (70–48%), as was the need for future surgery in the PRP-treated group. In both the groups the KOOS subscale, IKDC score, and WOMAC score improved, but values of VAS and KOOS symptoms exceeding MCID (minimally important clinical difference) were significantly elevated in the PRP group [96].

28.4.6 Bone Marrow Venting Procedures (BMVP) and Mesenchymal Stem Cells

Mesenchymal stem cells (MSC) are pluripotent cells, as they can differentiate into other specific cell types, like adipocytes, osteoblasts, and chondrocytes. Regardless of their differentiation potential, they support healing effect by regulating tissue homeostasis, remodeling, and neovascularization. They also have the ability to migrate toward the site of injury. MCS release cytokines and growth factors induce paracrine and autocrine activity [66, 95, 134]. Paracrine effects of MCS are responsible for angiogenesis by releasing vascular endothelial growth factor (VEGF) and hepatocyte growth factor (HGF) as well as immunosuppression of lymphocytes and peripheral blood mononuclear cells by releasing prostaglandin E2, leukemia inhibitor factor, and kynurenine [135]. MCS can be isolated from bone marrow (BM), periosteum, trabecular bone, adipose tissue, synovial membrane, skeletal muscle, and teeth. First isolation of MCS from bone marrow was reported in late 1960s, and bone marrow remains as a major source [95, 136]. BM healing potential is outlined during meniscal repair with concomitant ACL repair, where drilling tunnels in femur and tibia also release bone marrow with progenitor cells and growth factors [137, 138]. A potential mechanism leading to regeneration and repair of injured meniscus may involve differentiation of MSC into desired tissue, production of growth factors, and fusion with meniscus cells [135]. Animal study on MSC has presented good outcomes in the treatment of meniscal injuries. Limited studies on human menisci are also available, suggesting that stem cells may have the potential to support meniscal regeneration in humans.

The in vivo study on eight equine menisci performed by Ferris et al. compares the treatment with bone marrow-derived mesenchymal stem cells (BMSC) combined with fibrin to fibrin alone. Constructs were implanted subcutaneously in mice. The BMSC group demonstrated significantly improved vascularization, decreased thickness in histological examination, and increased total bonding as compared to control group [139]. Driscoll et al. performed a study on 18 rabbits with full-thickness cylindrical defect in the avascular meniscus zone. In the right knee, marrow was released from the bone into the joint using a 2.4 mm Kirchner wire. The left knee constituted a control group, without drilling. After 1, 4, and 12 weeks, medial meniscus was examined histologically, immunohistologically, and histomorphometrically. In the BM group, a better tissue quality was observed and a larger field of damaged meniscus was covered by regenerative tissue than in the control group, but no statistically significant differences were recorded at 12-week end point. Higher concentrations of IGF-1, TGF-beta, and PDGF were found in the regenerated tissue [138]. Tarafter et al. used bovine menisci in an in vivo study of healing avascular meniscus tears using fibrin glue with connective tissue growth factor (STGF, chemotactic, and profibrogenic agent) or transforming growth factor beta 3 (chondrogenic factor) to recruit synovial mesenchymal stem cells and form fibrous matrix as well as facilitate chondrogenic remodeling [140].

Clinical trials by Dean et al. [137] have provided high-quality evidence for the efficacy of BMVP in augmenting the rate of meniscal healing after repair. The failure rate was similar between meniscal repair with BMVP augmentation (12.9%) and meniscal repair plus ACL reconstruction (7.8%). Kaminski et al. carried out a prospective, randomized, double-blind, parallel group, placebo-controlled study to support the hypothesis of BM improving meniscal healing as assessed by a second-look arthroscopy. Twenty patients underwent meniscus repair only while another 20 received surgery with concomitant BMVP of the intercondylar notch; 100% menisci in the BMVP group were healed as compared to 76% in the control group. In both the groups, patients showed an improvement in pain score (VAS and KOOS) with no significant difference between groups. Functional outcomes (IKDC, WOMAC, KOOS) were significantly better in the BMVP group [141]. Piontek et al. analyzed 2-year follow-up of clinical and MRI results in 53 patients with meniscal tear in the red-white and white-white zones treated by arthroscopy and ChondroGide Collagen Membrane with BM injection. They observed significantly better outcomes in IKDC, Lysholm, and Barret score (86.8%) as compared to preoperative data. MRI showed no meniscal tear in 76% of operated menisci [142].

Interestingly, adipose tissue-isolated stem cells were also used in meniscal repair augmentation. Pak et al. injected left patient knee with grade II meniscal tear with adipose tissue stem cells (ASC). The adipose tissue was harvested from subcutaneous layer of the lower abdominal area, and ASC was extracted through enzymatic digestion. At 3 months after the injection, MRI showed complete absence of meniscus injury, and patient-reported outcomes were significantly improved [135].

28.4.7 Treatment Options

28.4.7.1 Acute Meniscal Tears

An acute meniscus tear (AMT) is a consequence of knee injury, with the patient usually recalling the circumstances. An acute injury is usually accompanied by sudden pain, swelling, and other complaints. AMT often involves concomitant damage to knee structures [71]. The PRICE protocol (protection, rest, ice, compression, elevation) should be applied at the onset of an AMT, with MRI and X-ray recommended to exclude other lesions and arrive at a final diagnosis.

Many factors will influence the final (operative or nonoperative) treatment offered: age, activity level, expectations, location of meniscus tear, tissue quality, concomitant injury, etc. [67]. Conservative treatment (physiotherapy, exercise, anti-inflammatory pharmacotherapy, intra-articular injections) is recommended for symptom duration of less than 3 months without mechanical symptoms (locking). Otherwise, an arthroscopic meniscal repair should be considered [67, 71, 143]. The major exception is a locked knee when urgent arthroscopic surgery is indicated [143].

An arthroscopic meniscal surgery may take on the following forms: meniscectomy, meniscal repair, or meniscal reconstruction [67]. Meniscectomy is reserved for tears located in the avascular zone, otherwise meniscal repair by outside-in, inside-out, or all-inside technique should be undertaken.

As more evidence is accumulated, biological augmentation may improve the likelihood of meniscal healing after surgical repair. Simple, almost costless and safe techniques such as trephination, synovial, and meniscal rasping as well as BMVP may be an attractive option to be applied during arthroscopy.

28.4.7.2 Chronic Meniscal Lesions

The mechanism of degenerative meniscal lesions is still unknown. In all likelihood, it is related to obesity, aging, and osteoarthritis [67, 71]. Clinical trials have shown arthroscopy to be as effective as placebo in the treatment of chronic meniscal lesions [144, 145].

Nonoperative treatment (physiotherapy, exercise, anti-inflammatory pharmacotherapy, intraarticular injections) and X-ray (AP + lateral + Schuss view) for at least 3 months is the first-line strategy in degenerative lesions. If treatment fails and patient presents with symptoms, the diagnosis should be verified by means of MRI, and a non-urgent arthroscopic meniscal repair may be considered. An exception would be advanced structural osteoarthritis, when arthroscopic meniscal surgery is not indicated unless mechanical symptoms are present. In such case early treatment of arthritis is recommended [67, 143, 146].

Chronic meniscal tears are still a bit of a mystery. They tend to be a part of knee degenerative disease, and no definitive treatment is established. We believe these patients may benefit from percutaneous procedures, carrying very little risk when compared to surgery. PRP in particular is already quite well documented as playing a positive role in the treatment of knee osteoarthritis. At this point multicenter clinical trials are necessary to verify PRP efficacy in meniscal lesions treatment (Fig. 28.3).

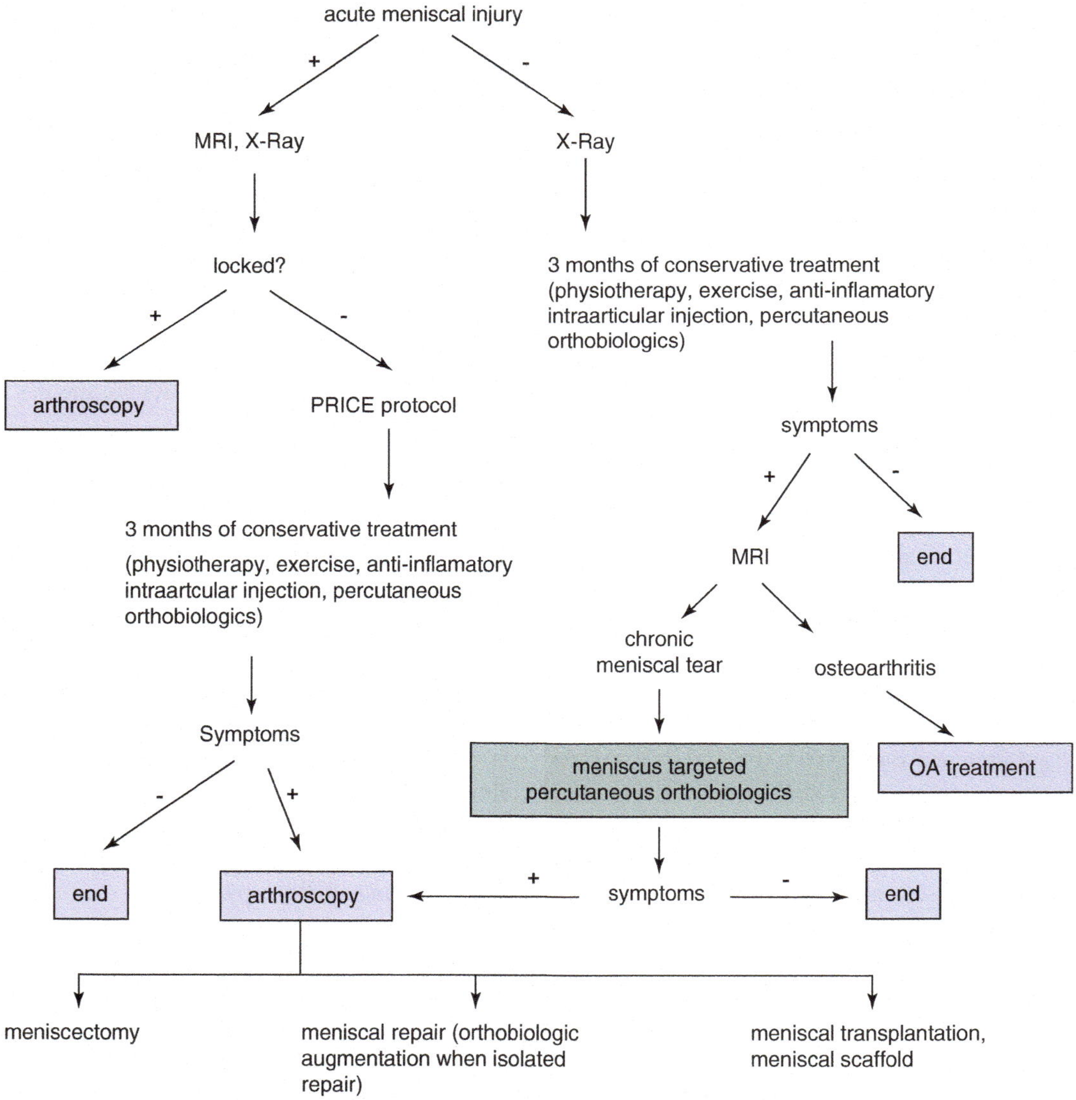

Fig. 28.3 Modification of ESSKA and BASK algorithm on the meniscal lesion treatment, including the use of orthobiologics

28.4.7.3 Future Treatment Options

In the future, meniscal surgery will involve younger and more active patients with higher expectation levels. The challenges of meniscal repair will still focus on the limited blood supply and high degree of meniscal tissue fragmentation. Meniscal transplants or scaffolds will play a clearly defined role, while blood- and cell-based techniques still require further evaluation. The development of meniscal repair devices may also improve the healing rates to a great extent.

In summary, meniscectomy should no longer constitute the first-line treatment. The knowledge of the meniscus biology has improved and the biological options to augment repairs have obtained evidence, thus synovial/meniscal abrasion as well as bone marrow stimulation techniques should be applied when feasible. The nonoperative treatment for degenerative tears should be considered and may include percutaneous procedures such as PRP. Further research is necessary to gather high-quality evidence.

28.5 Current Application of Stem Cell Therapy in Orthopedics and Sports Medicine

There is a growing interest in orthopedics and sports medicine with the use of innovative biological therapies where traditional conservative or operative therapies have failed to achieve success. The International Society for Cellular Therapy proposes minimal criteria to define human MSC. First, MSC must be plastic-adherent when maintained in standard culture conditions. Second, MSC must express CD105, CD73, and CD90 and lack expression of CD45, CD34, CD14 or CD11b, CD79alpha or CD19, and HLA-DR surface molecules [147]. Third, MSC must differentiate to osteoblasts, adipocytes and chondroblasts in vitro. Recently, as per Arnold Caplan, it is more appropriate to call MSCs as medicinal signaling cells, as these cells in vivo respond to the injury or disease by secreting bioactive factors that has immunomodulatory effect, providing promising therapeutic options [148].

The application of MSCs could facilitate the healing mechanism of tissues with limited healing potential and vascularity such as tendons, cartilage, meniscus, and ligaments. The term stem cell has been overused based on the consensus of the expert's opinion [149]. It is recommended that the use of minimally manipulated cell products and tissue-derived culture-expanded cells be referred to as cell therapy, and the nature of these treatments be clearly understood. Basic science research affirmed proof of concept that MSC therapy downregulates inflammation and produces an analgesic effect. Few studies show promising long-term clinical results for cartilage injuries and ligaments tears. As such, there is a continued need for high-quality basic science and clinical investigation into the safety and efficacy of cell-based therapies. The DOSES tool for describing cell therapies must be utilized by clinicians, researchers, regulators, and industry professionals to improve transparency and to allow clinicians and patients to understand the characteristics of current and future cell preparations [150]. It is recommended that physicians and institutions offering biological therapies establish patient registries for surveillance and quality assessments.

28.5.1 Cell-Based Therapies

Various therapeutic protocols involving the use of MSCs have been developed for clinical applications, and they have demonstrated the potential for enhancing regenerative processes for a many condition. These cells may be isolated from a variety of tissues such as the muscle, periosteum, synovium, bone marrow, and adipose tissue. Bone marrow aspirate concentrate (BMAC) is classified through the US Food and Drug Administration (FDA) as a 361 product, and hence, it is not subjected to premarket review and approval. The regulatory foundation of European Union (EU) similar to the US system, processes such as centrifugation, are considered as minimal manipulation. BMAC has progenitor cells and growth factors with reparative, homing, and trophic properties causing them to migrate to areas of damage. Once at the site of injury, they release numerous factors that can help in healing and inflammation modulation. Recently, Cassano et al. found an increased concentration of interleukin 1 receptor antagonist (IL-1RA), which, in combination with the other constituents, may provide anti-inflammatory and immunomodulatory effects [151]. Adipose-derived stromal cell therapy, also known as an adipose stromal vascular fraction (ASC), has gained recent popularity as a minimally manipulated product. Adipose tissue, which is typically structured with consistent vascularity, has been increasingly recognized as a reliable source of these cells; also in comparison to BMAC, it has the advantage of procuring much larger source for MSCs.

28.5.2 Osteoarthritis

Few studies have demonstrated patient safety and improved clinical outcomes after BMAC treatment for OA; however, there is a paucity of high-level studies or randomized trials with joint osteoarthritis.

Adipose-derived stromal cell therapy, also known as adipose stromal vascular fraction (ASC) therapy, has gained recent popularity as a treatment. Compared with BMAC, adipose tissue has been reported to have larger quantities of progenitor cells. An RCT demonstrated a significant reduction in Western Ontario and McMaster Universities Osteoarthritis Index (WOMAC), an improvement in Lysholm score, and significant pain reduction (VAS) [152]. Although promising, these studies have been insufficient to conclude the efficacy of ASC therapy to adopt it into standard practices.

28.5.3 Focal Osteochondral Injuries

Gobbi et al. [153] in a prospective study concluded that the repair of full-thickness cartilage injury in the knee with a HA-BMAC provides good to excellent clinical outcomes at long-term follow-up in the treatment of small to large lesions, single or multiple lesions, and lesions in one or two compartments, as well as in cases of associated lesion treatment. While good outcomes can be expected among patients more than 45 years of age, outcomes may be comparatively more successful in younger patients.

In our experience based on the quantification of colony-forming units (CFUs) in 25 patients, we did not find any correlation between the clinical outcomes and the number of CFUs.

An intriguing explanation for these results may come from the new vision of MSC recently proposed by Caplan as "medicinal signaling cells." According to this concept, MSCs, rather than participating in tissue formation, work as site-regulated "drugstores" in vivo by releasing trophic and immunomodulatory factors and are activated by local injury. They hypothesize that the harvesting procedure from the iliac crest may be enough to activate the MSC and allow for the establishment of a regenerative microenvironment within the defect site [154].

28.5.4 Tendon Injuries

In the setting of rotator cuff repair, there are few studies using bone marrow cells (BMAC) to augment the healing rate. One case–control study using BMAC sourced from posterior iliac crest showed significant improvement in healing outcomes and reduced number of re-tears determined by ultrasound and MRI at 10 years follow-up [155]. However, another study showed no significant difference in clinical scores at 6 months using BMAC sourced from the ipsilateral humeral head.

28.5.5 Ligament Injuries

The injection of autologous bone marrow concentrate and PRP using fluoroscopic or arthroscopic guidance with good clinical outcomes and MRI showing the ACL healing was documented in patients with partial and complete ACL tears with less than 1-cm retraction [156]. Gobbi et al. [157] concluded that primary ACL repair combined PRP and BMAC to treat select cases of knee instability secondary to incomplete ACL rupture demonstrated good long-term outcomes in athletes, with high rates of restoration of knee stability and returned to preinjury athletic activities.

28.5.6 Meniscal Injuries

Clinical studies using cellular therapies for meniscal repair are currently limited. An RCT found statistically significant meniscus growth on MRI at 24 weeks post-injection, as well as better functional and clinical outcomes using expanded autologous bone marrow mesenchymal stem cells injected percutaneously in knees [158]. A clinical study reported the repair of a grade II meniscal tear following a percutaneous injection of autologous adipose stem cell (ASCs) along with PRP, hyaluronic acid, and $CaCl_2$ [159].

The use of mesenchymal stem cells to stimulate the regeneration of meniscal tissue appears to be a promising approach to restore as much meniscal tissue as possible [160]. However, these regenerative technologies still need to be optimized.

28.6 Growth Factors for the Treatment of Cartilage Injuries

The degenerative process of the articular cartilage affects almost everyone. The reasons that cause its degradation are the aggressions caused by articular trauma and because the cartilage is under pressure that may be excessive.

The avascularity of the articular cartilage, the limited chondrocytes in a mature tissue, and the inability to migrate to the injured site provoke a slow cartilage healing and, in many cases, a permanent cartilage defect [161]. Under physiological conditions, the application of mechanical force to the joint results in increased proteoglycan synthesis and collagen synthesis may also increase if shear forces increase, especially in the superficial zone [162].

Understanding beforehand the biological processes of the tissue repair, the use of biological therapies based on signaling proteins is recommendable and useful. It is well known that the platelets have a major role in hemostasis, inflammation, and proliferation for remodeling and tissue healing. In addition, platelets have an angiogenic power to deliver molecules into the damaged tissue. This inherent healing potential has made some authors use plasma rich in growth factors (PRGF) for the treatment of cartilage injuries.

Growth factors have a proliferative, differentiative, and anti-inflammatory effect. The platelet-rich plasma (PRP) has been shown to have a strong positive effect on chondrocyte proliferation in vitro, observed either in a monolayer or three-dimensional environment. There is less concordance in the effect of PRP on chondrocyte differentiation, but PRP treatment seems to increase proteoglycan and collagen type II synthesis and could also induce the expression of chondrocyte differentiation proteins such as aggrecan and Sox9 [163]. PRP also released diminished multiple inflammatory IL-1 beta-mediated effects on human osteoarthritic chondrocytes, including inhibition of NF-κB activation [164]. It should also be noted that some PRP formulations could be pro-inflammatory, and the presence of concentrated leukocytes increased the levels of catabolic and pro-inflammatory signaling molecules.

Due to these properties of inherent healing potential, the use of PRP for cartilage injuries has been widely studied. In particular, a study performed in 808 patients with knee pathology who were treated with three intra-articular PRP injections showed at 6 months statistically significant differences between pretreatment and follow-up values for pain, stiffness, and functional capacity in the WOMAC index; pain and total score, distance and daily life activities in the Lequesne index; the VAS pain score; and the SF-36 physical health domain improving in function and quality of life [165]. The same procedure was performed in 205 patients, and at 12 months statistically significant differences between pretreatment and follow-up values for the same parameters confirmed the effectiveness of the treatment.

Two case studies of full-thickness knee cartilage injuries were published, treated with an autologous-made scaffold consisting of hyaline cartilage chips combined with a clot of mixed plasma poor-rich in platelets [166]. They reported successful outcomes with good function and ability to return to high-level soccer. Moreover, the same group performed a study in sheep where the same technique was successfully applied [167]. A histological and immunohistochemical analysis demonstrated that this technique was able to restore hyaline cartilage with adequate presence of type II collagen and minimum of type I collagen.

This novel autologous-made matrix consisting of hyaline cartilage chips combined with mixed plasma poor-rich in platelets clot, and plasma rich in growth factors (PRGF) in liquid stage provided excellent clinical, functional, and MRI-based (cartilage repair quality and quantity) outcomes in young, active individuals with full-thickness cartilage or osteochondral defects. This technique seems an excellent alternative for cartilage injuries, as it can be performed in very active, young individuals as a single surgery, is cheap, has no intolerance or rejection potential, and has demonstrated histological and immunohistochemical characteristics very similar to healthy articular cartilage in animal studies [167, 168] (Fig. 28.4).

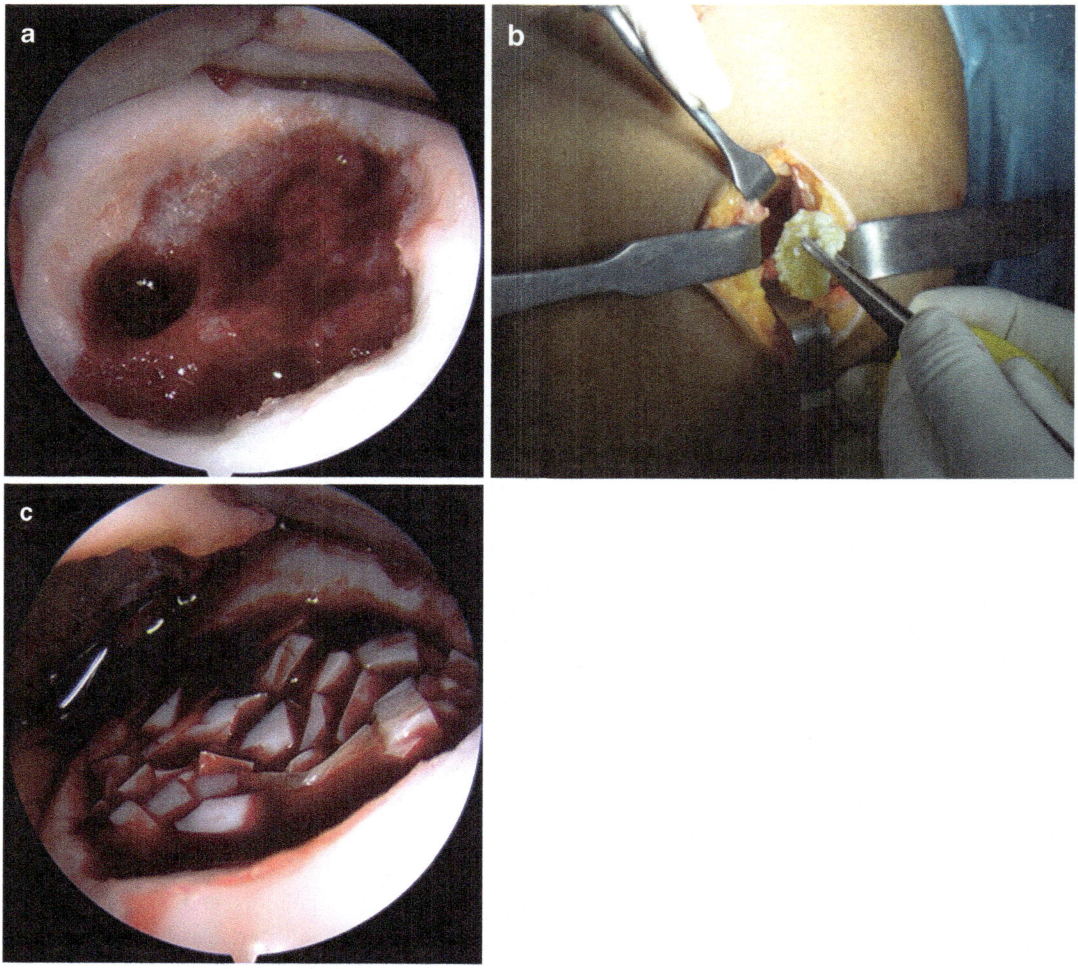

Fig. 28.4 Composition of figures demonstrating the initial injury and surgical treatment. (**a**) Intraoperative picture demonstrating the debrided defect in the lateral femoral condyle. (**b**) Intraoperative picture demonstrating the autologous matrix before implantation. (**c**) Arthroscopic view of the filled defect at the end of the procedure

References

1. Nguyen RT, Borg-Stein J, McInnis K. Applications of platelet-rich plasma in musculoskeletal and sports medicine: an evidence-based approach. PM R. 2011;3(3):226–50.
2. Zhu Y, Yuan M, Meng HY, Wang AY, Guo QY, Wang Y, et al. Basic science and clinical application of platelet-rich plasma for cartilage defects and osteoarthritis: a review. Osteoarthritis Cartilage. 2013;21(11):1627–37.
3. Cavallo C, Roffi A, Grigolo B, Mariani E, Pratelli L, Merli G, et al. Platelet-rich plasma: the choice of activation method affects the release of bioactive molecules. Biomed Res Int. 2016;2016:6591717.
4. Stiles CD. The molecular biology of platelet-derived growth factor. Cell. 1983;33(3):653–5.
5. Boakye LA, Ross KA, Pinski JM, Smyth NA, Haleem AM, Hannon CP, et al. Platelet-rich plasma increases transforming growth factor-beta1 expression at graft-host interface following autologous osteochondral transplantation in a rabbit model. World J Orthop. 2015;6(11):961–9.
6. Park SI, Lee HR, Kim S, Ahn MW, Do SH. Time-sequential modulation in expression of growth factors from platelet-rich plasma (PRP) on the chondrocyte cultures. Mol Cell Biochem. 2012;361(1–2):9–17.
7. Wu CC, Chen WH, Zao B, Lai PL, Lin TC, Lo HY, et al. Regenerative potentials of platelet-rich plasma enhanced by collagen in retrieving pro-inflammatory cytokine-inhibited chondrogenesis. Biomaterials. 2011;32(25):5847–54.
8. Fice MP, Miller JC, Christian R, Hannon CP, Smyth N, Murawski CD, et al. The role of platelet-rich plasma in cartilage pathology: an updated systematic review of the basic science evidence. Arthroscopy. 2019;35(3):961–76.e3.
9. Narcisi R, Quarto R, Ulivi V, Muraglia A, Molfetta L, Giannoni P. TGF beta-1 administration during ex vivo expansion of human articular chondrocytes in a serum-free medium redirects the cell phenotype toward hypertrophy. J Cell Physiol. 2012;227(9):3282–90.
10. Re'em T, Kaminer-Israeli Y, Ruvinov E, Cohen S. Chondrogenesis of hMSC in affinity-bound TGF-beta scaffolds. Biomaterials. 2012;33(3):751–61.
11. Yin Z, Yang X, Jiang Y, Xing L, Xu Y, Lu Y, et al. Platelet-rich plasma combined with agarose as a bioactive scaffold to enhance cartilage repair: an in vitro study. J Biomater Appl. 2014;28(7):1039–50.
12. Pereira RC, Scaranari M, Benelli R, Strada P, Reis RL, Cancedda R, et al. Dual effect of platelet lysate on human articular cartilage: a maintenance of chondrogenic potential and a transient proinflammatory activity followed by an inflammation resolution. Tissue Eng Part A. 2013;19(11–12):1476–88.
13. Lee HR, Park KM, Joung YK, Park KD, Do SH. Platelet-rich plasma loaded hydrogel scaffold enhances chondrogenic differentiation and maturation with up-regulation of CB1 and CB2. J Control Release. 2012;159(3):332–7.
14. Dohan Ehrenfest DM, Rasmusson L, Albrektsson T. Classification of platelet concentrates: from pure platelet-rich plasma (P-PRP) to leucocyte- and platelet-rich fibrin (L-PRF). Trends Biotechnol. 2009;27(3):158–67.
15. Dohan Ehrenfest DM, Bielecki T, Jimbo R, Barbe G, Del Corso M, Inchingolo F, et al. Do the fibrin architecture and leukocyte content influence the growth factor release of platelet concentrates? An evidence-based answer comparing a pure platelet-rich plasma (P-PRP) gel and a leukocyte- and platelet-rich fibrin (L-PRF). Curr Pharm Biotechnol. 2012;13(7):1145–52.
16. Mishra A, Harmon K, Woodall J, Vieira A. Sports medicine applications of platelet rich plasma. Curr Pharm Biotechnol. 2012;13(7):1185–95.
17. Bielecki T, Dohan Ehrenfest DM, Everts PA, Wiczkowski A. The role of leukocytes from L-PRP/L-PRF in wound healing and immune defense: new perspectives. Curr Pharm Biotechnol. 2012;13(7):1153–62.
18. Cavallo C, Filardo G, Mariani E, Kon E, Marcacci M, Pereira Ruiz MT, et al. Comparison of platelet-rich plasma formulations for cartilage healing: an in vitro study. J Bone Joint Surg Am. 2014;96(5):423–9.
19. Moojen DJ, Everts PA, Schure RM, Overdevest EP, van Zundert A, Knape JT, et al. Antimicrobial activity of platelet-leukocyte gel against Staphylococcus aureus. J Orthop Res. 2008;26(3):404–10.
20. Di Martino A, Di Matteo B, Papio T, Tentoni F, Selleri F, Cenacchi A, et al. Platelet-rich plasma versus hyaluronic acid injections for the treatment of knee osteoarthritis: results at 5 years of a double-blind, randomized controlled trial. Am J Sports Med. 2019;47(2):347–54.
21. Connell DA, Schneider-Kolsky ME, Hoving JL, et al. Longitudinal study comparing sonographic and MRI assessments of acute and healing hamstring injuries. AJR Am J Roentgenol. 2004;183:975–84.
22. de Jesus JO, Parker L, Frangos AJ, et al. Accuracy of MRI, MR arthrography, and ultrasound in the diagnosis of rotator cuff tears: a meta-analysis. AJR Am J Roentgenol. 2009;192:1701–7.
23. Warden SJ, Kiss ZS, Malara FA, et al. Comparative accuracy of magnetic resonance imaging and ultrasonography in confirming clinically diagnosed patellar tendinopathy. Am J Sports Med. 2007;35:427–36.
24. Setayesh K, Villarreal A, Gottschalk A, et al. Treatment of muscle injuries with platelet-rich plasma: a review of the literature. Curr Rev Musculoskelet Med. 2018;11:635–42.
25. Hussain N, Johal H, Bhandari M. An evidence-based evaluation on the use of platelet rich plasma in orthopedics—a review of the literature. SICOT J. 2017;3:57.
26. Yan R, Gu Y, Ran J, et al. Intratendon delivery of leukocyte-poor platelet-rich plasma improves healing compared with leukocyte-rich platelet-rich

plasma in a rabbit Achilles tendinopathy model. Am J Sports Med. 2017;45:1909–20.
27. Rossi LA, Molina Rómoli AR, Bertona Altieri BA, et al. Does platelet-rich plasma decrease time to return to sports in acute muscle tear? A randomized controlled trial. Knee Surg Sports Traumatol Arthrosc. 2017;25:3319–25.
28. Mishra AK, Skrepnik NV, Edwards SG, et al. Efficacy of platelet-rich plasma for chronic tennis elbow: a double-blind, prospective, multicenter, randomized controlled trial of 230 patients. Am J Sports Med. 2014;42:463–71.
29. Dragoo JL, Wasterlain AS, Braun HJ, et al. Platelet-rich plasma as a treatment for patellar tendinopathy: a double-blind, randomized controlled trial. Am J Sports Med. 2014;42:610–8.
30. Boesen AP, Hansen R, Boesen MI, et al. Effect of high-volume injection, platelet-rich plasma, and sham treatment in chronic midportion Achilles tendinopathy: a randomized double-blinded prospective study. Am J Sports Med. 2017;45:2034–43.
31. Maffulli N, Longo UG, Loppini M, et al. Tissue engineering for rotator cuff repair: an evidence-based systematic review. Stem Cells Int. 2012;2012:418086.
32. Andia I, Maffulli N. Use of platelet-rich plasma for patellar tendon and medial collateral ligament injuries: best current clinical practice. J Knee Surg. 2015;28:11–8.
33. Franceschi F, Papalia R, Franceschetti E, et al. Platelet-rich plasma injections for chronic plantar fasciopathy: a systematic review. Br Med Bull. 2014;112:83–95.
34. Saltzman BM, Jain A, Campbell KA, et al. Does the use of platelet-rich plasma at the time of surgery improve clinical outcomes in arthroscopic rotator cuff repair when compared with control cohorts? A systematic review of meta-analyses. Arthroscopy. 2016;32:906–18.
35. Filardo G, Di Matteo B, Kon E, et al. Platelet-rich plasma in tendon-related disorders: results and indications. Knee Surg Sports Traumatol Arthrosc. 2018;26:1984–99.
36. Mirzatolooei F, Alamdari MT, Khalkhali HR. The impact of platelet-rich plasma on the prevention of tunnel widening in anterior cruciate ligament reconstruction using quadrupled autologous hamstring tendon: a randomised clinical trial. Bone Joint J. 2013;95-B:65–9.
37. Terada S, Ota S, Kobayashi M, et al. Use of an antifibrotic agent improves the effect of platelet-rich plasma on muscle healing after injury. J Bone Joint Surg Am. 2013;95:980–8.
38. Delos D, Maak TG, Rodeo SA. Muscle injuries in athletes: enhancing recovery through scientific understanding and novel therapies. Sports Health. 2013;5:346–52.
39. A Hamid MS, Mohamed Ali MR, Yusof A, et al. Platelet-rich plasma injections for the treatment of hamstring injuries: a randomized controlled trial. Am J Sports Med. 2014;42:2410–8.
40. Sheth U, Dwyer T, Smith I, et al. Does platelet-rich plasma lead to earlier return to sport when compared with conservative treatment in acute muscle injuries? A systematic review and meta-analysis. Arthroscopy. 2018;34:281–288.e1.
41. Hamilton B, Tol JL, Almusa E, et al. Platelet-rich plasma does not enhance return to play in hamstring injuries: a randomised controlled trial. Br J Sports Med. 2015;49:943–50.
42. Grassi A, Napoli F, Romandini I, et al. Is platelet-rich plasma (PRP) effective in the treatment of acute muscle injuries? A systematic review and meta-analysis. Sports Med. 2018;48:971–89.
43. Hoffmann A, Gross G. Tendon and ligament engineering in the adult organism: mesenchymal stem cells and gene-therapeutic approaches. Int Orthop. 2007;31(6):791–7.
44. Sánchez M, Delgado D, Sánchez P, et al. Platelet rich plasma and knee surgery. Biomed Res Int. 2014;2014:890630.
45. Woo SL, Abramowitch SD, Kilger R, et al. Biomechanics of knee ligaments: injury, healing, and repair. J Biomech. 2006;39(1):1–20.
46. Caplan AI, Dennis JE. Mesenchymal stem cells as trophic mediators. J Cell Biochem. 2006;98(5):1076–84.
47. Ekdahl M, Wang JH, Ronga M, Fu FH. Graft healing in anterior cruciate ligament reconstruction. Knee Surg Sports Traumatol Arthrosc. 2008;16(10):935–47.
48. Zhang J, Middleton KK, Fu FH, et al. HGF mediates the anti-inflammatory effects of PRP on injured tendons. PLoS One. 2013;8(6):e67303.
49. Kia C, Baldino J, Bell R, Ramji A, et al. Platelet-rich plasma: review of current literature on its use for tendon and ligament pathology. Curr Rev Musculoskelet Med. 2018;11(4):566–72.
50. Madry H, Kohn D, Cucchiarini M. Direct FGF-2 gene transfer via recombinant adeno-associated virus vectors stimulates cell proliferation, collagen production, and the repair of experimental lesions in the human ACL. Am J Sports Med. 2013;41:194–202.
51. Marui T, Niyibizi C, Georgescu HI, et al. Effect of growth factors on matrix synthesis by ligament fibroblasts. J Orthop Res. 1997;15:18–23.
52. Hildebrand KA, Woo SL-Y, Smith DW, et al. The effects of platelet derived growth factor-BB on healing of the rabbit medial collateral ligament: an in vivo study. Am J Sports Med. 1998;26:549–54.
53. Fleming BC, Spindler KP, Palmer MP, et al. Collagen-platelet composites improve the biomechanical properties of healing anterior cruciate ligament grafts in a porcine model. Am J Sports Med. 2009;37:1554–63.
54. Zhao JG, Zhao L, Jiang YX, et al. Platelet-rich plasma in arthroscopic rotator cuff repair: a meta- analysis of randomized controlled trials. Arthroscopy. 2015;31(1):125–35.
55. Figueroa D, Figueroa F, Calvo R, et al. Platelet-rich plasma use in anterior cruciate ligament surgery:

systematic review of the literature. Arthroscopy. 2015;31(5):981–8.
56. Komatsu DE, King L, Gurevich M, et al. The in vivo impact of leukocyte injections on normal rat Achilles tendons: potential detriment to tendon morphology, cellularity, and vascularity. Am J Orthop (Belle Mead NJ). 2018;47(10).
57. Xu Z, Yin W, Zhang Y, et al. Comparative evaluation of leukocyte- and platelet-rich plasma and pure platelet-rich plasma for cartilage regeneration. Sci Rep. 2017;7:43301.
58. Magnussen RA, Flanigan DC, Pedroza AD, et al. Platelet rich plasma use in allograft ACL reconstructions: two-year clinical results of a MOON cohort study. Knee. 2013;20(4):277–80.
59. Vogrin M, Rupreht M, Crnjac A, et al. The effect of platelet-derived growth factors on knee stability after anterior cruciate ligament reconstruction: a prospective randomized clinical study. Wien Klin Wochenschrift. 2010;122(S2):91–5.
60. Vadalà A, Iorio R, De Carli A, et al. Platelet-rich plasma: does it help reduce tunnel widening after ACL reconstruction? Knee Surg Sports Traumatol Arthrosc. 2013;21(4):824–9.
61. Rupreht M, Vogrin M, Hussein M. MRI evaluation of tibial tunnel wall cortical bone formation after platelet-rich plasma applied during anterior cruciate ligament reconstruction. Radiol Oncol. 2013;47(2):118–24.
62. Di Matteo B, Loibl M, Andriolo L, et al. Biologic agents for anterior cruciate ligament healing: a systematic review. World J Orthop. 2016;7(9):592–603.
63. Anitua E, Sánchez M. A new biological approach to Orthopedic surgery and sports medicine. 1st ed. Madrid: Team Work Media; 2013.
64. Khan KM, Scott A. Mechanotherapy: how physical therapists' prescription of exercise promotes tissue repair. Br J Sports Med. 2009;43(4):247.
65. Kelly JD, IV, editor. Meniscal injuries [Internet]. New York: Springer New York; 2014 [cited 2019 Aug 22]. http://link.springer.com/10.1007/978-1-4614-8486-8.
66. Chirichella PS, Jow S, Iacono S, Wey HE, Malanga GA. Treatment of knee meniscus pathology: rehabilitation, surgery, and orthobiologics. PM R. 2019;11(3):292–308.
67. Doral MN, Bilge O, Huri G, Turhan E, Verdonk R. Modern treatment of meniscal tears. EFORT Open Rev. 2018;3:260–8.
68. Makris EA, Hadidi P, Athanasiou KA. The knee meniscus: structure–function, pathophysiology, current repair techniques, and prospects for regeneration. Biomaterials. 2011;32:7411–31.
69. Cooper DE, Arnoczky SP, Warren RF. Meniscal repair. Clin Sports Med. 1991;10:529–48.
70. LaPrade RF, Arendt EA, Getgood A, Faucett SC, editors. The menisci [Internet]. Berlin: Springer; 2017 [cited 2019 Aug 22]. http://link.springer.com/10.1007/978-3-662-53792-3.
71. Hulet C, Pereira H, Peretti G, Denti M, editors. Surgery of the meniscus [Internet]. Berlin: Springer; 2016 [cited 2019 Aug 22]. http://link.springer.com/10.1007/978-3-662-49188-1.
72. Wadhwa V, Omar H, Coyner K, Khazzam M, Robertson W, Chhabra A. ISAKOS classification of meniscal tears—illustration on 2D and 3D isotropic spin echo MR imaging. Eur J Radiol. 2016;85:15–24.
73. Anderson AF, Irrgang JJ, Dunn W, Beaufils P, Cohen M, Cole BJ, et al. Interobserver reliability of the International Society of Arthroscopy, Knee Surgery and Orthopaedic Sports Medicine (ISAKOS) classification of meniscal tears. Am J Sports Med. 2011;39:926–32.
74. Anderson AF. The ISAKOS classification of meniscal tears. ISAKOS Newsletter. 2010;14:11–3.
75. Snoeker BAM, Bakker EWP, Kegel CAT, Lucas C. Risk factors for meniscal tears: a systematic review including meta-analysis. J Orthop Sports Phys Ther. 2013;43:352–67.
76. Hwang B-Y, Kim S-J, Lee S-W, Lee H-E, Lee C-K, Hunter DJ, et al. Risk factors for medial meniscus posterior root tear. Am J Sports Med. 2012;40:1606–10.
77. Jones JC, Burks R, Owens BD, Sturdivant RX, Svoboda SJ, Cameron KL. Incidence and risk factors associated with meniscal injuries among active-duty US military service members. J Athl Train. 2012;47:67–73.
78. Baker BE, Peckham AC, Pupparo F, Sanborn JC. Review of meniscal injury and associated sports. Am J Sports Med. 1985;13:1–4.
79. Nielsen AB, Yde J. Epidemiology of acute knee injuries: a prospective hospital investigation. J Trauma. 1991;31:1644–8.
80. Lauder TD, Baker SP, Smith GS, Lincoln AE. Sports and physical training injury hospitalizations in the army. Am J Prev Med. 2000;18:118–28.
81. Ma JZ, Cui SF, Hu F, Lu QJ, Li W. Incidence and characteristics of meniscal injuries in cadets at a military school, 2013-2015. J Athl Train. 2016;51:876–9.
82. Steadman JR, Matheny LM, Singleton SB, Johnson NS, Rodkey WG, Crespo B, et al. Meniscus suture repair: minimum 10-year outcomes in patients younger than 40 years compared with patients 40 and older. Am J Sports Med. 2015;43:2222–7.
83. Hauser RA, Phillips HJ, Maddela H. Platelet rich plasma prolotherapy as first-line treatment for meniscal pathology. Pract Pain Manag. 2010;10.
84. Beaty JH, Canale ST, Campbell WC. Campbell's operative orthopaedics. [Internet]. Philadelphia: Elsevier Mosby; 2013 [cited 2019 Aug 22]. https://nls.ldls.org.uk/welcome.html?ark:/81055/vdc_100052194843.0x000001.
85. Smith BE, Thacker D, Crewesmith A, Hall M. Special tests for assessing meniscal tears within the knee: a systematic review and meta-analysis. Evid Based Med. 2015;20:88–97.

86. Hegedus EJ, Cook C, Hasselblad V, Goode A, McCrory DC. Physical examination tests for assessing a torn meniscus in the knee: a systematic review with meta-analysis. J Orthop Sports Phys Ther. 2007;37:541–50.
87. Pookarnjanamorakot C, Korsantirat T, Woratanarat P. Meniscal lesions in the anterior cruciate insufficient knee: the accuracy of clinical evaluation. J Med Assoc Thail. 2004;87:618–23.
88. Antunes LC, de Souza JMG, Cerqueira NB, Dahmer C, de Pinho Tavares BA, de Faria ÂJN. Evaluation of clinical tests and magnetic resonance imaging for knee meniscal injuries: correlation with video arthroscopy. Rev Bras Ortop. 2017;52:582–8.
89. Dai H, Huang Z, Chen Z, Liu J. Diagnostic accuracy of ultrasonography in assessing meniscal injury: meta-analysis of prospective studies. J Orthop Sci. 2015;20:675–81.
90. Shetty AA, Tindall AJ, James KD, Relwani J, Fernando KW. Accuracy of hand-held ultrasound scanning in detecting meniscal tears. J Bone Joint Surg. 2008;90-B:1045–8.
91. Lefevre N, Naouri JF, Herman S, Gerometta A, Klouche S, Bohu Y. A current review of the meniscus imaging: proposition of a useful tool for its radiologic analysis. Radiol Res Pract. 2016;2016:1–25.
92. Magee T, Williams D. 3.0-T MRI of meniscal tears. Am J Roentgenol. 2006;187:371–5.
93. Wong S, Steinbach L, Zhao J, Stehling C, Ma CB, Link TM. Comparative study of imaging at 3.0 T versus 1.5 T of the knee. Skelet Radiol. 2009;38:761–9.
94. Van Dyck P, Vanhoenacker FM, Lambrecht V, Wouters K, Gielen JL, Dossche L, et al. Prospective comparison of 1.5 and 3.0-T MRI for evaluating the knee menisci and ACL. J Bone Joint Surg Am. 2013;95:916–24.
95. Longo UG, Campi S, Romeo G, Spiezia F, Maffulli N, Denaro V. Biological strategies to enhance healing of the avascular area of the meniscus. Stem Cells Int. 2012;2012:1–7.
96. Kaminski R, Maksymowicz-Wleklik M, Kulinski K, Kozar-Kaminska K, Dabrowska-Thing A, Pomianowski S. Short-term outcomes of percutaneous trephination with a platelet rich plasma intrameniscal injection for the repair of degenerative meniscal lesions. A prospective, randomized, double-blind, parallel-group, placebo-controlled study. Int J Mol Sci. 2019;20:856.
97. Uchio Y, Ochi M, Adachi N, Kawasaki K, Iwasa J. Results of rasping of meniscal tears with and without anterior cruciate ligament injury as evaluated by second-look arthroscopy. Arthroscopy. 2003;19:463–9.
98. Arnoczky SP, Warren RF. The microvasculature of the meniscus and its response to injury. An experimental study in the dog. Am J Sports Med. 1983;11:131–41.
99. Gao JZ. [Experimental study on healing of old tear in the avascular portion of menisci in dogs]. Zhonghua Wai Ke Za Zhi. 1990;28:726–9, 782.
100. Fox JM, Rintz KG, Ferkel RD. Trephination of incomplete meniscal tears. Arthroscopy. 1993;9:451–5.
101. Zhang Z, Arnold JA. Trephination and suturing of avascular meniscal tears: a clinical study of the trephination procedure. Arthroscopy. 1996;12:726–31.
102. Nakhostine M, Gershuni DH, Anderson R, Danzig LA, Weiner GM. Effects of abrasion therapy on tears in the avascular region of sheep menisci. Arthroscopy. 1990;6:280–7.
103. Cisa J, Basora J, Madarnas P, Ghibely A, Navarro-Quilis A. Meniscal repair by synovial flap transfer. Healing of the avascular zone in rabbits. Acta Orthop Scand. 1995;66:38–40.
104. Yamazaki K, Tachibana Y. Vascularized synovial flap promoting regeneration of the cryopreserved meniscal allograft: experimental study in rabbits. J Orthop Sci. 2003;8:62–8.
105. Henning CE, Lynch MA, Clark JR. Vascularity for healing of meniscus repairs. Arthroscopy. 1987;3:13–8.
106. Shelbourne KD, Gray T. Meniscus tears that can be left in situ, with or without trephination or synovial abrasion to stimulate healing. Sports Med Arthrosc Rev. 2012;20:62–7.
107. Hutchinson I, Rodeo S, Perrone G, Murray M. Can platelet-rich plasma enhance anterior cruciate ligament and meniscal repair? J Knee Surg. 2014;28:019–28.
108. Chrysanthou C, Laliotis N, Galanis N, Paraskevas G, Potoupnis M, Sayegh F, et al. Meniscal repair using fibrin clot from autologous blood: description of the surgical technique. JRPMS. 2018;02:89–94.
109. Chahla J, Kennedy NI, Geeslin AG, Moatshe G, Cinque ME, DePhillipo NN, et al. Meniscal repair with fibrin clot augmentation. Arthrosc Tech. 2017;6:e2065–9.
110. Kemmochi M, Sasaki S, Takahashi M, Nishimura T, Aizawa C, Kikuchi J. The use of platelet-rich fibrin with platelet-rich plasma support meniscal repair surgery. J Orthop. 2018;15:711–20.
111. Sidelmann JJ, Gram J, Jespersen J, Kluft C. Fibrin clot formation and lysis: basic mechanisms. Semin Thromb Hemost. 2000;26:605–18.
112. Jang SH, Ha JK, Lee DW, Kim JG. Fibrin clot delivery system for meniscal repair. Knee Surg Relat Res. 2011;23:180–3.
113. Sethi PM, Cooper A, Jokl P. Technical tips in orthopaedics: meniscal repair with use of an in situ fibrin clot. Arthroscopy. 2003;19:1–4.
114. Zhang S, Matsushita T, Kuroda R, Nishida K, Matsuzaki T, Matsumoto T, et al. Local administration of simvastatin stimulates healing of an avascular meniscus in a rabbit model of a meniscal defect. Am J Sports Med. 2016;44:1735–43.
115. Arnoczky SP, Warren RF, Spivak JM. Meniscal repair using an exogenous fibrin clot. An experimental study in dogs. J Bone Joint Surg Am. 1988;70:1209–17.

116. Henning CE, Lynch MA, Yearout KM, Vequist SW, Stallbaumer RJ, Decker KA. Arthroscopic meniscal repair using an exogenous fibrin clot. Clin Orthop Relat Res. 1990:64–72.
117. van Trommel MF, Simonian PT, Potter HG, Wickiewicz TL. Arthroscopic meniscal repair with fibrin clot of complete radial tears of the lateral meniscus in the avascular zone. Arthroscopy. 1998;14:360–5.
118. Ra HJ, Ha JK, Jang SH, Lee DW, Kim JG. Arthroscopic inside-out repair of complete radial tears of the meniscus with a fibrin clot. Knee Surg Sports Traumatol Arthrosc. 2013;21:2126–30.
119. Yaltirik M, Koray M, Kocaelli H, Ofluoglu D. Platelet-rich plasma in trauma patients. In: Gözler S, editor. Trauma in dentistry [Internet]. IntechOpen; 2019 [cited 2019 Aug 23]. https://www.intechopen.com/books/trauma-in-dentistry/platelet-rich-plasma-in-trauma-patients.
120. Niewczas P, Kotela A, Łęgosz P, Pirko-Kotela K, Sarzyńska S, Starczyńska M. Use of platelet-rich plasma in orthopaedics and traumatology. Med Stud. 2016;1:63–8.
121. Alves R, Grimalt R. A review of platelet-rich plasma: history, biology, mechanism of action, and classification. Skin Appendage Disord. 2018;4:18–24.
122. Cozma CN, Raducu L, Jecan CR. Platelet rich plasma—mechanism of action and clinical applications. J Clin Investig Surg. 2016;1:41–6.
123. Dhurat R, Sukesh M. Principles and methods of preparation of platelet-rich plasma: a review and author's perspective. J Cutan Aesthet Surg. 2014;7:189.
124. Ishida K, Kuroda R, Miwa M, Tabata Y, Hokugo A, Kawamoto T, et al. The regenerative effects of platelet-rich plasma on meniscal cells *in vitro* and its *in vivo* application with biodegradable gelatin hydrogel. Tissue Eng. 2007;13:1103–12.
125. Pujol N, Tardy N, Boisrenoult P, Beaufils P. Long-term outcomes of all-inside meniscal repair. Knee Surg Sports Traumatol Arthrosc. 2015;23:219–24.
126. Kaminski R, Kulinski K, Kozar-Kaminska K, Wielgus M, Langner M, Wasko MK, et al. A prospective, randomized, double-blind, parallel-group, placebo-controlled study evaluating meniscal healing, clinical outcomes, and safety in patients undergoing meniscal repair of unstable, complete vertical meniscal tears (bucket handle) augmented with platelet-rich plasma. Biomed Res Int. 2018;2018:1–9.
127. Griffin JW, Hadeed MM, Werner BC, Diduch DR, Carson EW, Miller MD. Platelet-rich plasma in meniscal repair: does augmentation improve surgical outcomes? Clin Orthop Relat Res. 2015;473:1665–72.
128. Dai W-L, Zhang H, Lin Z-M, Shi Z-J, Wang J. Efficacy of platelet-rich plasma in arthroscopic repair for discoid lateral meniscus tears. BMC Musculoskelet Disord. 2019;20:113.
129. Zhang H, Chen S, Qiu M, Zhou A, Yan W, Zhang J. Lateral meniscus allograft transplantation with platelet-rich plasma injections: a minimum two-year follow-up study. Knee. 2018;25:568–76.
130. Everhart JS, Cavendish PA, Eikenberry A, Magnussen RA, Kaeding CC, Flanigan DC. Platelet-rich plasma reduces failure risk for isolated meniscal repairs but provides no benefit for meniscal repairs with anterior cruciate ligament reconstruction. Am J Sports Med. 2019;47:1789–96.
131. Blanke F. Percutaneous injections of platelet rich plasma for treatment of intrasubstance meniscal lesions. Muscles Ligaments Tendons J [Internet]. 2015 [cited 2019 Aug 23]. http://www.mltj.org/common/php/portiere.php?ID=9a59ca680004bb9e0b27d767bf19dc91.
132. Betancourt JP, Murrell WD. Leukocyte-poor platelet-rich plasma to treat degenerative meniscal tear: a case report. J Clin Orthop Trauma. 2016;7:106–9.
133. Strümper R. Intra-articular injections of autologous conditioned serum to treat pain from meniscal lesions. Sports Med Int Open. 2017;1:E200–5.
134. Koch M, Hammer S, Fuellerer J, Lang S, Pfeifer C, Pattappa G, et al. Bone marrow aspirate concentrate for the treatment of avascular meniscus tears in a one-step procedure—evaluation of an in vivo model. IJMS. 2019;20:1120.
135. Pak J, Lee JH, Lee SH. Regenerative repair of damaged meniscus with autologous adipose tissue-derived stem cells. Biomed Res Int. 2014;2014:1–10.
136. Pak J, Lee JH, Park KS, Jeon JH, Lee SH. Potential use of mesenchymal stem cells in human meniscal repair: current insights. OAJSM. 2017;8:33–8.
137. Dean CS, Chahla J, Matheny LM, Mitchell JJ, LaPrade RF. Outcomes after biologically augmented isolated meniscal repair with marrow venting are comparable with those after meniscal repair with concomitant anterior cruciate ligament reconstruction. Am J Sports Med. 2017;45:1341–8.
138. Driscoll MD, Robin BN, Horie M, Hubert ZT, Sampson HW, Jupiter DC, et al. Marrow stimulation improves meniscal healing at early endpoints in a rabbit meniscal injury model. Arthroscopy. 2013;29:113–21.
139. Ferris D, Frisbie D, Kisiday J, McIlwraith CW. *In vivo* healing of meniscal lacerations using bone marrow-derived mesenchymal stem cells and fibrin glue. Stem Cells Int. 2012;2012:1–9.
140. Tarafder S, Gulko J, Sim KH, Yang J, Cook JL, Lee CH. Engineered healing of avascular meniscus tears by stem cell recruitment. Sci Rep. 2018;8:8150.
141. Kaminski R, Kulinski K, Kozar-Kaminska K, Wasko MK, Langner M, Pomianowski S. Repair augmentation of unstable, complete vertical meniscal tears with bone marrow venting procedure: a prospective, randomized, double-blind, parallel-group, placebo-controlled study. Arthroscopy. 2019;35:1500–1508.e1.
142. Piontek T, Ciemniewska-Gorzela K, Naczk J, Jakob R, Szulc A, Grygorowicz M, et al. Complex meniscus tears treated with collagen matrix wrapping and

bone marrow blood injection: a 2-year clinical follow-up. Cartilage. 2016;7:123–39.
143. Abram SGF, Beard DJ, Price AJ, BASK Meniscal Working Group. Arthroscopic meniscal surgery: a national society treatment guideline and consensus statement. Bone Joint J. 2019;101-B:652–9.
144. Katz JN, Brophy RH, Chaisson CE, de Chaves L, Cole BJ, Dahm DL, et al. Surgery versus physical therapy for a meniscal tear and osteoarthritis. N Engl J Med. 2013;368:1675–84.
145. Sihvonen R, Paavola M, Malmivaara A, Itälä A, Joukainen A, Nurmi H, et al. Arthroscopic partial meniscectomy versus sham surgery for a degenerative meniscal tear. N Engl J Med. 2013;369:2515–24.
146. Beaufils P, Becker R, Kopf S, Englund M, Verdonk R, Ollivier M, et al. Surgical management of degenerative meniscus lesions: the 2016 ESSKA meniscus consensus. Knee Surg Sports Traumatol Arthrosc. 2017;25:335–46.
147. Dominici M, Le Blanc K, Mueller I, Slaper-Cortenbach I, Marini F, Krause D, et al. Minimal criteria for defining multipotent mesenchymal stromal cells. The International Society for Cellular Therapy position statement. Cytotherapy. 2006;8(4):315–7.
148. Caplan AI. Mesenchymal stem cells: time to change the name! Stem Cells Transl Med. 2017;6(6):1445–51.
149. Chu CR, Rodeo S, Bhutani N, Goodrich LR, Huard J, Irrgang J, et al. Optimizing clinical use of biologics in orthopaedic surgery: consensus recommendations from the 2018 AAOS/NIH U-13 conference. J Am Acad Orthop Surg. 2019;27(2):e50–63.
150. Murray IR, Chahla J, Safran MR, Krych AJ, Saris DBF, Caplan AI, et al. International expert consensus on a cell therapy communication tool: DOSES. J Bone Joint Surg Am. 2019;101(10):904–11.
151. Cassano JM, Kennedy JG, Ross KA, Fraser EJ, Goodale MB, Fortier LA. Bone marrow concentrate and platelet-rich plasma differ in cell distribution and interleukin 1 receptor antagonist protein concentration. Knee Surg Sports Traumatol Arthrosc. 2018;26(1):333–42.
152. Jones IA, Wilson M, Togashi R, Han B, Mircheff AK, Thomas Vangsness C Jr. A randomized, controlled study to evaluate the efficacy of intra-articular, autologous adipose tissue injections for the treatment of mild-to-moderate knee osteoarthritis compared to hyaluronic acid: a study protocol. BMC Musculoskelet Disord. 2018;19(1):383.
153. Gobbi A, Whyte GP. Long-term clinical outcomes of one-stage cartilage repair in the knee with hyaluronic acid-based scaffold embedded with mesenchymal stem cells sourced from bone marrow aspirate concentrate. Am J Sports Med. 2019;47(7):1621–8.
154. Caplan AI, Correa D. The MSC: an injury drugstore. Cell Stem Cell. 2011;9(1):11–5.
155. Hernigou P, Flouzat Lachaniette CH, Delambre J, Zilber S, Duffiet P, Chevallier N, et al. Biologic augmentation of rotator cuff repair with mesenchymal stem cells during arthroscopy improves healing and prevents further tears: a case-controlled study. Int Orthop. 2014;38(9):1811–8.
156. Centeno CJ, Pitts J, Al-Sayegh H, Freeman MD. Anterior cruciate ligament tears treated with percutaneous injection of autologous bone marrow nucleated cells: a case series. J Pain Res. 2015;8:437–47.
157. Gobbi A, Whyte GP. Long-term outcomes of primary repair of the anterior cruciate ligament combined with biologic healing augmentation to treat incomplete tears. Am J Sports Med. 2018;46(14):3368–77.
158. Vangsness CT Jr, Farr J 2nd, Boyd J, Dellaero DT, Mills CR, LeRoux-Williams M. Adult human mesenchymal stem cells delivered via intra-articular injection to the knee following partial medial meniscectomy: a randomized, double-blind, controlled study. J Bone Joint Surg Am. 2014;96(2):90–8.
159. Pak J, Chang JJ, Lee JH, Lee SH. Safety reporting on implantation of autologous adipose tissue-derived stem cells with platelet-rich plasma into human articular joints. BMC Musculoskelet Disord. 2013;14:337.
160. Pak J, Lee JH, Park KS, Park M, Kang LW, Lee SH. Current use of autologous adipose tissue-derived stromal vascular fraction cells for orthopedic applications. J Biomed Sci. 2017;24(1):9.
161. Snyder TN, Madhavan K, Intrator M, Dregalla RC, Park D. A fibrin/hyaluronic acid hydrogel for the delivery of mesenchymal stem cells and potential for articular cartilage repair. J Biol Eng. 2014;8:10. https://doi.org/10.1186/1754-1611-8-10.
162. Anitua E, Sanchez M. A new biological approach to orthopaedic surgery and sports medicine. Madrid: Vitoria Team Work Media; 2013.
163. Infante A, Rubio-Azpeitia E, Sánchez P, Alberdi R, Rodriguez CI, Andia I. Platelet rich plasma and culture configuration affect the matrix forming phenotype of bone marrow stromal cells. Tissue Eng Regen Med. 2017;14:567–77.
164. van Buul GM, Koevoet WL, Kops N, et al. Platelet-rich plasma releasate inhibits inflammatory processes in osteoarthritic chondrocytes. Am J Sports Med. 2011;39(11):2362–70.
165. Wang-Saegusa A, Cugat R, Ares O, Seijas R, Cusco X, Garcia-Balletbo M. Infiltration of plasma rich in growth factors for osteoarthritis of the knee short-term effects on function and quality of life. Arch Orthop Trauma Surg. 2011;131(3):311–7.
166. Cugat R, Alentorn-Geli E, Steinbacher G, et al. Treatment of knee osteochondral lesions using a novel clot of autologous plasma rich in growth factors mixed with healthy hyaline cartilage chips and intra-articular injection of PRGF. Case Rep Orthop. 2017;2017:8284548. https://doi.org/10.1155/2017/8284548.
167. Dominguez Perez JM, Fernandez-Sarmiento JA, Aguilar Garcia D, et al. Cartilage regeneration using a novel autologous growth factors-based matrix for

full-thickness defects in sheep. Knee Surg Sports Traumatol Arthrosc. 2019;27(3):950–61. https://doi.org/10.1007/s00167-018-5107-z.

168. Cugat R, Alentorn-Geli E, Navarro J, Cuscó X, Steinbacher G, Seijas R, Álvarez-Díaz P, Barastegui D, Laiz P, Samitier G, García-Balletbó M. A novel autologous-made matrix using hyaline cartilage chips and platelet-rich growth factors for the treatment of full-thickness cartilage or osteochondral defects: preliminary results. J Orthop Surg (Hong Kong). 2020;28(1):2309499019887547.

29 ARIF (Arthroscopic Reduction and Internal Fixation) Around the Elbow

E. Guerra, A. Marinelli, G. Bettelli, M. Cavallo, A. Ritali, and R. Rotini

29.1 Introduction

Arthroscopy of the elbow is a relatively recent surgical procedure. Although the first experience described in the literature dates back to the 80s, it is only in the last 15 years that a real and increasing interest can be seen with the inclusion of series of patients [1] and case reports that describe the research for new indications.

Intra-articular fractures, by their definition, should be anatomically reduced with extreme accuracy besides being fixed in a stable manner. Arthroscopy has already shown its usefulness in all the joints, by improving the visual field of the joint surface with a minimally invasive surgical approach.

Besides several case reports in the literature on single fractures, in 2010 Savoie et al. [1, 2] performed the first overview on this innovative elbow arthroscopy technique.

The literature shows little scientific evidence about the various indications for arthroscopy of the elbow [3]. These indications include fractures of the radial head, capitellum, trochlea, and coronoid.

This chapter addresses the various articular fractures of the elbow, where arthroscopy can nowadays be considered to be a real help. The most important technical aspects are summarized in the light of the literature and the authors' personal experience.

29.2 Fractures of the Capitulum humeri and Trochlea (Shear Fracture)

Fractures of the capitulum humeri and trochlea are rare fractures that alter the joint considerably. Even when they are not the result of high energy trauma, they produce severe stiffness and instability in the elbow, if they are not immediately recognized and treated adequately.

Various classifications try to group the various morphologies and determine correct treatment algorithms (Bryan and Morrey 1985 [4], McKee 1996 [5], Ring 2003 [6], Dubberley 2006 [7]). Anatomical reduction is necessary to restore the joint anatomy and the correct tension of the external ligament compartment.

29.2.1 In the Literature

Only a few cases have been described. Feldmann [8] reported two cases of fracture with thin osteochondral fragments (Type 2 fracture, Regan and

E. Guerra (✉) · A. Marinelli · G. Bettelli
M. Cavallo · A. Ritali · R. Rotini
Istituto Ortopedico Rizzoli, Bologna, Italy
e-mail: enrico.guerra@ior.it; alessandro.marinelli@ior.it; graziano.bettelli@ior.it; marco.cavallo@ior.it; alice.ritali@ior.it; roberto.rotini@ior.it

M. T. Hirschmann et al. (eds.), *ESSKA Instructional Course Lecture Book*,
https://doi.org/10.1007/978-3-662-61264-4_29

Morrey). Having ascertained the absence of combined joint instability, this author decided for the simple removal of the fragments by arthroscopy using two approaches, anteromedial and anterolateral.

In 2002, Hardy [9] described reduction and fixation of a Hahn-Steinthal fracture (Type I, Regan and Morrey) achieved arthroscopically, by three different anterolateral approaches. The metal screw, in the subchondral bone must be tilted from lateral to medial on the frontal plane, to avoid the radial nerve.

In 2009, Mitani [10] published a new clinical case with interesting practical advice. By two simple anteromedial and anterolateral portals, he used the arthroscope together with the probe to reduce the displaced osteochondral fragment; maintaining the reduction with the probe from the anterolateral portal, he performed fixation with two metal screws in a posteroanterior direction.

The following year Kuryjama [11] went a step further by attempting arthroscopic reduction and fixation (ARIF) of two more complex cases (Type IIIA Dubberley) through two portals (anterolateral and midlateral). In one of the two cases the operation was transformed into open surgery, albeit with an incision of only a few centimeters.

29.2.2 Surgical Technique in our Experience

From 2000 to 2017 about 51 type I or type II shear fractures were treated in our department by open reduction and internal fixation in 43 cases, by miniopen technique in 5 cases and all arthroscopic in 3 cases. Our experience with arthroscopic treatment started in 2004 with 3 type III fractures in which we performed fragment removal. In the last 2 years our indications were widened to include strictly selected type I and type II fractures (8 cases).

All the patients underwent preoperative CT of the elbow that is essential to define the fracture morphology and to find medial fracture lines directed toward the trochlea or impacted fractures with osteochondral fragments deformity (so-called elbow Hill–Sachs lesions) which can make the reduction more difficult.

In open surgery, the Kocher approach extended proximally (Extensile Kocher approach) with posterolateral subluxation maneuvers, enables easy control over both the anterior articular compartment (with access to the medial trochlea) and the posterior one (to treat impacted lesions).

The capitellum and trochlea fractures that come to our attention are apparently simple injuries. The CT nearly always shows more medial fracture lines (toward the trochlea) or impact lesions with deformation of the osteochondral fragments (elbow Hill–Sachs lesions) that make reduction difficult. In arthroscopic surgery, the fracture must be well visualized in the anterior compartment and the posterolateral gutter (Fig. 29.1). Therefore, if arthroscopic treatment is selected, it is not sufficient in our opinion to perform only the anterior or posterolateral portals, but it is necessary to move the arthroscope several times, before performing fixation, which is a very complex procedure.

It is common to find an intraoperative lesion of the external collateral ligament complex, which, in open surgery can be repaired.

Another aspect to take into consideration is the direction of the fixation. We strongly advocate anterograde fixation, with screws and pins made of polylactic acid. In this direction compression fixation can be performed by sinking the screws under the cartilage plane, perpendicularly to the fracture lines. If the ARIF technique is chosen screws that enter posteriorly are needed in order to avoid risks to the radial nerve. Therefore, the screws are made of metal, and making thinner fractures stable (Type 2) will be difficult.

These reasons suggest restricting arthroscopic treatment of capitellum and trochlea fractures to rare cases that fulfill the following criteria:

- Type I and II fractures without posterior depression.
- Type III fractures.
- Absence of combined ligament lesions.

For the recommended surgical technique, the patient is placed in a lateral position. Insufflate sterile saline solution repeatedly to drain the hematoma before starting surgery (useful tip in the arthroscopic treatment of all intra-articular fractures). Through three arthroscopic approches (antero medial, antero lateral and proximal antero lateral), appropriate joint shaving and lesion planning can be performed, by keeping the arthroscope in the medial portals and working through the two lateral portals. Some authors recommend placing the elbow in extension to facilitate reduction. In our opinion, extension reduces the space to work, so we prefer to keep flexion at 90° and operate with the two lateral approaches. After performing temporary reduction and fixation,

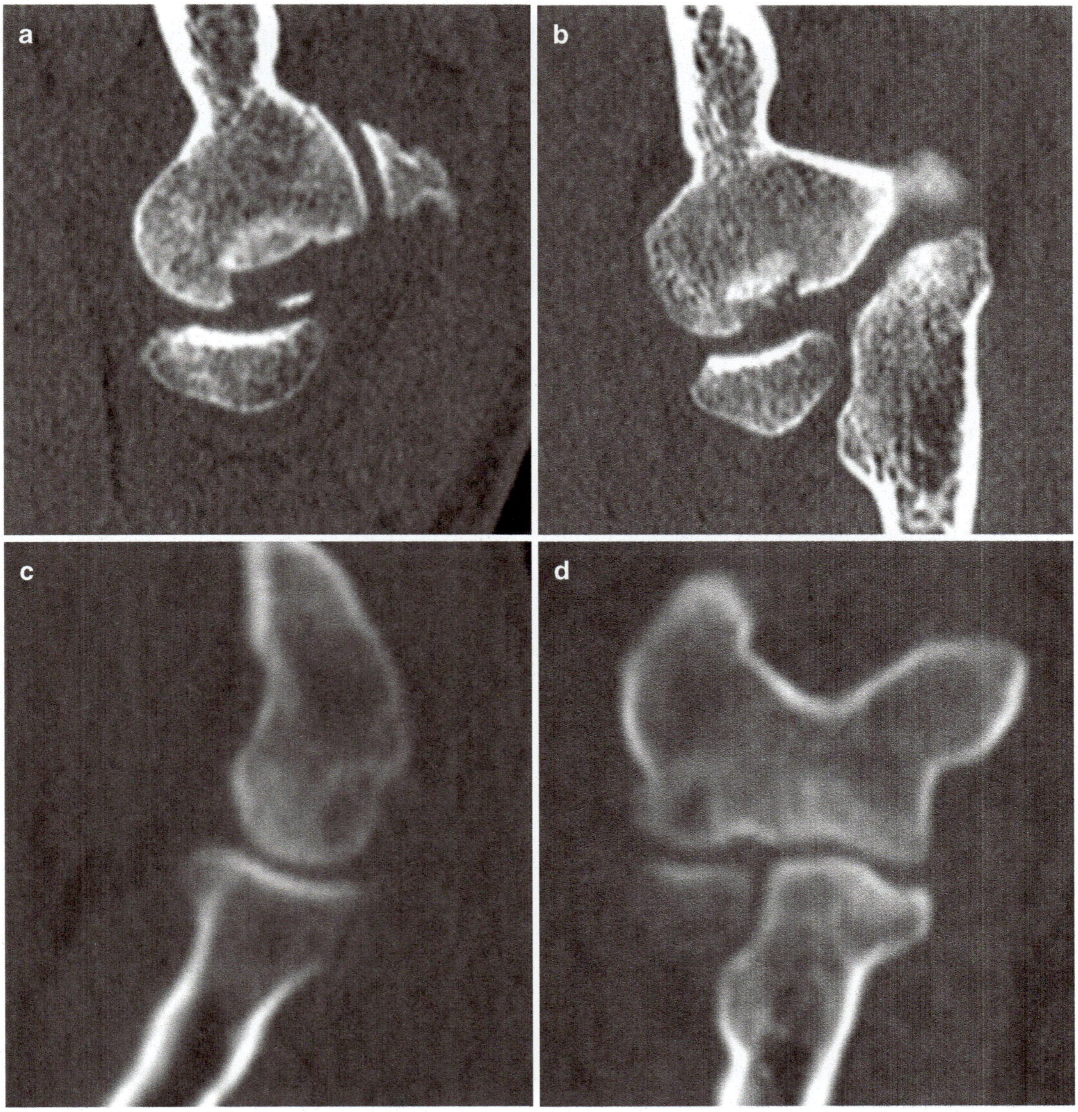

Fig. 29.1 Impacted capitellum fracture. Thirty-six-year-old patient, right elbow. CT scan image of a rare impacted fracture of the posterior face of the capitellum before (**a**, **b**) and after (**c**, **d**) reduction and fixation. Drawing (**e**) of the arthroscopic portals used to perform ARIF of the fracture. Examination of the anterior joint compartment allowed to remove the intra-articular fractured tip of the coronoid. In order to visualize the fracture it was necessary to reach the posterolateral gutter placing the scope in the posterolateral portal (**f**). Once the fracture has been reduced by a probe through the midlateral portal (**g**), fixation has been performed by a temporary percutaneous K wire (**h**) and by a resorbable pin (**h**, **i**) (RSB implant, Hit Medica, Lima Corporate)

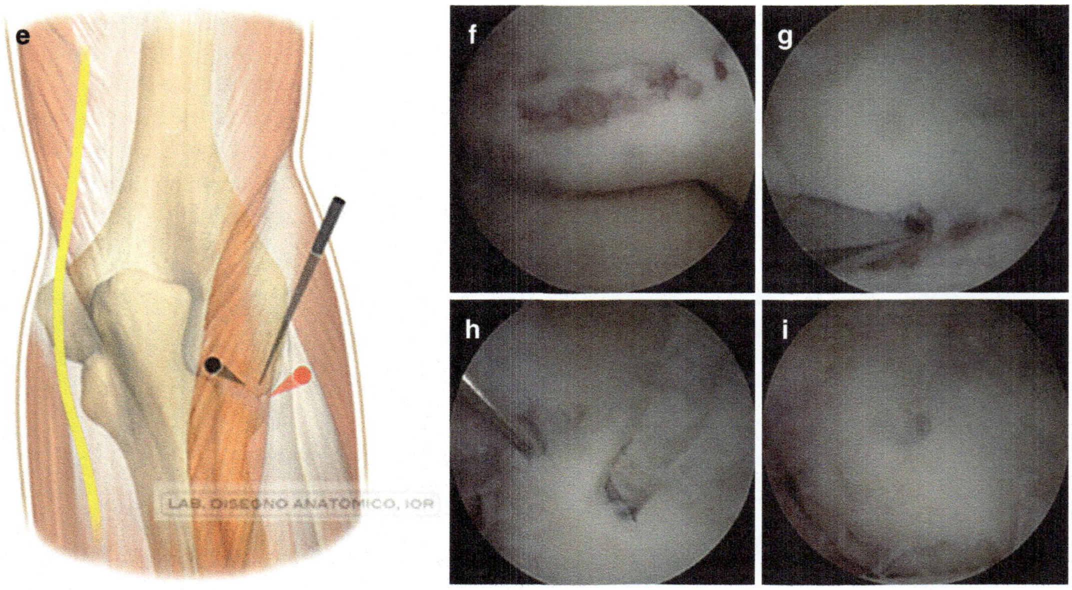

Fig. 29.1 (continued)

the fracture must be explored posterolaterally. We also recommended exploring the posterior compartment to drain the hematoma and check for any posterior loose bodies (posterolateral and posterocentral arthroscopic approaches). By the posterolateral portals it will be thus possible to go down posterolaterally to the posterior humeroradial joint (using the palpator and shaver through the midlateral approach). At this point, by bringing the arthroscope back anteromedially under image intensifier guidance, percutaneous fixation can be performed with cannulated screws, in a posteroanterior direction (enlarging the midlateral approach).

In our five cases, we preferred to end the operation in open surgery, with a small incision that joins the anteromedial portal to the midlateral one (ideally following the incision by the Kocher approach). This miniopen surgery enabled us to perform fixation with resorbable screws and pins, in an anteroposterior direction, without putting the radial nerve at risk.

Treatment was completely arthroscopic with fragments removal in three type III cases. Also in these cases we deem mandatory to explore by the arthroscope all the joint compartments, after having accurately examined the fracture comminution by CT scan, in order to reduce the risk of leaving debris.

We have concluded ARIF in only two cases: One type II where the fragment was so thin that only an osteosuture was possible and one type I fracture where the fragment was quite at its place, thick but unstable (by two cannulated screws). A small incision posteriorly on the capitulum by the same technique described for the osteosutures and screw fixation of the coronoid fracture, (see later).

The last case, apart from the presented series, is a rare impacted fracture of the capitellum (Osborne-Cotteril lesion) combined with a coronoid tip fracture (Fig. 29.1). By arthroscopy it was possible to remove the coronoid fragment (working in the anterior compartment), to raise the impacted osteochondral fragment and fix it with resorbable pins (working in the posterolateral gutter). In this case arthroscopy displayed all of its efficacy, reducing surgical aggressiveness at a minimum.

At the end of fixation or debridement, articular stability is evaluated (possible also arthroscopically [12]). Faced with doubt about the stability, we recommend exploring, and possibly repairing, the lateral collateral ligament.

29.3 Coronoid Fractures

The coronoid plays a key role in elbow joint stability. Fractures were classified into three types according to their size by Regan and Morrey [13] in 1989 and only recently have new more complex classifications been devised [13, 14] to include possible morphologies of the fragments connected to the type of injury that can produce them.

Larger fractures are caused by a direct posterior injury, whereas a posterolateral or posteromedial distortion mechanism has been identified for fractures of the apex and medial surface, respectively (sublime tubercle insertion site of the anterior bundle of the medial collateral ligament) [14].

Reduction and fixation of coronoid fractures is necessary to restore the anterior and medial elbow stability that was lost with the injury.

When combined with fractures of the radial head, which require prosthetic replacement, after radial head excision the coronoid fracture can be reached through Kocher's lateral approach. Conversely, when the fracture is isolated, reaching and exposing the coronoid requires wide approaches (anterior, anteromedial or medial), which are aggressive and not simple to perform [15].

29.3.1 In the Literature

There are only two articles in the literature.

Liu [16] in 1996 showed two cases of coronoid tip fracture, which after conservative treatment produced pain and joint stiffness. Arthroscopic removal of the fracture fragment is decisive.

But the first real experience was described by Adams [17] in 2007. Two of the seven fractures described had fragments that were too small to be fixed. In four cases arthroscopic-assisted fixation (ARIF) was performed, whereas in one case open surgery was needed to perform a stronger fixation, by dedicated plate. In three of the seven cases, reconstruction of the lateral collateral ligament (LUCL) was needed.

29.3.2 Surgical Technique in our Experience

As for capitellum fractures, coronoid fractures are very rarely isolated. Mostly, they are combined with radial head or olecranon fractures. In these cases, open surgery, necessary to treat combined fractures, cannot be replaced by arthroscopic treatment of the coronoid.

Conversely, isolated fractures of the coronoid can be treated arthroscopically. From January 2000 to July 2017, 13 of the 21 isolated coronoid fractures treated by the authors were treated arthroscopically. Four cases were treated with reduction and fixation with wires alone, three with cannulated screws as well as K wires, five with one or two osteosuture and one case with osteosuture combined with K wires. In five patients the evaluation under anesthesia revealed a posterolateral instability after the coronoid synthesis and a collateral repair were needed.

With the patient in a lateral position, and after having washed repeatedly with needle and saline solution, the anterior arthroscopic portals are made (anteromedial, anterolateral, and anteromedial or lateroproximal). Having removed the hematoma the arthroscope is inserted into the anterolateral portal to assess the fracture well. With a motorized instrument and thermal ablator the surfaces of the fragments are exposed. The retractor in the proximal anterior portal (medial or lateral) is fundamental in this phase to keep the joint space open, thus permitting working with a lower inflow pressure. The joint capsule is constantly lacerated and retracted, together with the fragment/s of the fracture. A high pressure of infusion will lead to an early extra-articular swelling, making surgery gradually more difficult and dangerous.

Through the "combined effect" of the retractor (from the proximal portal) and the probe (from the anteromedial portal) the larger articular fragments are put back in place, thus maintaining the capsular insertion, whereas the smaller ones can be removed. At this point, it is useful to expose the dorsal surface of the ulna with a small incision, so that the skin and the subcutaneous tissue do not interfere with the instruments required for the fixation.

According to the size of the fragments, two different fixation techniques can be used:

- cannulated screws and/or K wires
- osteosuture

Cannulated screws and/or K wires (Fig. 29.2): After redislocating the intra-articular fracture with the lever from the proximal portal, K wires are drilled from the posterior cortex of the ulna, keeping the arthroscope in the anterolateral

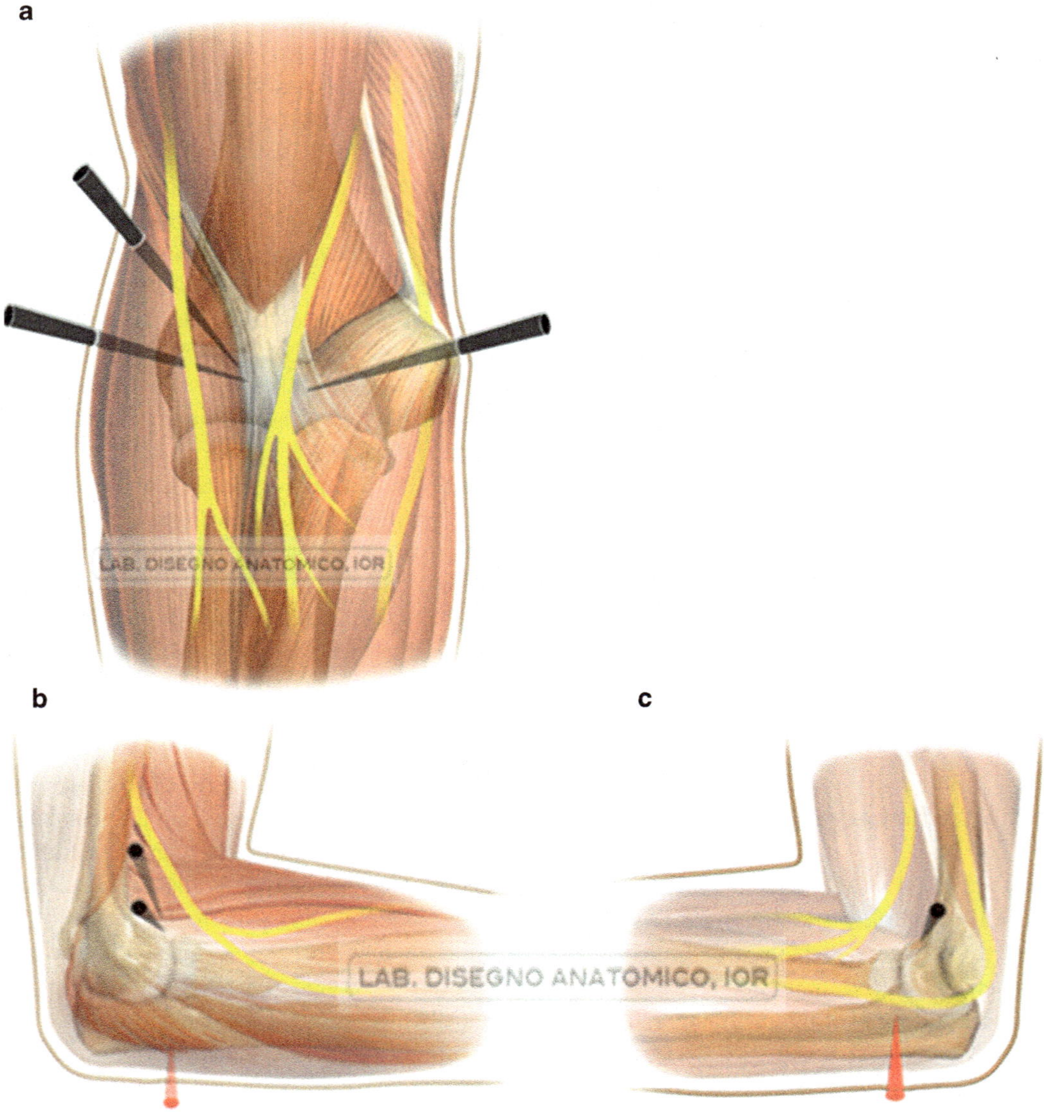

Fig. 29.2 Coronoid fracture. ARIF of a coronoid fracture: (**a**–**c**) Drawing of the anteromedial, anterolateral, and proximal anterolateral arthroscopic portals. In red the path of the percutaneous fixation (a small skin incision is advised to avoid possible K wire impingement); (**d**) CT scan of the fracture is routinely performed to study the fracture morphology and to plan the surgical steps; (**e**, **f**) – intraoperative X-ray checking of the temporary fixation by K wires and of the definitive one by K wire and cannulated screw; intraoperative images: the fracture is approached by the scope in the anterolateral portal, the retractor in the proximal anterolateral portal and the shaver in the anteromedial one (**g**); at least two K wires are placed out-in under the fracture fragments (**h**); while the fracture reduction is held, the wires are advanced behind the fragment (**i**) while protecting their tips to prevent damage to the vascular and nervous structures. If the fragment size is adequate, fixation can be performed exploiting the wires by one or more cannulated screws (**j**, **k**, **l**)

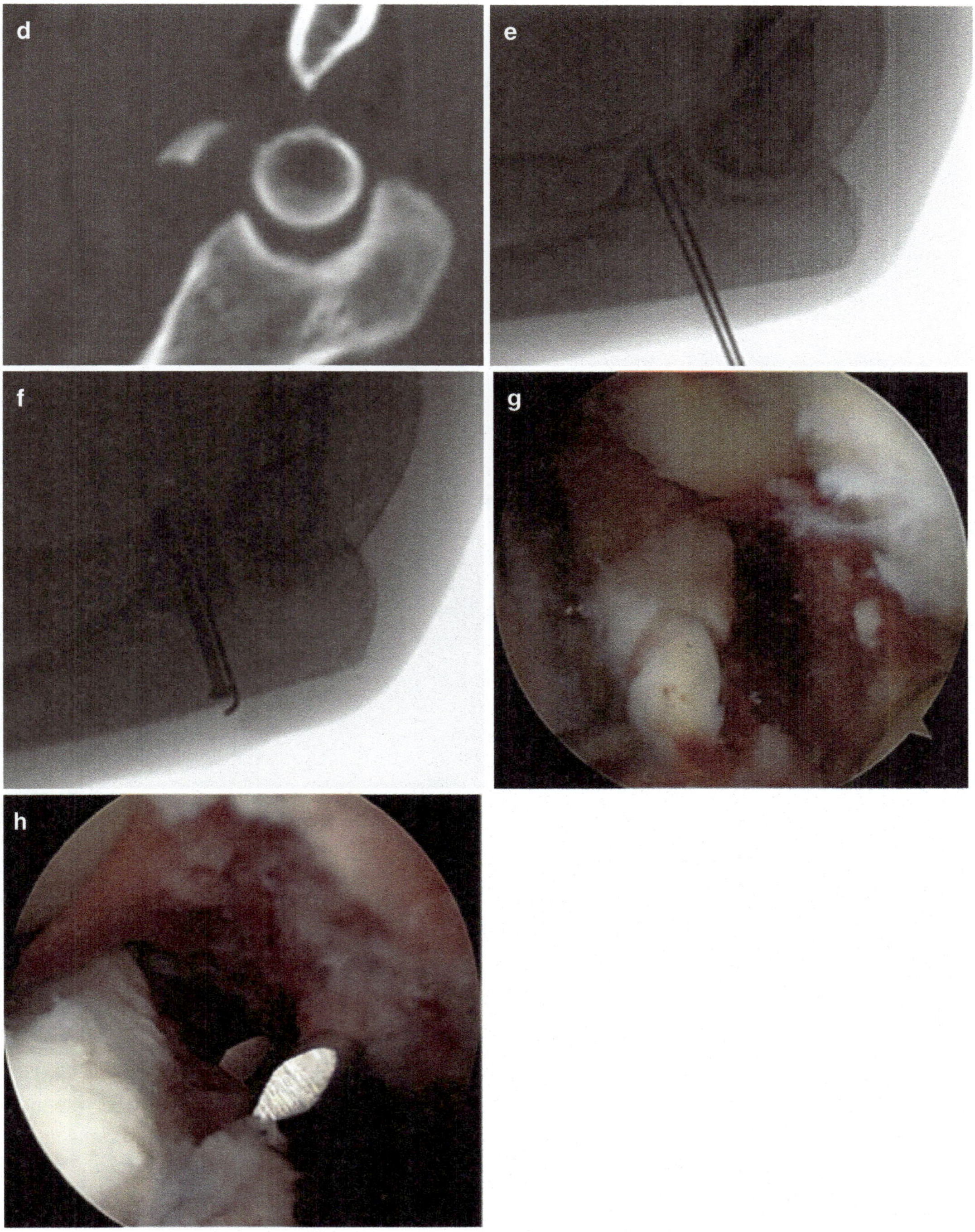

Fig. 29.2 (continued)

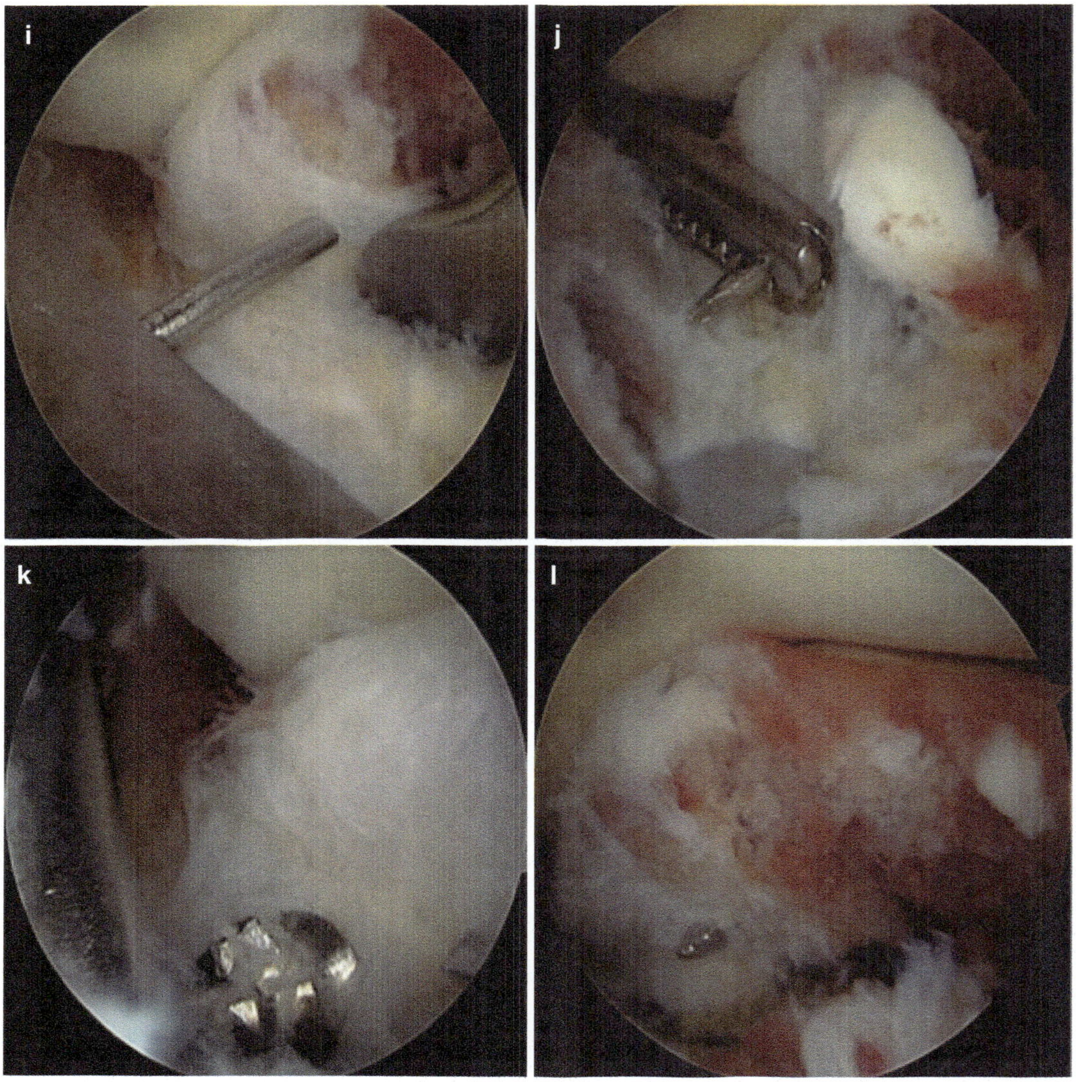

Fig. 29.2 (continued)

portal and checking its exit from the base of the fractured coronoid (Fig. 29.2h). This action is made safer and repeatable by the use of an aiming device for cruciate ligament surgery; a small-sized tip device must be used, because it has to enter through the anteromedial portal, and a bulky tip might impinge in the brachial muscle. The intraoperative radiographic checking is useful to evaluate the direction of the wires, especially if the freehand technique is chosen.

Having placed the first K wire, the others are placed (at least two to achieve rotational stability of the fixation).

After slightly retracting the wires, until the tip goes into the medullary bone, the fracture is reduced with the lever by the proximal portal, and with an arthroscopic grasper by the anteromedial portal.

While maintaining reduction (pushing strongly the fragments against the anterior surface of the trochlea that works as a mold), the wires are pushed forward again, checking that they come out anteriorly to the fragments.

When the size of the fragment allows, a cannulated screw, 3.5 mm in diameter, can be placed on one of the K wires. It is cautious to hold the tip of the intra-articular K wire firm with a Kocher, while inserting the cannulated drill and the screw, to prevent the wire from being pushed anteriorly, crossing dangerously the anterior brachial muscle (Fig. 29.2l–n).

Osteosuture: this is chosen when the fragments are too small and numerous to be fixed. This fixation will not be as stable as the previous one, but it enables the correct tension of the anteromedial joint capsule to be maintained, while scarring takes place. Often this technique also enables small bone fragments to consolidate.

To contain the joint capsule with suture thread, the suture passer commonly used for suturing rotator cuff lesions is extremely useful. The work portal is always anteromedial, whereas the arthroscope one remains anterolateral. Once again the retractor through the accessory proximal portal plays a fundamental role.

The vector suture is replaced by a reinforced double-zero suture (Orthocord, Depuy-Mitek or Hi-Fi Conmed Linvatec or Fiberwire Arthrex…).

Having placed the suture thread through the joint capsule (immediately behind the fragments of the coronoid tip), the first out-in hole is made at the base of the coronoid with a K wire 1.4 mm in diameter. Having removed the thread, a spinal needle (18 GA 3.50 IN/1.2 mm × 90 mm spinal needle) is inserted by which a vector thread (single-filament 1 mm in diameter), which having been recovered from the anteromedial portal, will take the first head of the osteosuture through the ulna, posteriorly. By inserting the second head using the same technique, the osteosuture can be closed on the posterior cortex, guiding the fracture fragments with the probe (Fig. 29.3).

Regardless of the ARIF technique chosen, the fixation must be stable upon palpation and flexion-extension tests of the elbow, to reduce the period of postoperative immobilization to a minimum. Therefore, in our cases we always supplemented screw fixation or osteosuture by K wiring.

At the end of the synthesis, the elbow wasn't deemed stable in five cases by X-ray stress tests.

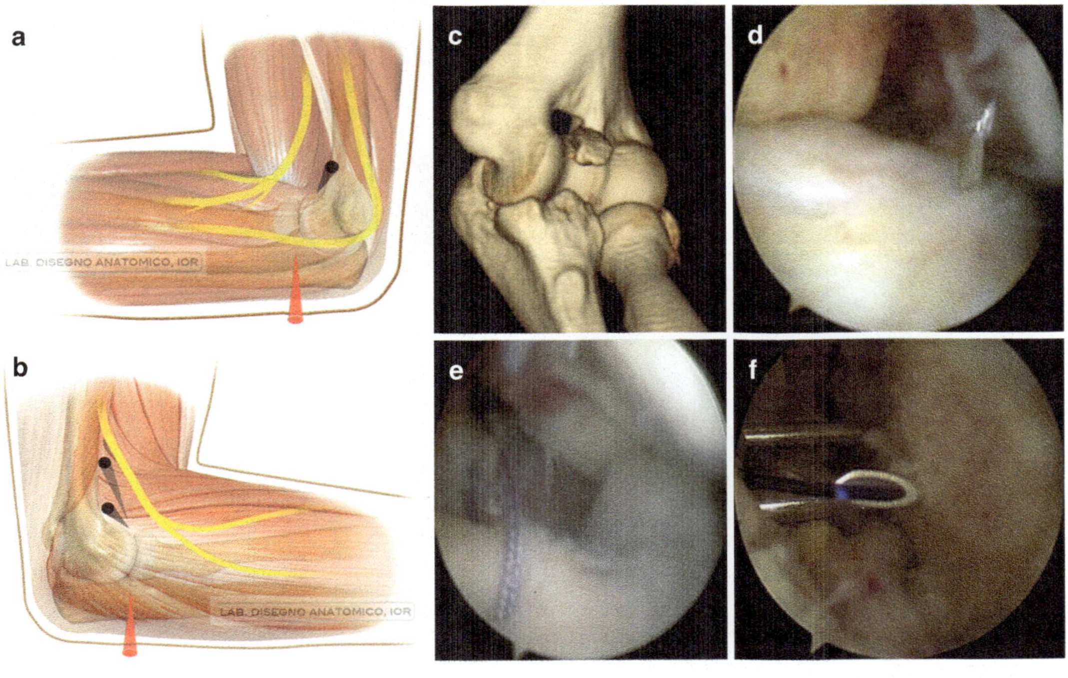

Fig. 29.3 Osteosuture of a coronoid fracture. The portals to perform osteosuture are the same as for K wires or screw fixation (**a**, **b**). Preoperative CT scan (**c**) shows a displaced fracture, suggesting joint derangement. By placing the scope in the anterolateral portal it is possible to perform an ostheosuture as described in the text (**d**–**i**), eventually reinforced by K wires (**j**, **k**)

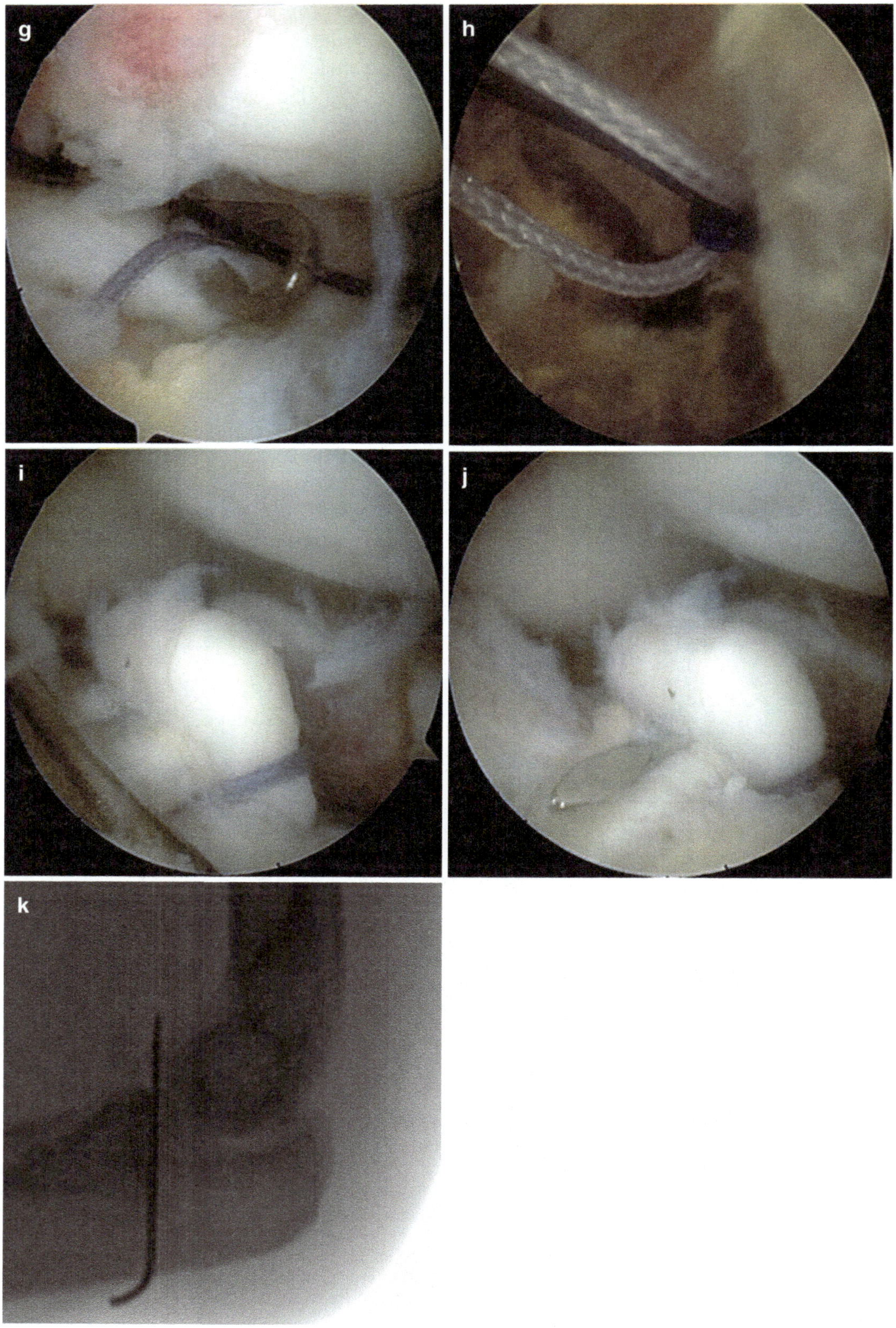

Fig. 29.3 (continued)

In the first two cases, we decided to repair the lateral collateral ligaments by a small incision on the lateral epicondyle. In the last three cases, we proceeded with a posterolateral arthroscopic-assisted capsular plication (as described for the combined radial head and coronoid lesions) invented by Van Riet. All cases resulted stable after the plication and the open ligament repairs were not necessary.

29.4 Radial Head Fractures

Radial head fractures, extremely common, are classified into four types by Mason and Johnston and divided further into simple and complex, according to possible combined lesions [17]. The option of conservative or surgical treatment depends on the number of fragments, their displacement, whether the fracture involves the olecranon and/or coronoid and if there are ligament lesions. When surgery is the choice, the surgeon has to decide among radial head excision, reduction and fixation of the fracture, or prosthetic replacement. It has been shown that ORIF or the prosthetic replacement of the radial head enables a better recovery of articular stability [18, 19] and therefore will certainly be the best choice when there is a combined lesion of the medial collateral ligament. Conversely, an isolated fracture of the radial capitellum can be treated by the simple excision of the fragments (if they interfere with the passive joint range) or by full radial head excision (if more than 50% of the surface is involved).

29.4.1 In the Literature

The first arthroscopic treatment was described in 2004 [20] for a fracture of the surgical neck of the proximal radius of a child, which was reduced by a manual maneuver and fixed by percutaneous wiring.

In 2006, Rolla [21] published a short series of six fractures of the radial head (II, III and IV types according to Mason) reduced and fixed with a percutaneous screw. The author used his own surgical technique, and recommended reducing the fracture by working in the anterior compartment, and moving in the posterolateral gutter for arthroscopic fixation.

Fourteen cases were collected by Michels [22] the following year, all Mason type II with a mean follow-up of 5.6 years and results ranging from good to excellent, matching those of open surgery. For this series the author managed ARIF by the use of only two portals (anterolateral and posterolateral) besides a small incision to insert the screws.

The elbow and wrist ESSKA [23, 24] committee showed on specimen studies that all the radial head surface is approachable and that modified anteroinferior portals are more effective to perform a correct radial head fracture ARIF.

29.4.2 Surgical Technique in our Experience

In our center arthroscopic treatment of isolated fractures of the radial head began in 2007. Until now 21 cases have been treated arthroscopically (7 ARIF, 8 partial removals of the fragments, 3 radial head excisions and 3 simple reductions, without fixation).

29.4.2.1 Arthroscopic Reduction Internal Fixation (Arif) for Mason Type II Fractures

The first stage consists of removing the intra-articular hematoma and visualizing the fracture in the anterior compartment. We perform three approaches routinely: anteromedial (for the arthroscope), anterolateral (for the tools), and proximal anterolateral (for the retractor). The fracture is reduced by using alternately the probe from the anterolateral portal and proximal anterolateral, by pronosupination movements. Having achieved reduction, the fragments must be stabilized with K wires, after choosing the position in pronosupination to hold for fixation.

The working position to perform screw fixation may vary. In our experience we divided the fractures according to the position of the fracture fragment/s in relation to the safe zone (part of the radial head that does not come in contact with the small sigmoid notch). Dividing the radial head ideally into two halves in neutral pronosupination we have the lateral half (which contains the Safe Zone) and the medial one (Fig. 29.4).

Fractures of the lateral half can be fixed by holding the position used for reduction, by placing the forearm in pronation. The retractor and the probe hold reduction and keep the workspace open. An accessory lateral portal is directed at the radial head and a small 5-mm cannula is placed in the joint. The cannula is important to protect the soft tissues from the rotating tools (K wire, drill, screwdriver) as well as to prevent the thin K wire, used to insert the screw, from bending or breaking. The K wire is inserted through the cannula. If the fracture appears to be stable the fixation procedure is performed (measurement, drilling, screw), otherwise other percutaneous K wires should be placed (outside the cannula) to hold the fragment still while the drill produces the hole for the screw (Fig. 29.5).

Fractures of the lateral half can also be fixed by working in the [20] the posterolateral gutter, by opening the posterolateral and midlateral portals to place alternately the arthroscope and the work tools. The forearm will have to be progressively placed in supination, until the fracture can be visualized. The procedure for the fixation is the same as that seen in the previous position (Fig. 29.5).

Conversely, when the fracture involves the medial half of the radial head (Fig. 29.5) pronosupination cannot put the fragment to be fixed in the correct place. In this case arthroscopic fixation can be performed by the anteromedial portal by placing the arthroscope in the anterolateral one. The work cannula is even more important to protect the soft tissues.

The ARIF described is certainly more difficult than fixation in open surgery, but offers the numerous advantages of arthroscopy. For example in four of the seven cases treated surgically we found small loose osteochondral fragments not visible by preoperative CT that certainly would not be found in open surgery.

However, choosing the length of the screws is more difficult because it is not easy to perform an intraoperative radiographic check with the tools in place; Generally, the screws range from 14 to 18 mm long and in case of doubt it is better to choose a shorter screw and check at the end of fixation, without risking a loss of reduction or bending the K wires in an attempt to get a satisfactory radiographic view.

The instruments should be chosen carefully so that the drill and the screwdriver of the 2.5-mm diameter screws are not too short, especially when fixation is performed by the anteromedial portal. If these tools are not available, the arthroscopic cannula can be cut on the serving table, before inserting it inside the joint.

29.4.2.2 Simple Arthroscopic Reduction

In three cases of Mason fracture type II, after debriding the fracture, reduction was easy. The reduced fragment on the remaining intact part of

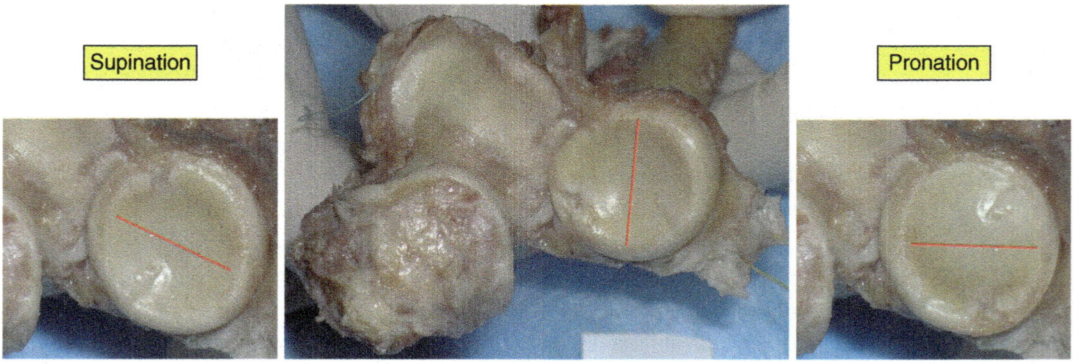

Fig. 29.4 Cadaver specimen. Radial head in full supination, in neutral position and in full pronation. Fractures involving the side of the radial head opposite to the safe zone are more difficult to fix through the direct lateral portal

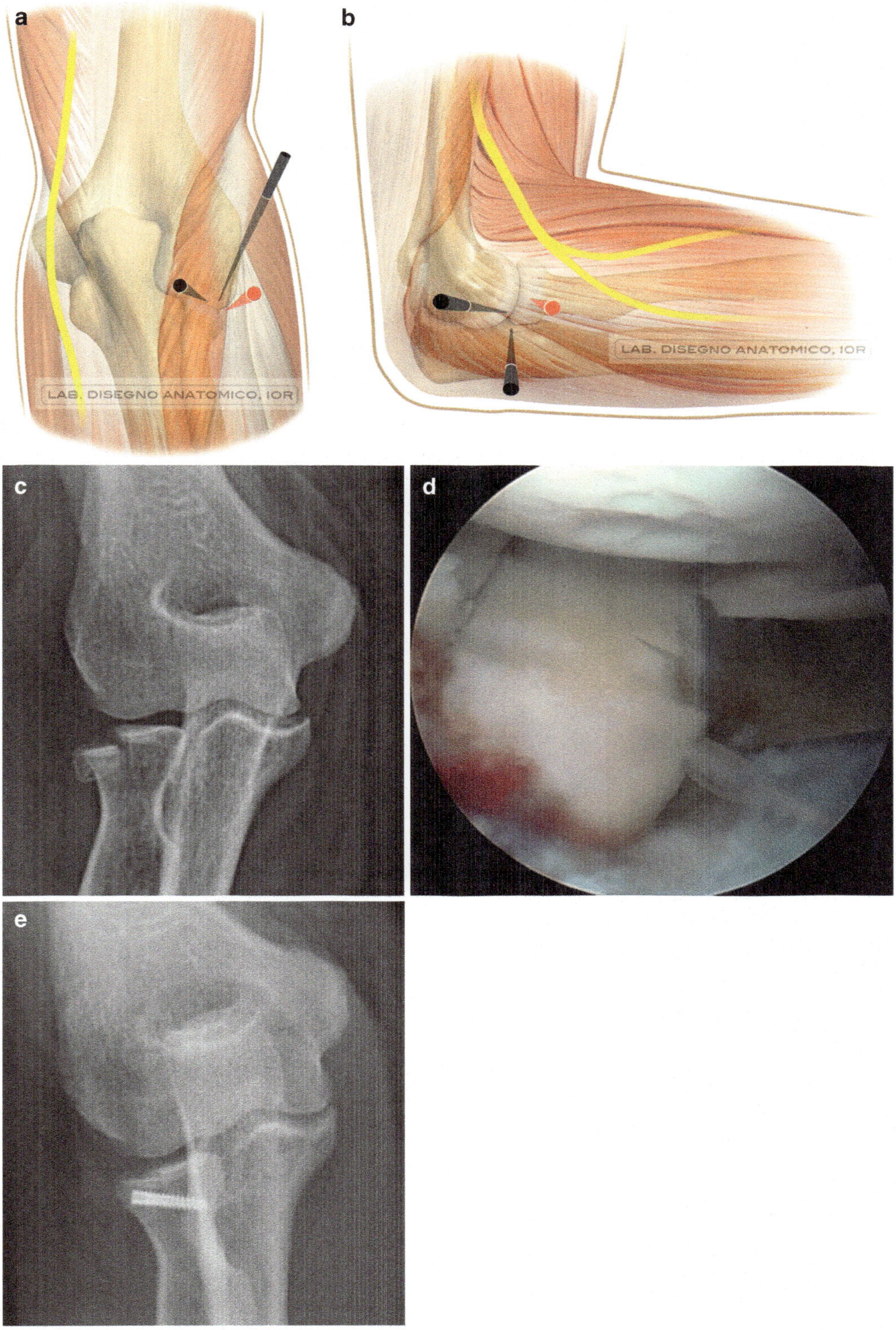

Fig. 29.5 Different fixation modes for radial head fractures. In the posterolateral gutter (**a**–**e**) and in the anterior compartment (**f**–**j**) for radial head fractures involving the lateral half, fixation will take place through a direct accessory portal (in red); in the anterior compartment (**k**–**r**) for fractures of the medial side of the radial head, fixation will be done through the anteromedial portal (in red)

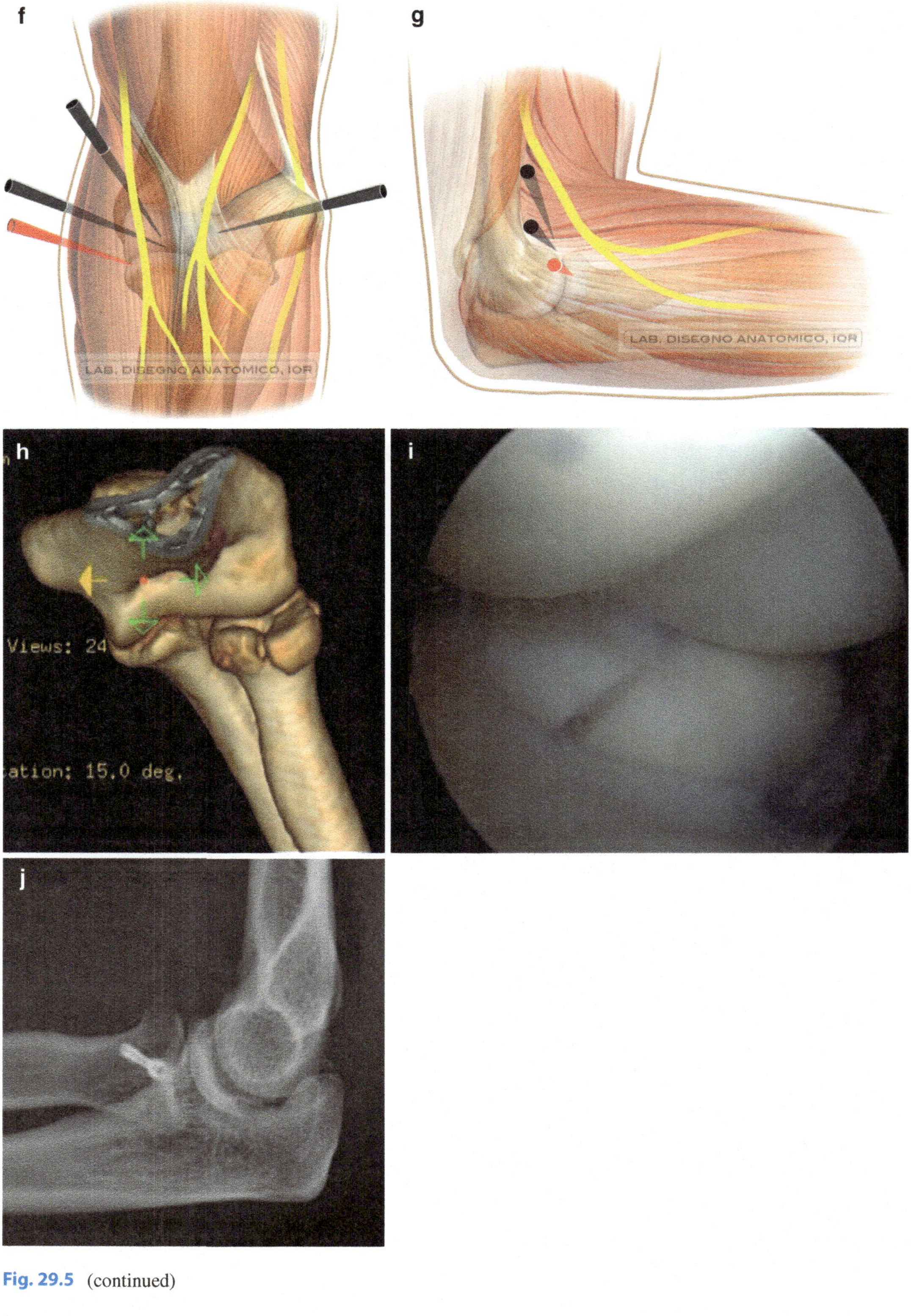

Fig. 29.5 (continued)

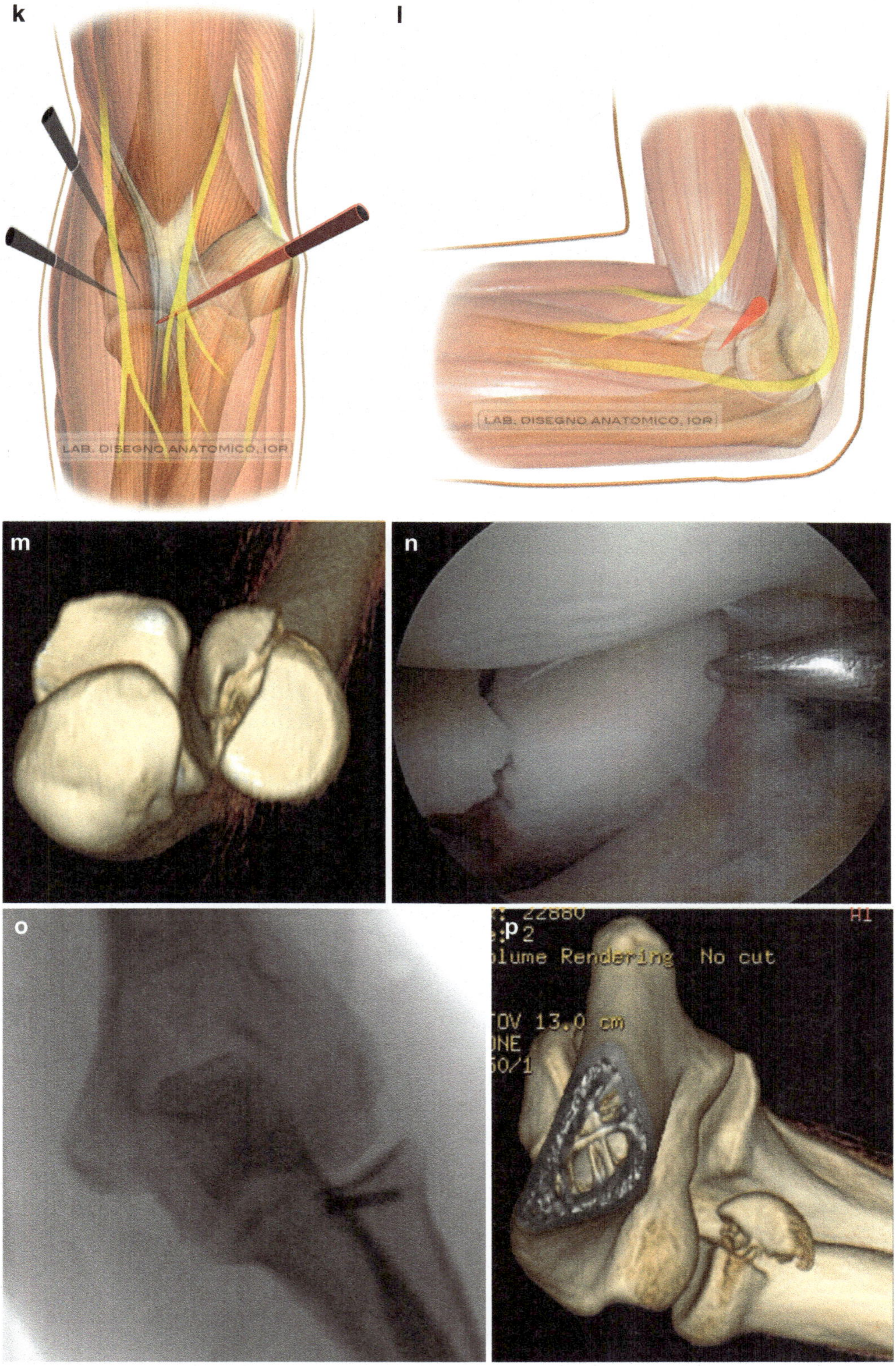

Fig. 29.5 (continued)

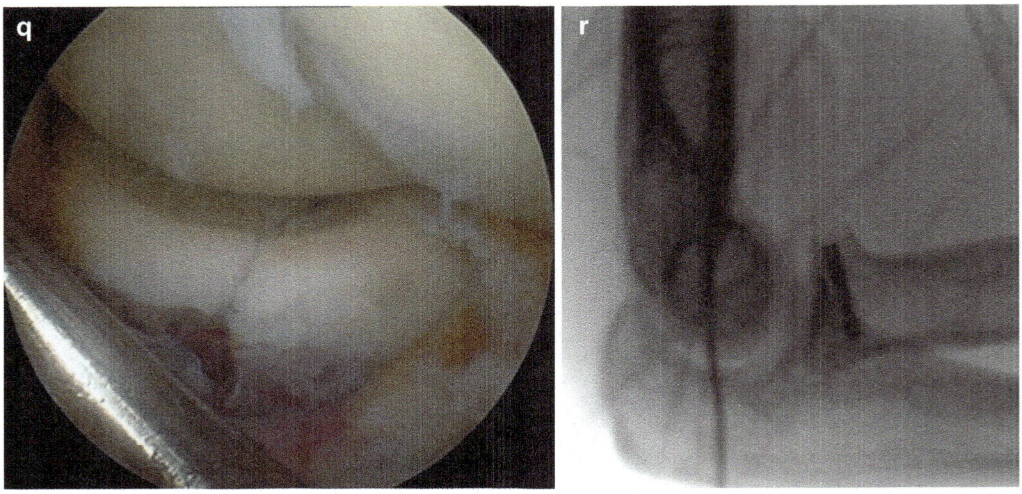

Fig. 29.5 (continued)

the radial head was firmly kept in place by the annular ligament, which the arthroscopic technique leaves intact.

After several stability tests we decided to avoid further surgical steps; all cases had a favorable outcome and full, swift recovery.

29.4.2.3 Arthroscopic Fragment Removal

In fractures with more comminution, when more than 50% of the radial head is still in site, fixation is not reliable and prosthetic replacement can be excessive.

In these cases, arthroscopic exploration enables removal of the fragments and ample joint debridement, without invalidating articular stability with the surgical approach. It is performed in the anterior compartment (by anteromedial, anterolateral, and proximal anterolateral approaches) or in the posterolateral gutter (by the posterolateral and midlateral approaches).

Arthroscopy can also be used to assess the articular stability of the ulno-humeral joint [12], which is important in decision-making about radial head prosthesis.

29.4.2.4 Arthroscopic Radial Head Removal

When the comminution does not enable fixation, the elbow is stable, and the patient is not so young, resection of the radial head is indicated, which can be performed by arthroscopy.

After removing the fragments in the anterior compartment, resection of the radial head is precise and easy by inserting the burr through the midlateral portal while the arthroscope is still in the anteromedial portal. The radial head is cut at the level of the superior margin of the intact annular ligament. Shortening the proximal radius as little as possible without impairing the annular ligament helps to hold the tension of the lateral collateral compartment (Fig. 29.6).

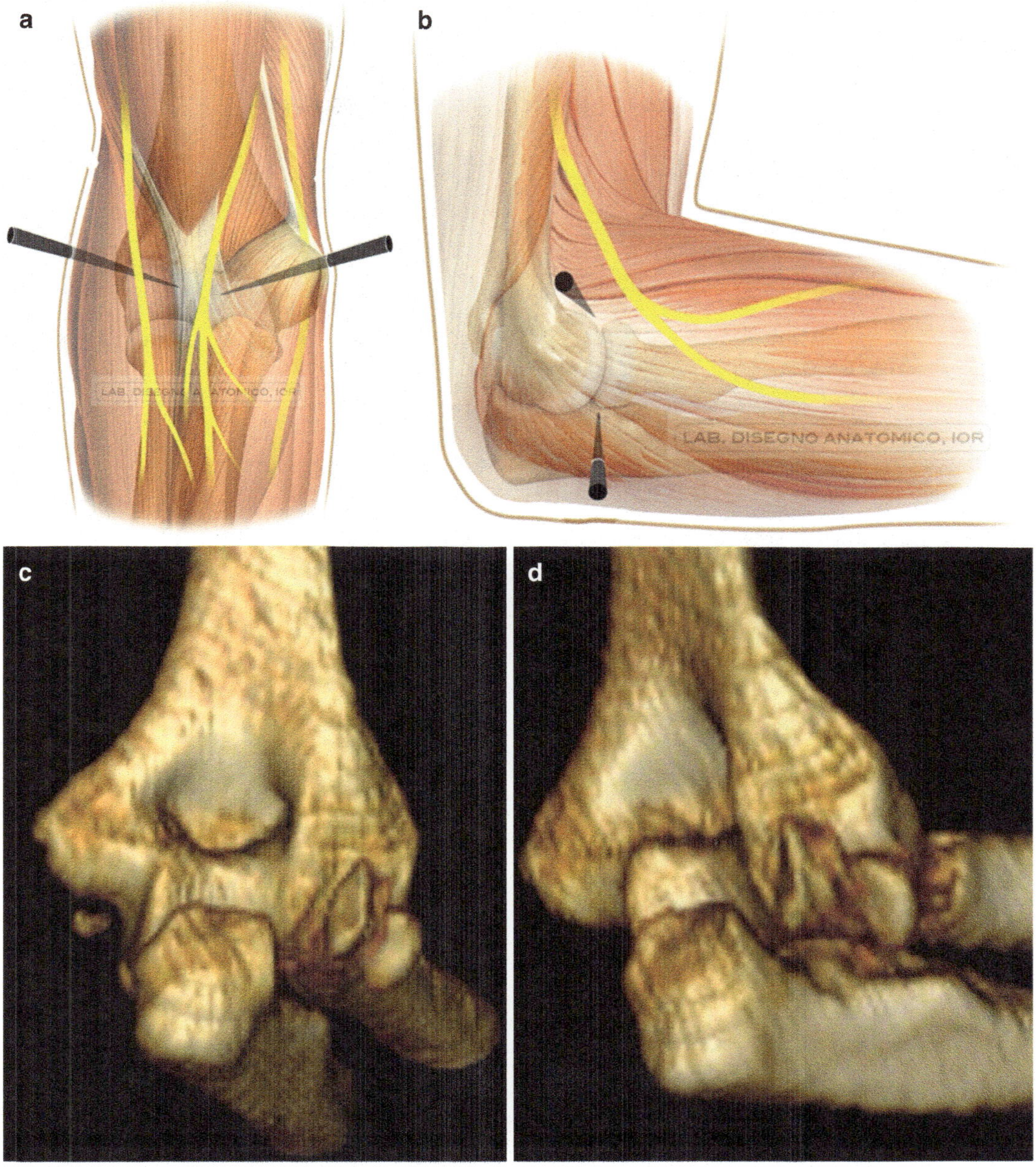

Fig. 29.6 Radial head removal. Drawing of the anteromedial, anterolateral, and midlateral arthroscopic portals (**a**, **b**) TC scan of the comminuted radial head fracture in an elderly woman (**c**, **d**), representing an indication for radial head excision, performed arthroscopically through anteromedial, anterolateral, and midlateral portals (**e**). Radiograph of the radial head excision (**f**, **g**)

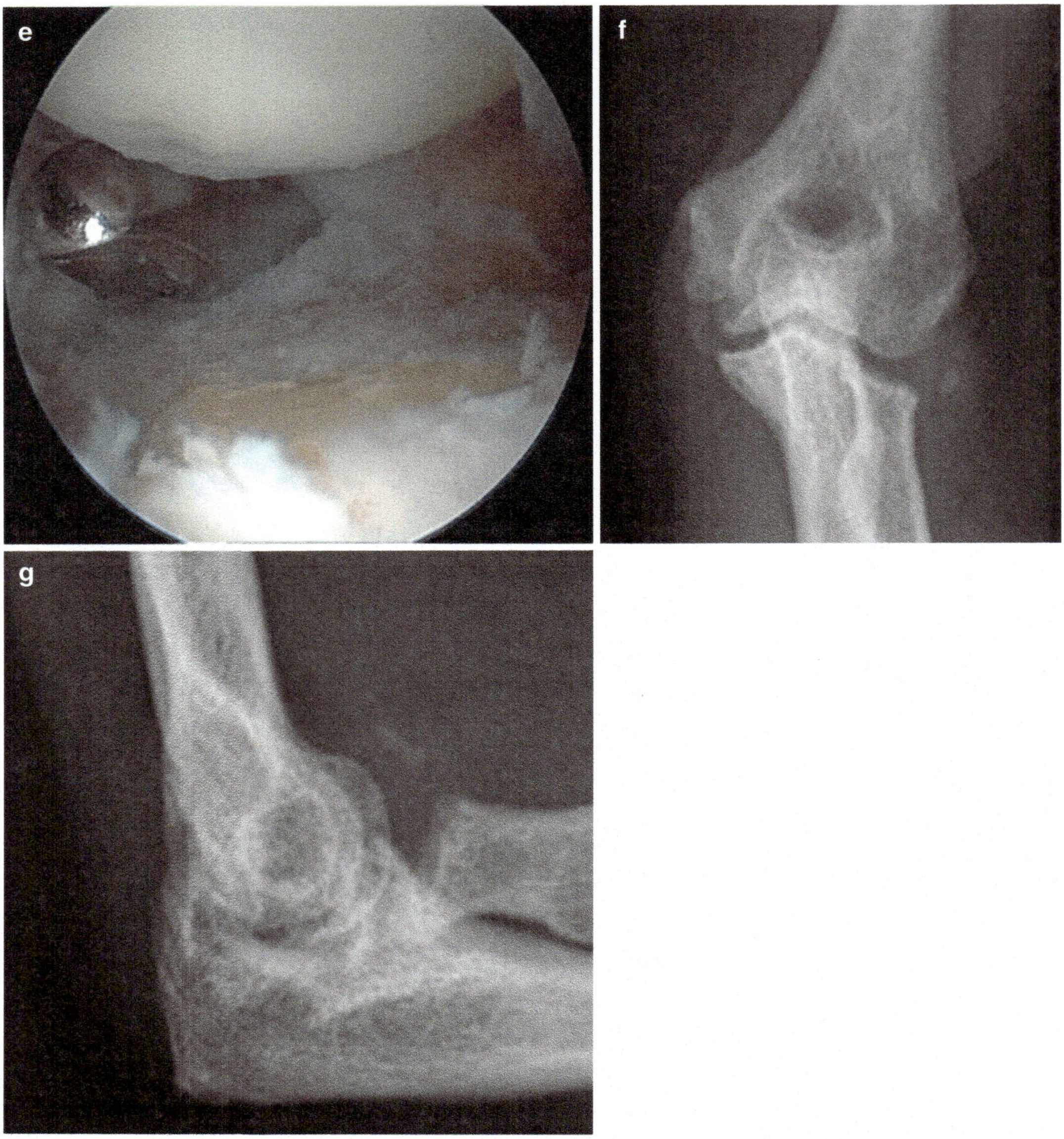

Fig. 29.6 (continued)

29.5 Combined Radial Head and Coronoid Fractures (Terrible Triad)

We treated arthroscopically seven cases of elbow dislocation and combined radial head and coronoid fracture (terrible triad). All cases where really selected with a fractures pattern that could be an indication of ARIF.

By arthroscopy we followed carefully the path of the radial head fracture, (removing in three cases or reducing and fixing the fragments in four cases), and performed an ARIF of the coronoid (by k Wires and screws as we have described. At the end of the synthesis the elbow wasn't deemed stable in five cases by dynamic tests. We proceed with a posterolateral arthroscopic-assisted capsular plication (Fig. 29.7). All five

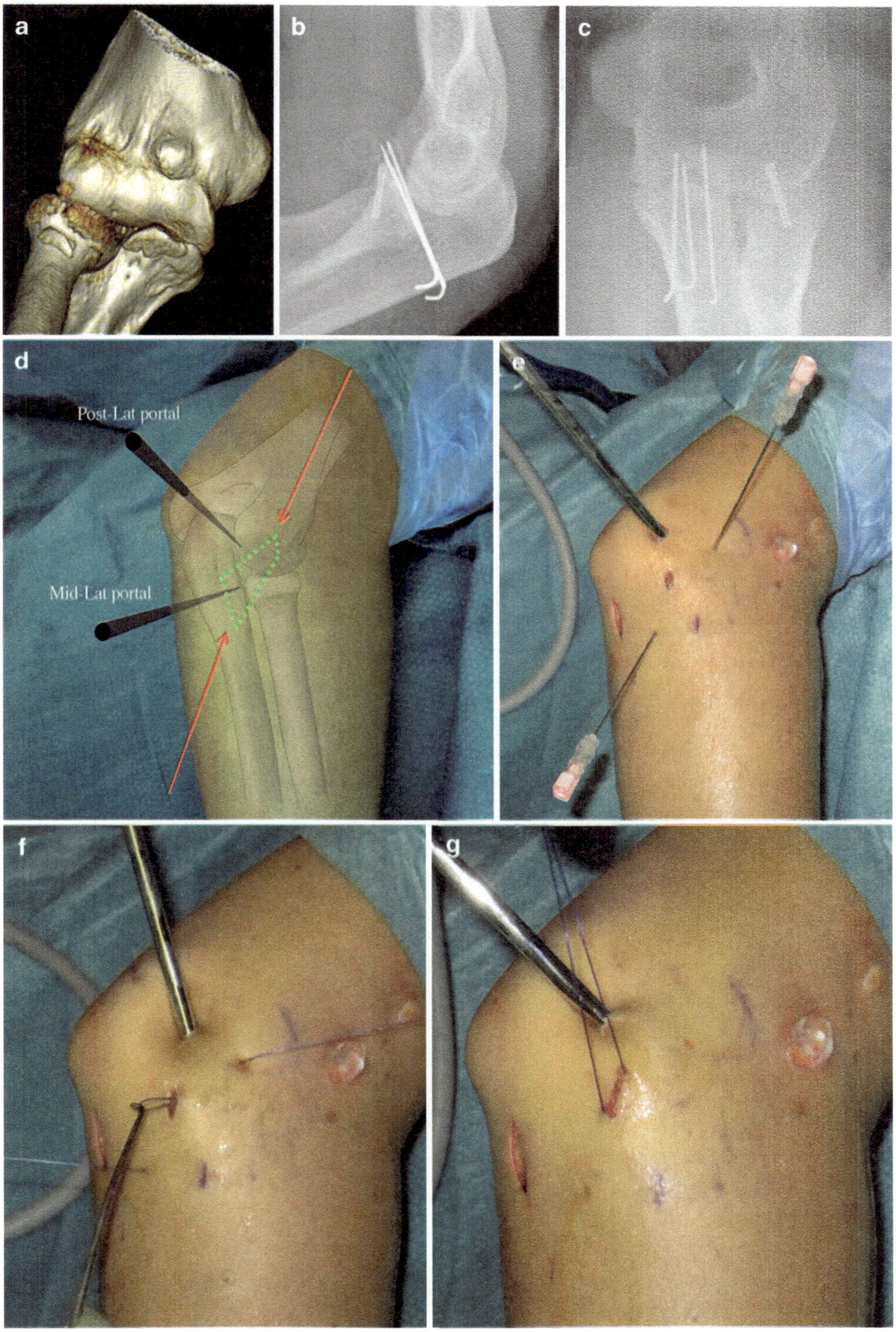

Fig. 29.7 Posterolateral plication after surgical ARIF of radial head and coronoid in Terrible triad: CT scan images (**a**) and intraoperative X-rays (**b**, **c**) of the radial head and coronoid fracture. The scope is in through the posterolateral portal while the midlateral portal is needed to retrieve the sutures. These sutures are passed percutaneously by two spinal needles inserted in the direction of the fibers of the Lateral Ulnar Collateral Ligament (green area in **d**) as shown (**d**–**g**)

elbows resulted stable after the plication and the open ligament repairs were not necessary.

29.6 Complications

No neurological or vascular lesions were recorded.

There were two cases of postoperative stiffness. One Manson II fracture occurred with extension deficit, which was treated again after 9 months by soft tissue release and arthroscopic removal of the screw. The screw was in place, the fracture healed, and the stiffness was connected to the reactive fibrosis of the anterior capsule. The soft tissue release enabled the full recovery. The second is the case of heterotopic ossifications as a sequela of the terrible triad treated by arthroscopy.

29.7 Conclusions

The indications for arthroscopic surgery have become wider and more perfected, over the last two decades, and provide new tools to better address various diseases: one example is the joint fracture treatment which has witnessed the move from surgical debridement to arthroscopic reduction and fixation (ARIF).

The impetus to strive for this difficult but interesting evolution comes from the need to reduce the surgical trauma caused by exposing and reducing articular fractures, which even now give high sequela rates over time.

If 10 years ago ARIF was a future possibility, today it is becoming a reality which, with its advantages and limits (see Table 29.1), is on a par with open surgery.

In this chapter we have tried to summarize the state of the art in the light of our experience. The various surgical techniques described are still not perfectly reproducible, and the surgeon must adapt them to suit each patient. If the feeling is that of a promising road to go down, the two complications that we have highlighted teach us that arthroscopy is also not exempt from the risk of postoperative stiffness. The number of cases is still too small and more in-depth studies are required to assess the real cost/benefit relationship of arthroscopic treatment of articular fractures.

Table 29.1 Advantages and limits of ARIF technique

Advantages
– Minimally invasive
– Better control of the reduction and stability of the fixation
– Draining of the hematoma and removal of small fragments in the recesses
– Does not preclude conversion into open surgery
Limits
– Current lack of dedicated instruments (aiming device, screwdriver and long cannulated drill, arthroscopic cannulae
– Possible need to have to change the patient's position if open surgery is required
– Need for precise selection of the surgical indication, excluding beforehand cases that require repair/reconstruction of the collateral ligaments
– Technique still in evolution: although the removal of small articular fragments and radial head excision can also be performed by surgeons with limited experience, conversely ARIF requires deep knowledge of traumatology and of open and arthroscopical elbow surgery

A strict selection of the surgical indication is indispensable; currently we can indicate the following conditions for arthroscopic treatment:

- Fractures of the radial head: Mason type 2—3 fractures (no combined ligament lesions).
- Isolated fractures of the coronoid.
- Fractures of the capitulum humeri (no combined ligament lesions).

Only case reports are found for the arthroscopic treatment of combined fractures of the radial capitellum and coronoid, other articular fractures (inter or supra-condyloid) or lesions of the lateral collateral ligament [25]. These cases are to be left in the hands of more expert surgeons of the sector, while waiting for further technical development and significant results.

References

1. Kelly EW, Morrey BF, O'Driscoll SW. Complications of elbow arthroscopy. J Bone Joint Surg Am. 2001;83(1):25–34.
2. Peden JP, Savoie FH, Field LD. Chapter 17: arthroscopic treatment of elbow fractures. In: The elbow and wrist—AANA advanced artrhoscopy. Philadelphia: Saunders; 2010. p. 136–43.
3. Yeoh KM, King GJW, Faber KJ, Glazebrook MA, Athwal GS. Systematic review evidence-based indications for elbow arthroscopy. Arthroscopy. 2012;28(2):272–82.
4. Bryan RS, Morrey BF. Fractures of the distal humerus. In: Morrey BF, editor. The elbow and its disorders. Philadelphia: WB Saunders; 1985. p. 325–33.
5. McKee MD, Jupiter JB, Bamberger HB. Coronal shear fractures of the distal end of the humerus. J Bone Joint Surg Am. 1996;78:49–54.
6. Ring D, Jupiter J, Gulotta L. Articular fractures of the distal part of the humerus. J Bone Joint Surg Am. 2003;85:232–8.
7. Dubberley JH, Faber KJ, Macdermid JC, Patterson SD, King GJ. Outcome after open reduction and internal fixation of capitellar and trochlear fractures. J Bone Joint Surg Am. 2006;88(1):46–54.
8. Feldman MD. Arthroscopic excision of type II capitellar fractures. Arthroscopy. 1997;13(6):743–8.
9. Hardy P, Menguy F, Guillot S. Arthroscopic treatment of capitellum fracture of the humerus. Arthroscopy. 2002;18(4):422–6.
10. Mitani M, Nabeshima Y, Ozaki A, Mori H, Issei N, Fujii H, Fujioka H, Doita M. Arthroscopic reduction and percutaneous cannulated screw fixation of a capitellar fracture of the humerus: a case report. J Shoulder Elbow Surg. 2009;18(2):e6–9. Epub 2008 Nov 25.
11. Kuriyama K, Kawanishi Y, Yamamoto K. Arthroscopic-assisted reduction and percutaneous fixation for coronal shear fractures of the distal humerus: report of two cases. J Hand Surg Am. 2010;35(9):1506–9. Epub 2010 Aug 21.
12. Hsu JW, Gould JL. The emerging role of elbow arthroscopy in chronic use injuries and fracture care. Hand Clin. 2009;25:305–21.
13. Regan NM, Morrey BF. Classification and treatment of coronoid process fractures. Orthopaedics. 1992;15(7):345–53.
14. O'Drisoll SW, Jupiter JB, Cohen MS, Ring D, McKee MG. Difficult elbow fractures: pearls and pitfalls. Instr Course Lect. 2003;52:113–34.
15. Pollock JW, Brownhill J, Ferreira L, McDonald CP, Johnson J, King G. The effect of anteromedial facet fractures of the coronoid and lateral collateral ligament injury on elbow stability and kinematics. J Bone Joint Surg Am. 2009;91(6):1448–58.
16. Liu SH, Henry M, Bowen R. Complications of type I coronoid fractures in competitive athletes: report of two cases and review of the literature. J Shoulder Elbow Surg. 1996;5(3):223–7.
17. Adams JE, Merten SM, Steinmann SP. Arthroscopic-assisted treatment of coronoid fractures. Arthroscopy. 2007;23(10):1060–5.
18. van Riet RP, Van Glabbeek F, Morrey BF. Radial head fracture. In: Morrey BF, editor. The elbow and its disorders. 4th ed. Philadelphia: Saunders Elsevier; 2009. p. 359–81.
19. Pike JM, Athwal GS, Faber KJ, King GJW. Radial head fractures—an update. J Hand Surg. 2009;34A:557–65.
20. Dawson FA, Inostroza F. Arthroscopic reduction and percutaneous fixation of a radial neck fracture in a child. Arthroscopy. 2004;20(Suppl 2):90–3.
21. Rolla PR, Surace MF, Bini A, Pilato G. Arthroscopic treatment of fractures of the radial head. Arthroscopy. 2006;22(2):233.e1–6.
22. Michels F, Pouliart N, Handelberg F. Arthroscopic management of Mason type 2 radial head fractures. Knee Surg Sports Traumatol Arthrosc. 2007;15(10):1244–50. Epub 2007 Jul 17.
23. Cucchi D, Guerra E, Luceri F, Lenich A, Nicoletti S, Randelli P, Wirtz DC, Eygendaal D, Arrigoni P, ESSKA Elbow and Wrist Committee 2016–2018. A combination of an anteromedial, anterolateral and midlateral portals is sufficient for 360° exposure of the radial head for arthroscopic fracture fixation. Knee Surg Sports Traumatol Arthrosc. 2019;27(1):319–25.
24. Cucchi D, Arrigoni P, Luceri F, Menon A, Guerra E, Müller LP, Burger C, Eygendaal D, Wegmann K, ESSKA Elbow and Wrist Committee 2016–2018. Modified anteromedial and anterolateral elbow arthroscopy portals show superiority to standard portals in guiding arthroscopic radial head screw fixation. Knee Surg Sports Traumatol Arthrosc. 2019;27(10):3276–83.
25. Shaun Holt M, Savoie FH III, Field LD, Ramsey JR. Arthroscopic management of elbow trauma. Hand Clin. 2004;20:485–95.

Intra-articular Osteotomies After Tibial Head Fractures

30

Karl-Heinz Frosch

Malreduced tibial plateau fractures often lead to pain and can be accompanied by instability, deviation of the mechanical axis, restricted mobility, and constant wear of the joint [1]. The main reasons for malreduction after tibial head fracture are insufficient visualization of the fractured joint surface or insufficient fixation with secondary loss of reduction [1]. It has been demonstrated, that through standard approaches only 30–40% of the joint surface can be visualized [2]. With standard approaches and intraoperative fluoroscopy around 30% of lateral tibial plateau fractures are not sufficiently reduced, especially in the posterolateral quadrant [3]. In bicondylar fractures the "posterolateral-central segment" is involved in 85% of all cases [4] and cannot be visualized by fluoroscopy [5] nor by a lateral standard approach [2]. Remaining steps of more than 5 mm in the posterolateral quadrant of the tibial head are associated with a worse clinical result [1, 6].

The complexity of the different pathologies of tibial head fractures requires comprehensive and standardized preoperative analysis and planning. A standardized clinical examination is used in conjunction with the radiological imaging. After a thorough clinical exam radiological evaluation with long leg X-ray, CT scan, MRI, and lateral slope views are necessary in most cases of posttraumatic malreduction after tibial head fractures. Intra-articular and extra-articular deformities should be distinguished. It is essential to differentiate between ligamentous and pseudoligamentous instabilities. In the case of intra-articular malreduction, bony defects, steps, and gaps must be accurately identified and localized during preoperative planning. The correct surgical approach can only be chosen after an in-depth analysis of the posttraumatic malreduction and a detailed planning of the operative procedure. Prior to the osteotomy an arthroscopy is performed to evaluate cartilage, remaining intra-articular malreduction and the status of the menisci. To be successful, a direct view into the affected articular surface is necessary. Extended approaches with osteotomy of the medial and/or lateral femoral epicondyle play an increasing role in this context [1, 2, 7]. The surgical approach should allow an intra-articular osteotomy with anatomical reconstruction of the articular surface and osteosynthetic stabilization. Intra-articular osteotomies of the tibial plateau can achieve good long-term results. In some cases, irreparable damage to the articular surface, or already pronounced osteoarthritis, make an artificial joint replacement necessary. Furthermore, in cases of additional loss of the meniscus at the side of the fracture or age higher than 65 years the

K.-H. Frosch (✉)
Department of Trauma and Orthopaedic Surgery, University Medical Center Hamburg-Eppendorf, Hamburg, Germany
e-mail: unfallchirurgie@uke.de

M. T. Hirschmann et al. (eds.), *ESSKA Instructional Course Lecture Book*,
https://doi.org/10.1007/978-3-662-61264-4_30

implantation of a total knee arthroplasty should be considered.

Whenever possible and reasonable the knee joint should be preserved.

References

1. Frosch KH, Krause M, Frings J, Drenck T, Akoto R, Müller G, Madert J. Posttraumatic deformities of the knee joint: intra-articular osteotomy after malreduction of tibial head fractures. Unfallchirurg. 2016;119(10):859–76.
2. Krause M, Krüger S, Müller G, Püschel K, Frosch KH. How can the articular surface of the tibial plateau be best exposed? A comparison of specific surgical approaches. Arch Orthop Trauma Surg. 2019;139:1369. [Epub ahead of print]
3. Meulenkamp B, Martin R, Desy N, Duffy P, Korley R, Puloski S, Buckley R. Incidence, risk factors, and location of articular malreductions of the tibial plateau. J Orthop Trauma. 2017;31(3):146–50.
4. Krause M, Preiss A, Muller G, et al. Intraarticular tibial plateau fracture characteristics according to the "Ten segment classification". Injury. 2016;47(11): 2551–7.
5. Krause M, Preiss A, Meenen NM, et al. Fracturoscopy is superior to fluoroscopy in the articular reconstruction of complex tibial plateau fractures—an arthroscopy assisted fracture reduction technique. J Orthop Trauma. 2016;30(8):437–44.
6. Solomon LB, Stevenson AW, Lee YC, et al. Posterolateral and anterolateral approaches to unicondylar posterolateral tibial plateau fractures: a comparative study. Injury. 2013;44:1561–8.
7. Krause M, Müller G, Frosch KH. [Extended medial and extended lateral approach for tibial plateau fractures]. Oper Orthop Traumatol. 2019;31:127–142.

Preoperative Planning

31

Adrian Błasiak, Wojciech Solecki,
and Olivier Verborgt

31.1 Introduction

The goal of this video is to present preoperative planning of reverse shoulder arthroplasty.

The number of RSA performed worldwide is increasing with time and the long-term outcomes are encouraging. Overall survivorship reaches 91–93% at minimum 10-year follow-up [1, 2].

The goal of preoperative planning in RSA is an assessment of anatomical or pathological conditions of the glenoid and proximal humerus for accurate sizing and placing the implants.

The most common indication for RSA are conditions which are contraindications to anatomic prosthesis like arthritis with cuff disease, rheumatoid arthritis, failed cuff repair, arch insufficiency, failed arthroplasty, failed HHR, failed anatomic arthroplasty, posttraumatic conditions, acute fracture (4-part), malunion or nonunion, posttraumatic sequelae, instability, and tumors.

Electronic Supplementary Material The online version of this chapter (https://doi.org/10.1007/978-3-662-61264-4_31) contains supplementary material, which is available to authorized users.

A. Błasiak (✉) · W. Solecki
Department of Orthopedics, St Luke's Hospital, Bielsko-Biała, Poland
e-mail: blasiak@lukasza.pl

O. Verborgt
Department of Orthopaedic Surgery and Traumatology, AZ Monica, Antwerp, Belgium
e-mail: olivier.verborgt@azmonica.be

Currently RSA is the most common solution of all kind of shoulder replacement in Europe.

31.2 Positioning Principles

Glenosphere positioning is crucial. It determines the center of rotation and biomechanical traits. Malposition of the glenosphere can lead to various complications such as dislocation, scapular notching, decreased range of motion, and component loosening.

Main reasons for malposition are inaccurate assessment of pathologic anatomy, incorrect choice of implant and/or positioning of the implant to correct pathology, inaccurate execution of the preoperative plan at the time of surgery [3–5]. Overall complications rate of RSA is around 16% of all operated patients [6]. Instability, periprosthetic fracture, infection and component loosening make up over 81% of all complications. Sixty percent of them are biomechanical problems resulting from implant malposition and periprosthetic fractures. This means that better preoperative planning could prevent complications in 10% of all operated patients [6].

Patients undergoing revision surgeries after failed osteosynthesis of proximal humerus, hemiarthroplasty, anatomic or reverse prosthesis are the other group in which preoperative planning is so important. Preoperative assessment of deformity, implant selection, accuracy of implant

M. T. Hirschmann et al. (eds.), *ESSKA Instructional Course Lecture Book*,
https://doi.org/10.1007/978-3-662-61264-4_31

placement, and bone grafting consideration can save many complications. Due to a three-dimensional character of deformities, both of glenoid and humeral head preoperative planning should be based on CT scan, instead of plain X-rays. Preoperative planning applies to both standard and patient-specific instrumentation.

31.3 Patient Selection

Patients who require advanced preoperative planning with use of a CT scan are all revision cases and selected cases of primary RSA. Selection should be based on a modified Walch classification of glenoid deformity in transverse plane, and Favard's classification in the oblique coronal plane to distinguish a group which would need advance preoperative planning [7, 8]. Types A2, B2, B3, C in Walch classification and E3 in Favard's classification are the indications to precise preoperative CT analysis with 3D reconstruction. In these cases sole intraoperative glenoid assessment can be misleading and result in baseplate malposition. Glenoid types B1, D, E1, and E2 should be considered when combined with an anterior or posterior shoulder subluxation.

31.4 Baseplate Positioning

In general precise preoperative planning should be considered especially regarding the glenoid, which is deformed in almost 40% patients qualified for the RSA [9]. 2D CT scan still remains the basic tool in pre-op planning, however 3D reconstructions seem to be more reliable and are superior to subjective intraoperative landmarks such like "subchondral smile" [10–13]. It is crucial that the baseplate size fits the anatomical size of the glenoid and should not be oversized neither in pre-op planning nor intraoperatively. The baseplate should be implanted in inferior part of the glenoid. To achieve this position intraoperatively it is important to reveal and identify the scapular pillar. The lower ridge of the baseplate should be aligned with the inferior glenoid neck. The position of the baseplate in transverse plane should be perpendicular to the long axis of the scapula, not parallel to the glenoid surface, which is very often deformed and retroverted. However, it is important to keep in mind that in the glenoid with a severe bone loss, placing the baseplate in slight retroversion saves part of the bony bed during rimming and provides better bone support. In coronal-oblique plain the baseplate should be placed 10 or at least zero degrees inferiorly—this decreases a risk of inferior notching. Baseplate should be supported by native bone in at least 50% of its surface, usually in the inferior part of the glenoid due to inferior tilt (subchondral smile) [14]. If the native bone is missing, auto or allogenic grafts or special implants can be used to fill in the gap. In case of autologous grafts, trabecular bone from the humeral head is used. In case where there is not enough bone, iliac crest graft can be used. Rotational orientation of the base plate influences the position of fixating screws. Drill holes orientation in the 11–5 o'clock axis provides more stable screw fixation to the scapula than drilling in the 12–6 o'clock axis [15]. When using two fixating screws, the superior one should be oriented superiorly, toward the coracoid base and the inferior one toward scapular pillar but perpendicular to the peg. This decreases the risk of notching, erosion, and implant destabilization. While the size of the glenosphere is determined by the size of glenoid and implanted baseplate, its' position can be modified by increasing the inferior eccentricity to optimize the range of motion and avoid notching.

31.5 Humeral Implant Positioning

The humeral head should be either cut according to the guidelines of the surgical method, different in inlay and onlay implants, or a bit less—it can be cut more in the later part of the surgery. The optimal position is 10–20 degrees of retroversion. In case of the external rotators deficit, the lack of external rotation can be diminished by reducing the retroversion angle. Increasing the humeral neck-shaft angle can optimize range of motion and decrease notching.

31.6 Conclusions

Positioning of the glenoid implant is crucial in the following aspects: version, tilt, position, rotation, screws placement, and bone support. On the humeral head side, the height of the cut and retroversion are the main factors that influence the outcome. The augmented reality is a new solution in an experimental phase and perhaps may become more popular in the future.

References

1. Bacle G, Nove-Josserand L, Garaud P, et al. Long-term outcomes of reverse total shoulder arthroplasty: a follow-up of a previous study. J Bone Joint Surg Am. 2017;99:454–61.
2. Cuff DJ, Pupello DR, Santoni BG, et al. Reverse shoulder arthroplasty for the treatment of rotator cuff deficiency: a concise follow-up, at a minimum of 10 years, of previous reports. J Bone Joint Surg Am. 2017;99:1895–9.
3. Iannotti JP, Greeson C, Downing D, et al. Effect of glenoid deformity on glenoid component placement in primary shoulder arthroplasty. J Shoulder Elbow Surg. 2012;21:48–55.
4. Hendel MD, Bryan JA, Barsoum WK, et al. Comparison of patient-specific instruments with standard surgical instruments in determining glenoid component position: a randomized prospective clinical trial. J Bone Joint Surg Am. 2012;94:2167–75.
5. Iannotti J, Baker J, Rodriguez E, et al. Three-dimensional preoperative planning software and a novel information transfer technology improve glenoid component positioning. J Bone Joint Surg Am. 2014;96:e71.
6. Bohsali KI, Bois AJ, Wirth MA. Complications of shoulder arthroplasty. J Bone Joint Surg Am. 2017;99:256–69.
7. Bercik MJ, Kruse K, Yalizis M, Gauci M-O, Chaoui J, Walch G. A modification to the Walch classification of the glenoid in primary glenohumeral osteoarthritis using three-dimensional imaging. J Shoulder Elbow Surg. 2016;25(10):1601–6.
8. Sirveaux F, Favard L, Oudet D, Huquet D, Walch G, Mole D. Grammont inverted total shoulder arthroplasty in the treatment of glenohumeral osteoarthritis with massive rupture of the cuff. Results of a multicentre study of 80 shoulders. J Bone Joint Surg Br. 2004;86:388–95.
9. Frankle MA, Teramoto A, Luo ZP, Levy JC, Pupello D. Glenoid morphology in reverse shoulder arthroplasty: classification and surgical implications. J Shoulder Elbow Surg. 2009;18:874–85.
10. Dilisio MF, Warner JJ, Walch G. Accuracy of the subchondral smile and surface referencing techniques in reverse shoulder arthroplasty. Orthopedics. 2016;39:e615–20.
11. Verborgt O, De Smedt T, Vanhees M, et al. Accuracy of placement of the glenoid component in reversed shoulder arthroplasty with and without navigation. J Shoulder Elbow Surg. 2011;20:21–6.
12. Scalise JJ, Codsi MJ, Bryan J, et al. The influence of three-dimensional computed tomography images of the shoulder in preoperative planning for total shoulder arthroplasty. J Bone Joint Surg Am. 2008;90:2438–45.
13. Iannotti JP, Weiner S, Rodriguez E, et al. Three-dimensional imaging and templating improve glenoid implant positioning. J Bone Joint Surg Am. 2015;97:651–8.
14. Formaini NT, Everding NG, Levy JC, et al. The effect of glenoid bone loss on reverse shoulder arthroplasty baseplate fixation. J Shoulder Elbow Surg. 2015;24:e312–9.
15. Parsons BO, Gruson KI, Accousti KJ, Klug RA, Flatow EL. Optimal rotation and screw positioning for initial glenosphere baseplate fixation in reverse shoulder arthroplasty. J Shoulder Elbow Surg. 2009;18:886–91.

Inlay Patellofemoral Arthroplasty

32

Geert Pagenstert

32.1 Introduction

Isolated arthroplasty of the patellofemoral joint has been invented more than 30 years ago [1, 2]. However, it's use is still discussed controversial [3, 4]. Poor clinical outcomes and high failure rates have been reported for patellofemoral arthroplasty (PFA) in the past [2, 3, 5, 6–8].

Concerns with the early designs of the trochlear component have been believed to be a major reason for failures [4]. Since the invention of new implant designs, PFA has produced more consistent outcomes and regained relevance in clinical practice [9, 10].

Currently available trochlear implant designs can be divided into inlay and onlay designs [4, 11]. Inlay design trochlear components are implanted minimally deep to the surrounding cartilage after creation of a bone bed within the native trochlea. Onlay design trochlear components replace the whole anterior compartment by using the same anterior cutting procedure known from total knee arthroplasty.

First generation inlay designs have been associated with higher failure rates compared to second-generation onlay designs [2–4, 6–8, 11]. Therefore, onlay design trochlear components have been considered the gold standard for the last several years [4, 11]. However, with the invention of a new second-generation inlay design, which allows for individualized and anatomic trochlear resurfacing, a much better implant became available. Advantages of the new inlay designs include no overstuffing of the patellofemoral joint, no impingement or contact to the retinacular soft tissues, and increased implant stability [9, 12–14].

G. Pagenstert (✉)
University of Basel, Clarahof Clinic of Orthopaedic Surgery, Merian-Iselin Hospital, Swiss Olympic Medical Center, Basel, Switzerland
e-mail: geert.pagenstert@unibas.ch

32.2 Indications and Contraindications

PFA is indicated in patients with isolated disabling patellofemoral pain and the presence of patellofemoral osteoarthritis (grade III–IV Kellgren–Lawrence [15]) or chondral destruction (grade III-IV Outerbridge [16]) refractory to non-surgical treatment and/or failed prior.

Patellofemoral instability and leg deformities are relative contraindications and need to be addressed during PFA as has been described elsewhere. The tuberosity should be transferred if the tibial tuberosity trochlear groove distance is over 15–20 mm, and/or the Caton-Deschamps Index [17] is over 1.3. The femoral malalignment should be corrected if mechanical valgus over 5° or excessive internal femoral torsion of more than 20° to the normal values where found [18].

M. T. Hirschmann et al. (eds.), *ESSKA Instructional Course Lecture Book*,
https://doi.org/10.1007/978-3-662-61264-4_32

Contraindications for PFA were inflammatory arthropathy, progressive chondrocalcinosis of the menisci and femorotibial cartilage, chronic regional pain syndrome, active infection, and symptomatic tibiofemoral OA with pain during activities of daily living. Mild osteoarthritic changes in the tibiofemoral joint without symptoms can be neglected. Trochlea dysplasia is not a contraindication for inlay PFA because bone-bed preparation is adapted to act as deepening trochleoplasty [19].

32.3 Implant Design and Surgical Technique

The inlay PFA (HemiCAP® Wave) incorporates a cobalt chrome trochlear component that is connected to a titanium bone anchoring socked via a taper interlock, and an all-polyethylene patella component. This system intends to replicate joint biomechanics by intraoperative joint surface mapping, three-dimensional socket reaming, and implantation of a matching, contoured trochlear inlay component. Eight implant sizes with varying offsets are available which allows for a patient-specific geometry match (Fig. 32.1).

A dynamic leg holder is recommended for easy flexion adjustments during the procedure and a tourniquet can be used. A medial parapatellar surgical approach without eversion of the patella is recommended. With the knee in 20–30 degrees of flexion the patella can be retracted by temporary K-wires. An offset drill guide is used to establish a working axis to the central trochlear articular surface and to confirm trochlear defect coverage. In the presence of a dysplastic trochlea with a central spur, the spur is removed by a rongeur to allow the offset guide to rest on the anterior cortex of the femur with its superior feet. The inferior feet of the guide should not impinge at the posterior cruciate ligament. Once the superior and inferior drill guide feet were aligned with the trochlear orientation, a guide pin is advanced into the bone. To determine the proper implant geometry, the superior/inferior and the medial/lateral offsets were measured using specific instrumentation to measure the depth of the trochlear groove and the height of the sagittal curve. In case of a flat trochlea dysplasia, the deepest groove will be renamed despite the flat measurement and the curvature set to the anterior cortex of the femur. According to the plan, the implant bed is reamed three-dimensionally with the aid of

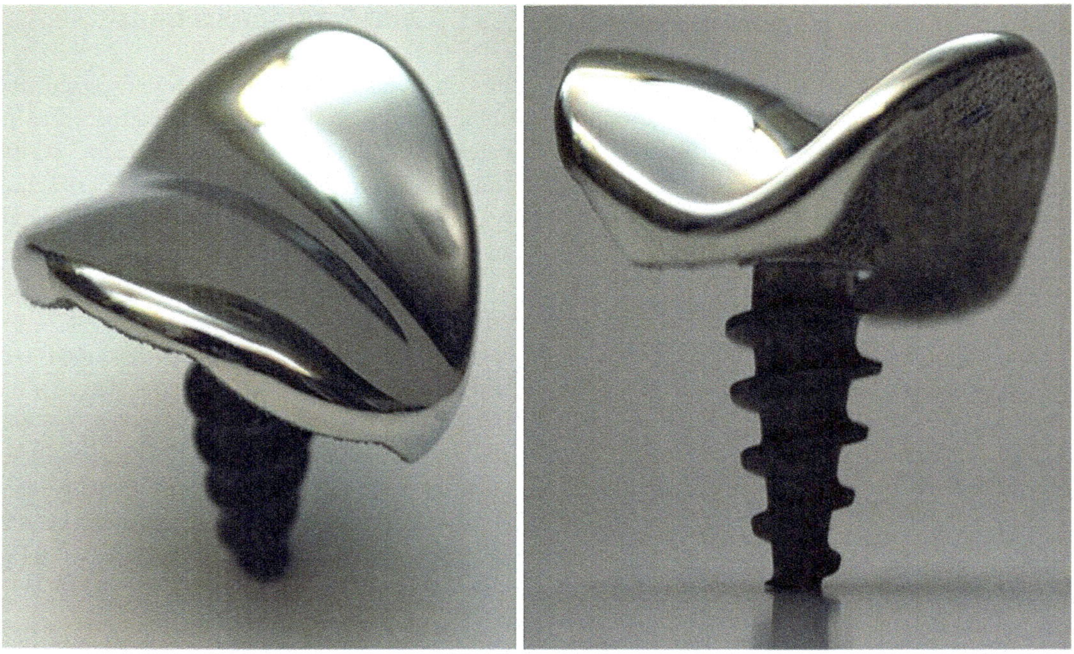

Fig. 32.1 Second-generation inlay trochlear design (HemiCAP® Wave, Arthrosurface, Franklin, MA, USA). (Reprinted with kind permission from Arthrosurface)

a guide block. The screw fixation socked bearing a conus is then advanced into the bone and the trochlear component is fixed to the conus using an impactor. Debridement of patellar osteophytes, lateral facetectomy, and circular denervation can be performed as necessary. Resurfacing of the patella is recommended in patellofemoral incongruence caused by patellar dysplasia, or in the presence of large subchondral bone defects. To replace the patellar surface the thickness of the patella is measured, and the surface resected using a saw aiming for a bone block preservation of more than 12 mm thickness. An asymmetric whole surface all-poly with three pegs along with cemented fixation is recommended to remove the painful margins of the patella.

32.4 Postoperative Rehabilitation

Patients with isolated PFA are allowed immediate full weight-bearing and free range of motion using two crutches as needed during the first 2–6 weeks. In case of osteotomies of the tibial tubercle or the femur, partial weight-bearing according to the protocol is adjusted. Lateral retinacular lengthening or reconstruction of the medial patellofemoral ligament usually need restriction of weight-bearing as well. We use continuous passive range of motion and compression cooling for our patients.

32.5 Outcome of Inlay Patellofemoral Arthroplasty

There is just evidence growing for this inlay PFA implant. Imhoff et al. [20]. published a paper in 2019 including 2 and 5 years results counting only isolated PFA. All patients with concomitant surgical procedures have been excluded (app. 50%). Clinical and radiographic results were assessed in 32 patients at the 2-year follow-up and in 24 patients at the 5-year follow-up. Patients converted to TKA were included in the risk factor and survival analysis. Both showed significant improvements at the 2- and 5-year follow-up compared to preoperative values. No significant difference was observed between the 2-year and 5-year results. Pain and function showed significant improvements after 2 and 5 years, whereas improvements in the stiffness subscale reached significance at 2 years alone. At the 5-year follow-up, 20 out of 24 patients (83%) were satisfied with the procedure: 7 patients (29%) rated themselves "excellent," 8 patients (33%) rated themselves "good," 5 patients (21%) rated themselves "fair," and 4 patients (17%) rated themselves "poor." No significant progression of tibiofemoral OA according to the Kellgren–Lawrence grading was observed and no significant change in patellar height according to the Caton-Deschamps Index was seen. No evidence of periprosthetic loosening, cyst formation, or implant subsidence was found when comparing AP and lateral radiographs of the ones which were taken immediately after implantation to the ones at the 5-year follow-up. Six patients underwent TKA during the study period, with a mean time to conversion of 27 ± 13 months. One patient suffered from an allergic reaction to chrome and nickel resulting in progressive synovitis and stiffness and five patients suffered from persistent knee pain without radiographic evidence of progressive tibiofemoral arthritis. There were no statistical significant differences in patient demographics such as age and BMI in the failure group. The overall survival rate was 91% at 2 years and 83% at 5 years.

Patel et al. [21] evaluated the outcome of 16 consecutive patients after a mean follow-up of 24 months and found a statistically significant improvement in clinical outcomes, however, no significant improvement was observed for range of motion and Short Form-36. Radiographically, only one patient had progression of OA and no patient was converted to total knee arthroplasty.

The outcome of 19 knees in 15 patients after a mean follow-up of 35 months was evaluated in another study by Zicaro et al. [22]. Significant improvements were observed for all outcome measures, and no progression of OA was observed. Two patients were converted to TKA because of persistent pain.

Laursen [23] reported results on 18 patients who were followed prospectively for 1 year; of those, 11 were followed for 2 years. The patella was resurfaced in 7 of the 18 (39%) patients.

Significant improvements were observed for clinical and functional outcomes using the American Knee Society Subjective Score (AKSS) with an improvement in AKSS of more than 20 points in 91% of the patients. However, significant progression of OA in the medial tibiofemoral and patellofemoral compartment was observed. Implant survival rate was analyzed at 6 years postoperatively using the National Joint Replacement Register of Denmark. Within 6 years, a total of 5 implants were revised to TKA. The high revision rate reported by Laursen does not correspond to the experience of the other studies and may be explained with a different algorithm for indication and treatment, but also underlines the crucial need for preoperative patient selection.

32.6 Comparing Inlay and Onlay Patellofemoral Arthroplasty

Feucht et al. compared current onlay and inlay designs in isolated PFA [24]. Based on the theoretical advantages of an inlay design, it was hypothesized that an inlay design will produce better clinical results and less progression of tibiofemoral osteoarthritis (OA) compared to an onlay design.

Only patients who underwent isolated PFA were included ($n = 64$). An onlay trochlear design (Journey™ PFJ, Smith & Nephew, Andover, MA, USA) was used in 15 patients and 49 patients received isolated implantation of the inlay design (HemiCAP® Wave). Since the patients were not randomized preoperatively, a matched-pair analysis was conducted in order to minimize selection bias. Matching criteria were age (±5 years), gender, body mass index (±5 kg/m^2), and follow-up period (±3 months).

In this series, patellofemoral resurfacing was performed in five patients within each group (33%). Postoperative rehabilitation was identical for both groups. Patients performed partial weight-bearing with 20 kg for 2 weeks, followed by progression of weight-bearing with 20 kg per week. Full range of motion was allowed immediately.

Both implants significantly improved functional outcome scores and pain, without significant differences between both groups. In addition, no significant difference between both implants was found with regard to the reoperation rate, which was low in both groups. None of the patients with an inlay component required reoperation because of patellofemoral maltracking or mechanical patellofemoral complications such as catching, snapping, or clunking. The authors concluded that the development of the second-generation inlay component has resolved design-specific complications of first-generation inlay designs and can be considered a valuable alternative to currently used onlay designs, with the theoretical advantages of an inlay design component.

Progression of tibiofemoral OA is the most common reason for failure of PFA using modern prosthetic designs [25, 26]. An interesting finding of the study was that none of the patients with an inlay component showed progression of tibiofemoral osteoarthritis (OA), whereas more than half of the patients in the onlay group demonstrated progression of medial and/or lateral tibiofemoral OA. The hypothesis for this observation is the more anatomic approach of the inlay design that better reproduces the complex kinematics of the patellofemoral joint, by preventing soft tissue irritation due to overstuffing.

References

1. Mckeever DC. Patellar prosthesis. J Bone Joint Surg Am. 1955;37-A:1074–84.
2. Blazina ME, Fox JM, Del Pizzo W, Broukhim B, Ivey FM. Patellofemoral replacement. Clin Orthop Relat Res. 1979;144:98–102.
3. Leadbetter WB. Patellofemoral arthroplasty in the treatment of patellofemoral arthritis: rationale and outcomes in younger patients. Orthop Clin North Am. 2008;39(3):363–80.
4. Lustig S, Magnussen RA, Dahm DL, Parker D. Patellofemoral arthroplasty, where are we today? Knee Surg Sports Traumatol Arthrosc. 2012;20(7):1216–26.
5. Arciero RA, Toomey HE. Patellofemoral arthroplasty. A three- to nine-year follow-up study. Clin Orthop Relat Res. 1988;236:60–71.

6. van Wagenberg JM, Speigner B, Gosens T, de Waal MJ. Midterm clinical results of the autocentric II patellofemoral prosthesis. Int Orthop. 2009;33(6):1603–8.
7. Charalambous CP, Abiddin Z, Mills SP, Rogers S, Sutton P, Parkinson R. The low contact stress patellofemoral replacement: high early failure rate. J Bone Joint Surg Br. 2011;93(4):484–9.
8. Board TN, Mahmood A, Ryan WG, Banks AJ. The Lubinus patellofemoral arthroplasty: a series of 17 cases. Arch Orthop Trauma Surg. 2004;124(5):285–7.
9. Imhoff AB, Feucht MJ, Meidinger G, Schottle PB, Cotic M. Prospective evaluation of anatomic patellofemoral inlay resurfacing: clinical, radiographic, and sports-related results after 24 months. Knee Surg Sports Traumatol Arthrosc. 2015;23(5):1299–307.
10. Walker T, Perkinson B, Mihalko WM. Patellofemoral arthroplasty: the other unicompartmental knee replacement. J Bone Joint Surg Am. 2012;94(18):1712–172.
11. Lonner JH, Bloomfield MR. The clinical outcome of patellofemoral arthroplasty. Orthop Clin North Am. 2013;44(3):271–80.
12. Davidson PA, Rivenburgh D. Focal anatomic patellofemoral inlay resurfacing: theoretic basis, surgical technique, and case reports. Orthop Clin North Am. 2008;39(3):337–46.
13. Cannon A, Stolley M, Wolf B, Amendola A. Patellofemoral resurfacing arthroplasty: literature review and description of a novel technique. Iowa Orthop J. 2008;28:42–8.
14. Provencher M, Ghodadra NS, Verma NN, Cole BJ, Zaire S, Shewman E, Bach BR Jr. Patellofemoral kinematics after limited resurfacing of the trochlea. J Knee Surg. 2009;22(4):310–6.
15. Kellgren JH, Lawrence JS. Radiological assessment of osteo-arthrosis. Ann Rheum Dis. 1957;16(4):494–502.
16. Outerbridge RE. The etiology of chondromalacia patellae. J Bone Joint Surg Br. 1961;43-B:752–7.
17. Caton J, Deschamps G, Chambat P, et al. Patella infera. Apropos of 128 cases. Rev Chir Orthop Reparatrice Appar Mot. 1982;68:317–25.
18. Borus T, Brilhault J, Confalonieri N, Johnson D, Thienpont E. Patellofemoral joint replacement, an evolving concept. Knee. 2014;21(Suppl 1):S47–50.
19. Pagenstert G, Liebensteiner M. Isolated patellofemoral arthroplasty. Arthroskopie. 2015;28(3):220–8. https://doi.org/10.1007/s00142-015-0029-y.
20. Imhoff AB, Feucht MJ, Bartsch E, Cotic M, Pogorzelski J. High patient satisfaction with significant improvement in knee function and pain relief after mid-term follow-up in patients with isolated patellofemoral inlay arthroplasty. Knee Surg Sports Traumatol Arthrosc. 2019;27:2251–8.
21. Patel A, Haider Z, Anand A, et al. Early results of patellofemoral inlay resurfacing arthroplasty using the HemiCap wave prosthesis. J Orthop Surg (Hong Kong). 2017;25(1):2309499017692705.
22. Zicaro JP, Yacuzzi C, Astoul Bonorino J, et al. Patellofemoral arthritis treated with resurfacing implant: clinical outcome and complications at a minimum two-year follow-up. Knee. 2017;24:1485–91.
23. Laursen JO. High mid-term revision rate after treatment of large, full-thickness cartilage lesions and OA in the patellofemoral joint using a large inlay resurfacing prosthesis: HemiCAPWave(R). Knee Surg Sports Traumatol Arthrosc. 2017;25:3856–61.
24. Feucht MJ, Cotic M, Beitzel K, et al. A matched-pair comparison of inlay and onlay trochlear designs for patellofemoral arthroplasty: no differences in clinical outcome but less progression of osteoarthritis with inlay designs. Knee Surg Sports Traumatol Arthrosc. 2017;25:2784–91.
25. Dahm DL, Kalisvaart MM, Stuart MJ, Slettedahl SW. Patellofemoral arthroplasty: outcomes and factors associated with early progression of tibiofemoral arthritis. Knee Surg Sports Traumatol Arthrosc. 2014;22(10):2554–9.
26. Tarassoli P, Punwar S, Khan W, Johnstone D. Patellofemoral arthroplasty: a systematic review of the literature. Open Orthop J. 2012;6:340–7.

Conservative Treatment Approaches of Patellar and Achilles Tendinopathies

33

Goktug Firatli, Yunus Emre Ozdemir, and Baris Kocaoglu

33.1 Patellar Tendinopathy

33.1.1 Introduction

Formerly known as "jumper's knee," patellar tendinopathy gives rise to considerable functional deficit and disability in recreational as well as professional athletes. It can affect their performance, cause trouble in their sports carrier, and even can cause to end it. With the help of the diagnostic tests which are ultrasonography (USG), magnetic resonance imagining (MRI), and X-Ray, the diagnosis of tendinopathy is mainly based on the clinical examination [1].

Nowadays, therapeutic protocols are preferred by experience rather than scientific evidence. Moreover, current evidences make us able to change our minds about previous doctrines and dogmatic belief on tendon overuse. Surprisingly, histologic and biochemical results have indicated that the underlying pathology of tendinopathy is not an inflammatory tendinitis but a degenerative tendinosis. Therefore, pain in chronic patellar tendinopathy is not caused by inflammatory process, but its exact origin is still unknown. In the light of molecular evidences, rehabilitation with eccentric exercises should be more important than the anti-inflammatory protocols when it comes to conservative management. The surgery should be preferred when the conservative therapy is not enough for recovery. However, wide spectrum of the surgical procedures and absence of the randomized studies, the effectivity of the surgical treatment of the patellar tendinopathy is still under debate. Based on the pathophysiology and molecular mechanisms of the pain in the patellar tendinopathy, new treatment strategies should be planned in the future.

33.1.2 Anatomy and Definition of Patellar Tendinopathy

The extension of the common tendon of insertion of the quadriceps femoris muscle, patellar tendon, extends to the tibial tuberosity from the inferior pole of the patella. It has approximately 3 cm width in the coronal plane and 4–5 mm thickness in the sagittal plane. Macroscopically it appears bright, fibrous, and white.

Contribution of blood supply to patellar tendinopathy is a common belief [2, 3]. The anastomotic ring in the thin layers of loose connective tissue covering the dense fibrous expansion of the

G. Firatli
Faculty of Medicine, Acibadem University, Istanbul, Turkey
e-mail: info@stargardtdisease.com

Y. E. Ozdemir · B. Kocaoglu (✉)
Department of Orthopedics and Traumatology, Faculty of Medicine, Acibadem University, Istanbul, Turkey
e-mail: info@acibadem.edu.tr

M. T. Hirschmann et al. (eds.), *ESSKA Instructional Course Lecture Book*,
https://doi.org/10.1007/978-3-662-61264-4_33

rectus femoris constitutes the patellar tendon vascularization. The major arteries are the medial inferior genicular, lateral inferior genicular, lateral superior genicular, and the anterior tibial recurrent artery [4, 5]. The proximal posterior side of the tendon is the most commonly affected by patellar tendinopathy.

It's widely accepted that the patellar tendon has a "relatively avascular osteotendinous junction." There is an "avascular zone between ligament and bone" in the distal attachment of the tendon to tuberosity of tibia, the proximal attachment is adjacent to the inferior half of the patella and the infrapatellar fat pad, which are both highly vascularized. Hence the proximal patellar tendon is well vascularized. However, blood flow at rest and activity does not necessarily overlap each other. Patellar tendon vasculature at rest and activity would be possible by the recent technical advances [6].

The stretching can cause corruption of the arrangement of the fibrils. During the sportive activities, the particular load causes the fibrils to become more parallel and the tendon has a relatively linear response to mechanical stress. Beyond this limit lengthening, micro failures can occur [7]. The mesh structure of the collagen fibers fails. With even further elongation, the elastic failure of fibers themselves, combined with shear failure, causes macroscopic damage [8].

33.1.3 Epidemiology

Patellar tendinopathy can affect a wide variety of sports branches like basketball, volleyball, soccer, football, running even in the military, etc. There are a lot of intrinsic or extrinsic risk factors that have been described in musculoskeletal overuse injuries. More specifically, patellar tendinopathy is very common in the elite athletes of volleyball probably due to intensity of training on jumping performance, and ankle and knee joint dynamics. Also, current literature mostly says that patellar tendinopathies are more common in males than females.

33.1.4 Pathophysiology

Like other chronic tendinopathies such as Achilles tendinopathy or extensor tendinopathy of the elbow, patellar tendinopathy is basically caused by tendon overload. Cumulative microtrauma occurs due to failure of coherence between collagen fibers, which is caused by repeated strain of the tendon, beyond its elastic capacity.

Tendency to injury is inevitable as a result of low metabolic rate of tendon when it comes to increased demand for raw materials like collagen and matrix to repair of the tissue. This is the main cause of the vicious cycle, which then results with the further reduction of repair capacity and more predispositions to injury. The final result of this overload mechanism or failed healing response is the formation of a tendinosis area within the tendon, which is as indicated by the proposed nomenclature of a noninflammatory condition. The predisposition of the posterior tendon fibers within the patellar tendon is still unclear.

The precise origin of pain caused by patellar tendinopathy remains unclear but it's clear by the evidences that chronic patellar tendinopathy is not an inflammatory condition. Peritendinous pain receptor activation may be the cause of the symptoms.

The inferior pole impingement of the patellar tendon is an alternative hypothesis to chronic overload hypothesis, which is widely accepted. However, there are a lot of studies that say the opposite of each other so the impingement hypothesis is a scientifically weak hypothesis [3].

33.1.5 Diagnosis

The usual presentation of pain in the patellar tendinopathies is anterior knee pain which worsens with prolonged knee flexion. Pain starts mostly insidious, but often patients can notice it during or after sportive activity. The proximal insertion of patellar tendon to patella is the generally certain location of pain. At the beginning of the disease the pain starts after the end of the activity, and as the disease progresses, pain may be experienced at the beginning of specific activities or even throughout their sport activity. When this happens, patellar tendinopathy can affect their performance. In severe cases, patient feels pain during daily activities or at rest. Several scoring systems for knee pathology are used in the literature but most of them fail to detect the specific deficits of athletes with patellar tendinopathy.

Physical findings are generally parallel to patellar tendinopathy. The most consistent finding is localized tenderness at the inferior patellar pole [9]. Decline squatting is a good functional testing for patellar tendon [10]. The number of pain-free decline squats is generally low. Patellofemoral pain syndrome or Hoffa impingement is one of the most important differential diagnoses. Sometimes, these conditions can be seen even together.

Plain X-rays can be a good option to diagnose bony abnormalities and occasional neurotendinous calcification. Technological advancement makes us able to get more detailed visualization of the tendons, bones, etc. However, the issue is to decide which imaging modality is the best choice and its clinical relevance of detected abnormalities.

Due to the alignment of the patellar tendon is superficially and in parallel with the skin surface, it is well suited for ultrasonographic evaluation [11]. Hypoechogenic zone often associated with tendon thickening due to disorganization of collagen fibers. In advanced tendinosis, small areas of hyperreflectivity or intratendinous clefts can be observed.

The good correlation of imaging and histopathological findings does not necessarily correspond to a good clinical correlation or guidance for therapy. Tendon imaging has been used for several purposes, ranging from screening modality to surgical indication and postoperative monitoring guidance. However, recent studies have questioned some of these assumed qualities of tendon imaging.

They can be used in the screening of athletes to establish individual tendon prevention programs, as athletes with increased risk can be identified, or they can be used to confirm the athlete's symptoms so that therapeutic decisions can be made.

With color and power Doppler evaluation made us obtaining an estimation of intratendinous blood flow [12]. In patellar and Achilles tendinopathy, color Doppler ultrasonography could characterize the neovascularization and this increased blood flow in symptomatic tendons. Ultrasonographic effects of different treatments need to be established in longitudinal studies.

The USG as the first line investigation for its lower cost, availability, direct clinical correlation, and possibility of adding blood flow evaluation through Doppler technique, and MRI can be hold up for additional anatomical view as differential diagnosis or preoperative evaluation is required.

33.1.6 Therapy

The deficiency of the knowledge of the pathophysiologic events and the pain mechanisms about the patellar tendinopathy can be the reason for the different treatment methods. Conservative treatment before surgical treatment has been preferred for long years [13]. The current trend in therapeutic approach for patellar tendinopathy focuses the requirement for a more comprehensive approach with emphasis on strengthening exercises in contrast to the previous literature that may be caused by lack of studies about the conservative treatment options. Strengthening could be the critical point in a more pathophysiology-based management of patellar tendinopathy because the missing healing response is the key element of this tendinopathy.

33.1.6.1 Conservative Management

Correction of Intrinsic and Extrinsic Risk Factors

Training Errors

It has been known by evidences that training conditions like ground selections, training intensity, style, frequency, etc. are extremely important about this tendinopathy.

Flexibility

Mobility limitations are one of the most important reasons of the tendinopathies (REF), and the flexibility of the muscles is very important for the mobility of a joint (REF); Witvrouw et al. [14], found that flexibility of quadriceps and hamstring muscles can be the only reason of this injury. Therefore, correction of limited flexibility of the responsible muscles by corrective exercises is a very logical option.

Biomechanical Abnormality

It's been hypothesized that intrinsic risk factors like foot hyperpronation, pes planus or cavus, forefoot varus or valgus, hindfoot varus or valgus, tibia vara, genu valgum or varum, patellofemoral malalignment, femoral neck anteversion, and leg length discrepancies can play role in the biomechanical derangement in patellar tendinopathy but unfortunately there is no evidence in the literature which proves this theory. But of course, if an apparent biomechanical abnormality exists in a patient with patellar tendinopathy, correction of this could be logical because it doesn't mean that lack of evidence is equal evidence of the opposite.

Symptomatic Approach

Relative Rest

The tendinopathy results from mechanical overload, therefore decreasing the overload by giving a break to the activity can cause relief of these firing mechanisms. That does not mean complete immobilization; moreover, complete immobilization causes thinner and disoriented collagen fibers, decreased blood volume which results to tendon atrophy.

Nonsteroidal Anti-Inflammatory Drugs (NSAID)

Anti-inflammatory medication for an injury, which originates from degenerative, noninflammatory causes, should be questioned. There is no evidence about supportive effect of NSAIDs on chronic tendinopathy. There is an isolated study on the patient's acute tendon pain, reveals a positive effect of NSAIDs but still the place of pain in the overuse-related tendinopathy is questionable. Currently, the histopathology of acute tendon pain remains unclear. NSAIDs can also have additional effects than simply anti-inflammatory or analgesic effects [15]. There are some studies which have proved the potential favorable effects of NSAIDs in tendon healing while others have reported deleterious mechanisms of NSAIDs in tendons. Still, in the clinical management of chronic tendinopathy, the use of an NSAID can hide symptoms by its analgesic effect and consequently prevent optimum therapeutic management. Therefore, until further evidence of exact effects of NSAIDs in tendinopathy is revealed, their use in patellar tendinopathy is not evidence based.

Corticosteroids

Corticosteroid application in the tendinopathy treatment is a popular issue [16]. There are a lot of studies on this topic, some of these say it causes short-term pain relief but some of these say there is no positive effect. The increased risk of tendon rupture is a fact because strengthening is an important issue that has to be regained. Nevertheless, as patellar tendinopathy is a noninflammatory condition and corticosteroids can impair collagen synthesis and tendon strength, usage of corticosteroids needs to be rethought.

Ice Application

Icing causes vasoconstriction and by this, it causes neovascularization within tendinosis, and as a consequence it decreases leakage of blood and protein. Still, there is no precise protocol, which includes the parameters like time, duration, frequency, and repetition. Due to masking of the pain effect by icing, avoidance of usage before sport participation would be logical.

Local Physiotherapeutic Modalities

There are a lot of studies about the beneficial effects of the different physical therapy strategies about the treatment of patellar tendinopathy, including, fine needling, electrotherapy, electromagnetic fields, ultrasound, and laser therapy (Figs. 33.1, 33.2 and 33.3) [17]. Increase of collagen synthesis and tensile strength of the tendon have been showed by studies. Therefore, the local application of physical modalities is still debatable.

Extracorporeal Shock Wave Therapy

An ESWT session consists of the application of shock waves, which are sonic pulses generating high stress forces in tissue, which we better know this modality as a successful treatment method for urolithiasis. Analgesic process, the dissolution of calcific deposits, and the stimulation of a tissue regeneration process are known mechanisms of action of this therapy and the positive results of its use in patellar tendinopathy are supported by some studies [18]. Recently, the efficiency of ESWT was demonstrated in a randomized, double-blind, placebo-controlled

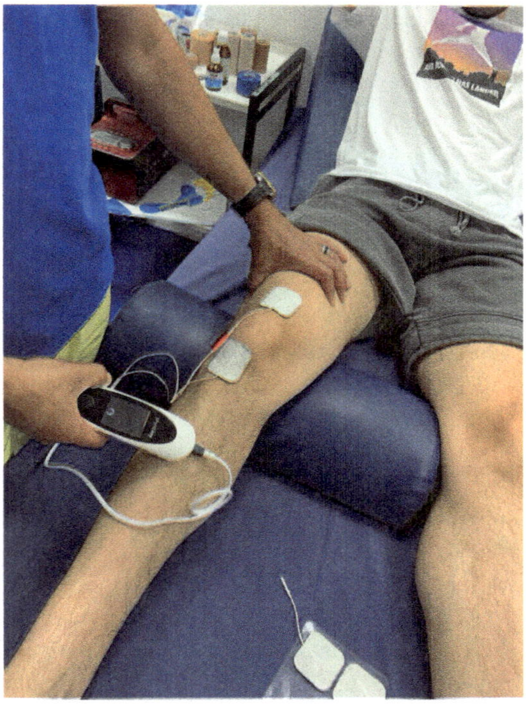

Fig. 33.2 Electrotherapy

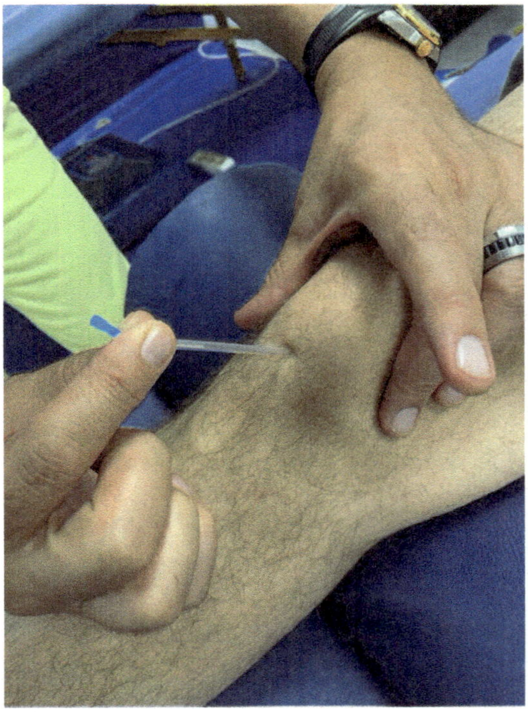

Fig. 33.1 Patellar tendon needling

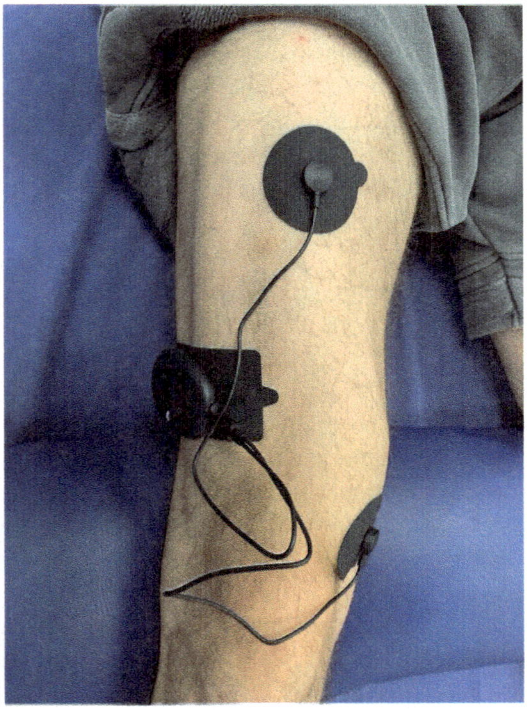

Fig. 33.3 Magnetic field therapy

trial in the short-term management of chronic patellar tendinopathy [19]. Further studies seem justified and warranted to clarify the contradictory results in other insertional tendinopathies and evaluate long-term effects and the relative effectiveness of ESWT for patellar tendinopathy compared with other therapeutic approaches.

Autologous Blood Injection

Augmentation of tendon healing through collagen regeneration and the stimulation of a well-ordered angiogenic response is the principle of this method by providing cellular and humoral mediators. However, there are no perfect models for tendinopathy, and clinical application is unreliable.

Mesenchymal Stem Cells

Not only their ability to differentiate and to directly participate in the regeneration process but also the immune modulation and trophic activities may be the most important therapeutic effect of mesenchymal stem cells (MSCs). As they arrive on sites of inflammation or tissue injury, they start to secrete immunomodulatory and trophic agents such as cytokines and growth factors that re-establish physiological homeostasis. Combined with the relative easy process of isolation and expansion, all these factors have made the MSCs very useful in recent years for clinical applications [20].

Rehabilitation

Due to heterogeneity in every single step of the diagnosis, therapy, patient selection, program design, results about the success rate have variety, there is no strong evidence that one precise physical therapy program is superior to others, still it is truth that rehabilitation of the afflicted muscle tendon is the cornerstone of tendinopathy management. Mostly, strength training especially eccentric exercise training is become the key element in the treatment of chronic tendinopathy but unfortunately most of the studies are about the Achilles tendinopathy.

Unfortunately, the mechanisms through which eccentric exercise can alter pain in chronic tendinopathy remain still unclear. There are some in vivo studies that show the increased metabolic activity and increased formation of collagen type I in response to acute exercise of peritendinous tissue [21]. Therefore, scientifically, it's impossible to say that one exercise program is superior to others in treatment of patellar tendinopathy.

33.1.7 Conclusion

Patellar tendinopathy is a common and important problem. Clinical examination and history are generally enough however technological advancement of the imaging techniques are helping to physician. The therapeutic regimen should be shifted from anti-inflammatory approaches to a more compete rehabilitation. Pain in tendinopathy patients is still unclear. If the conservative therapy cannot relieve the pain, surgical procedure can be applied. There are different surgical techniques but the real effect of surgery is still contentious. Pathophysiology-based new emerging techniques may lead to better curative or preventive regimens in the future.

33.2 Achilles Tendinopathy

33.2.1 Introduction

Achilles tendinopathy is a common condition, particularly in running dominant sports. It is a chronic syndrome, which is characterized by the pain and thickening in the Achilles tendon. The prevalence of Achilles tendinopathy is 52% in former runners, and the annual incidence is 7–9% in current runners. This syndrome is a summation of several pathologies and is different from rupture or partial rupture. Onset is generally subtle and chronic, although in some cases a patient may present with acute tendinopathy [22].

There is no worldwide accepted classification system. If the symptoms last longer than 3 months, the term "tendinitis" is not precisely fit to the situation because it has to be addressed to degenerative structural changes (tendinosis) within the tendon, not to the inflammation, which is rarely present in most cases.

Discrimination of tendinosis from paratendonitis is hard and not possible in most cases and these two are generally seen together. Still efforts should be made to diagnose the source of pain.

33.2.2 Anatomy and Definition of Achilles Tendinopathy

The Achilles tendon is the biggest and strongest tendon in the human body. The tendon is very capable of absorbing strong forces. It originates from a distal confluence of the gastrocnemius and soleus muscle and inserts at the bottom of the calcaneus.

A typical tendon structure consists of thin, cylindrical cells and an extracellular matrix. The cells of the tendon, commonly tenocytes tenoblasts, are responsible for the synthesis of all of the components of the extracellular matrix. Inside the matrix we find bundles of type I collagen and elastin. This type-I collagen is responsible for the strength of the tendon. Between the collagen there is a ground substance located which is made up of proteoglycans and glycosaminoglycans [23].

The Achilles tendon is surrounded by paratenon and by this it can move freely between surrounding tissue. The paratenon includes a layer of cells and is responsible for the blood supply of the tendon. The layers that are placed under the paratenon are the epitenon, which is a thin membrane and the endotenon, which surrounds the collagen fibers which results in bundles.

The blood supply of the tendon is low, as it has small numbers of blood vessels in all sections but especially 4–6 cm proximal of calcaneus. Lower vascularity may be the reason of slow healing rate following trauma.

Males have greater maximum rupture force and stiffness with a larger cross-sectional area than females. Younger individuals have greater tensile rupture stress and lower stiffness.

33.2.3 Epidemiology

The Achilles tendon has a cumulative lifetime injury incidence of approximately 24% in athletes. Running-related injuries have a prevalence between 11 and 85% or 2.5–59 injuries per 1000 h of running [24]. Results from one study cite the frequency of Achilles tendinopathy to be 1–2% in elite adolescent athletes [25]. Another study cited the frequency of injury as 9% in recreational athletes [22]. The lifetime injury incidence of 2.35 per 1000 is strongly associated with sporting activities [26]. This incidence increases in older men.

33.2.4 Pathophysiology

Achilles tendinopathy is basically caused by tendon overload. Cumulative microtrauma occurs due to failure of coherence between collagen fibers, which is caused by repeated strain of the tendon, beyond its tendons elastic capacity [27, 28].

As in other tendinopathies, tendency to injury is inevitable as a result of low metabolic rate of tendon when it comes to increased demand for raw materials like collagen and matrix to repair of the tissue [29]. This is the main cause of the vicious cycle which then results with the further reduction of repair capacity and more predisposition to injury. The final result of this overload mechanism or failed healing response is the formation of a tendinosis area within the tendon, which is as indicated by the proposed nomenclature of a noninflammatory condition.

The causes and mechanisms of Achilles tendinopathy (AT) can be divided into intrinsic and extrinsic factors. The intrinsic factors include anatomic factors, age, sex, metabolic dysfunction, foot cavity, dysmetria, muscle weakness, imbalance, gastrocnemius dysfunction, anatomical variation of the plantaris muscle, tendon vascularization, torsion of the Achilles tendons, slippage of the fascicle, and lateral instability of the ankle. And extrinsic factors include mechanical overload, constant effort, inadequate equipment, obesity, medications improper footwear, insufficient warming or stretching, hard training surfaces, and direct trauma, among others.

Strong and flexible type I collagen fibers are the main component of the Achilles tendon and it is covered by elastin rich paratenon which is a thin layer of connective tissue and it penetrates into the tendon, keeping the collagen bundles together while allowing movement between them [30].

The difference between tendinosis and tendinitis is that in tendinosis there are degenerative changes in the tendon's structure and the sheath, which makes the tendon more vulnerable to breaking.

Healthy tendons are almost avascular. Forming of abnormal vessels, neovascularization, is one feature of Achilles tendinopathy [31]. It is hypothesized that pain in chronic midportion Achilles tendinopathy is caused by neovascularization. The midportion Achilles tendon and the paratendon tissues have greater postcapillary venous filling pressures but there is no difference between Achilles tendinopathy and normal tendon tissue.

33.2.5 Diagnosis

Pain is the main symptom of Achilles tendinopathy but the main mechanism is the chronically deranged healing response nature, even in acute cases. In most cases pain appears at the beginning and at the end of a training session, relatively comfortable in between. As the pathologic process progresses, pain can extend to exercise, and, in further cases, it can even affect daily activities.

Detailed clinical examination is the best way to diagnose. Both legs are exposed from above the knees and the patient was examined during standing and prone. The foot and the heel should be inspected for any malalignment, deformity, and obvious asymmetry in the tendons size, localized thickening, Haglund heel, and any previous scars. The AT should be palpated for tenderness, heat, thickening, nodule, and crepitation. The tendons excursion is estimated to determine any tightness. The "painful arc" sign helps to distinguish between tendon and paratenon lesions. In paratendinopathy, the area of maximum thickening and tenderness remains fixed in relation to the malleoli from full dorsiflexion to plantarflexion, whereas lesions within the tendon move with ankle motion. There is often a discrete nodule, whose tenderness significantly decreases or disappears when the tendon is put under tension.

Although plain soft tissue radiography is not the imaging modality of choice in tendon disorders nowadays, it still took its place in diagnosing associated or incidental bony abnormalities. It can be taken more extensive information could be obtained about the internal morphology of tendon and the surrounding anatomy by magnetic resonance imaging (MRI). It is a useful tool to assess the different stages of chronic degeneration and differentiation between paratendinopathy and tendinopathy of the main body of the tendon.

When it comes to tendon incomplete rupture, MRI is superior to ultrasound (US). However, very high amount of extensive information coming from MRI has to be interpreted in correlation to the patient clinic before making any recommendation. Ultrasonography is bit of more operator-dependent, but it correlates well with histopathologic findings, and specifically in Europe, it took its place as a first imaging method. Thickening of the AT can be detected easily with both methods. So, US can be used as a first diagnostic method and an additional magnetic resonance study may be needed if US remains unclear and, together with the clinical diagnosis, decision of surgery can be taken more effectively. One important advantage of US is the interactive facility, which helps to provoke symptom by probes compression on the pathologic area. Concerning the high specificity and sensitivity of US, like MRI, it has a relatively high incidence of false positive findings.

33.2.6 Therapy

33.2.6.1 Conservative Management

Noninvasive Methods

Noninvasive methods such as relative rest or modification of activity, orthotics, heel lifts, massage, hot and cold compresses, strengthening exercises, ultrasound, and nonsteroidal anti-inflammatory drugs (NSAID) or oral corticosteroid can be applied as a first line treatment. NSAIDs has been questioned about its effectiveness because of prostaglandin inflammatory mediator absence in AT [32].

Corticosteroids Injections

Corticosteroids are a group of medications that contain cortisone. They relieve pain by reducing the inflammation that occurs in a diseased tendon. There is a controversy about the use of these injections in Achilles tendinosis since there is no inflammatory process. In some studies, cortisone injection gives short-term pain relief but in some other studies there is no pain relief after the injection.

Eccentric Training

The eccentric training program designed by Alfredson et al. [33] improve tendon healing by enhancing the tendon volume and signal intensity which is thought to be a response to trauma. But after a 12-week program, size and appearance of the tendon returns to normal on ultrasound and magnetic resonance imaging (MRI). With longer periods, eccentric loading program of the Achilles tendon, muscle tendon unit length will be increased and resistance of tendon to load will be increased overtime. Damage to abnormal blood vessel and the nerves may be the mechanism of repetitive eccentric loading on eliminating pain in the tendon concluded by Alfredson et al. [34] with the 12-week program, it has produced 90% good results with midportion, 30% good results in insertional Achilles tendinosis (Fig. 33.4).

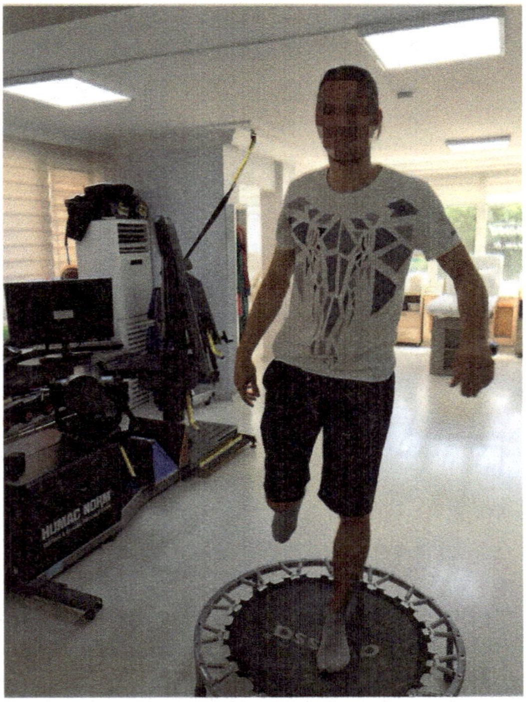

Fig. 33.4 Proprioception training

Extracorporeal Shock Wave Therapy

The extracorporeal shock wave therapy (ESWT) is another treatment option for Achilles tendinosis (Fig. 33.5). There are two treatment strategies: first one is the low energy treatment which is three weekly sessions without local anesthesia or intravenous anesthesia and second one is the high energy treatment which is a one session but with local or intravenous anesthesia. Repeated shock wave to the affected area causes microtrauma which is then followed by neovascularization.

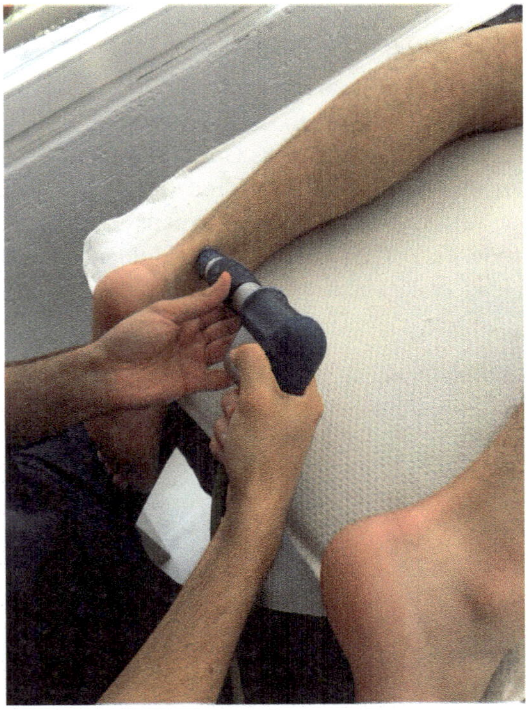

Fig. 33.5 ESWT

Emerging blood flow stimulates tissue healing which results with relief of pain. It can also block afferent pain receptor functioning and increase nitric oxide synthase. This treatment strategy seems beneficial and may have a place in the treatment of Achilles tendinosis [35].

Low-Level Laser Therapy

Low-level laser therapy produces effects on a diseased tendon like enhanced adenosine triphosphate production, enhanced cell function, and increased protein synthesis [36]. It also reduces inflammation, increases collagen synthesis, and promotes angiogenesis. In a study by Stergioulas et al. [35], it was established that Achilles tendinosis patients who underwent eccentric exercises together with low-level laser therapy demonstrated decreased pain intensity, morning stiffness, tenderness to palpation, active dorsiflexion, and crepitus with no side effects in comparison with the patients who underwent eccentric exercises only. However, the data to confirm the efficiency of low-level laser therapy is still inadequate for the treatment of Achilles tendinosis.

Other Additional Methods

There are other methods that increase blood circulation. One of them is Graston method, which is performed by a metal rod (Fig. 33.6). It is mostly useful for tendon and soft tissue mobilization. Tecar therapy is another additional method. It is endogenous thermotherapy based on the principle of capacitive and resistive energy transfer that has an effect within the tendon, activating body's natural repairing and anti-inflammatory processes (Fig. 33.7). During those therapies, athletes shouldn't lose their cardiovascular condition. At this situation, anti-gravity treadmill helps patients to continue their cardiovascular form (Fig. 33.8).

Platelet Rich Plasma

In chronic Achilles tendinosis, there is no inflammation or paucity of platelets. Activated platelets begin to produce cytokines and granules, which followed, by producing of the growth factors that support the healing process. Higher number of concentration of platelets through injection to the tissue increases the healing possibility by triggering revascularization of the injured tendon. Although the current literature doesn't say that PRP is the treatment of choice in AT, emerging evidences suggest that patient may improve by PRP treatment. However, the rate of improvement not superior is to physical therapy or placebo [37].

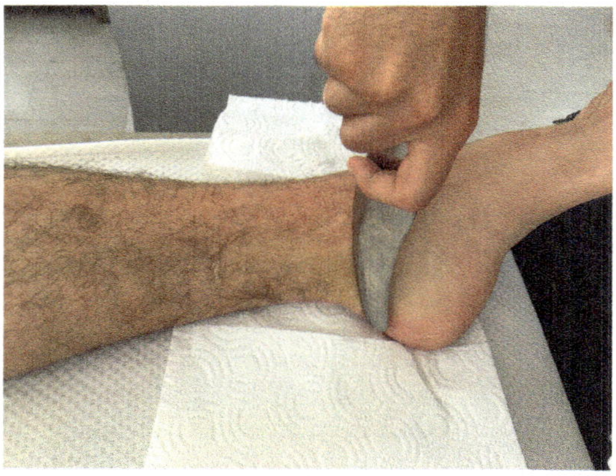

Fig. 33.6 Graston therapy

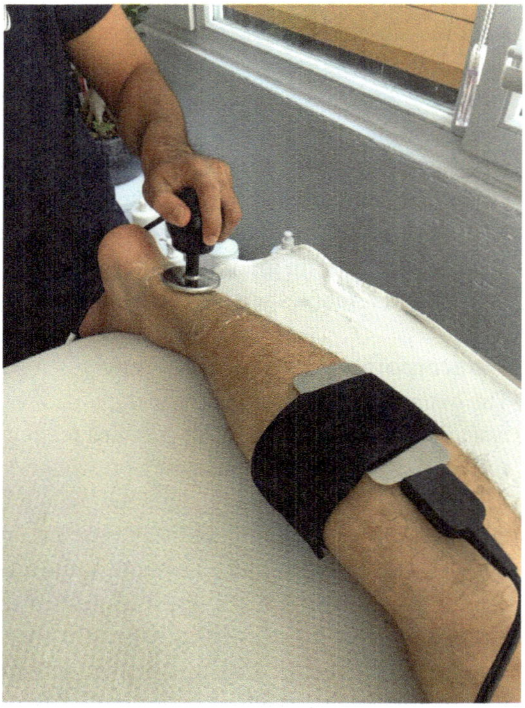

Fig. 33.7 Tecar therapy

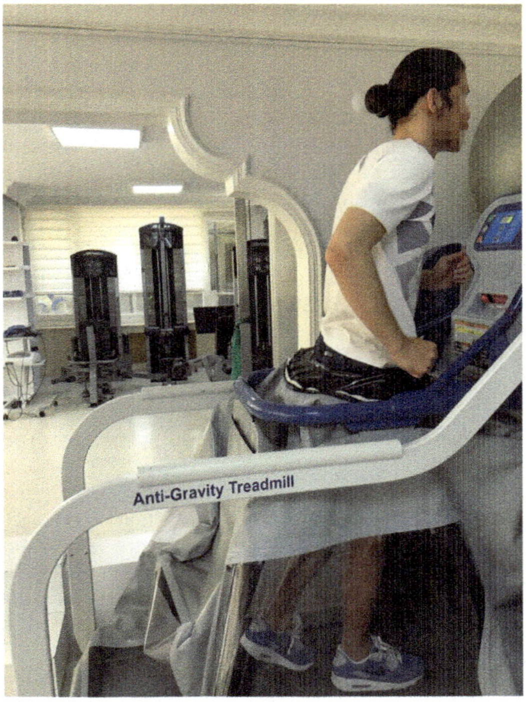

Fig. 33.8 Anti-gravity treadmill

33.2.6.2 Rehabilitation

Rehabilitation for an Achilles tendon rupture helps to regain strength and flexibility in the tendon and leg. It can be done at home or in a gym.

Rehabilitation program may include:

- Stretching and flexibility exercises.
- Strengthening exercises.
- Endurance activities, such as riding a stationary bicycle.
- Coordination and/or agility training.

Recovery varies among people. It depends on how severe the tendon injury is and whether you complete your program. Giving time and energy to a rehab program will speed recovery and help prevent future injury.

33.2.7 Conclusion

There are diverse conservative and surgical treatment strategies for Achilles tendinosis, which emphasizes the lack of the gold standard of the treatments. Mechanism of action for the ideal treatment is still controversial. Conservative measures such as corticosteroid injection reduces inflammation, but on the other hand eccentric training lengthens muscle tendon unit. ESWT or PRP stimulates neovascularization. Surgical measures include tendon microtenotomy, tendon debridement, and paratenon stripping [38].

References

1. Khan KM, Maffulli N, Coleman BD, Cook JL, Taunton JE. Patellar tendinopathy: some aspects of basic science and clinical management. Br J Sports Med. 1998;32(4):346–55.
2. Ferretti A, Ippolito E, Mariani P, et al. Jumper's knee. Am J Sports Med. 1983;11:58–62.
3. McLoughlin RF, Raber EL, Vellet AD, et al. Patellar tendinitis: MR features, with suggested pathogenesis and proposed classification. Radiology. 1995;197:843–8.
4. Scapinelli R. Blood supply of the human patella. J Bone Joint Surg Br. 1967;49:563–70.
5. Scapinelli R. Studies on the vasculature of the human knee joint. Acta Anat (Basel). 1968;70:305–31.
6. Astrom M, Westlin N. Blood flow in the normal Achilles tendon assessed by laser Doppler flowmetry. J Orthop Res. 1994;12:246–52.
7. Józsa L, Kannus P. Human tendons, vol. 576. Champaign: Human Kinetics; 1997.
8. O'Brien M. Functional anatomy and physiology of tendons. Clin Sports Med. 1992;11:505–20.
9. King JB, Cook JL, Khan KM, et al. Patellar tendinopathy. Sports Med Arthrosc Rev. 2000;8:86–95.
10. Purdam CR, Cook JL, Hopper DM, Khan KM. Discriminative ability of functional loading tests for adolescent jumper's knee. Phys Ther Sport. 2003;4(1):3–9.
11. Hodgson RJ, O'Connor PJ, Grainger AJ. Tendon and ligament imaging. Br J Radiol. 2012;85(1016):1157–72.
12. Yang X, Pugh ND, Coleman DP, Nokes LDM. Are Doppler studies a useful method of assessing neovascularization in human Achilles tendinopathy? A systematic review and suggestions for optimizing machine settings. J Med Eng Technol. 2010;34(7–8):365–72.
13. Cook JL, Khan KM, Purdam CR. Conservative treatment of patellar tendinopathy. Phys Ther Sport. 2001;2(2):54–65. https://doi.org/10.1054/ptsp.2001.0069.
14. Witvrouw E, Danneels L, Asselman P, D'Have T, Cambier D. Muscle flexibility as a risk factor for developing muscle injuries in male professional soccer players. Am J Sports Med. 2003;31(1):41–6.
15. Schwartz A, Watson JN, Hutchinson MR. Patellar tendinopathy. Sports Health. 2015;7(5):415–20.

16. Andres BM, Murrell GAC. Treatment of tendinopathy: what works, what does not, and what is on the horizon. Clin Orthop Relat Res. 2008;466(7):1539–54.
17. Rudavsky A, Cook J. Physiotherapy management of patellar tendinopathy (jumper's knee). J Physiother. 2014;60(3):122–9.
18. van Leeuwen MT, Zwerver J, van den Akker-Scheek I. Extracorporeal shockwave therapy for patellar tendinopathy: a review of the literature. Br J Sports Med. 2009;43(3):163–8.
19. Liao C-D, Xie G-M, Tsauo J-Y, Chen H-C, Liou T-H. Efficacy of extracorporeal shock wave therapy for knee tendinopathies and other soft tissue disorders: a meta-analysis of randomized controlled trials. BMC Musculoskelet Disord. 2018;19(1):278.
20. Abat F, Alfredson H, Cucchiarini M, Madry H, Marmotti A, Mouton C, de Girolamo L. Current trends in tendinopathy: consensus of the ESSKA basic science committee. Part I: biology, biomechanics, anatomy and an exercise-based approach. J Exp Orthop. 2017;4(1):18.
21. Kjaer M, Langberg H, Skovgaard D, Olesen J, Bülow J, Krogsgaard M, Boushel R. In vivo studies of peritendinous tissue in exercise. Scand J Med Sci Sports. 2000;10(6):326–31.
22. Li H-Y, Hua Y-H. Achilles tendinopathy: current concepts about the basic science and clinical treatments. Biomed Res Int. 2016;2016:6492597.
23. Screen HRC, Birk DE, Kadler KE, Ramirez F, Young MF. Tendon functional extracellular matrix. J Orthop Res. Author manuscript; available in PMC 2016 Jun 1. Published in final edited form as: J Orthop Res. 2015 Jun; 33(6): 793–799.
24. Olewnik Ł, Wysiadecki G, Podgórski M, Polguj M, Topol M. The plantaris muscle tendon and its relationship with the Achilles tendinopathy. Biomed Res Int. 2018;2018:9623579.
25. Dakin SG, Newton J, Martinez FO, Hedley R, Gwilym S, Jones N, Reid HAB, Wood S, Wells G, Appleton L, Wheway K, Watkins B, Carr AJ. Chronic inflammation is a feature of Achilles tendinopathy and rupture. Br J Sports Med. 2018;52(6):359–67.
26. Martin RL, Chimenti R, Cuddeford T, Houck J, Matheson JW, McDonough CM, Paulseth S, Wukich DK, Carcia CR. Achilles pain, stiffness, and muscle power deficits: midportion Achilles tendinopathy revision 2018. J Orthop Sports Phys Ther. 2018;48(5):A1–A38.
27. Traina F, Perna F, Ruffilli A, Mazzotti A, Meliconi R, Berti L, Faldini C. Surgical treatment of insertional Achilles tendinopathy: a systematic review. J Biol Regul Homeost Agents. 2016;30(4 Suppl 1):131–8.
28. Hubbard MJ, Hildebrand BA, Battafarano MM, Battafarano DF. Common soft tissue musculoskeletal pain disorders. Prim Care. 2018;45(2):289–303.
29. Albano D, Messina C, Usuelli FG, De Girolamo L, Grassi M, Maccario C, Bignotti B, Tagliafico A, Sconfienza LM. Magnetic resonance and ultrasound in achilles tendinopathy: predictive role and response assessment to platelet-rich plasma and adipose-derived stromal vascular fraction injection. Eur J Radiol. 2017;95:130–5.
30. Murphy M, Rio E, Debenham J, Docking S, Travers M, Gibson W. Evaluating the progress of mid-portion Achilles tendinopathy during rehabilitation: a review of outcome measures for self-reported pain and function. Int J Sports Phys Ther. 2018;13(2):283–92.
31. Baltes TPA, Zwiers R, Wiegerinck JI, van Dijk CN. Surgical treatment for midportion Achilles tendinopathy: a systematic review. Knee Surg Sports Traumatol Arthrosc. 2017;25(6):1817–38.
32. Astrom M, Westlin N. No effect of piroxicam on Achilles tendinopathy: a randomized study of 70 patients. Acta Orthop Scand. 1992;63(6):631–4.
33. Alfredson H, Pietila T, Jonsson P, Lorentzon R. Heavy-load eccentric calf muscle training for the treatment of chronic Achilles tendinosis. Am J Sports Med. 1998;26(3):360–6.
34. Alfredson H, Ohberg L, Forsgren S. Is vasculo-neural in- growth the cause of pain in chronic Achilles tendinosis? An investigation using ultrasonography and colour Doppler, immunohistochemistry, and diagnostic injections. Knee Surg Sports Traumatol Arthrosc. 2003;11(5):334–8.
35. Lake JE, Ishikawa SN. Conservative treatment of Achilles tendinopathy: emerging techniques. Foot Ankle Clin. 2009;14(4):663–74.
36. Stergioulas A, Stergioula M, Aarskog R, Lopes-Martins RA, Bjordal JM. Effects of low-level laser therapy and eccentric exercises in the treatment of recreational athletes with chronic Achilles tendinopathy. Am J Sports Med. 2008;36(5):881–7.
37. de Jonge S, de Vos RJ, Weir A, et al. One-year follow-up of platelet-rich plasma treatment in chronic Achilles tendinopathy: a double-blind randomized placebo-controlled trial. Am J Sports Med. 2011;39(8):1623–9.
38. Lopez RGL, Jung H-G. Achilles tendinosis: treatment options. Clin Orthop Surg. 2015;7(1):1.

Tendinopathy: From Basic Science to Return to Play

34

F. Abat, U. G. Longo, B. Kocaoglu, F. G. Usuelli, L. Lempainen, A. Jiménez-García, G. Stelitano, G. Firatli, and R. D'Ambrosi

34.1 Basic Science and Diagnosis of Tendinopathy

Tendinopathy is a common clinical problem which affects a substantial portion of recreational and professional athletes and those in many occupations involving repetitive work [1].

Tendon injuries, which represent approximately 50% of all sports injuries, can occur in any tendon. It is often at the level of or near its insertion where there is the area of major mechanical stress concentration [2]. The most commonly involved tendons are the rotator cuff (particularly supraspinatus) tendons in the shoulder, the forearm extensor and flexor tendons in the forearm, the patella tendon in the knee, and the Achilles tendon in the ankle as they are more exposed to repeated loads, shear and compressive forces [3].

The term "*tendinopathy*" describes the clinical features in and around tendons which include activity-related pain, swelling, focal tendon tenderness, decreased strength and movement in the affected area associated with decreased exercise tolerance and function of the limb, up to total rupture [4].

The histologically descriptive terms "*tendinosis*" (a degenerative pathological condition with a lack of inflammatory change) and "*tendonitis*" or "*tendinitis*" (implying an inflammatory process associated to degenerative injury) should be used only after histopathological confirmation. The pathogenic mechanisms underlying the onset of tendinopathies are still unclear [5].

Historically, inflammation has been thought of as the central pathological process in tendon disorders, but histological studies of surgical

F. Abat (✉)
Department of Orthopaedic Sports Medicine, ReSport Clinic, Blanquerna Faculty of Health Science, Ramon Llull University, Barcelona, Spain
e-mail: abat@resportclinic.com

U. G. Longo · G. Stelitano
Department of Orthopaedic and Trauma Surgery, Campus Bio-Medico University, Rome, Italy

Centro Integrato di Ricerca (CIR), Campus Bio-Medico University, Rome, Italy

B. Kocaoglu
Department of Orthopedics and Traumatology, Faculty of Medicine, Acibadem University, Istanbul, Turkey

F. G. Usuelli
IRCCS Istituto Ortopedico Galeazzi, Milan, Italy

L. Lempainen
Sports Trauma Research Unit, Mehiläinen NEO Sports Hospital, Turku, Finland

A. Jiménez-García
Department of Strength and Conditioning, ReSport Clinic, Blanquerna Faculty of Health Science, Ramon Llull University, Barcelona, Spain

G. Firatli
Faculty of Medicine, Acibadem University, Istanbul, Turkey

R. D'Ambrosi
Humanitas San Pio X, Milan, Italy

M. T. Hirschmann et al. (eds.), *ESSKA Instructional Course Lecture Book*,
https://doi.org/10.1007/978-3-662-61264-4_34

specimens have consistently shown the presence of degenerative lesions, either absent of or with a minimal inflammatory component [6].

The most widely shared hypothesis sees inflammation's contribution only in the early phases of disease. Currently, mechanical overload and excessive mechanical stress on the muscle–tendon unit seem to play a key role in the onset and perpetuation of tendon degeneration even though a full understanding of the biomechanical basis for tendinopathy is still lacking and needs to evolve [3].

Histological changes in tendinopathies have been widely described [7]. Macroscopically normal tendon is white, brilliant and has a fibroelastic consistency. Affected tendons lose their normal sparkling white appearance and become gray or brown, amorphous, thinner and softer [8]. The typical thickening in the degenerated regions can be diffuse, fusiform, or nodular [9]. Microscopic histopathological changes include loss of the parallel orientation of collagen fibers along with a decrease in collagen fiber diameter and in the overall density collagen. There is also increased overall cellularity, increased deposition of mucoid ground substance and proteoglycans as well as the proliferation of new randomly oriented blood vessels. Moreover, an increase in type III (reparative) collagen fibers is usually described [10]. All these reflect a failure of the native tendon healing process.

Depending on the histopathological alterations, different theories on tendinopathy etiopathogenesis have been hypothesized.

The mechanical theory places overuse injury at the center of the pathologic process. The excessive load to which the tendon is exposed may cause repeated microinjuries that lead to biological alterations of ground substance and tenocytes with subsequent mechanical breakdown of the loaded tendon. The increase in E2 prostaglandin and B4 leukotriene production seems to be mainly responsible for degenerative process. The affected tendons lose their mechanical properties, resulting in a reduction of the tendon cross-sectional area over which muscular forces are transmitted thereby making them more susceptible to failure [11].

The vascular theory would explain the onset of tendinopathy as a consequence of an inadequate vascular supply during mechanical activities due to the presence of intratendinous avascular areas as occurs in the Achilles tendon or extensors tendon of the elbow [12]. In contrast to the vascular theory, a new pathogenic hypothesis is being put forth. It postulates that physical training could create a localized hyperthermia condition, causing a decrease in tenocyte survival [13].

The neuronal response to repetitive tendon microtrauma seems to be involved. In degenerated tendons, a high level of nervous mediators (such as glutamate, calcitonin, P-peptide) and small nerve ingrowth are widely noticed [14]. Finally, disuse has also been identified as tending to alter tendon properties. Denervation and immobilization have both been found to decrease tendon stiffness and reduce final tissue strength and, at the same time, inactivity and unloading could have an effect on tendon collagen homeostasis dysregulation [13–15].

Some individuals are more susceptible to developing tendinopathy than others who have similar levels of physical activity [16]. This predisposition derives from the interaction between several risk factors identified in two large categories, extrinsic and intrinsic factors. Among the intrinsic factors, individual's genetic characteristics must be considered. The ABO blood group and tendon molecular structure were suggested as possible predisposing factors. Gender is another genetic expression key. Women seem to have less tendinopathy than men, thanks to the protective role of estrogens. Estrogenic protection is supported by the evidence that tendon ruptures are almost exclusively described after the onset of menopause [16, 17]. Increased age is another important intrinsic risk factor and certainly the prevalence of tendinopathy seems to increase with age. Age-related intratendinous changes such as the reduction in proteoglycans and an increase in cross-links between collagen fibers make tendons stiffer and less capable of tolerating load [18]. Body composition has recently been linked to tendinopathy. A greater waist circumference and high levels of adipose tissue suggest increased risk to the onset of tendinopathy. Ligamentous laxity, articular hypermobility, muscular stiffness or weakness, malalignment of the lower extremity, and limitation of joint mobility also has to be mentioned. Finally, the association between tendinopathy and several pathological conditions has been demonstrated [19]. Endocrine-metabolic diseases such as obesity, diabetes mellitus, hypertension, increased serum lipids, and hyperuricemia seem to have a positive association with the pathology [20]. Other diseases that have been found to be associated with tendinopathy include systemic diseases, neurological conditions, infectious diseases, chronic renal failure, psoriasis, systemic lupus erythematosus, hyperparathyroidism, and hyperthyroidism [21].

The main important extrinsic risks factors include mechanical overuse linked to sports activities like training errors (excessive distance, intensity, hill work, erroneous running technique, fatigue) and the use of several drugs (fluroquinolone antibiotics, statins, oral contraceptives, and locally injected corticosteroids) [22, 23]. Environmental conditions such as cold weather during outdoor training, faulty footwear and equipment, inadequate training surfaces or frequent changes in playing surface have been found to increase the prevalence of tendinopathy [19–23].

The clinical history and a physical examination are essential to making a diagnosis of tendinopathy. Clinically, tendinopathy is characterized by pain, swelling (diffuse or localized), and impaired physical performance. Pain is the cardinal symptom that usually occurs at the beginning of the training session or a short while afterwards. In advanced cases, it may interfere with the activities of daily living. Clinical examination is the best diagnostic tool and presupposes a careful valuation of the overall anatomical structures involved, and the use of specific tests to elicit pain and tenderness. Radiological imaging has a secondary role and it is used as diagnostic support. Ultrasound is considered the most appropriate and advantageous imaging modality for routine clinical evaluation despite it being operator dependent. MRI studies should be performed only if the ultrasound scan remains unclear.

34.1.1 Achilles Tendinopathy

Achilles tendinopathy is a clinical syndrome characterized by pain and swelling in and around the Achilles tendon associated with impaired physical performance [24]. The typical patient affected by Achilles tendinopathy is the so-called "*middle-age weekend warrior,*" a recreational athlete who practices sports, like running, with explosive accelerations and eccentric loads located on the lower limb [25]. The etiology of Achilles tendinopathy remains debatable and is likely caused by the interaction of intrinsic and extrinsic factors. In addition to the ones analyzed for tendinopathy etiopathogenesis in general, there are other specific factors responsible for the onset of the Achilles tendon disease. Intrinsic factors include an anatomical foot alteration like hypo-hyperpronation. It is often associated with ankle misalignment, varus or valgus hindfoot and forefoot, pes cavus or flat foot, tendon vascularity, weakness of as well as the lack of flexibility of the gastrocnemius–soleus complex and lateral ankle instability [26]. Excessive loading of the tendon is considered the major extrinsic causative factor for Achilles tendinopathy. Free radical damage occurring on reperfusion after ischemia, hypoxia, hyperthermia, and impaired tenocyte apoptosis has been linked to tendinopathy [27]. In a case-control study, subjects with painful Achilles tendinopathy had a lipid profile characteristic of dyslipidemia [28]. The use of local corticosteroid injections and of systemic antibiotics (in particular fluoroquinolones) has shown an increase in the development of the disease [29]. Achilles tendon pathology can be subdivided into acute and chronic tendinopathy, including the simple forms of tendinosis up to total rupture of the tendon.

Chronic tendinopathies are painful clinical conditions commonly found in athletes, often middle-aged male runners even though they can also affect sedentary subjects. They are typically associated with overuse damage and this would explain their greater incidence in athletes. However, 30% of patients with chronic tendinopathy do not participate in sports activities. Other pathogenetic mechanisms responsible of the chronic damage have to be found. Metabolic and vascular imbalances seem to play a crucial role in the onset of the disease.

Chronic Achilles tendinopathy can be categorized as insertional or non-insertional. They are two distinct disorders with different underlying pathophysiologies and options.

Non-insertional tendinopathies (also known as "*tendinopathy of the main body of the Achilles tendon*" or "*midportion Achilles tendinopathy*") are caused by an inflammatory cellular response that occurs inside the tendon structure. They are associated with microcirculatory alterations and edema that can progress, in the chronic phase of the pathology, toward the formation of fibrosis and exudate [30].

Pain is the most common clinical symptom. In athletes, pain typically occurs at the beginning and end of a training session, with a period of diminished discomfort in between. As the condition progresses, pain may occur with even minor exertion, and may interfere with activities of daily living. Clinical examination is the best diagnostic tool. The patient is examined while standing and prone with both legs exposed from above the knees. The tendon appears diffusely swollen and edematous, and tenderness is usually greatest 2–6 cm proximal to the tendon insertion [31]. The most widely used diagnostic tests for non-insertional Achilles tendinopathies are the *Royal London Hospital Test* and the *Painful Arc test.* In the first one, once the tester has elicited local tenderness by palpating the tendon with the ankle in neutral position, the patient is asked to actively dorsiflex and plantarflex the ankle. With the ankle in maximum dorsiflexion and in maximum plantarflexion, the portion of the tendon originally found to be tender is palpated again. The Painful arc test, instead, helps the surgeon to distinguish between tendon and paratenon lesions. In paratendinopathy, the area of maximum thickening and tenderness remains fixed in relation to dorsi- to plantarflexion [32]. Again, the *Victorian Institute of Sports Assessment—Achilles* (VISA-A) questionnaire can be used to evaluate the severity of Achilles Tendinopathy. It covers the domains of pain, function, and activity and has a total score of 100. An asymptomatic patient would score 100 [33]. Ultrasonography (Fig. 34.1), though operator dependent, represents the primary imaging method to make the final diagnosis thanks to its interactive capability. Grey scale ultrasonography is associated with color or power Doppler to detect neovascularity [34].

Only if ultrasonography remains unclear, should magnetic resonance imaging (MRI) be performed. MRI gives more detailed information about the internal morphology of the tendon, surrounding bone, and soft tissues. Because of its high sensitivity in detecting incomplete tendon ruptures, the MRI data should be interpreted with caution and correlated to the patient symptoms before starting any treatments. However, both US and MRI show damaged tissue as focal or diffuse thickening of the Achilles tendon with focal hypoechoic areas.

34.1.2 Patellar Tendinopathy

Patellar tendinopathy is a painful condition of the knee caused by small tears on the patellar tendon, usually localized in its proximal region.

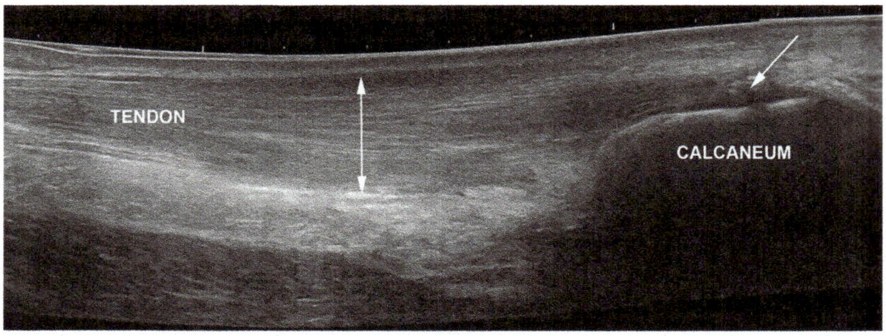

Fig. 34.1 Ultrasound image of the Achilles tendon in longitudinal view. Note the hypoechogenic area of the tendon (black zone inside the tendon), calcification (arrow) as well as a thickened tendon (double arrow)

It mainly occurs in sports which require strenuous jumping such as volleyball, track (long and high jump), and basketball. For this reason, patellar tendinopathy is also known as "*Jumper's knee*." This condition is a knee extensor mechanism overuse injury caused by repetitive mechanical stress to which the tendon is primarily exposed during knee extension [35]. The inferior pole of the patella, in correspondence of patellar tendon insertion, is the component of the knee extensor mechanism mostly involved. Less frequently, the injury is localized at the level of the quadriceps tendon insertion to the superior pole of patella and where the patellar tendon inserts into the tibial tuberosity. However, considering that most cases of Jumper's knee are due to problems on the patellar tendon insertion in the inferior pole of patella, the term patellar tendinopathy is used interchangeably. Patellar tendinopathy has a male predominance and usually affects adolescent athletes to those in their third decade and up [35]. The pathogenic mechanism underlying the disease includes the coexistence of several extrinsic and intrinsic factors. Overload on the knee extensor is the most important extrinsic factor which predisposes to the onset of patellar tendinopathy. Repetitive activities such as jumping, landing, acceleration, deceleration, and cutting cause microscopic changes within the tendon at high loads that causes progressive weakness and eventually leads to failure. Other extrinsic factors are the excessive frequency of training, the hardness of the ground on which sport is practiced, and the athletes' level of performance. On the other hand, intrinsic factors include joint misalignment, ligamentous laxity, abnormal patella height, quadriceps muscle weakness, and extreme hamstring muscles stiffness [36].

The diagnosis of patellar tendinopathy is mainly made through a patient's clinical history and physical examination. Anterior knee pain is the main symptom. Patients usually refer to well-localized pain on the inferior pole of the patella that is exacerbated by prolonged sitting, squatting, and stair climbing. Sudden tendon pain occurs with loading and usually stops almost immediately when the load is removed. Sometimes, patients even feel pain at rest. Physical examination presupposes a thorough evaluation of the entire lower extremity in order to identify the relevant abnormalities in the hip, knee, and ankle/foot region. Atrophy or reduced strength in antigravity muscles, including the gluteus maximus, quadriceps, and calf is often observed. Pain is elicited through palpation of the proximal portion of the tendon or by the complete extension of the leg. A positive *decline squat test* allows the surgeon to make a diagnosis of patellar tendinopathy. To do one, the patient performs a squat with a single leg, flexing the knee up to 30° and keeping the contralateral leg extended. In this way, the mechanical load is primarily exerted on the patellar tendon exacerbating the onset of symptoms [37].

The Victorian Institute of Sports Assessment —Patella (VISA-P) *questionnaire* specifically measures the severity of patellar tendinopathy. It covers the domains of pain, function, and activity. Scores are summed to give a total out of 100. An asymptomatic person would score 100. VISA-P can be used to assess the severity of symptoms as well as to monitor outcomes [38].

Currently, patellar tendinopathy is classified into five different stages according to the onset of pain in relation to physical activity: Stage 0: absence of painful symptoms; stage I: rare pain without performance limitation; stage II: moderate pain during sport without performance limitation (normal performance); stage III: pain with initial qualitative or quantitative limitation of performance (reduced training intensity); stage IV: pain with significant changes in sports performance; stage V: pain in everyday life with the impossibility of practicing sport. Ultrasound (Fig. 34.2) and magnetic resonance imaging (MRI) are widely accepted as first choice diagnostic techniques. Both can be used to detect abnormalities in the patellar tendon itself. Ultrasound is noninvasive, repeatable, accurate, and provides a dynamic image of the knee structure. Ultrasound images show the loss of tendon normal echogenicity, tendon thickening and irregularity, intratendinous calcifications and erosions localized primarily in the inferior pole of the patella. The use of the color Doppler makes

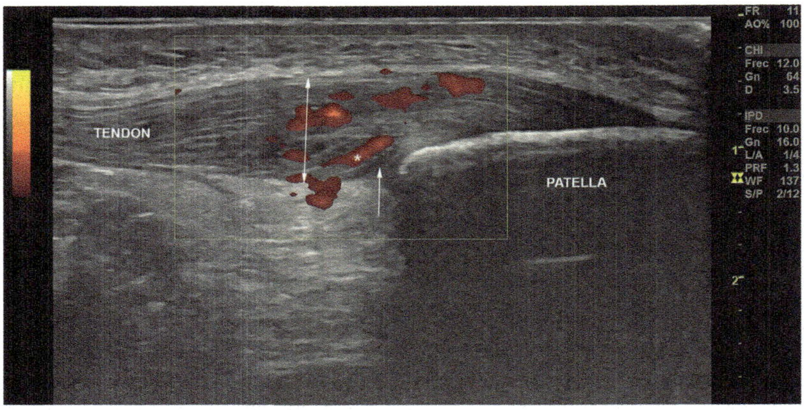

Fig. 34.2 High definition ultrasound image of the patellar tendon in longitudinal view. Observe the hypoechogenic area of the tendon (arrow) with hypervascular ingrowth (*) as well as a thickened tendon (double arrow) and with involvement of the Hoffa fad pad

for visualization of the vascular neoformations in proximity to *Hoffa's* fat pad (also called the infrapatellar adipose *body*) [39]. Tardive changes such as elongation of the involved pole of the patella, calcification and increased density within the patellar tendon matrix are usually viewable after 6 months of symptoms.

The MRI shows, preferentially in sagittal sections, thickening of the patellar tendon along with foci of increased signal intensity in the affected region. A CT and bone scan may also be used in the initial stages of the disease even though they are not usually indicated. It is important to highlight that the radiological assessment must be considered only as a diagnostic support since the diagnosis of patellar tendinopathy cannot ignore the patient's clinical history and physical examination.

34.2 Traditional Conservative Treatment for Achilles and Patellar Tendinopathy

34.2.1 Achilles Tendinopathy

34.2.1.1 Noninvasive Methods

Noninvasive methods such as relative rest or a modification of activity, orthotics, heel lifts, massage, hot and cold compresses, strengthening exercises, ultrasound, and nonsteroidal anti-inflammatory drugs (NSAID) or oral corticosteroids can be applied as a first line treatment. The use of NSAIDs has been questioned as to their effectiveness because of the prostaglandin inflammatory mediator absence in Achilles tendinopathy (AT) [40].

34.2.1.2 Corticosteroid Injections

Corticosteroids are a group of medications that contain cortisone. They relieve pain by reducing the inflammation that occurs in a diseased tendon. There is controversy around the use of these injections in Achilles tendinosis since there is no inflammatory process. In some studies, cortisone injections bring about short-term pain relief. However, there is no pain relief after the injection according to some studies.

34.2.1.3 Eccentric Training

The eccentric training program designed by Alfredson et al. [41] improves tendon healing by enhancing the tendon's volume and the signal intensity that is thought to be a response to trauma. But after a 12-week program, the size and appearance of the tendon returns to normal in ultrasound and magnetic resonance imaging (MRI). With an extended eccentric loading program of the Achilles tendon, muscle–tendon unit length will be increased and the resistance of tendon to load will be increased overtime. Repetitive eccentric exercise could be the mechanism to eliminate pain in the tendon due to abnormal blood vessels and the nerves with the 12-week program as concluded by Alfredson et al. [42]. It has produced 90% good results with the midportion and 30% good results in insertional Achilles tendinosis.

34.2.1.4 Extracorporeal Shock Wave Therapy

Extracorporeal shock wave therapy (ESWT) is another treatment option for Achilles tendinosis (Fig. 34.3). There are two treatment strategies. The first one is the low-energy treatment strategy. It consists of three weekly sessions without local anesthesia or intravenous anesthesia. The second one is the high-energy treatment of one session but with local or intravenous anesthesia. Repeated shock waves to the affected area cause microtrauma that is then followed by neovascularization. Emerging blood flow stimulates tissue healing that results in relief of pain. It can also block afferent pain receptor functioning and increase nitric oxide synthase. This treatment strategy seems to be beneficial and may have a place in the treatment of Achilles tendinosis [43].

34.2.1.5 Low-Level Laser Therapy

Low-level laser therapy produces effects in a diseased tendon-like enhanced adenosine triphosphate production, enhanced cell function, and increased protein synthesis. It also reduces inflammation, increases collagen synthesis, and promotes angiogenesis. In a study by Stergioulas et al. [44], it was established that Achilles tendinosis patients who underwent eccentric exercises together with low-level laser therapy demonstrated decreased pain intensity, morning stiffness, tenderness to palpation, active dorsiflexion, and crepitus with no side effects in comparison to the patients who took up eccentric exercises exclusively. However, the data to confirm the efficacy of low-level laser therapy is still inadequate for the treatment of Achilles tendinosis.

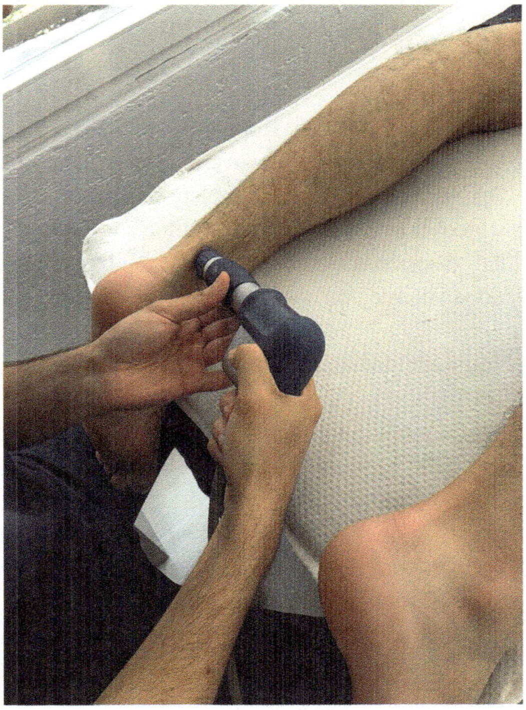

Fig. 34.3 Extracorporeal shock wave therapy (ESWT) for Achilles tendinosis

34.2.1.6 Other Additional Methods

There are other methods that increase blood circulation. One of them is the Graston method. It is carried out with a metal rod (Fig. 34.4). It is mostly useful for tendon and soft tissue mobilization. The Tecar therapy is another method. It is endogenous thermotherapy based on the principle of capacitive and resistive energy transfer having an effect within the tendon, activating the body's natural repair and anti-inflammatory processes (Fig. 34.5). During those therapies, athletes should work at maintaining their cardiovascular form. In this situation, the antigravity treadmill helps patients with that maintenance.

34.2.1.7 Rehabilitation

Rehabilitation for an Achilles tendon rupture aids in regaining strength and flexibility in the tendon and leg. It can be done at home or in a gym.

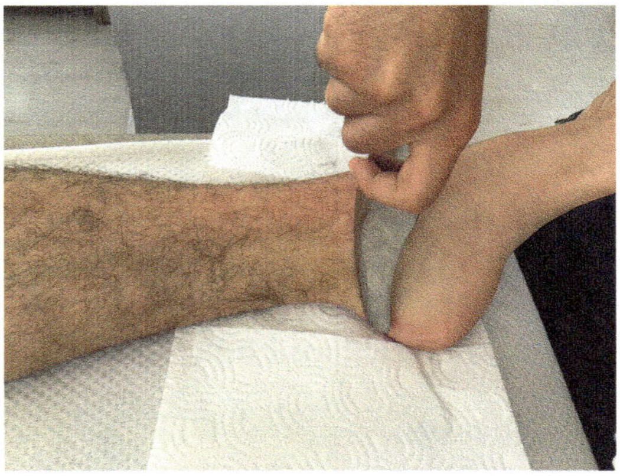

Fig. 34.4 Graston method in Achilles tendinopathy

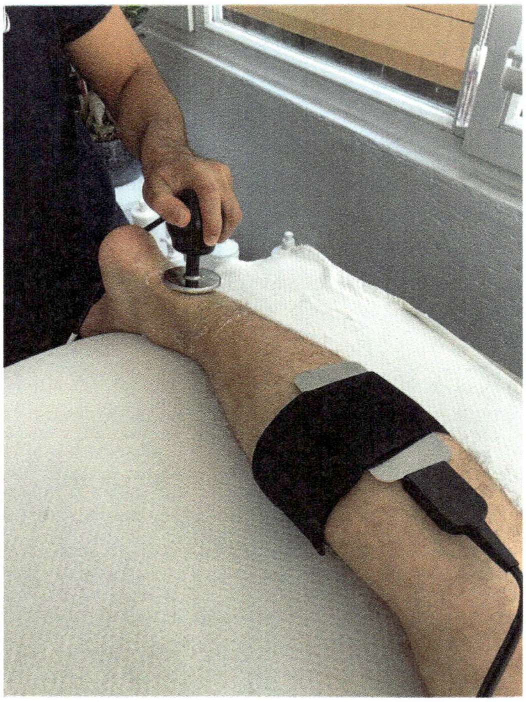

Fig. 34.5 Application of Tecar therapy in Achilles tendon

The rehabilitation program may include:

- Stretching and flexibility exercises
- Strengthening exercises
- Endurance activities, such as riding a stationary bicycle
- Coordination and/or agility training

Recovery varies among people. It depends on how severe the tendon injury is and whether they complete your program. Giving time and energy to a rehab program will speed recovery and help prevent future injury.

34.2.2 Patellar Tendinopathy

34.2.2.1 Correction of Intrinsic and Extrinsic Risk Factors

Training Errors

Training conditions like ground selection, intensity, style, and frequency are extremely important and well-studied in the literature.

Flexibility

Mobility limitations are one of the most important reasons behind tendinopathies, and the flexibility of the muscles is very important for the mobility of a joint. Witvrouw et al. [45] found that the lack of flexibility of the quadriceps and hamstring muscles may be the reason for this injury. Therefore, the correction for the limited flexibility of the responsible muscles with corrective exercises is a very logical option.

Biomechanical Abnormality

It has been hypothesized that intrinsic risk factors like foot hyperpronation, pes planus or cavus, forefoot varus or valgus, hindfoot varus or valgus, tibia vara, genu valgum or varum, patellofemoral malalignment, femoral neck anteversion, and leg length discrepancies play a role in biomechanical derangement in patellar tendinopathy. Unfortunately, there is no evidence in the literature which proves this theory. But of course, if an apparent biomechanical abnormality exists in a patient with patellar tendinopathy, correction of this could be logical.

34.2.2.2 Symptomatic Approach

Relative Rest

Tendinopathy results from mechanical overload. Therefore, decreasing the overload relieve the pain. That does not mean complete immobilization. Moreover, complete immobilization causes thinner and disoriented collagen fibers, and decreased blood volume that result in tendon atrophy.

Nonsteroidal Anti-inflammatory Drugs (NSAID)

The administration of anti-inflammatory medication for a degenerative injury (noninflammatory causes) should be questioned. There is no evidence on the supportive effect of NSAIDs in chronic tendinopathy. There is an isolated study on acute tendon pain. Currently, the histopathology of acute tendon pain remains unclear. NSAIDs can also have additional effects other than simply anti-inflammatory or analgesic effects [46]. Some studies have proven the potential favorable effects of NSAIDs in tendon healing while others have reported on deleterious mechanisms of NSAIDs in tendons. Still, in the clinical management of chronic tendinopathy, the use of an NSAID can hide symptoms due to its analgesic effect and consequently prevent optimum therapeutic management. Therefore, until further evidence of exact effects of NSAIDs in tendinopathy is revealed, their use in patellar tendinopathy is not evidence based.

Corticosteroids

Corticosteroid use in tendinopathy treatment is a topical issue [47]. There are a lot of studies of this topic. Some of them say that they provide short-term pain relief, but others say there is no positive effect. The increased risk of tendon rupture is a fact to be considered. Nevertheless, due to patellar tendinopathy being a noninflammatory condition and as corticosteroids can impair collagen synthesis and tendon strength, the use of corticosteroids needs to be rethought.

Ice Application

Cryotherapy causes vasoconstriction and neovascularization within the tendinosis. Consequently, it decreases blood and protein leakage. Still, there is no precise protocol that includes parameters like duration, frequency, and repetition. Due to the masking of the pain effect caused by icing, avoiding using it before sport participation would be logical.

34.2.2.3 Local Physiotherapeutic Modalities

There are many studies on the beneficial effects of the different physical therapy strategies for the treatment of patellar tendinopathy. They include fine needling, electrotherapy, electromagnetic fields, ultrasound, and laser therapy. An increase in collagen synthesis and the tensile strength of the tendon has been described in some studies. As such, the local application of physical modalities is still debatable.

Ultrasound-Guided Galvanic Electrolysis Technique (USGET)

In recent years, the ultrasound-guided galvanic electrolysis technique (USGET) has been described in the scientific literature as giving the good results as seen yielded in the treatment of refractory tendon injuries in comparison to other previous conservative treatments (Fig. 34.6) [48].

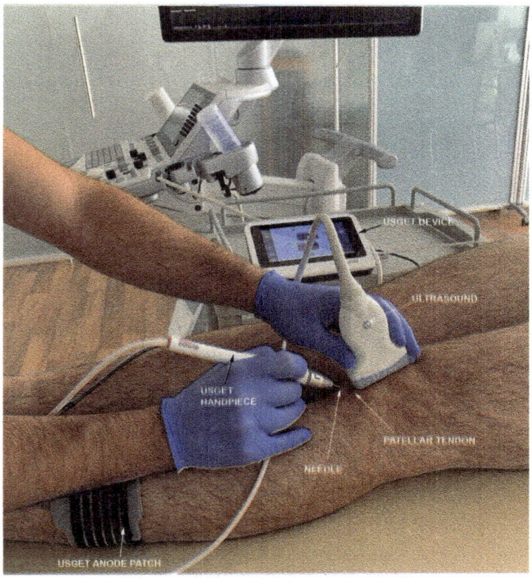

Fig. 34.6 Ultrasound-guided galvanic electrolysis technique (USGET) on patellar tendon. Use of ultrasound is mandatory to ensure the correct application

USGET is a nonthermal electrochemical ablation with a cathodic flow to the clinical focus of tendon degeneration. This treatment produces a dissociation of water, salts, and amino acids in the extracellular matrix that creates new molecules through ionic instability. The organic reaction, which occurs in the tissue around the cathodic needle causes a localized inflammation in the region dealt with. It produces an immediate activation of an inflammatory response and overexpression of the activated gamma receptor for peroxisome proliferation (PPAR-gamma). Furthermore, it acts to inhibit the action of IL-1, TNF, and COX-2, mechanisms of tendon degeneration through the direct inhibitory action of factor NFKB that facilitates phagocytosis and tendon regeneration [49].

Extracorporeal Shock Wave Therapy

An ESWT session consists of the application of shock waves, which are sonic pulses generating high stress forces in tissue. This modality is better known as a successful treatment method for urolithiasis. The analgesic process, the dissolution of calcific deposits and the stimulation of a tissue regeneration process are the known mechanisms of action of this therapy and positive results with its use in patellar tendinopathy is supported by some studies [50]. The efficacy of ESWT was recently demonstrated in a randomized, double-blind, placebo-controlled trial of the short-term management of chronic patellar tendinopathy [50]. Further studies seem justified to clarify the contradictory results in other insertional tendinopathies and evaluate the long-term effects and the relative effectiveness of ESWT for patellar tendinopathy compared with other therapeutic approaches.

Rehabilitation

Due to heterogeneity in every single step of the diagnosis, therapy, patient selection, program design, and the results relative to the success rate are varied [51]. There is no strong evidence that one precise physical therapy program is superior to others. Still, it is true that rehabilitation of the afflicted muscle tendon is the cornerstone of tendinopathy management. Mostly strength training, especially eccentric exercise training, is becoming the key element in the treatment of chronic tendinopathy. Unfortunately, most of the studies are of Achilles tendinopathy.

The mechanisms through which eccentric exercise can alter pain in chronic tendinopathy remain still unclear. There are some in vivo studies that show increased metabolic activity and the increased formation of collagen type I in response to acute exercise of peritendinous tissue [52]. Therefore, it is scientifically impossible to say that one exercise program is superior to another in the treatment of patellar tendinopathy.

34.3 Orthobiologics in Management of Achilles and Patellar Tendinopathy

34.3.1 Achilles Tendinopathy

34.3.1.1 Growth Factors

Growth factors like the transforming growth factor-β (TGF-β), vascular endothelial growth factor (VEGF), platelet-derived growth factor (PDGF), and insulin-like growth factor (IGF-I) are signal molecules involved in the process of proliferation, differentiation, cell chemotaxis, and synthesis of the extracellular matrix. These factors are produced by tenocytes and white blood cells and are released by platelets during the process of degranulation. In the case of a tendon injury, numerous growth factors are involved in the activation and regulation of the cellular responses [53].

34.3.1.2 Transforming Growth Factor–β

TGF-β1 regulates cellular migration and proliferation and can increase the synthesis of collagen type I and III in tendon-derived cells. Moreover, TGF-β1 is overexpressed in tendon in the early postinjury period. Promising results have been obtained using TGF- β1 complementary DNA-transduced BMSCs grafts, injections of TGF-β, and delivery of TGF-β by adenovirus-modified muscle grafts in rat Achilles tendon models [54, 55].

Maeda et al. in 2011 [56] showed that the interruption of tendon continuity in an acute injury can cause a loss of tensile loading, resulting in the destabilization of the extracellular matrix and releasing excessively high levels of active TGF-β that lead to tenocyte death. Jorgenses and Katzel demonstrated, in an Achilles tendon model, that mannose-6-phosphate can reduce latent TGF-β activation, which results in an increase in elastin production and increased strain and peak stress failure [57, 58]. Recently, Potter et al. evaluated the role of TGF-β1 in regulating tendon extracellular matrix after acute exercise in rats. That work showed that TGF-β1 signaling is necessary for the regulation of tendon cross-link formation as well as collagen and lysyl oxidase gene transcription in an exercise-dependent manner. Target therapy with TGF-β can increase the mechanical strength of the healing Achilles tendon through the regulation of collagen synthesis, upregulation of cross-link formation, and enhanced matrix remodeling [59].

34.3.1.3 Vascular Endothelial Growth Factor

VEGF-mRNA plays a key role in neovascularization around the repair site. In fact, in vitro studies showed an increased peak at days 7–10 but returned to baseline by day 14 [59]. In an Achilles tendon model, VEGF gene therapy increased TGF-β gene expression, and exogenous VEGF appears to increase tensile strength [60].

Recently, Tempfer et al. stopped VEGF-A signaling using a local injection of Bevacizumab in a rat model with a complete Achilles tendon rupture. After the treatment, angiogenesis was found to be significantly reduced in the Bevacizumab-treated repair tissue. It was accompanied by significantly a reduced cross-sectional area, improved matrix organization, increased stiffness and in Young's modulus, and maximum load and stress [61, 62].

34.3.1.4 Platelet-Derived Growth Factor

PDGF is a basic protein composed of two subunits, an A and a B chain, that exist in three different isoforms (PDGF-AA, PDGF-BB, and PDGF-AB). Each isoform acts as a chemotactic agent during inflammation and helps to increase type I collagen synthesis and induce TGF-β1 expression and IGF-I [63]. An in vitro study demonstrated that the addition of exogenous PDGF increases the expression of type I collagen of the tenocytes.

Thomopoulos showed, in vivo, that a sustained delivery of PDGF-BB via a fibrin matrix led to an increase in cell density, cell proliferation, and type I collagen mRNA expression. Additionally, a fibrin/heparin delivery system demonstrated that PDGF-BB improved tendon function but not tendon structure [64, 65].

34.3.1.5 Insulin-Like Growth Factor

IGF-I is one of the three single-chain polypeptides belonging to the IGF family (IGF-I, IGF-II, and insulin). The expression of this molecule increases during wound healing, and its absence is thought to impair dermal repair [66]. Kurtz reported promising results using IGF-I to increase the rate of healing in the transected rat Achilles tendon [67]. Following transection, each tendon was treated with 25 mg of a recombinant variant form of IGF-I. It showed a positive effect on healing within 24 h after the transection and addition of IGF-I. This effect continued up until the tenth and last measurement on day 15.

34.3.1.6 Platelet-Rich Plasma

Platelet-rich plasma (PRP) is the plasma fraction of blood containing concentrated platelets and white blood cells. Due to its autologous nature, PRP is inherent, safe, and provides a natural conductive scaffold containing several growth factors [53].

A new classification regarding the contents and the role of different PRP was published in 2009 [68]. The classification separates the products in accordance with the cell's content (mostly leukocytes) and the fibrin architecture.

PRP was divided into four main families:

- Pure platelet-rich plasma, or leukocyte-poor platelet-rich plasma, is a preparation without leukocytes and with a low-density fibrin network after activation. It can be used as a liquid solution or in an activated gel form. The gel form is often used during surgery and can be injected. Many methods of preparation exist, particularly using cell separators (continuous flow plasmapheresis) even though this method is too involved to be used easily in daily practice.
- Leukocyte and platelet-rich plasma is a preparation with leukocytes and with a low-density fibrin network after activation. It can be used as a liquid solution or in an activated gel form. Most commercial systems belong to this family, and several protocols have been developed in the last few years. It requires the use of specific kits that allow for minimum handling of the blood samples and maximum standardization of the preparations.
- Pure platelet-rich fibrin, or leukocyte-poor platelet-rich fibrin, is a preparation without leukocytes and with a high-density fibrin network. This product only exists in a strongly activated gel form and cannot be injected or used like traditional fibrin glues. However, it can be handled like a real solid material for other applications because of its strong fibrin matrix. Its main inconvenience remains its cost and relative complexity in comparison to the other forms of platelet-rich fibrin.
- Leukocyte and platelet-rich fibrin products are preparations with leukocytes and with a high-density fibrin network. These products only

exist in a strongly activated gel form and cannot be injected or used like traditional fibrin glues. However, because of their strong fibrin matrix, they can be handled like a real solid material for other applications.

The clinical use of PRP in Achilles tendinopathies is still debated and the current literature is conflicting. A review published in 2018 by Lin et al. compared the effectiveness of autologous blood-derived product (ABP) injection with that of a placebo (sham injection or no injection or physiotherapy alone) in patients with Achilles tendinopathy [69]. A total of seven articles were included. The ABP injection and placebo revealed equal effectiveness in the Victorian Institute of Sports Assessment-Achilles questionnaire (VISA-A) improvement score at 4–6, 12, 24, and 48 weeks. In a meta-regression, there was no association between the change in the VISA-A score and duration of symptoms at 4–6 weeks (short term), 12 weeks (medium term), and 24 weeks (long term). The authors concluded that ABP injection was not more effective than a placebo in Achilles tendinopathy and that no association was found between the therapeutic effects and duration of symptoms [69].

Filardo et al. [70] analyzed four papers dealing with the use of PRP for Achilles tendon ruptures that highlighted that no beneficial effects of PRP administration during and/or immediately after tendon suturing were reported. It is worth noting that Schepull [71] hypothesized that PRP addition could even be detrimental in tissue healing because no biomechanical advantages and lower performance were reported in PRP patients with respect to the "suture-alone" group.

34.3.1.7 Adipose-Derived Stem Cells

In recent years, adipose-derived stem cells (ADSCs) have been the focus of several clinical and preclinical studies on tendon regeneration. The growing interest in them is mainly due to their high numbers in the human body (ADSCs are 5% of the nucleated cells in adipose tissue), the simplicity of harvesting and their rapid expansion and high proliferative potential [72, 73]. These cells can differentiate into different lines, such as adipocytes, chondrocytes, osteoblasts, hepatocytes, pancreatic cells, muscle cells, and neuron-like cells both in vitro and in vivo [72].

In tendon tissue, ADSCs can enhance the gene expression profile of the cartilage oligomeric matrix protein (COMP), an extracellular matrix protein. It is present primarily in cartilage. COMP is crucial to the binding and organization of collagen fibrils [72]. The use of ADSCs for the treatment of pathologic tendon conditions has been widely investigated in experimental animal models. The results have been encouraging. ADSCs can induce tenocyte differentiation, overexpressing the bone morphogenetic protein 12 gene [73].

Usuelli et al. first described the use of ADSCs to treat human non-insertional Achilles tendinopathy in comparison to PRP injections (28 patients in ADSCs group and 28 in PRP group). At final follow-up, there were no clinical (Visual Analog Scale pain, the VISA-A, the American Orthopaedic Foot and Ankle Society Ankle-Hindfoot Score, and the Short Form-36 [SF-36]) or imaging (MRI and ultrasonography -US) differences between the two groups. Neither were any serious side effects nor adverse events observed during the follow-up period. Both treatments were effective, but patients treated with ADSCs obtained faster results and they should be taken into consideration for patients who require an earlier return to daily activities [74].

Moreover, a significant increase in tendon thickness, measured using magnetic resonance ($P = 0.013$) and ultrasound ($P = 0.012$) and a power Doppler signal ($P = 0.027$), was seen. There was no significant difference between the pre- and posttreatment cross-sectional area, signal intensity, and echotexture ($P > 0.217$). None of the pretreatment parameters was a predictor of treatment outcome ($P > 0.104$). There was excellent agreement for tendon thickness measurements between magnetic resonance and ultrasound (intraclass correlation coefficient = 0.986) [75].

34.3.1.8 Peripheral Blood Mononuclear Cells

Recently, several studies highlighted peripheral blood mononuclear cells (PBMNCs) (monocytes/macrophages and lymphocytes) as a new generation of regenerative autologous cell concentrates as monocytes and macrophages promote tissue repair and regeneration [76].

In fact, monocytes and macrophages have a degree of plasticity comparable to that of marrow stem cells. They also have multiple action mechanisms [28], an angiogenic action thanks to the release of VEGF [77], a regenerative action through the release of growth factors, cytokines, and messenger molecules [78]. Furthermore, a recent study affirmed that osteo-inductive action is characteristic of monocyte populations rather than stem cells populations. They can activate resident MSCs through a paracrine effect and the release of exosomes [79]. They also have an anti-inflammatory and immune-modulatory action through the polarization of macrophages M1 in M2 [32] in injured tissues with a healing delay. Most of the macrophages are activated in the M1 state (degenerative inflammatory), whereas polarization in M2 (macrophages activated in anti-inflammatory regenerative state) allows for the regeneration of the injured or inflamed tissues.

Sugg et al. [80] performed a tenotomy and repair of the Achilles tendons of adult rats and evaluated changes in the macrophage phenotype (M1/M2) and related genes of both the extracellular matrix and the epithelial-mesenchymal transition pathways for a period of 4 weeks. The results suggest that changes in the phenotype of macrophages and the activation of epithelial-mesenchymal transition-related programs probably contribute first to the degradation of the injured tissue and then to the subsequent repair of the tendon tissue. The results also confirmed that the sequential transition between the M1 and M2 phenotypes supports the dual function of macrophages in the degradation and repair of damaged tendon tissue.

To date, no clinical studies have been reported in the literature. However, autologous cell therapy with injection monocytes could represent new perspectives. Moreover, it is not very invasive and has a solid scientific rationale in the treatment of tendinopathy. Moreover, the use of PBMNCs could be used as a complement during surgical procedures as biological augmentation to enhance the healing process, improve surgical outcomes, and reduce complication rates.

34.3.1.9 Bone Marrow Aspirate Concentrate

BMAC is the result of different density gradient centrifugations of bone marrow aspirated from the iliac crest [81]. This aspirate has a concentration of nucleated cells of less than 0.01%, and its role is to deliver MSCs to the injured tendon [82]. This procedure concentrates the mononucleated cells, hematopoietic stem cells, and platelets in one layer and the red blood cells in another. The efficacy of cells contained in BMAC is to modulate the healing response of the pathologic tendon by controlling inflammation, reducing fibrosis, and recruiting other cells, including tenocytes and MSCs [83].

Broese demonstrated, in vitro, an increase in cell proliferation in Achilles tendon scaffolds seeded with bone marrow aspirate [84]. Stein first reported outcomes in patients with sport-related Achilles tendon ruptures treated via open repair augmented with BMAC injection. A total of 27 patients treated with open repair and BMAC injection were reevaluated at a mean follow-up of 29.7 months and no re-ruptures were noted. Of those patients, 92% returned to their sport at 5.9 months. No soft tissue masses, bone formation, or tumors were observed in the operated extremity [85].

34.3.1.10 Scaffolds

Several natural and synthetic materials have recently been analyzed with the aim to promote cellular growth and provide mechanical support for tendon repair. The ideal scaffold for the Achilles tendon should allow a natural and fast bridging of tendinous defects as well as organized collagen-rich tissue with complete incorporation of the material within 8 weeks, returning functionality to the same. Moreover, the scaffold should release chemotactic factors to promote the recruitment of progenitor cells [53, 86].

Polyhydroxyalkanoates is a material that possesses several of the above qualities. It is part of the family of biopolymers consisting of polyesters produced in nature by microorganisms to store energy and carbon. These materials, poly-3-hydroxybutyrate-co-3-hydroxyhexanoate (PHBHHx) in particular, are compatible with many mesenchyme-derived cell types and have adaptable mechanical properties along with delayed biodegradability [87]. A study by Webb and colleagues reported how tendon repair using a PHBHHx scaffold was mechanically and histologically superior in comparison to controls [87].

Another type of scaffold involves the use of decellularized tendon tissue, which maintains the native characteristics and preserves more than 90% of the proteoglycans and growth factors. In vitro, the decellularized tendon slices were able to facilitate repopulation and the attachment of fibroblasts. Farnebo et al. [88], analyzing the use of decellularized grafts in rats, demonstrated an enhancement of the mechanical properties and a reduced immune response.

Decellularized porcine tendon can also be recellularized with human tenocytes [89]. An acellular human dermal allograft (GraftJacket; Wright Medical Technology, Inc., Arlington, TN, USA) reported significant improvement in mechanical strength and stiffness in biomechanical tests. In in vivo studies, patients treated with GraftJacket showed a desirable return-to-activity time without complications [90]. Recently, interest has also increased around xenografts. They seem to improve tendon strength if compared with isolated repair. The most used tissue is porcine small intestinal submucosa (SIS) [91]. Preclinical studies reported on the ability of SIS to remodel the tendon. SIS retains several growth factors, including VEGF, TGF- β, and fibroblast growth factors. They likely contribute to the behavior and migration of cells into the scaffold [48, 49]. Moreover, SIS is subject to a rapid degradation, with 60% of the mass lost after 30 days and complete degradation within 90 days. After complete degradation, the extracellular matrix looks very similar to native tissue in terms of vascularity and organization. A strength of SIS is its ability to recruit marrow-derived cells involved in the remodeling and repair process [92].

34.3.1.11 FARG (Foot and Ankle Reconstruction Group) Algorithm for Use of Biologics for Achilles Tendinopathy

We created an algorithm for the use of biologics for Achilles tendinopathy based on our clinical experience. In developing the FARG (foot and ankle reconstruction group) algorithm for Achilles tendinopathy [53], we were inspired by the MRI-based classification of tendinopathy described by Oloff et al. [93], and we categorized symptomatic patients according to their level of sporting activity:

- sport-active patients (sports activity at least 2 times a week)
- nonathletic patients (sports activity <2 times a week)

The treatment scheme is shown in Table 34.1. It is noteworthy that the major differences concern grades 1 and 2 tendinopathy in which,

Table 34.1 Treatement options in achilles tendinopathy

Achilles tendinopathy grade	Sport-active patients	Nonathletic patients
Grade 0: Hypertrophy, with homogeneous signal	Conservative treatment	Conservative treatment
Grade 1: Hypertrophy, with isolated signal changes in <25% of tendon	Biologic treatment[b]	Conservative treatment
Grade 2: Hypertrophy, with signal changes in >1 area, or diffuse changes in >25% of tendon	Stripping[a] + biologic treatment[b]	Biologic treatment
Grade 3: Severe hypertrophy, <50% tendon signal changes, with interstitial tear	Stripping[a] + biologic treatment[b]	Stripping + biologic treatment
Grade 4: Severe thickening, >50% of tendon with abnormal signal, partial tendon tear	FHL transfer ± biologic treatment[b]	FHL transfer ± biologic treatment

[a]Stripping technique as described by Maffulli and colleagues [94]
[b]Authors' preferred biologic treatments are ADSCs and PBMNCs injections

considering the lower functional request, the nonathletic patient can probably benefit more from less-invasive treatments.

To get satisfactory results in the treatment of Achilles tendinopathy with biological treatments, three goals need to be achieved [53]:

1. Identify the most appropriate biological tools
2. Achieve a strong level of evidence
3. Create evidence-based and personalized treatment protocols

In fact, Achilles tendinopathies are a challenge for orthopedic surgeons, particularly so considering the scarce tendency to healing and that patients are often young with a high-functional demand. In recent years, several studies have focused on biologics for the treatment of Achilles tendinopathy with preliminary good to excellent results [53]. Despite the encouraging results, there is still a huge variability in biological treatments and a wide spectrum of techniques and technologies available with no standardized protocols. Combining imaging with clinical features might be the key to arriving at a protocol for the use of biologics for the treatment of Achilles tendinopathy. Considering this, we have described our recently published protocol [53].

34.3.2 Patellar Tendinopathy

34.3.2.1 Platelet-Rich Plasma

The use of PRP for patellar tendinopathy has been reported in 19 papers as reported in the review published by Filardo et al. [70]. All but two PRP were used as a conservative injective treatment for the management of tendinopathy not responsive to other previous therapeutic attempts. All papers performing a surgical procedure were randomized controlled trials (RCTs), whereas only 4 out of 17 papers dealing with conservative management were RCTs.

The studies describing the intraoperative PRP application were authored by De Almeida et al. [95] and Seijas et al. [96], who injected PRP in the patellar tendon gap site after ACL reconstruction. In both trials, the results were in favor of the PRP group. Better pain control was documented in the initial post-op phases [95, 96] and, at the 6-month follow-up. The MRI evaluation also showed better tissue healing at the harvest site after PRP administration [95]. Looking at conservative treatment, the literature showed overall good results, but the heterogeneous therapeutic protocols differ in terms of number of injections performed and time interval between administrations. Some authors performed a single injection. It was followed by a second one in some cases only when a poor clinical outcome was reported, whereas other authors opted for a multiple injection regimen (2 or even 3 injections) ab initio. In most of the published studies, the injection treatment was followed by a rehabilitation program. Two RCTs [95, 96] investigated the correlation between clinical results and the number of PRP administrations, with controversial conclusions. In both studies, 40 patients were included and randomized to receive one or two PRP injection at two-week intervals. Kaux et al. [97] failed to show any significant beneficial effect related to the 2-injection protocol, whereas Zayni et al. [98] documented superior clinical outcome in patients treated with multiple PRP injections. Up to now, the low number of patients evaluated in these trials does not allow for drawing any reliable conclusions on the usefulness of multiple- vs. single-injection protocols. The other published RCTs compared PRP injections versus external shock wave therapy (ESWT) [99] and dry needling [100]. In the study authored by Vetrano et al. [99], 46 patients were randomized to receive either two PRP injections (at 2-week interval) or three weekly sessions of ESWT. The overall results were positive, but the best outcome was obtained in the PRP group. Those in the PRP group experienced more significant pain reduction and greater functional recovery at 6 and 12 months after treatment. In the trial by Dragoo et al. [100], 23 patients were included and randomized to receive a single PRP injection or dry needling alone. The authors documented that, at 12 weeks of follow-up, only the PRP group presented with a statistically significant improvement in pain and functional scores. These differences were not maintained at the final 26-week evaluation when the clinical outcomes were comparable between groups. However, it was significantly better in both cases than at the basal evaluation. The positive results described in said RCTs were confirmed by lower-quality studies. They reported encouraging results for PRP therapy in all cases.

34.3.2.2 Bone Marrow Aspirate Concentrate

Pascual-Garrido et al. [101] reported on the clinical results of a case series of ultrasound-guided BMAC injection for refractory patella tendinitis unresponsive to nonoperative treatment. Their report included eight patients (four males and four females) aged between 14 and 35 years. The study reported a significant improvement in pain, daily living activity scores, knee-related quality of life, and functional knee scores (International Knee Documentation Committee (IKDC) and the Knee Injury and Osteoarthritis Outcome Score (KOOS)) in seven out of eight patients treated with ultrasound-guided BMAC injection. Seven out of eight patients stated they would have the procedure again and categorized the outcome of their treatment as excellent. In this study, the number of nucleated cells in the BMA was 37×10^3 and it reached to 45×10^3 after concentration.

34.3.2.3 Hyaluronic Acid

High molecular weight hyaluronic acid has been reported to have an anti-inflammatory effect in addition to promoting tendon healing at the bone–tendon interface as well as tissue regeneration [102]. The current literature reports only a level IV study of 50 patients with patellar tendinopathy with no improvement after a minimum 2-month course of nonsurgical treatment. Patients were treated with a mean of two injections of hyaluronic acid and reported positive effects on recovery. High-quality evidence regarding this treatment is still lacking. More studies are needed to determine the efficacy of this treatment option, which remains at an investigational stage.

34.3.2.4 Sclerosing Agents

Neovascularization is a phenomenon that plays a key role in the pathophysiology of patellar tendinopathy. It is present in 60–80% of patients with pain [36]. The aim of sclerosing agents is to inhibit vessel formation and vessel collapse that have already formed and destroy the accompanying vasa nervorum, which has a denervating effect.

Alfredson [103] reported a considerable reduction in pain during activity following an ultrasound-guided injection of a sclerosing agent (5 mg/mL polidocanol) to the paratenon in his study. It indicates that sclerosing agents can reduce pain.

Additionally, Hoksrud et al. [104] administered an ultrasound-guided injection of polidocanol (10 mg/mL) into the paratenon in patients with painful chronic patellar tendinopathy and found a substantial difference in the Victorian Institute of Sport Assessment-P score in the group treated with a sclerosing agent versus a placebo. However, more than one-third of the group treated with sclerosing agents underwent surgery for pain in a subsequent study of the same group with a longer follow-up (44 months) [105]. Therefore, the usefulness of sclerosing agents remains unclear, and the agents still are at an experimental stage.

34.3.2.5 Additional Treatments

Various other treatments have been examined in level I studies. Glyceryl trinitrate delivers nitric oxide, which has exhibited a role in fibroblast proliferation, collagen synthesis, and the contraction of collagen lattices. Macrophage angiogenic activity, which is important for wound healing also depends on nitric oxide synthase, and nitric oxide synthase activity is upregulated in tendinopathy [36].

Steunebrink in 2013 [105] assessed whether continuous topical glyceryl trinitrate treatment (GTN) improved outcomes in patients with chronic patellar tendinopathy when compared to eccentric training alone. Randomized double-blind, placebo-controlled clinical trial comparing a 12-week program of using a GTN or placebo patch in combination with eccentric squats on a decline board. Measurements were performed at baseline, 6, 12, and 24 weeks. The primary outcome measure was the Victorian Institute of Sports

Assessment-Patella (VISA-P) questionnaire. VISA-P scores for both groups improved over the study period to 75.0 ± 16.2 and 80.7 ± 22.1 at 24 weeks. The results showed a significant effect for time ($p < 0.01$) but no effect for treatment × time ($p = 0.80$). The mean visual analogue scores for pain during sports for both groups increased over the study period to 6.6 ± 3 and 7.8 ± 3.1. Those results showed a significant effect for time ($p < 0.01$) but no effect for treatment × time ($p = 0.38$). Patient satisfaction showed no difference between the GTN and placebo groups ($p = 0.25$) after 24 weeks but did show a significant difference over time ($p = 0.01$). Three patients in the GTN group reported some rash.

Stasinopoulos and Warden [106, 107] each conducted a randomized study on the effectiveness of low-intensity pulsed ultrasonography and found that this modality provided no benefit compared with eccentric exercises for the management of patellar tendinopathy. These findings are supported by an earlier study by Giombini et al. [108] that showed that hyperthermia was more effective than low-intensity pulsed ultrasonography for the treatment of patellar tendinopathy. All these modalities remain at an investigational stage and are not recommended for patellar tendinopathy management.

34.4 Surgical Treatments of Achilles and Patellar Tendinopathy

34.4.1 Achilles Tendinopathy

34.4.1.1 Indications for Surgery

There are no absolute indications for surgical treatment in Achilles tendinopathy. Often the pain comes gradually and is first tolerated pretty well. If Achilles tendinopathy makes training impossible or symptoms reoccur after rest, proper conservative treatment surgery can be the last treatment option [109]. If surgery is considered, the decision to operate must be done individually and the operation scheduled for when best suited for the athlete. Often enough, the symptoms have lasted more than 6 months before the operation is performed. It is important to know that conservative management is unsuccessful even in 24–45.5% of patients with Achilles tendinopathy [110, 111].

34.4.1.2 Non-insertional Achilles Tendinopathy

In Achilles tendinopathy, the aim of the surgery is to relieve the pain and stimulate tendon healing. The pain in non-insertional Achilles tendinopathy can have several reasons. For example, peritendinous edema, thickened crural fascia, adhesions, tendinosis, partial tearing, and adherent plantaris tendon can be the reason for non-insertional Achilles tendinopathy. Sometimes there is only one reason for chronic pain and sometimes the pain is developed because of a combination of these factors.

All these reasons may be an indication for operation. Using an open surgical technique, the crural fascia covering the Achilles tendon is opened longitudinally. Kager's triangle is freed on both sides and fibrotic adhesions are removed. A fascial incision is continued proximally. Good hemostasis is very important. Excessive pathological blood neovessels locating ventrally to the Achilles tendon can be cut and cauterized. In tendinosis, longitudinal tenotomies may be needed to remove soft degenerative nodules. Sometimes in tendinosis, the so-called microtenotomy technique with Topaz radiofrequency may be needed as well. In partial Achilles tears, suturing or fascia augmentation may be used to repair the ruptured and scarred area. Pain because of an adherent plantaris tendon is often resolved by doing liberation and a simple resection of part of the plantaris tendon.

34.4.1.3 Insertional Achilles Tendinopathy

Insertional Achilles tendinopathy is a frequent cause of chronic heel pain in athletes [112]. Chronic and disabling symptoms can be a result of the prominence of the posterosuperior corner of the calcaneus and an irritated retrocalcaneal bursa [113]. Sometimes, intratendinous calcifications and a partial insertional tear can also aggravate symptoms [114].

In the operation, the posterosuperior corner of the calcaneus is resected as well as the inflamed retrocalcaneal bursa. Intratendious calcifications are removed. If the insertional tear is large, the tendon may also need suture anchor fixation or even graft reinforcement. The endoscopic technique is increasingly used nowadays for the excision of a prominent calcaneus corner [115].

Postoperative rehabilitation after common Achilles tendinopathy operations

Sutures 10–12 days
First 1–2 weeks limited weightbearing, crutches, elastic bandage allowing light ankle movements
Then gradually increasing weight with help of crutches, important to increase stress for the Achilles tendon and calcaneus using a step-by-step rehabilitation protocol
Aqua training after 3 weeks
Stationary cycling, spinning, and cross trainer after 4–6 weeks
After pain-free cycling, proceed to Alter-G treadmill running and walking
Progressive return to sports-specific exercise without pain, usually 3–6 months

The patients are often encouraged to weightbear soon after surgery. If there is a big partial tear or augmentation and suturing or suture anchor fixation is needed, then early protection with a cast or orthoses is often required. Then, more careful postoperative rehabilitation is followed.

34.4.1.4 Results of Surgery

The end results following Achilles tendinopathy operations are usually good in general. According to Khan et al. and Traina et al., the overall success rates after surgery were 83.5% in non-insertional tendinopathy and 89.6% in insertional tendinopathy [116, 117]. It is important to note that careful patient selection is an essential factor relating to good surgical results. Moreover, the experience of orthopedic surgeons has its own effect on the result. One needs to see and examine many athletes and tendon problems to be able to determine which disorders require surgery and which ones heal with conservative means.

34.4.1.5 Complications

Using proper surgical techniques and taking potential risk factors (good planning, patient selection, tissue handling, postoperative wound control) into consideration, the number of operative-related complications (infection, hematoma) can be reduced [118]. However, severe complications may also occur like skin necrosis. They call for significant plastic surgery repair to cover skin defects using vascularized graft.

34.4.2 Patellar Tendinopathy

34.4.2.1 Indications for Surgery

Like in Achilles tendinopathy, there are no absolute indications for surgery in patellar tendinopathy. If high-quality conservative treatment has failed and MRI or ultrasound reveals a partial patellar tendon rupture/large tendinosis area (tendinotic nodule) and scar, surgery can be considered.

34.4.2.2 Surgical Technique

There is no consensus as to the optimal surgical technique to use. Surgery can be done using an open procedure via vertical or horizontal incision or by using the arthroscopic technique.

In open surgery, the paratenon is excised and the tendon structure is opened longitudinally so that the tendinotic area can be removed from the posterior side of the proximal patellar tendon. The lower edge of the bony patella is also removed and then flattened [119]. The arthroscopic procedure is also possible in this Jumper's knee operation [119, 120]. Debridement and excision of the pathological tissue is done by shaving and vaporization. The microtenotomy technique with Topaz radiofrequency can also be used.

Sometimes the tendinotic area is more distally located [121]. Intratendinous calcifications can be a reason for the patellar tendinopathy, too.

34.4.2.3 Postoperative Rehabilitation

Very similar postoperative guidelines can be used after patellar tendinopathy surgery like in the Achilles surgery. The patient is encouraged to do light early mobilizations and practice full range-of-motion. It is very important is to achieve vastus medialis activation during early rehabilitation.

34.4.2.4 Results of Surgery

Surgery is not a “quick fix” for patellar tendinopathy. If after failed conservative treatment and the decision to operate has been taken, the surgeon must advise the patient about the possibly long rehabilitation process and told not to be too optimistic about the result [122–124]. Even though the symptomatic benefit is very likely to occur after surgery, the return to sport cannot always be guaranteed. If the previous sport level is achieved, it can take several months and even 1 year in some cases.

34.5 Return to Play After Achilles and Patellar Tendon Injury

In the process of tendon lesion treatment, the diagnostic phase [51] is as important as the therapeutic phase [48]. Of course, making for optimum Return to Play [125] and the subsequent Return to Performance are equally critical.

With the establishment of the Ardent et al. in Return to Play consensus as of 2016 [125], different levels are stratified according to the individual objective of each person in terms of rehabilitation. The goal is common regardless of whether we are talking about a professional athlete, an amateur athlete or just an active person. The aim is to return to the initial levels prior to the injury [126].

At the end of the last century, Alfredson et al. [41] had already proposed a rehabilitation program based on high-load eccentric exercise. In an antithesis to this proposal, heavy-slow resistance training (HSRT) arose [127] and was subsequently advocated for in a relatively review [128]. With a combination of different exercises with eccentric and concentric components along with a progression proposal, the last program proposed by Silbernagel & Crossley was defined [129].

As a result of these programs, a multitude of studies arose that attempted to validate the most appropriate program for a correct rehabilitation. Thus, we find those that compare the Alfredson Program vs the Silberganel Protocol, from which no definitive data was obtained [130]. On the other hand, there are studies in which the Alfredson Program vs HSRT were compared and no conclusive data was obtained from either [131]. Some studies have also been conducted to analyze the differences between concentric and eccentric exercises in the rehabilitation process, but no global consensus was arrived at in it either [132].

Finally, the main idea is defined by the impossibility of determining a unique and effective program. Therefore, the design of a program based on the individual characteristics of each individual (injury, progression, treatment, functional requirements, and expectations) must take precedence.

There is no doubt that eccentric work is not for everyone [133] even though it has been shown to be beneficial in many cases [134]. Similarly, it is worth noting the known beneficial effect of isometric work in the management of pain caused by the injury [135]. Therefore, opting for one or another method would lead to eliminating the possibility, right from the start, of using countless different stimuli in pursuit of a correct recovery. This is even more so the case when we are talking about a process that lasts no less than 12 weeks, thus demonstrating the need to provide constant stimuli.

The readjustment process must have an adequate progression in which the tendon assimilates the different loads gradually. The patient needs demanding situations in which the tendon needs to perform actions similar to the activity to be readapted to in a final phase of the process [136]. In this way, very high force peaks have been seen in actions such as the jump that are also generated in a very short time. Thus, in the final stages, the objective in patellar or Achilles tendinopathies should be to look for actions such as those described.

In addition to the stretching-shortening and velocity cycle, one of the elements that causes the tendon the most stress is the work with eccentric overload. Since its implementation in a NASA program [137], the use of flywheels and conical pulleys has moved to the training field. Although not without reluctance, given the difficulty of its use both from the execution technique and from

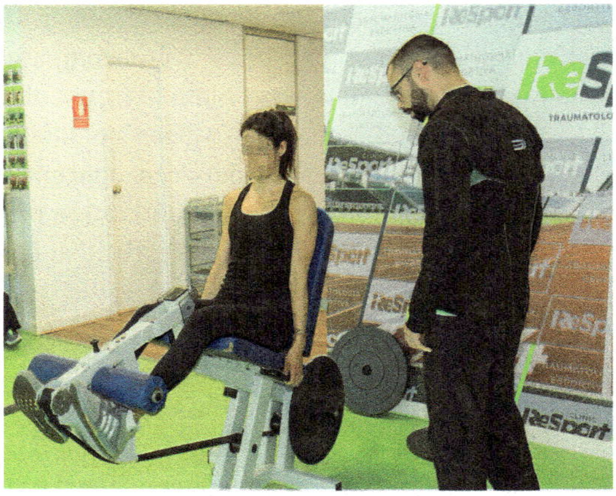

Fig. 34.7 Patient during eccentric exercises session. Note the use of isoinertial device. Execution technique and load management controlled by our strength and conditioning coach

the load management, this factor can be easily solved with qualified personnel (Fig. 34.7). The benefits of eccentric work have been demonstrated relative to the improvement in strength and hypertrophy [51, 138]. These two are necessary in tendinopathies when muscular atrophy is a factor [136]. There have been improvements in the implications that it may have on actions in team sports [139] as well as in direction changes [140]. This type of exercise has also proven beneficial for older people, in achieving an improvement in balance and mobility [141], more specifically, in patellar tendinopathies [142] and in terms of injury reduction [143].

All this will not come to fruition without proper planning of the process. For this, it is vital that the tendon regeneration processes as well as the individual characteristics of the case be taken into account. For this, the recording methods of both load management and the rating of perceived exertion (RPE) [144] should be used. In addition, it is fundamental to implement constant pain monitoring.

In conclusion, the importance of designing a program adapted to the individual characteristics of each case is stressed. This will not be possible without a coordinated work team and different competencies in medicine, physiotherapy, psychology, nutrition, and sports sciences.

References

1. Rees JD, Maffulli N, Cook J. Management of tendinopathy. Am J Sports Med. 2009;37(9):1855–67. https://doi.org/10.1177/0363546508324283.
2. Herring SA, Nilson KL. Introduction to overuse injuries. Clin Sports Med. 1987;6(2):225–39.
3. Del Buono A, Battery L, Denaro V, Maccauro G, Maffulli N. Tendinopathy and inflammation: some truths. Int J Immunopathol Pharmacol. 2011;24(1 Suppl 2):45–50.
4. Riley G. Tendinopathy—from basic science to treatment. Nat Clin Pract Rheumatol. 2008;4(2):82–9. https://doi.org/10.1038/ncprheum0700.
5. Dean BJF, Dakin SG, Millar NL, Carr AJ. Review: emerging concepts in the pathogenesis of tendinopathy. Surgeon. 2017;15(6):349–54. https://doi.org/10.1016/j.surge.2017.05.005.
6. Almekinders LC, Temple JD. Etiology, diagnosis, and treatment of tendonitis: an analysis of the literature. Med Sci Sports Exerc. 1998;30(8):1183–90.
7. Ruzzini L, Longo UG, Campi S, Maffulli N, Onetti Muda A, Denaro V. Adhesion and collagen production of human tenocytes seeded on degradable poly(urethane urea). Knee Surg Sports Traumatol Arthrosc. 2013;21(8):1834–40. https://doi.org/10.1007/s00167-012-2249-2.
8. Longo UG, Franceschi F, Ruzzini L, Rabitti C, Morini S, Maffulli N, Forriol F, Denaro V. Light microscopic histology of supraspinatus tendon ruptures. Knee Surg Sports Traumatol Arthrosc. 2007;15(11):1390–4.
9. Khan KM, Cook JL, Bonar F, Harcourt P, Astrom M. Histopathology of common tendinopathies. Update and implications for clinical management. Sports Med. 1999;27(6):393–408.
10. Maffulli N, Longo UG, Maffulli GD, Rabitti C, Khanna A, Denaro V. Marked pathological changes proximal and distal to the site of rupture in acute Achilles tendon ruptures. Knee Surg Sports Traumatol Arthrosc. 2011;19(4):680–7. https://doi.org/10.1007/s00167-010-1193-2.
11. Magnusson SP, Hansen P, Aagaard P, Brønd J, Dyhre-Poulsen P, Bojsen-Moller J, Kjaer M. Differential strain patterns of the human gastrocnemius aponeurosis and free tendon, in vivo. Acta Physiol Scand. 2003;177(2):185–95.
12. Ahmed IM, Lagopoulos M, McConnell P, Soames RW, Sefton GK. Blood supply of the Achilles tendon. J Orthop Res. 1998;16(5):591–6.
13. Wilson AM, Goodship AE. Exercise-induced hyperthermia as a possible mechanism for tendon degeneration. J Biomech. 1994;27(7):899–905.
14. Gibson W, Arendt-Nielsen L, Sessle BJ, Graven-Nielsen T. Glutamate and capsaicin-induced pain, hyperalgesia and modulatory interactions in human tendon tissue. Exp Brain Res. 2009;194(2):173–82. https://doi.org/10.1007/s00221-008-1683-3.

15. Maganaris CN, Narici MV, Almekinders LC, Maffulli N. Biomechanics and pathophysiology of overuse tendon injuries: ideas on insertional tendinopathy. Sports Med. 2004;34(14):1005–17.
16. Magra M, Maffulli N. Genetic aspects of tendinopathy. J Sci Med Sport. 2008;11(3):243–7.
17. Maffulli N, Waterston SW, Squair J, Reaper J, Douglas AS. Changing incidence of Achilles tendon rupture in Scotland: a 15-year study. Clin J Sport Med. 1999;9(3):157–60.
18. Maffulli N, Ewen SW, Waterston SW, Reaper J, Barrass V. Tenocytes from ruptured and tendinopathic Achilles tendons produce greater quantities of type III collagen than tenocytes from normal Achilles tendons. An in vitro model of human tendon healing. Am J Sports Med. 2000;28(4):499–505.
19. Cook JL, Kiss ZS, Khan KM, Purdam CR, Webster KE. Anthropometry, physical performance, and ultrasound patellar tendon abnormality in elite junior basketball players: a cross-sectional study. Br J Sports Med. 2004;38(2):206–9.
20. Longo UG, Petrillo S, Berton A, Spiezia F, Loppini M, Maffulli N, Denaro V. Role of serum fibrinogen levels in patients with rotator cuff tears. Int J Endocrinol. 2014;2014:685820. https://doi.org/10.1155/2014/685820.
21. Ames PR, Longo UG, Denaro V, Maffulli N. Achilles tendon problems: not just an orthopaedic issue. Disabil Rehabil. 2008;30(20–22):1646–50. https://doi.org/10.1080/09638280701785882.
22. Casparian JM, Luchi M, Moffat RE, Hinthorn D. Quinolones and tendon ruptures. South Med J. 2000;93(5):488–91.
23. Ferry ST, Dahners LE, Afshari HM, Weinhold PS. The effects of common anti-inflammatory drugs on the healing rat patellar tendon. Am J Sports Med. 2007;35(8):1326–33.
24. Longo UG, Ronga M, Maffulli N. Achilles tendinopathy. Sports Med Arthrosc Rev. 2018;26(1):16–30. https://doi.org/10.1097/JSA.0000000000000185.
25. Egger AC, Berkowitz MJ. Achilles tendon injuries. Curr Rev Musculoskelet Med. 2017;10(1):72–80. https://doi.org/10.1007/s12178-017-9386-7.
26. Kaufman KR, Brodine SK, Shaffer RA, Johnson CW, Cullison TR. The effect of foot structure and range of motion on musculoskeletal overuse injuries. Am J Sports Med. 1999;27(5):585–93.
27. Leadbetter WB. Cell-matrix response in tendon injury. Clin Sports Med. 1992;11(3):533–78.
28. Gaida JE, Alfredson L, Kiss ZS, Wilson AM, Alfredson H, Cook JL. Dyslipidemia in Achilles tendinopathy is characteristic of insulin resistance. Med Sci Sports Exerc. 2009;41(6):1194–7.
29. Järvinen TA, Kannus P, Paavola M, Järvinen TL, Józsa L, Järvinen M. Achilles tendon injuries. Curr Opin Rheumatol. 2001;13(2):150–5.
30. Chimenti RL, Cychosz CC, Hall MM, Phisitkul P. Current concepts review update: insertional Achilles tendinopathy. Foot Ankle Int. 2017;38(10):1160–9.
31. Hutchison AM, Evans R, Bodger O, Pallister I, Topliss C, Williams P, Vannet N, Morris V, Beard D. What is the best clinical test for Achilles tendinopathy? Foot Ankle Surg. 2013;19(2):112–7.
32. Longo UG, Berton A, Stelitano G, Madaudo C, Perna M, Ciuffreda M, Guarnieri A, Papalia R, Maffulli N, Denaro V. 2017 Marathon of Rome: anthropometry and sport profile in 350 runners and association with Achilles and patellar tendinopathy. Clin J Sport Med. 2018. https://doi.org/10.1097/JSM.0000000000000695.
33. Robinson JM, Cook JL, Purdam C, Visentini PJ, Ross J, Maffulli N, Taunton JE, Khan KM, Victorian Institute Of Sport Tendon Study Group. The VISA-A questionnaire: a valid and reliable index of the clinical severity of Achilles tendinopathy. Br J Sports Med. 2001;35(5):335–41.
34. van Schie HT, de Vos RJ, de Jonge S, Bakker EM, Heijboer MP, Verhaar JA, Tol JL, Weinans H. Ultrasonographic tissue characterisation of human Achilles tendons: quantification of tendon structure through a novel non-invasive approach. Br J Sports Med. 2010;44(16):1153–9.
35. Hägglund M, Zwerver J, Ekstrand J. Epidemiology of patellar tendinopathy in elite male soccer players. Am J Sports Med. 2011;39(9):1906–11.
36. Figueroa D, Figueroa F, Calvo R. Patellar tendinopathy: diagnosis and treatment. J Am Acad Orthop Surg. 2016;24(12):e184–92.
37. Malliaras P, Cook J, Purdam C, Rio E. Patellar tendinopathy: clinical diagnosis, load management, and advice for challenging case presentations. J Orthop Sports Phys Ther. 2015;45(11):887–98.
38. Maffulli N, Longo UG, Testa V, Oliva F, Capasso G, Denaro V. VISA-P score for patellar tendinopathy in males: adaptation to Italian. Disabil Rehabil. 2008;30(20–22):1621–4.
39. Hoksrud A, Ohberg L, Alfredson H, Bahr R. Color Doppler ultrasound findings in patellar tendinopathy (jumper's knee). Am J Sports Med. 2008;36(9):1813–20.
40. Aström M, Westlin N. No effect of piroxicam on Achilles tendinopathy. A randomized study of 70 patients. Acta Orthop Scand. 1992;63(6):631–4.
41. Alfredson H, Pietilä T, Jonsson P, Lorentzon R. Heavy-load eccentric calf muscle training for the treatment of chronic Achilles tendinosis. Am J Sports Med. 1998;26(3):360–6.
42. Alfredson H, Ohberg L, Forsgren S. Is vasculo-neural ingrowth the cause of pain in chronic Achilles tendinosis? An investigation using ultrasonography and colour Doppler, immunohistochemistry, and diagnostic injections. Knee Surg Sports Traumatol Arthrosc. 2003;11(5):334–8.
43. Lake JE, Ishikawa SN. Conservative treatment of Achilles tendinopathy: emerging techniques. Foot Ankle Clin. 2009;14(4):663–74. https://doi.org/10.1016/j.fcl.2009.07.003.
44. Stergioulas A, Stergioula M, Aarskog R, Lopes-Martins RA, Bjordal JM. Effects of low-level laser

therapy and eccentric exercises in the treatment of recreational athletes with chronic Achilles tendinopathy. Am J Sports Med. 2008;36(5):881–7. https://doi.org/10.1177/0363546507312165.
45. Witvrouw E, Danneels L, Asselman P, D'Have T, Cambier D. Muscle flexibility as a risk factor for developing muscle injuries in male professional soccer players. A prospective study. Am J Sports Med. 2003;31(1):41–6.
46. Schwartz A, Watson JN, Hutchinson MR. Patellar tendinopathy. Sports Health. 2015;7(5):415–20. https://doi.org/10.1177/1941738114568775.
47. Andres BM, Murrell GA. Treatment of tendinopathy: what works, what does not, and what is on the horizon. Clin Orthop Relat Res. 2008;466(7):1539–54. https://doi.org/10.1007/s11999-008-0260-1.
48. Abat F, Alfredson H, Cucchiarini M, Madry H, Marmotti A, Mouton C, Oliveira JM, Pereira H, Peretti GM, Spang C, Stephen J, van Bergen CJA, de Girolamo L. Current trends in tendinopathy: consensus of the ESSKA basic science committee. Part II: treatment options. J Exp Orthop. 2018;5(1):38. https://doi.org/10.1186/s40634-018-0145-5.
49. Abat F, Valles SL, Gelber PE, Polidori F, Stitik TP, García-Herreros S, Monllau JC, Sanchez-Ibánez JM. Molecular repair mechanisms using the intratissue percutaneous electrolysis technique in patellar tendonitis. Rev Esp Cir Ortop Traumatol. 2014;58(4):201–5. https://doi.org/10.1016/j.recot.2014.01.002.
50. Liao CD, Xie GM, Tsauo JY, Chen HC, Liou TH. Efficacy of extracorporeal shock wave therapy for knee tendinopathies and other soft tissue disorders: a meta-analysis of randomized controlled trials. BMC Musculoskelet Disord. 2018;19(1):278. https://doi.org/10.1186/s12891-018-2204-6.
51. Abat F, Alfredson H, Cucchiarini M, Madry H, Marmotti A, Mouton C, Oliveira JM, Pereira H, Peretti GM, Romero-Rodriguez D, Spang C, Stephen J, van Bergen CJA, de Girolamo L. Current trends in tendinopathy: consensus of the ESSKA basic science committee. Part I: biology, biomechanics, anatomy and an exercise-based approach. J Exp Orthop. 2017;4(1):18. https://doi.org/10.1186/s40634-017-0092-6.
52. Kjaer M, Langberg H, Skovgaard D, Olesen J, Bülow J, Krogsgaard M, Boushel R. In vivo studies of peritendinous tissue in exercise. Scand J Med Sci Sports. 2000;10(6):326–31.
53. Indino C, D'Ambrosi R, Usuelli FG. Biologics in the treatment of Achilles tendon pathologies. Foot Ankle Clin. 2019;24(3):471–93.
54. Hou Y, Mao Z, Wei X, et al. Effects of transforming growth factor-beta1 and vascular endothelial growth factor 165 gene transfer on Achilles tendon healing. Matrix Biol. 2009;28:324–35.
55. Kashiwagi K, Mochizuki Y, Yasunaga Y, et al. Effects of transforming growth factor-beta 1 on the early stages of healing of the Achilles tendon in a rat model. Scand J Plast Reconstr Surg Hand Surg. 2004;38:193–7.
56. Maeda T, Sakabe T, Sunaga A, et al. Conversion of mechanical force into TGFbeta- mediated biochemical signals. Curr Biol. 2011;21:933–41.
57. Jorgensen HG, McLellan SD, Crossan JF, et al. Neutralisation of TGF beta or binding of VLA-4 to fibronectin prevents rat tendon adhesion following transection. Cytokine. 2005;30:195–202.
58. Katzel EB, Wolenski M, Loiselle AE, et al. Impact of Smad3 loss of function on scarring and adhesion formation during tendon healing. J Orthop Res. 2011;29:684–93.
59. Potter RM, Huynh RT, Volper BD, et al. Impact of TGF-b inhibition during acute exercise on Achilles tendon extracellular matrix. Am J Physiol Regul Integr Comp Physiol. 2017;312:R157–64.
60. Boyer MI, Watson JT, Lou J, et al. Quantitative variation in vascular endothelial growth factor mRNA expression during early flexor tendon healing: an investigation in a canine model. J Orthop Res. 2001;19:869–72.
61. Zhang F, Liu H, Stile F, et al. Effect of vascular endothelial growth factor on rat Achilles tendon healing. Plast Reconstr Surg. 2003;112:1613–9.
62. Tempfer H, Kaser-Eichberger A, Lehner C, et al. Bevacizumab improves Achilles tendon repair in a rat model. Cell Physiol Biochem. 2018;46:1148–58.
63. Wurgler-Hauri CC, Dourte LM, Baradet TC, et al. Temporal expression of 8 growth factors in tendon-to-bone healing in a rat supraspinatus model. J Shoulder Elbow Surg. 2007;16:S198–203.
64. Thomopoulos S, Zaegel M, Das R, et al. PDGF-BB released in tendon repair using a novel delivery system promotes cell proliferation and collagen remodeling. J Orthop Res. 2007;25:1358–68.
65. Thomopoulos S, Das R, Silva MJ, et al. Enhanced flexor tendon healing through controlled delivery of PDGF-BB. J Orthop Res. 2009;27:1209–15.
66. Chetty A, Cao GJ, Nielsen HC. Insulin-like growth factor-I signaling mechanisms, type I collagen and alpha smooth muscle actin in human fetal lung fibroblasts. Pediatr Res. 2006;60:389–94.
67. Kurtz CA, Loebig TG, Anderson DD, et al. Insulin-like growth factor I accelerate functional recovery from Achilles tendon injury in a rat model. Am J Sports Med. 1999;27:363–9.
68. Dohan Ehrenfest DM, Rasmusson L, Albrektsson T. Classification of platelet concentrates: from pure platelet-rich plasma (P-PRP) to leucocyte- and platelet-rich fibrin (L-PRF). Trends Biotechnol. 2009;27:158–67.
69. Lin MT, Chiang CF, Wu CH, et al. Meta-analysis comparing autologous blood derived products (including platelet-rich plasma) injection versus placebo in patients with Achilles tendinopathy. Arthroscopy. 2018;34:1966–75.
70. Filardo G, Di Matteo B, Kon E, Merli G, Marcacci M. Platelet-rich plasma in tendon-related disorders: results and indications. Knee Surg Sports Traumatol Arthrosc. 2018;26(7):1984–99.
71. Schepull T, Kvist J, Norrman H, et al. Autologous platelets have no effect on the healing of human

Achilles tendon ruptures: a randomized single-blind study. Am J Sports Med. 2011;39:38–47.
72. Longo UG, Lamberti A, Petrillo S, et al. Scaffolds in tendon tissue engineering. Stem Cells Int. 2012;2012:517165.
73. Usuelli FG, D'Ambrosi R, Maccario C, et al. Adipose-derived stem cells in orthopaedic pathologies. Br Med Bull. 2017;124:31–54.
74. Usuelli FG, Grassi M, Maccario C, Vigano' M, Lanfranchi L, Alfieri Montrasio U, de Girolamo L. Intratendinous adipose-derived stromal vascular fraction (SVF) injection provides a safe, efficacious treatment for Achilles tendinopathy: results of a randomized controlled clinical trial at a 6-month follow-up. Knee Surg Sports Traumatol Arthrosc. 2018;26(7):2000–10.
75. Albano D, Messina C, Usuelli FG, De Girolamo L, Grassi M, Maccario C, Bignotti B, Tagliafico A, Sconfienza LM. Magnetic resonance and ultrasound in Achilles tendinopathy: predictive role and response assessment to platelet-rich plasma and adipose-derived stromal vascular fraction injection. Eur J Radiol. 2017;95:130–5.
76. Ogle ME, Segar CE, Sridhar S, et al. Monocytes and macrophages in tissue repair: implications for immunoregenerative biomaterial design. Exp Biol Med (Maywood). 2016;241:1084–97.
77. Barbeck M, Unger RE, Booms P, et al. Monocyte preseeding leads to an increased implant bed vascularization of biphasic calcium phosphate bone substitutes via vessel maturation. J Biomed Mater Res A. 2016;104:2928–35.
78. Caplan AI. New era of cell-based orthopedic therapies. Tissue Eng Part B Rev. 2009;15:195–200.
79. Henrich D, Seebach C, Verboket R, et al. The osteoinductive activity of bone-marrow-derived mononuclear cells resides within the CD141 population and is independent of the CD341 population. Eur Cell Mater. 2018;35:165–77.
80. Sugg KB, Lubardic J, Gumucio JP, et al. Changes in macrophage phenotype and induction of epithelial-to-mesenchymal transition genes following acute Achilles tenotomy and repair. J Orthop Res. 2014;32:944–51.
81. Salamanna F, Contartese D, Nicoli Aldini N, et al. Bone marrow aspirate clot: a technical complication or a smart approach for musculoskeletal tissue regeneration? J Cell Physiol. 2018;233:2723–32.
82. Hegde V, Shonuga O, Ellis S, et al. A prospective comparison of 3 approved systems for autologous bone marrow concentration demonstrated nonequivalency in progenitor cell number and concentration. J Orthop Trauma. 2014;28:591–8.
83. Imam MA, Holton J, Horriat S, et al. A systematic review of the concept and clinical applications of bone marrow aspirate concentrate in tendon pathology. SICOT J. 2017;3:58.
84. Broese M, Toma I, Haasper C, et al. Seeding a human tendon matrix with bone marrow aspirates compared to previously isolated hBMSCs—an in vitro study. Technol Health Care. 2011;19:469–79.
85. Stein BE, Stroh DA, Schon LC. Outcomes of acute Achilles tendon rupture repair with bone marrow aspirate concentrate augmentation. Int Orthop. 2015;39:901–5.
86. D'Ambrosi R, Ragone V, Comaschi G, Usuelli FG, Ursino N. Retears and complication rates after arthroscopic rotator cuff repair with scaffolds: a systematic review. Cell Tissue Bank. 2019;20(1):1–10.
87. Webb WR, Dale TP, Lomas AJ, et al. The application of poly (3-hydroxybutyrateco- 3-hydroxyhexanoate) scaffolds for tendon repair in the rat model. Biomaterials. 2013;34:6683–94.
88. Farnebo S, Woon CY, Bronstein JA, et al. Decellularized tendon-bone composite grafts for extremity reconstruction: an experimental study. Plast Reconstr Surg. 2014;133:79–89.
89. Lohan A, Stoll C, Albrecht M, et al. Human hamstring tenocytes survive when seeded into a decellularized porcine Achilles tendon extracellular matrix. Connect Tissue Res. 2013;54:305–12.
90. Lee DK. A preliminary study on the effects of acellular tissue graft augmentation in acute Achilles tendon ruptures. J Foot Ankle Surg. 2008;47:8–12.
91. Wisbeck JM, Parks BG, Schon LC. Xenograft scaffold full-wrap reinforcement of Krackow Achilles tendon repair. Orthopedics. 2012;35:e331–4.
92. Zantop T, Gilbert TW, Yoder MC, et al. Extracellular matrix scaffolds are repopulated by bone marrow-derived cells in a mouse model of Achilles tendon reconstruction. J Orthop Res. 2006;24:1299–309.
93. Oloff L, Elmi E, Nelson J, et al. Retrospective analysis of the effectiveness of platelet-rich plasma in the treatment of Achilles tendinopathy: pretreatment and posttreatment correlation of magnetic resonance imaging and clinical assessment. Foot Ankle Spec. 2015;8:490–7.
94. Longo UG, Ramamurthy C, Denaro V, et al. Minimally invasive stripping for chronic Achilles tendinopathy. Disabil Rehabil. 2008;30:1709–13.
95. de Almeida AM, Demange MK, Sobrado MF, Rodrigues MB, Pedrinelli A, Hernandez AJ. Patellar tendon healing with platelet-rich plasma: a prospective randomized controlled trial. Am J Sports Med. 2012;40(6):1282–8. https://doi.org/10.1177/0363546512441344.
96. Seijas R, Cuscó X, Sallent A, Serra I, Ares O, Cugat R. Pain in donor site after BTB-ACL reconstruction with PRGF: a randomized trial. Arch Orthop Trauma Surg. 2016;136(6):829–35. https://doi.org/10.1007/s00402-016-2458-0.
97. Kaux JF, Croisier JL, Forthomme B, Le Goff C, Buhler F, Savanier B, Delcour S, Gothot A, Crielaard JM. Using platelet-rich plasma to treat jumper's knees: exploring the effect of a second closely-timed infiltration. J Sci Med Sport. 2016;19(3):200–4. https://doi.org/10.1016/j.jsams.2015.03.006.
98. Zayni R, Thaunat M, Fayard JM, Hager JP, Carrillon Y, Clechet J, Gadea F, Archbold P, Sonnery Cottet B. Platelet-rich plasma as a treatment for chronic patellar tendinopathy: comparison of a single versus

two consecutive injections. Muscles Ligaments Tendons J. 2015;5(2):92–8.
99. Vetrano M, Castorina A, Vulpiani MC, Baldini R, Pavan A, Ferretti A. Platelet-rich plasma versus focused shock waves in the treatment of jumper's knee in athletes. Am J Sports Med. 2013;41(4):795–803. https://doi.org/10.1177/0363546513475345.
100. Dragoo JL, Wasterlain AS, Braun HJ, Nead KT. Platelet-rich plasma as a treatment for patellar tendinopathy: a double-blind, randomized controlled trial. Am J Sports Med. 2014;42(3):610–8. https://doi.org/10.1177/0363546513518416.
101. Pascual-Garrido C, Rolón A, Makino A. Treatment of chronic patellar tendinopathy with autologous bone marrow stem cells: a 5-year-followup. Stem Cells Int. 2012;2012:953510. https://doi.org/10.1155/2012/953510.
102. Muneta T, Koga H, Ju YJ, Mochizuki T, Sekiya I. Hyaluronan injection therapy for athletic patients with patellar tendinopathy. J Orthop Sci. 2012;17(4):425–31.
103. Hoksrud A, Ohberg L, Alfredson H, Bahr R. Ultrasound-guided sclerosis of neovessels in painful chronic patellar tendinopathy: a randomized controlled trial. Am J Sports Med. 2006;34(11):1738–46.
104. Hoksrud A, Bahr R. Ultrasound-guided sclerosing treatment in patients with patellar tendinopathy (jumper's knee): 44-month follow-up. Am J Sports Med. 2011;39(11):2377–80.
105. Steunebrink M, Zwerver J, Brandsema R, Groenenboom P, van den Akker-Scheek I, Weir A. Topical glyceryl trinitrate treatment of chronic patellar tendinopathy: a randomised, double-blind, placebo controlled clinical trial. Br J Sports Med. 2013;47(1):34–9.
106. Stasinopoulos D, Stasinopoulos I. Comparison of effects of exercise programme, pulsed ultrasound and transverse friction in the treatment of chronic patellar tendinopathy. Clin Rehabil. 2004;18(4):347–52.
107. Warden SJ, Metcalf BR, Kiss ZS, et al. Low intensity pulsed ultrasound for chronic patellar tendinopathy: a randomized, double blind, placebo-controlled trial. Rheumatology (Oxford). 2008;47(4):467–71.
108. Giombini A, Di Cesare A, Casciello G, Sorrenti D, Dragoni S, Gabriele P. Hyperthermia at 434 MHz in the treatment of overuse sport tendinopathies: a randomised controlled clinical trial. Int J Sports Med. 2002;23(3):207–11.
109. Kvist M. Achilles tendon injuries in athletes. Sports Med. 1994;18(3):173–201.
110. Paavola M, Kannus P, Paakkala T, Pasanen M, Järvinen M. Long-term prognosis of patients with Achilles tendinopathy. An observational 8-year follow-up study. Am J Sports Med. 2000;28(5):634–42.
111. Kvist H, Kvist M. The operative treatment of chronic calcaneal paratenonitis. J Bone Joint Surg Br. 1980;62(3):353–7.
112. van Dijk CN, van Sterkenburg MN, Wiegerinck JI, Karlsson J, Maffulli N. Terminology for Achilles tendon related disorders. Knee Surg Sports Traumatol Arthrosc. 2011;19(5):835–41.
113. Maffulli N, Saxena A, Wagner E, Torre G. Achilles insertional tendinopathy: state of the art. J ISAKOS. 2019;4:48–57.
114. Johansson KJ, Sarimo JJ, Lempainen LL, Laitala-Leinonen T, Orava SY. Calcific spurs at the insertion of the Achilles tendon: a clinical and histological study. Muscles Ligaments Tendons J. 2013;2(4):273–7.
115. Jerosch J, Schunck J, Sokkar SH. Endoscopic calcaneoplasty (ECP) as a surgical treatment of Haglund's syndrome. Knee Surg Sports Traumatol Arthrosc. 2007;15(7):927–34.
116. Khan WS, Malvankar S, Bhamra JS, Pengas I. Analysing the outcome of surgery for chronic Achilles tendinopathy over the last 50 years. World J Orthop. 2015;6(6):491–7. https://doi.org/10.5312/wjo.v6.i6.491.
117. Traina F, Perna F, Ruffilli A, Mazzotti A, Meliconi R, Berti L, Faldini C. Surgical treatment of insertional Achilles tendinopathy: a systematic review. J Biol Regul Homeost Agents. 2016;30(4 Suppl 1):131–8.
118. Paavola M, Orava S, Leppilahti J, Kannus P, Järvinen M. Chronic Achilles tendon overuse injury: complications after surgical treatment. An analysis of 432 consecutive patients. Am J Sports Med. 2000;28(1):77–82.
119. Lorbach O, Diamantopoulos A, Paessler HH. Arthroscopic resection of the lower patellar pole in patients with chronic patellar tendinosis. Arthroscopy. 2008;24(2):167–73. https://doi.org/10.1016/j.arthro.2007.08.021.
120. Coleman BD, Khan KM, Kiss ZS, Bartlett J, Young DA, Wark JD. Open and arthroscopic patellar tenotomy for chronic patellar tendinopathy. A retrospective outcome study. Victorian Institute of Sport Tendon Study Group. Am J Sports Med. 2000;28(2):183–90.
121. Sarimo J, Sarin J, Orava S, Heikkilä J, Rantanen J, Paavola M, Raatikainen T. Distal patellar tendinosis: an unusual form of jumper's knee. Knee Surg Sports Traumatol Arthrosc. 2007;15(1):54–7.
122. Khan WS, Smart A. Outcome of surgery for chronic patellar tendinopathy: a systematic review. Acta Orthop Belg. 2016;82(3):610–326.
123. Panni AS, Tartarone M, Maffulli N. Patellar tendinopathy in athletes. Outcome of nonoperative and operative management. Am J Sports Med. 2000;28(3):392–7.
124. Testa V, Capasso G, Maffulli N, Bifulco G. Ultrasound-guided percutaneous longitudinal tenotomy for the management of patellar tendinopathy. Med Sci Sports Exerc. 1999;31(11):1509–15.
125. Ardern CL, Glasgow P, Schneiders A, Witvrouw E, Clarsen B, Cools A, Gojanovic B, Griffin S, Khan KM, Moksnes H, Mutch SA, Phillips N, Reurink G, Sadler R, Silbernagel KG, Thorborg K, Wangensteen A, Wilk KE, Bizzini M. 2016 consensus statement on return to sport from the first world congress in sports physical therapy, Bern. Br J Sports Med. 2016;50(14):853–64. https://doi.org/10.1136/bjsports-2016-096278.

126. Habets B, van den Broek AG, Huisstede BMA, Backx FJG, van Cingel REH. Return to sport in athletes with midportion Achilles tendinopathy: a qualitative systematic review regarding definitions and criteria. Sports Med. 2018;48(3):705–23. https://doi.org/10.1007/s40279-017-0833-9.
127. Kongsgaard M, Reitelseder S, Pedersen TG, Holm L, Aagaard P, Kjaer M, Magnusson SP. Region specific patellar tendon hypertrophy in humans following resistance training. Acta Physiol (Oxf). 2007;191(2):111–21.
128. Malliaras P, Barton CJ, Reeves ND, Langberg H. Achilles and patellar tendinopathy loading programmes : a systematic review comparing clinical outcomes and identifying potential mechanisms for effectiveness. Sports Med. 2013;43(4):267–86. https://doi.org/10.1007/s40279-013-0019-z.
129. Silbernagel KG, Crossley KM. A proposed return-to-sport program for patients with midportion Achilles tendinopathy: rationale and implementation. J Orthop Sports Phys Ther. 2015;45(11):876–86. https://doi.org/10.2519/jospt.2015.5885.
130. Habets B, van Cingel REH, Backx FJG, Huisstede BMA. Alfredson versus Silbernagel exercise therapy in chronic midportion Achilles tendinopathy: study protocol for a randomized controlled trial. BMC Musculoskelet Disord. 2017;18(1):296. https://doi.org/10.1186/s12891-017-1656-4.
131. Beyer R, Kongsgaard M, Hougs Kjær B, Øhlenschlæger T, Kjær M, Magnusson SP. Heavy slow resistance versus eccentric training as treatment for Achilles tendinopathy: a randomized controlled trial. Am J Sports Med. 2015;43(7):1704–11. https://doi.org/10.1177/0363546515584760.
132. Couppé C, Svensson RB, Silbernagel KG, Langberg H, Magnusson SP. Eccentric or concentric exercises for the treatment of tendinopathies? J Orthop Sports Phys Ther. 2015;45(11):853–63. https://doi.org/10.2519/jospt.2015.5910.
133. Cook JL, Stasinopoulos D, Brismée JM. Insertional and mid-substance Achilles tendinopathies: eccentric training is not for everyone—updated evidence of non-surgical management. J Man Manip Ther. 2018;26(3):119–22. https://doi.org/10.1080/10669817.2018.1470302.
134. O'Neill S, Watson PJ, Barry S. Why are eccentric exercises effective for Achilles tendinopathy? Int J Sports Phys Ther. 2015;10(4):552–62.
135. Rio E, van Ark M, Docking S, Moseley GL, Kidgell D, Gaida JE, van den Akker-Scheek I, Zwerver J, Cook J. Isometric contractions are more analgesic than isotonic contractions for patellar tendon pain: an in-season randomized clinical trial. Clin J Sport Med. 2017;27(3):253–9. https://doi.org/10.1097/JSM.0000000000000364.
136. Scott A, Docking S, Vicenzino B, Alfredson H, Murphy RJ, Carr AJ, Zwerver J, Lundgreen K, Finlay O, Pollock N, Cook JL, Fearon A, Purdam CR, Hoens A, Rees JD, Goetz TJ, Danielson P. Sports and exercise-related tendinopathies: a review of selected topical issues by participants of the second international scientific tendinopathy symposium (ISTS) Vancouver 2012. Br J Sports Med. 2013;47(9):536–44. https://doi.org/10.1136/bjsports-2013-092329.
137. Berg HE, Tesch PA. Force and power characteristics of a resistive exercise device for use in space. Acta Astronaut. 1998;42(1–8):219–30.
138. Tesch PA, Fernandez-Gonzalo R, Lundberg TR. Clinical applications of iso-inertial, eccentric-overload (YoYo™) resistance exercise. Front Physiol. 2017;8:241. https://doi.org/10.3389/fphys.2017.00241.
139. Gonzalo-Skok O, Tous-Fajardo J, Valero-Campo C, Berzosa C, Bataller AV, Arjol-Serrano JL, Moras G, Mendez-Villanueva A. Eccentric-overload training in team-sport functional performance: constant bilateral vertical versus variable unilateral multidirectional movements. Int J Sports Physiol Perform. 2017;12(7):951–8. https://doi.org/10.1123/ijspp.2016-0251.
140. Núñez FJ, Santalla A, Carrasquila I, Asian JA, Reina JI, Suarez-Arrones LJ. The effects of unilateral and bilateral eccentric overload training on hypertrophy, muscle power and COD performance, and its determinants, in team sport players. PLoS One. 2018;13(3):e0193841. https://doi.org/10.1371/journal.pone.0193841.
141. Sañudo B, González-Navarrete Á, Álvarez-Barbosa F, de Hoyo M, Del Pozo J, Rogers ME. Effect of flywheel resistance training on balance performance in older adults. A randomized controlled trial. J Sports Sci Med. 2019;18(2):344–50.
142. Abat F, Gelber PE, Polidori F, Monllau JC, Sanchez-Ibañez JM. Clinical results after ultrasound-guided intratissue percutaneous electrolysis and eccentric exercise in the treatment of patellar tendinopathy. Knee Surg Sports Traumatol Arthrosc. 2015;23(4):1046–52. https://doi.org/10.1007/s00167-014-2855-2.
143. Gual G, Fort-Vanmeerhaeghe A, Romero-Rodríguez D, Tesch PA. Effects of in-season inertial resistance training with eccentric overload in a sports population at risk for patellar tendinopathy. J Strength Cond Res. 2016;30(7):1834–42. https://doi.org/10.1519/JSC.0000000000001286.
144. Foster C, Florhaug JA, Franklin J, Gottschall L, Hrovatin LA, Parker S, Doleshal P, Dodge C. A new approach to monitoring exercise training. J Strength Cond Res. 2001;15(1):109–15.

Printed by Printforce, the Netherlands